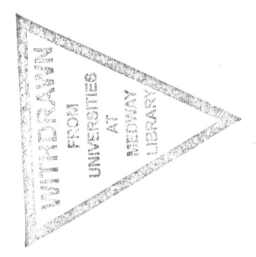

Interventional Cardiology

Companion DVD-ROM

This book is accompanied by a companion DVD with:

- 33 additional cases with video clips
- Table of Contents for DVD—

Case contributions by Drs. Di Mario and Tyczynski

Interventional Cardiology
Principles and Practice

EDITED BY

Carlo Di Mario, MD, PhD, FRCP, FACC, FSCAI, FESC

Professor of Cardiology
National Heart & Lung Institute Imperial College London
Consultant Cardiologist
Royal Brompton Hospital
Professor of Clinical Cardiology
Imperial College London
London
UK

George D. Dangas, MD, PhD, FACC, FSCAI, FESC, FAHA

Professor of Medicine
Director, Cardiovascular Innovation
Mount Sinai Medical Center
New York, NY
USA

Peter Barlis, MBBS, MPH, PhD, FCSANZ, FESC, FRACP

Associate Professor of Medicine
Faculty of Medicine, Dentistry & Health Sciences
The University of Melbourne
Consultant & Interventional Cardiologist
The Northern Hospital
Melbourne, VIC
Australia

Forewords by
Patrick W. Serruys, MD, PhD
and
Martin B. Leon, MD

(W) WILEY-BLACKWELL

A John Wiley & Sons, Ltd., Publication

This edition first published 2011 © 2011 by Blackwell Publishing Ltd

Blackwell Publishing was acquired by John Wiley & Sons in February 2007. Blackwell's publishing program has been merged with Wiley's global Scientific, Technical and Medical business to form Wiley-Blackwell.

Registered office: John Wiley & Sons, Ltd, The Atrium, Southern Gate, Chichester, West Sussex, PO19 8SQ, UK

Editorial offices: 9600 Garsington Road, Oxford, OX4 2DQ, UK

The Atrium, Southern Gate, Chichester, West Sussex, PO19 8SQ, UK

111 River Street, Hoboken, NJ 07030-5774, USA

For details of our global editorial offices, for customer services and for information about how to apply for permission to reuse the copyright material in this book please see our website at www.wiley.com/wiley-blackwell

The right of the author to be identified as the author of this work has been asserted in accordance with the UK Copyright, Designs and Patents Act 1988.

Designations used by companies to distinguish their products are often claimed as trademarks. All brand names and product names used in this book are trade names, service marks, trademarks or registered trademarks of their respective owners. The publisher is not associated with any product or vendor mentioned in this book. This publication is designed to provide accurate and authoritative information in regard to the subject matter covered. It is sold on the understanding that the publisher is not engaged in rendering professional services. If professional advice or other expert assistance is required, the services of a competent professional should be sought.

The contents of this work are intended to further general scientific research, understanding, and discussion only and are not intended and should not be relied upon as recommending or promoting a specific method, diagnosis, or treatment by physicians for any particular patient. The publisher and the author make no representations or warranties with respect to the accuracy or completeness of the contents of this work and specifically disclaim all warranties, including without limitation any implied warranties of fitness for a particular purpose. In view of ongoing research, equipment modifications, changes in governmental regulations, and the constant flow of information relating to the use of medicines, equipment, and devices, the reader is urged to review and evaluate the information provided in the package insert or instructions for each medicine, equipment, or device for, among other things, any changes in the instructions or indication of usage and for added warnings and precautions. Readers should consult with a specialist where appropriate. The fact that an organization or Website is referred to in this work as a citation and/or a potential source of further information does not mean that the author or the publisher endorses the information the organization or Website may provide or recommendations it may make. Further, readers should be aware that Internet Websites listed in this work may have changed or disappeared between when this work was written and when it is read. No warranty may be created or extended by any promotional statements for this work. Neither the publisher nor the author shall be liable for any damages arising herefrom.

Library of Congress Cataloging-in-Publication Data

Interventional cardiology: principles and practice / [edited by] Carlo Di Mario, George Dangas, Peter Barlis.
p. ; cm.
Includes bibliographical references.
ISBN 978-1-4051-7887-7
1. Coronary heart disease–Surgery. I. Di Mario, Carlo. II. Dangas, George D. III. Barlis, Peter.
[DNLM: 1. Cardiovascular Diseases–therapy. 2. Cardiac Surgical Procedures. 3. Cardiovascular Diseases–diagnosis. WG 166 I616 2009]
RD598I547 2009
617.4′12–dc22
2009013385

A catalogue record for this book is available from the British Library.

This book is published in the following electronic formats: ePDF 9781444319439; Wiley Online Library 9781444319446

Set in 9.5 on 12 pt Minion by Toppan Best-set Premedia Limited
Printed and bound in Singapore by Markono Print Media Pte Ltd

1 2011

Contents

Question and Answer contributions by Drs. Tayo
Addo and George D. Dangas.

Contributors

Alexandre Abizaid, MD, PhD
Chief of Coronary Interventions
Institute Dante Pazzanese of Cardiology
São Paulo
Brazil

Tayo Addo, MD
Assistant Professor of Medicine
Southwestern Medical Center
Dallas, TX
USA

Flavio Airoldi, MD
Director
Interventional Cardiology Unit
IRCCS Multimedica
Sesto San Giovanni (MI)
Italy

Andrew E. Ajani, MD, MBBS, FRACP, FJFICM
Associate Professor
Interventional Cardiologist
Director of Coronary Care Unit
Director of Physician Training
Royal Melbourne Hospital
Melbourne, VIC
Australia

Jiro Aoki, MD, PhD
Interventional Cardiologist
Division of Cardiology
Mitsol Memorial Hospital
Tokyo
Japan

Zoë Astroulakis, MBBS, MRCP
Clinical Research Fellow
Department of Cardiology
King's College London
James Black Centre
London
UK

Joseph Babb, MD
Professor of Medicine
Director, Interventional Cardiology Fellowship
Department of Cardiovascular Sciences
East Carolina University Brody School of Medicine
Greenville, NC
USA

Adrian P. Banning, MD, FRCP, FESC
Consultant Cardiologist
Department of Cardiology
John Radcliffe Hospital
Oxford
UK

Peter Barlis, MBBS, MPH, FCSANZ, FESC, FRACP, PhD
Associate Professor of Medicine
Faculty of Medicine, Dentistry & Health Sciences
The University of Melbourne
Consultant & Interventional Cardiologist
The Northern Hospital
Melbourne, VIC
Australia

Andreas Baumbach, MD, FRCP, FESC
Consultant Cardiologist
Bristol Heart Institute
University Hospitals Bristol
Bristol
UK

Elena Bonanno, MD
Assistant Professor Pathology
Department of Pathology
University of Rome Tor Vergata
Rome
Italy

Carlo Briguori, MD, PhD
Chief of Laboratory
Laboratory of Interventional Cardiology
Clinica Mediterranea
Naples
Laboratory of Interventional Cardiology
"Vita e Salute" University School of Medicine
Milan
Italy

Eric Brochet, MD
Cardiologist
Echocardiography Laboratory
Department of Cardiology
Bichat Hospital
Paris
France

Adriano Caixeta, MD, PhD
Postdoctoral Research Fellow
Center for Interventional Vascular Therapy
Columbia University Medical Center
Clinical Trial Center
Cardiovascular Research Foundation
New York, NY
USA

Estêvão C. de Campos Martins, MD
Interventional Cardio-Angiology Unit
GVM Hospitals of Care and Research
Cotignola (RA)
Italy

Fausto Castriota, MD
Interventional Cardio-Angiology Unit
GVM Hospitals of Care and Research
Cotignola (RA)
Italy

Alaide Chieffo, MD
Consultant Interventional Cardiologist
Invasive Cardiology Unit
San Raffaele Hospital
Milan
Italy

David J. Clark, MD, FRACP
Director of Interventional Research
Austin Hospital
Melbourne, VIC
Australia

Antonio Colombo, MD
San Raffaele Scientific Institute and EMO Centro
Cuore Columbus
Milan
Italy

Alberto Cremonesi, MD
Interventional Cardio-Angiology Unit
GVM Hospitals of Care and Research
Cotignola (RA)
Italy

George D. Dangas, MD, PhD, FACC, FESC, FSCAI, FAHA
Professor of Medicine
Director, Cardiovascular Innovation
Mount Sinai Medical Center
New York, NY
USA

Carlo Di Mario, MD, PhD, FRCP, FSCAI, FESC
Professor of Cardiology
National Heart & Lung Institute Imperial College London
Consultant Cardiologist
Royal Brompton Hospital
Professor of Clinical Cardiology
Imperial College London
London
UK

Germano Di Sciascio, MD, FACC, FESC
Professor of Cardiology
Department of Cardiovascular Sciences
Campus Bio-Medico University of Rome
Rome
Italy

John Edmond, MD, MRCP
Consultant Interventional Cardiologist
Bristol Heart Institute
University Hospitals Bristol
Bristol
UK

Albrecht Elsaesser, MD
Head of the Department of Cardiology
Heart Center
Oldenburg Medical Center
Oldenburg
Germany

Amir-Ali Fassa, MD
Interventional Cardiology Fellow
Cardiology Service
Geneva University Hospitals
Geneva
Switzerland

Ted Feldman, MD, FSCAI
Director, Cardiac Catheterization Laboratory
Cardiology Division
Evanston Hospital
Evanston, IL
USA

Giuseppe Ferrante, MD
Cardiologist
Institute of Cardiology
Catholic University of the Sacred Heart
Rome
Italy

Pim J. de Feyter, MD, PhD, FESC, FACC
Professor of Cardiac Imaging
Departments of Cardiology and Radiology
Erasmus MC University Medical Center
Rotterdam
The Netherlands

Francesca del Furia, MD
Research Fellow
Royal Brompton Hospital
London
UK

William J. van Gaal, MBBS, FRACP, MSc, FESC, FCSANZ
Director of Cardiology
The Northern Hospital
Epping, VIC
Australia

Philippe Généreux, MD
Clinical Instructor
Division of Cardiology
Center for Interventional Vascular Therapy
Columbia University Medical Center
New York, NY
USA

Bernard J. Gersh, MBChB, DPhil, FRCP, FACC
Professor of Medicine
The Division of Cardiovascular Diseases and Department
of Internal Medicine
Mayo Clinic and Mayo Foundation
Rochester, MN
USA

Anthony Gershlick, MBBS, BSc, FRCP
Professor of Interventional Cardiology
Glenfield Hospital
Leicester
UK

Shane Gieowarsingh, MBBS, MET
Master of Endovascular Techniques Fellow
Interventional Cardio-Angiology Unit
GVM Hospitals of Care and Research
Cotignola (RA)
Italy

Christian W. Hamm, MD
Medical Director
Heart and Thorax Center
Kerckhoff-Klinic
Bad Nauheim
Germany

Eric Heller, MD
Instructor in Clinical Medicine
Columbia University Medical Center
New York, NY
USA

Jonathan M. Hill, MD
Consultant Cardiologist
Department of Cardiology
King's Health Partners
London
UK

Dominique Himbert, MD
Cardiologist
Department of Cardiology
Bichat Hospital
Paris
France

Srinivas Iyengar, MD
Clinical Instructor
Division of Cardiology
New York-Presbyterian Hospital
Columbia University Medical Center
New York, NY
USA

Rohit Khurana, MD, MRCP
Department of Cardiology
Imperial College Health Trust
London
UK

Ajay J. Kirtane, MD, ScM
Assistant Professor of Clinical Medicine
Center for Interventional Vascular Therapy
Columbia University Medical Center
New York-Presbyterian Hospital
New York, NY
USA

Gerhard Koning, MSc
Senior Scientific Researcher
Division of Image Processing (LKEB)
Department of Radiology
Leiden University Medical Center
Leiden
The Netherlands

Neville Kukreja, MA, MRCP
Research Fellow
Lister Hospital
Stevenage
UK

Alexandra J. Lansky, MD
Associate Professor of Clinical Medicine
Columbia University Medical Center
Joint Chief Scientific Officer, Clinical Trial Center &
Director, Women's Cardiovascular Health Initiative
Cardiovascular Research Foundation
New York, NY
USA

Azeem Latib, MB, BCh
Interventional Cardiologist
Interventional Cardiology Unit
San Raffaele Scientific Institute
Milan
Italy

Martin B. Leon, MD
Professor of Medicine and Associate Director
Center for Interventional Vascular Therapy
Columbia University Medical Center
Founder & Chairman Emeritus
Cardiovascular Research Foundation
New York, NY
USA

Akiko Maehara, MD
Director of Intravascular Imaging &
Physiology Core Laboratories
Associate Director of MRI Core Laboratories
Cardiovascular Research Foundation
Assistant Professor, Columbia University Medical Center
New York, NY
USA

Valeria Magni, MD
Research Fellow
Invasive Cardiology Unit
San Raffaele Hospital
Milan
Italy

Amgad N. Makaryus, MD, FACC, FACP, FASE
Director of Cardiac CT and MRI
Department of Cardiology
North Shore University Hospital
NYU School of Medicine
Manhasset, NY
USA

Alessandro Mauriello, MD
Associate Professor of Pathology
Department of Pathology
University of Rome Tor Vergata
Rome
Italy

Roxana Mehran, MD
Associate Professor of Medicine
Columbia University College of Physicians and Surgeons
Director of Outcomes Research
Center for Interventional Vascular Therapy
Columbia University Medical Center
Joint Chief Scientific Officer
Cardiovascular Research Foundation
New York, NY
USA

Narbeh Melikian, MD, MRCP
Clinical Lecturer in Cardiology and Interventional
Cardiologist
Cardiology Department
King's College London School of Medicine and
King's College Hospital Foundation Trust
London
UK

Gary S. Mintz, MD
Chief Medical Officer
Cardiovascular Research Foundation
New York, NY
USA

Saidi A. Mohiddin, MBChB
Specialist Registrar in Cardiology,
Barts and The London NHS Trust
The London Chest Hospital
London
UK

Jeffrey W. Moses, MD
Professor of Medicine
Columbia University Medical Center
Director Center for Intravascular Therapy (CIVT)
Director Adult Cardiac Catheterization Laboratories
New York-Presbyterian Hospital
New York, NY
USA

Eugenia Nikolsky, MD, PhD
Columbia University Medical Center
Cardiovascular Research Foundation
New York, NY
USA
Rambam Health Care Campus
Heart Institute
Haifa
Israel

Annunziata Nusca, MD
Interventional Cardiologist
Department of Cardiovascular Sciences
Campus Bio-Medico University of Rome
Rome
Italy

Yoshinobu Onuma, MD
Research Fellow
Thoraxcenter
Erasmus Medical Center
Rotterdam
The Netherlands

Rikesh Patel, MD
Postdoctoral Residency Fellow
Department of Medicine
Columbia University Medical Center
New York-Presbyterian Hospital
New York, NY
USA

Stuart J. Pocock, PhD
Professor of Hygiene and Tropical Medicine
London School of Hygiene and Tropical Medicine
London
UK

Abhiram Prasad, MD, FRCP, FACC, FESC
Professor of Medicine
Consultant, Cardiac Catheterization Laboratory
The Division of Cardiovascular Diseases and Department
of Internal Medicine
Mayo Clinic and Mayo Foundation
Rochester, MN
USA

Francesca Pugliese, MD
Consultant Cardiac Radiologist
Cardiothoracic Centre Basildon University Hospital
Basildon
UK
Hon. Consultant
Royal Brompton Hospital and Imperial College Healthcare
Trust
London
UK
Clinical Researcher
Erasmus MC University Medical Center
Rotterdam
The Netherlands

Evelyn Regar, MD, PhD
Interventional Cardiologist
Thoraxcenter
Erasmus Medical Center
Rotterdam
The Netherlands

Johan H.C. Reiber, PhD
Professor of Medical imaging
Division of Image Processing (LKEB)
Department of Radiology
Leiden University Medical Center
Leiden
The Netherlands

Martin T. Rothman, FRCP, FACC, FESC
Professor of Interventional Cardiology
Director of Cardiac Research & Development
Barts and The London NHS Trust
The London Chest Hospital
London
UK

Giuseppe Sangiorgi, MD, FESC, FSCAI
Assistant Professor of Cardiology
Director, Cardiac Catheterization Laboratory
University of Modena
Department of Pathology
University of Rome
Italy

Carl Schultz, MD, PhD
Interventional Cardiologist
Department of Cardiology
Thoraxcentre
Erasmus Medical Center
Rotterdam
The Netherlands

Patrick W. Serruys, MD, PhD
Professor of Cardiology
Thoraxcenter
Erasmus Medical Center
Rotterdam
The Netherlands

Ulrich Sigwart, MD, FACC, EFESC, FRCP
Professor and Chairman Emeritus
Cardiology Service
Geneva University Hospitals
Geneva
Switzerland

Alex Sirker, MB, BChir, MRCP
Specialist Registrar in Cardiology and Clinical Research
Fellow
Department of Cardiology
King's College London
James Black Centre
London
UK

Luigi Giusto Spagnoli, MD
Professor of Pathology and Director
Pathology Department
University of Rome Tor Vergata
Rome
Italy

Neil Swanson, MBChB
Consultant Cardiologist
James Cook University Hospital
Middlesbrough
UK

Jun Tanigawa, MD, PhD
First Department of Internal Medicine
Osaka Medical College
Takatsuki, Osaka
Japan

Martyn R. Thomas, MD, MBBS, FRCP
Clinical Director
Cardiothoracic Centre and Consultant
Interventional Cardiologist
Cardiology Department
St Thomas' Hospital
London
UK

Leif Thuesen, MD, DMSc, FESC
Director, Cardiac Catheterization Laboratory
Department of Cardiology
Aarhus University Hospital
Skejby
Denmark

Santi Trimarchi, MD
Assistant Professor of Vascular Surgery
Department of Vascular Surgery
IRCCS Policlinico San Donato
San Donato Milanese
Milan
Italy

Joan C. Tuinenburg, MSc
Scientific Researcher
Division of Image Processing (LKEB)
Department of Radiology
Leiden University Medical Center
Leiden
The Netherlands

Pawel Tyczynski, MD, PhD
Cardiologist
Department of Coronary Artery Disease
Institute of Cardiology
Warsaw
Poland
Recipient of the EAPCI Training Grant in
Interventional Cardiology
Royal Brompton Hospital
London
UK

Alec Vahanian, MD, FESC, FACC
Head of Cardiology
Bichat Hospital
Paris
France

Marco Valgimigli, MD, PhD
Senior Interventional Cardiologist
Cardiovascular Institute
University of Ferrara
Ferrara
Italy

Gerald S. Werner, MD, FACC, FESC
Professor of Cardiology and Director
Cardiology & Intensive Care
Klinikum Darmstadt
Darmstadt
Germany

William Wijns, MD, PhD
Senior Interventional Cardiologist
Cardiovascular Center Aalst
Moorselbaan
Aalst
Belgium

Steven D. Wolff, MD, PhD
Director of Advanced Cardiovascular Imaging
Assistant Professor of Medicine and Radiology
Columbia University, College of Physicians and Surgeons
New York, NY
USA

Bryan P. Yan, MBBS, FRACP
Assistant Professor
Division of Cardiology, Prince of Wales Hospital
Department of Medicine & Therapeutics
The Chinese University of Hong Kong
Hong Kong
China

Gerald Yong, MBBS (Hons), FRACP
Interventional Fellow
Cardiology Division
Evanston Hospital
Evanston, IL
USA

Acknowledgements

In a time when interventional cardiology has become too complex to be mastered by one or even three individuals, we decided to involve the best scholars in the field to cover the various topics of this book: without their help we could not have achieved this final result.

Our masters have taught us more than to push catheters. They made us love our profession and love teaching: we are delighted that many of them also contributed to this textbook.

Our Fellows have told us with their questions and doubts that not everything can be found in the many existing textbooks and the Internet. They inspired us to embark in this endeavor and acted as a continuous source of inspiration to draw enough attention to practical details.

Finally, we have neglected our spouses and children to spend long hours in front of a computer screen. We are confident that our wives already understand us and we hope one day our children will see this textbook on the shelves of the family library, read some pages and forgive us.

Carlo Di Mario
George D. Dangas
Peter Barlis

Foreword

By Patrick W. Serruys

Interventional cardiology has grown dramatically since the early days of Andreas Gruntzig, and today coronary angioplasty is the most commonly performed intervention in medicine. It remains an impossible task for today's interventional cardiologist to stay abreast of all developments and Carlo Di Mario, George Dangas amd Peter Barlis must therefore be commended for assembling a distinguished field of experts who share their vast knowledge and experience in this rapidly changing field.

The importance of sound technique and an understanding of the principles of interventional cardiology cannot be overstated, and Part I provides crucial information for both the junior cardiologist starting on the long road of training in interventional cardiology, and the more seasoned experienced interventional cardiologist who will still find their knowledge enhanced. As we enter a new decade, the cath lab is increasingly becoming a high-tech environment as we strive to obtain the best results for our patients, and decisions are no long based on just plain 'luminography.' The editors must therefore be congratulated for providing an indispensable chapter on complementary imaging; techniques which still remain novel to many of us. The complexity of lesions being treated in the cath lab is ever increasing, and Part V provides essential reading on the fundamental aspects of treating these lesions, by operators dealing with lesions day in day out.

The wealth of information that this book provides means it will suitably grace any cath lab and personal library.

Patrick W. Serruys,
Thoraxcenter, Rotterdam, The Netherlands
2010

Foreword

By Martin B. Leon

For the past three decades the discipline of interventional cardiology has evolved from a simple balloon procedure, to a valued collection of lesser-invasive therapies, and currently into a clearly defined subspecialty that provides worthwhile treatment alternatives to millions of patients around the world each year. Importantly, the spirit of interventional cardiology has always embraced evolutionary change, with a strong emphasis on both technical expertise in the catheterization laboratory and clinical decision-making enhanced by evidence-based medicine. These are crucial times in the life history of interventional cardiology with many challenges, including the socioeconomic burdens of procedural therapies in many parts of the world. A vital component to preserve and grow the specialty requires a commitment to the education and training of the next generation of interventional physicians. In the past, most textbooks in interventional cardiology have focused on broad academic and clinical overviews or selective niche topics (e.g. chronic total occlusions or drug-eluting stents). The unique significance of "Interventional Cardiology: Principles and Practice" is that this is the first legitimate textbook which targets the education and training of young coronary interventionalists, spanning the range from fellows, to junior faculty, to clinical practitioners. Interestingly, the design and nature of the textbook also lends itself to a much wider readership; the expanding mass of healthcare professionals (e.g. cardiovascular nurses, technologists) who desire a formal updated reference text in the field of interventional cardiology.

The textbook, edited by Drs. Di Mario, Dangas and Barlis, is thoughtfully organized and provides an engaging balance of factual data and practical clinical insights. The authors are an amalgam of well known international thought leaders, next generation budding stars, and early stage interventionalists who have recently completed training experiences. This provocative blend of author expertise results in a textbook which certainly provides the necessary knowledge content from "brand name" individuals, but also allows a spirited digression into areas of practical clinical relevance which are of great importance to younger trainees. The chapter progression moves seamlessly from fundamental principles, to general and specific interventional techniques, to adjunctive pharmacology, to indications for treatment, to complications, and concludes with a worthwhile session on many of the seminal interventional clinical trials. The content is an admixture of standard topics required to master clinical interventional practice and many of the newest and most novel potential therapies of the future, such as transcatheter valve and cell-based therapies.

In the dynamic subspecialty of interventional cardiology, wherein rapid evolutionary and even revolutionary changes are expected in a telescoped time horizon (usually in very few years), there needs to be a comprehensive, modern era textbook which provides an educational and training experience for dedicated individuals who crave to master basic and advance skills or simply desire a formal in-depth introduction into the field. "Interventional Cardiology: Principles and Practice" nicely fills this critical gap and should be embraced as a major success, supporting and complementing the dynamism of the subspecialty.

Martin B. Leon,
Center for Interventional Vascular Therapy,
NewYork-Presbyterian Hospital/Columbia
University Medical Center,
New York, USA
2010

Preface

The idea for the generation of this book has been the continuous encouragement from the attendees of the Interventional Cardiology review courses we have been holding regularly both in the United States and Europe. The genesis of the subspecialty of cardiology has paralleled the exponential development of techniques and equipment to provide minimally invasive interventional therapies to patients with cardiovascular disease. The proper administration of such therapies requires a unique set of qualifications as well as special understanding of the disease entities and the interventions used. In many ways, this is not simply something in-between classic surgery and medical therapy, but demands skills and knowledge of both classic entities. The immediate therapeutic results and their relationship to rational hemodynamic and pathophysiologic algorithms attract the attention of both trainees and teachers for life. The fast pace of evidence based decision making is a challenge which requires continuous knowledge updates to all involved.

This subspecialty has been a recognized one in the United States since 1999 with the advent of the first Board Examination and the ensuing Certifications. Although other places of the world have not yet set up a formal teaching pathway, this should be expected soon, since this specialty is practiced widely everywhere. Therefore, a compre-

hensive review of this discipline is in high demand. We have been fortunate to have initiated the review courses in 1998 in the USA and in 2006 in Europe and have firmly believed all along that a written instruction should ideally complement the live teaching methods.

We are quite pleased to provide the present book to all those seeking initial or repeat certification in Interventional Cardiology. Furthermore, we would also encourage anyone outside the formal specialty (e.g. cardiac or vascular surgeons, radiologists, etc) who have keen interest in interventional therapies to complement their practical instruction with structured studying. We have worked with our review courses faculty in this task, and we would like to thank all of the co-authors for their contributions of carefully written narratives, illustrative figures, organized tables and inquisitive question-answer sections.

Finally, we would like to thank our Publisher for the high quality of the final product and once again thank our students, teachers and colleagues of the international community of academic interventional cardiologists for the continuous inspiration they have provided to us.

Carlo Di Mario
George D. Dangas
Peter Barlis

PART I

Principles and Techniques

CHAPTER 1

Interventional Cardiology Training

Carlo Di Mario[1], & Joseph Babb[2]

[1] Royal Brompton Hospital, London, UK

[2] East Carolina University Brody School of Medicine, Greenville, NC, USA

Introduction

The treatment of coronary artery disease has undergone rapid evolution, with many groundbreaking innovations introduced in the last years. Angioplasty is now the first option in the acute phase of myocardial infarction, allows rapid control and early discharge of patients with acute coronary syndromes, and has eroded the prevalent use of bypass surgery in stable angina and silent ischemia. The drastic reduction of restenosis observed with the use of drug eluting stents makes percutaneous revascularization a viable option in complex lesions, including multivessel and left main disease, with ongoing clinical trials of comparison with surgery. Interventional cardiology has expanded its field of application from coronary arteries to structural heart disease and other degenerative atherosclerotic changes such as peripheral artery disease. If laser and directional atherectomy have almost disappeared from the therapeutic armamentarium, other devices such as Rotablator, cutting balloon, filters, and thromboaspiration devices have become a welcome addition in selected cases as preparation to balloon dilatation and stent implantation. Aspirin and heparin were the only options available 15 years ago and are now complemented or substituted by a variety of antiplatelet and antithrombin agents. Another important

change transforming the practice of interventional cardiology has been the increasing pressure of healthcare systems, forcing interventionalists to use strict interpretation of guidelines for indications, meticulously document procedures and complications in databases open to review from health providers and the general public, acquire management skills to optimize resource utilization, motivate and enhance performance of the team, build stable referral networks.

Specific mandatory training is implemented in few countries around the world. With these few exceptions, all cardiologists but also many other medical specialists (radiologists, cardiac and vascular surgeons) are legally entitled to perform percutaneous interventional procedures after successful completion of training in their main specialty without any specific knowledge and experience in the interventional field. In this chapter, the different reality of interventional training in Europe and the United States is examined to help Fellows understand the similarities and differences and to stimulate growth and improvement on both sides of the Atlantic.

Principles of Medical Training Applied to Interventional Cardiology

As for most doctors, the three cornerstones of the training required for a successful interventionalist are knowledge, professional skills and professionalism. The most knowledgeable cardiologist with a complete background spanning from pathophysiology

Interventional Cardiology, First Edition. Edited by Carlo Di Mario, George D. Dangas, Peter Barlis.
© 2010 Blackwell Publishing Ltd. Published 2010 by Blackwell Publishing Ltd.

of coronary artery disease to the results of the most recent trials will be unable to work safely if s/he has not achieved sufficient practical experience of a variety of procedures, assisted and coached by qualified supervisors. Similarly, a physician combining good theoretical knowledge and hands-on experience can still be inefficient and dangerous if s/he does not use in his/her practice respect and human compassion towards his/her patients and does not have the ability to select and motivate his/her team. Training in interventional cardiology must pay attention to these three complementary essential aspects of the education process and must develop reliable methods of assessment to certify the progress made and indicate the additional steps required to become an independent professional. As the undergraduate and postgraduate medical education is different in the various countries also the curriculum of Interventional Cardiology training must adapt to the different background which explains differences among countries. In this chapter we limited our observations to Europe and the United States.

The State of Interventional Cardiology Training in Europe

The training of specialists in interventional cardiology is not formally regulated in any European countries. Most countries, however, offer a period of one to two years' training in interventional cardiology and the appointment of cardiologists expected to carry out angioplasties and other interventional procedures is in practice restricted at a level of interviews/local credentials required by hospitals to candidates who prove they have successfully completed this training. Still, no official certificates with binding legal value are issued. The official approval of a new Specialty called Interventional Cardiology requires a direct decision of the National Governments since this legislation is demanded to individual countries. The European Community only checks compatibility with the principles governing the community of member states. One such principle is the promotion of free movement of workers, including professionals. It is understandable, therefore, that the European Commission, the Government of the Union, seeks advice from a body representing all

the Medical Colleges of the Member states, called UEMS (European Union of Medical Specialists). This supernational representation has allowed in the past a radical review of the denomination and duration of training in the different post-graduate medical Specialty areas. The complexity of the process required, involving the consultation of all the Departments of Health and Education, Universities and Medical Colleges, is one of the factors explaining the reluctance to introduce too frequent new changes. In most European countries, cardiology training is constituted by a period of training in internal medicine (1–2 years) and 3–4 years' training in Cardiology, covering the different invasive and non-invasive fields. The ability to perform diagnostic coronary angiography and right and left cardiac catheterization is still part of the general training for all Cardiologists in most European countries, with a minimum number of procedures often indicated in the curriculum of trainees in general cardiology. This is reflected by the Core Curriculum in Cardiology, recently published by the Education Committee of the European Society of Cardiology [1]. In the Curriculum a minimum of 300 catheterizations as first operator is required. For diagnostic catheterization (right and left, with coronary angiography and left ventriculography) the level required (III) implies that the trainee is able to "independently perform the procedure unaided" at the end of his/her training. Also percutaneous interventions are part of the techniques required, with a lower number (50) and a Level II which indicates "practical experience but not as independent operator". The Core Curriculum, promoted and implemented by the European Society of Cardiology and recently updated, implicitly recognizes that percutaneous interventions are part of a different Subspecialty training.

To promote the application of the Curriculum and issue the Diploma of European Cardiologist, a certificate not required to practice in individual countries but helpful to move across different European countries, a permanent body joining the expertise provided by the European Society of Cardiology and the authority of the UEMS has been created. This permanent Committee, called European Board of the Specialty in Cardiology, has already endorsed the concept that practice of activities like interventional cardiology, electrophysiology and pacing, cardiovascular imaging, require a specific and additional training and has set the general rules regulating its organization, devolving to each individual Working Group or Association the development of the specific educational content of the programs.

The European Curriculum and Syllabus

After several meetings between members of the ESC WG of Interventional Cardiology and the chairmen of the national interventional societies, a Committee was nominated to finalize a Curriculum and Syllabus for interventional cardiology training in Europe. The final document has been published in EuroIntervention in 2006 [2]. The intention of the curriculum is to identify an educational process for specialists in interventional cardiology in Europe. The curriculum mandates a two-year program divided into four semesters, with the trainee starting to prepare the patient for the intervention, including diagnostic angiography, and assist the supervisor or another experienced interventionalist performing the angioplasty procedure. It was recommended that the trainee starts working as primary operator for simple angioplasties under close supervision and assists in the most complex angioplasty procedures (bifurcations, thrombus containing lesions, chronic occlusions, diffuse disease, severe calcifications, etc.) till s/he reaches a level of confidence allowing him/her to work as primary and independent operator in both simple and complex coronary interventional procedures. Apprenticeship learning is defined as the mainstay of the training process in interventional cardiology. Candidates are required to be involved in procedure planning, assessment of indications and contraindications, and specific establishment of the individual patient risks based on clinical and angiographic characteristics. The performance of supervised angioplasty procedures is regulated with the goal of a progressive increase of the candidate involvement and direct handling of angioplasties of increasing complexity. A parallel formal learning is also required, ensuring that the candidate achieves sufficient knowledge of all the subjects included in the Syllabus. Trainees are required to attend at least 30 full days (240 hours) in two years of accredited formal sessions locally, nationally or abroad, including attendance of study

days and post graduate courses, national and international courses in Interventional Cardiology, including live courses. Distance learning through journals, textbooks and the Internet is also encouraged and certified. In the Curriculum it is indicated that all trainees must be exposed by the training program to research in interventional cardiology.

It is a formidable challenge to ensure homogeneous high standard training when no central European government can enforce it and in the absence of any legal recognition of this training. The solution proposed by EBSC and approved by the EAPCI and most National Interventional Cardiological Societies and interventional groups is the development of web based platforms dedicated to subspecialty training, with the scientific and educational content determined by EAPCI within a general scheme valid for all the Subspecialties approved by EBSC [3]. The platform is currently under development and will offer to the trainee the possibility to document attendance of accredited formal training courses and to record their catheter lab based procedures [4]. The website will ask for mandatory reports of Directly Observed Procedures, appraisal from the program director, a 360 degrees assessment involving medical colleagues but also nurses, radiographers, technicians and patients. The final judgment should report the trainee's ability to interact with cath lab staff and colleagues, attention to minimize patient risk and attitude to discuss complex procedures with more expert colleagues, ability to make independent appropriate choices and cope with emergency situations. No final summative examination is envisioned at the end of the training, but multiple choice questions (MCQ) are embedded into a first section testing theoretical knowledge and covering all items included in the Syllabus, and a second series of MCQ in present under "Skills", using real or simulated clinical cases to appraise practical experience.

Training centers are asked to fulfill technical and staffing requirements such as having an independent interventional cardiology unit, allowing the trainee to follow the patient from the beginning to the completion of the interventional treatment, having a volume of at least 800 coronary angioplasties per year including acute coronary syndromes and primary angioplasty for acute myocardial infarction. At least two certified supervisors must be available, with an experience of at least 1,000 coronary interventions and more than five years experience mainly dedicated to interventional cardiology.

These activities have already promoted changes de facto or via a legal governmental approval of the training programs of interventional cardiology in most European countries. A final year of subspecialist training after a common trunk of three years in general cardiology has been adopted in most countries, with an additional year of fellowship encouraged. The emphasis posed by the EAPCI and the National groups of interventional cardiology on education and training [5] has gained the consensus of all the components within cardiology. Trainees enthusiastically subscribe to the dedicated courses organized for fellows, modeled after similar initiatives of the US Society for Cardiac Angiography and Interventions. Europe, the cradle of modern interventional cardiology, is being reinvigorated to ensure this tradition is continued by competent and dedicated physicians, sharing common knowledge, skills and professionalism throughout Europe.

The State of Interventional Cardiology Training in the USA

The development of training and education in interventional cardiology in the United States followed a path similar to that in Europe. Initial training in percutaneous transluminal coronary angioplasty (PTCA) occurred via attendance at a live demonstration course in Zurich given by Dr. Andreas Gruentzig and his colleagues. At that time (late 1970s, very early 1980s), there was only one manufacturer of PTCA equipment in the USA. Initially they would not sell equipment to hospitals unless the operator had a diploma from attendance at a Gruentzig course and the hospital had Institutional Review Board (IRB) approval to perform PTCA. As the procedure gained acceptance and Dr. Gruentzig moved from Zurich to Emory University in Atlanta, Georgia, more "Courses in Angioplasty" began to appear and more companies began selling PTCA equipment. With this, the requirement for IRB approval of the procedure disappeared and certification of an

individual as "PTCA competent" was left to the discretion of individual hospital credentialing committees.

PTCA became accepted very quickly as an appropriate alternative to coronary artery bypass grafting (CABG) for a select number of patients. Add to this the pioneering work of Dr. Geoffrey Hartzler in late 1980 in performing "direct" angioplasty (as he termed it) in acute myocardial infarction, and the impetus to expand the field of angioplasty was very strong indeed. On the job training through attendance at live demonstration courses and preceptorships rapidly expanded the number of physicians performing angioplasty. PTCA procedures were, by necessity, performed only in hospitals which had an open heart surgery program as the requirement for urgent CABG due to coronary dissection or acute closure was not infrequent in this pre-stent, pre-glycoprotein 2b/3a era. Since a large proportion of these hospitals with on-site CABG and PTCA programs were teaching hospitals with training programs in cardiology, exposure to PTCA became a regular part of basic cardiology training. The core training program in cardiology consisted of three years of internal medicine training followed by three years of cardiology training. This three-year cardiology program covered all aspects of non-invasive and invasive cardiology. As a result, new graduates of programs having PTCA on site began to be certified by their program directors as being capable of performing PTCA.

In this early era, there was no nationally specified curriculum of training in interventional cardiology and, as a result, this process was essentially an unstructured apprenticeship. The graduates of these programs were products of a highly varied educational experience, some with excellent cognitive as well as technical exposure and some with limited cognitive and/or technical exposure.

As the field grew and patient and technical complexity increased, programs began to electively add an additional year of training for persons wishing to pursue careers in interventional cardiology. According to survey results, by 1993 approximately half of the then approved cardiology training programs were requiring an additional year of training if graduates wished certification in interventional procedures [6].

This rapid growth led both The Society for Cardiovascular Angiography and Interventions and The American College of Cardiology to discuss in the early 1990s a means to structure and codify the interventional cardiology training process. An added impetus was the concern that patient outcomes might be compromised by low volume operators with limited training, especially if performing in low volume hospitals. This was supported by several publications which showed a clear relationship between lower operator volumes and increased rates of emergency coronary artery bypass surgery in both the pre-stent and stent eras [7,8].

As a result, a group of interventional leaders began conversation with the American Board of Internal Medicine (ABIM), the American Board of Medical Specialties (ABMS), and the Accreditation Council for Graduate Medical Education (ACGME) about creating a new subspecialty of interventional cardiology. It is requisite that all these bodies interact in order to create a new medical specialty, designate an approved training pathway, and offer certification of competence in that specialty.

In order to recognize a new specialty area, the ACGME requires the following criteria be met:

1. The new specialty signifies the differentiation of a new specialty based on major new concepts in medical science.

2. The new specialty is based on substantial advancement in medical science. The necessary training must be sufficiently complex or extended that it is not feasible to include it in established training programs.

3. There will be sufficient interest and resources available to establish the critical mass of quality training programs with long term commitments for successful integrating of the graduates in the health care system nationally.

4. The new discipline is recognized as legitimate and significant by the medical profession in general and the closely related specialties in particular for a consensus of the training required to perform in this new field.

5. That training in the new field is recognized as the single pathway to the competent preparation of a practitioner in this discipline.

Additionally, the ACGME requires that a number of other criteria be fulfilled to warrant a new training pathway. Detailed information on these requirements is available on the ACGME website. [9] As is evident, the creation of a new accredited subspecialty is a highly structured and codified process requiring much thought, effort, and coordination with other specialty areas. As a result of these extensive discussions, in 1999 the ACGME began reviewing and certifying training programs in interventional cardiology.

In addition to these ACGME training requirements, the ABIM had to find, amongst other things, that the specified body of knowledge is testable and objectively assessable. In 1999, the ABIM created a Certificate of Added Qualification in Interventional Cardiology (now simply called Certification in Interventional Cardiology), and the first examinations were given in the autumn of that year. To be eligible, a candidate had to hold a valid existing board certification in internal medicine and cardiovascular diseases. The candidate then applied through either the practice pathway (no formal interventional fellowship) or the training pathway (with formal interventional fellowship) meeting specified procedural requirements. The practice pathway ended with the 2003 examination. Thereafter, all applicants had to qualify via the training pathway with graduation from an ACGME approved interventional fellowship experience. The reason for this somewhat complex interweaving of eligible training pathways was to allow existing practitioners without formal interventional training to take IC boards until the training pipeline was established.

The IC examination is a timed multiple choice format examination given over two days. At the present, the question content is divided as follows:

- Case selection 25%
- Procedural techniques 25%
- Imaging 15%
- Pharmacology 15%
- Basic science 15%
- Miscellaneous 5%

Detailed information on content is available on the ABIM website [10] At the time of writing, the ABIM is preparing to utilize simulation in upcoming examinations in order to more adequately assess examinees technical skills and intra-procedure decision making.

Training and education are living processes undergoing constant evolution. In 2004 the ACGME promulgated new educational guidelines for all graduate medical education programs in the US and specified that all training had to comply with the six core competencies which are part of the Outcomes Project. These are:

- Medical Knowledge (MK)
- Patient Care (PC)
- Practice Based Learning and Improvement (PBLI)
- Systems Based Practice (SBP)
- Professionalism (P)
- Interpersonal and Communication Skills (ICS)

Details regarding these, procedural exposure, conferencing, research, and other ACGME requirements are available at their website [11].

As a result of these highly structured and codified requirements, training and credentialing in the US has achieved a high standard of excellence. The requirement of a structured didactic curriculum along with case conferences, basic science, conferences, morbidity and mortality conferences, and a required research project assure each trainee of a comprehensive and intensive training experience. The trainee is accepted in the program for one purpose only—to educate him/her. The notion of an unstructured apprenticeship built around clinical service to the mentor is no longer acceptable.

The next challenge to be faced is how to accommodate training for non-coronary interventions and structural heart disease within the existing framework. Note that according to the existing training documents, current IC training is specifically focused on coronary intervention. Adding this to the existing IC curriculum would require additional conversations with the ACGME, ABIM, and ABMS as they would have to agree to this plan according to the criteria enumerated above. Regardless of the outcome of these discussions, some form of formal, structured education beyond coronary intervention seems both likely and necessary.

In summary, the process of training and credentialing in interventional cardiology in the United States has evolved into a highly structured and codified process. Such training was initially obtained in the context of the basic three-year curriculum in cardiology and then developed into an additional year of training at many institutions but without clearly outlined expectations of didactic or clinical content. These unstructured apprenticeships then evolved into the current system of ACGME approved training in interventional cardiology beginning in 1999. In the same year, the ABIM began administering written examinations in interventional cardiology to provide "board certification" in the sub-sub-specialty. Until 2003 one could take these examinations via the practice pathway which required no formal training in IC but substantial experience. Thereafter, only graduates of ACGME approved IC programs were eligible for these examinations which provide a 10-year time-limited certification. At the end of that time, the applicant must re-take the examinations to maintain certification. As the field of IC continues to evolve, it seems highly likely that the current guidelines will be modified to include specified training in non-coronary interventions and/or structural heart disease with curricula and certifying examinations to match.

Conclusion

Interventional cardiovascular practice remains a dynamic, evolving and demanding subspecialty of cardiology which requires significant personal commitment to training and significant system resources to provide properly structured training. The evolution of similar systems in Europe suggests that this formalized process is superior to unstructured apprenticeships/fellowships and there may come a day when a truly international program of training and certification may be available.

References

1. http://www.escardio.org/education/coresyllabus/Pages/core-curriculum.aspx.
2. Di Mario C, Di Sciascio G, Dubois-Randé LG, Michels R, Mills P. Curriculum and syllabus for interventional cardiology subspecialty training in Europe. EuroInterv 2006; 31–36.
3. Lopez-Sendon J, Mills P, Weber H, Michels R, Di Mario C, Filippatos G, Heras M, Fox K, Merino J, Pennell DJ, Sochor H, Ortoli J on behalf of the Coordination Task Force on Sub-speciality

Accreditation of the European Board for the Speciality of Cardiology. Recommendations on sub-speciality accreditation in Cardiology. Eur Heart J 2007; **28**(17): 2163–2171. Epub August 3, 2007.

4. http://www.escardio.org/communities/EAPCI/news/Pages/accreditation-status-june08.aspx.

5. Wijns W., Di Mario C. EAPCI: Presidential Criss–Cross. The transfer of office between EAPCI Presidents. EuroInterv 2009; **5**: 293–297.

6. Cheitlin MD, Langdon LO. Certification in interventional cardiology: How far have we come? What remains to be done? Journal of Interventional Cardiology 1995; **8**: 339–341.

7. Jollis JG, Peterson ED, Nelson CL, *et al.* Relationship between physicians and hospital coronary angioplasty volume and outcome in elderly patients. Circulation 1997; **95**: 2485–2491.

8. McGrath PD, Wennberg DE, Dickens JD Jr, *et al.* Relation between operator and hospital volume and outcomes following percutaneous coronary interventions in the era of the coronary stent. Journal of the American Medical Association 2000; **284**: 3139–3144.

9. http://www.acgme.org/acWebsite/about/ab_ACGMEPoliciesProcedures.pdf.

10. http://www.abim.org/pdf/blueprint/icard_cert.pdf.

11. http://www.acgme.org.

CHAPTER 2

Atherogenesis and Inflammation

Giuseppe Sangiorgi[1], Alessandro Mauriello[2], Santi Trimarchi[3],
Elena Bonanno[2], & Luigi Giusto Spagnoli[2]

[1] Cardiac Catheterization Laboratory, University of Modena, Italy
[2] University of Rome Tor Vergata, Rome, Italy
[3] IRCCS Policlinico San Donato, Milanese, Italy

Introduction

Atherosclerosis and its clinical consequences are the leading cause of death in Western nations. Mechanisms that lead to the formation of the atherosclerotic plaque are numerous. Atherosclerosis, by now considered a chronic inflammatory disease, begins in young age and progresses slowly for decades [1–3]. The clinical symptoms of atheroma occur in adult age and usually involve plaque rupture and thrombosis [4–6].

The risk of major thrombotic and thromboembolic complications of atherosclerosis appears to be related more to the stability of atheromatous plaques than to the extent of disease [7,8]. Stable angina is associated with smooth fibrous coronary-artery plaques (stable plaque), whereas unstable angina, acute myocardial infarction (AMI), and sudden cardiac death are almost invariably associated to destabilisation of plaques [9]. Similarly, in patients with carotid-artery atherosclerotic disease, plaque irregularity and rupture are closely associated with cerebral ischemic events, and patients with irregular or ulcerated plaque demonstrate a higher risk of ischemic stroke irrespective of the degree of luminal stenosis [10].

Many efforts have been recently performed to identifying plaques at high risk of disruption leading to thrombosis, generally defined as "vulnerable plaques" [5,9]. Several data sustain the hypothesis that some morphologic and molecular markers identifying unstable plaques could be expressed during plaque vulnerability. As shown by a number of anatomical and clinical studies, these vulnerable plaques, are associated with rupture and thrombosis, as compared to the stable ones covered by a thin fibrous cap and show an extensive inflammatory infiltrate [11,12].

Unlike the stable plaque that shows a chronic inflammatory infiltrate, the vulnerable and ruptured plaque is characterised by a chronic inflammation [13,12]. There are a large number of studies showing that "active" inflammation mainly involves T-lymphocytes and macrophages which are activated toward a pathway of inflammatory response, secrete cytokines and lytic enzymes which in turn cause thinning of the fibrous cap, predisposing to plaque rupture. Recent research has furnished new insight into the molecular mechanisms that cause transition from a stable to an unstable phase of atherosclerosis and points to inflammation as the playmaker in the events leading to plaque destabilization.

A current challenge is to identify morphological and molecular markers able to discriminate stable plaques from vulnerable ones allowing the stratification of "high risk" patients for acute cardiac and

Interventional Cardiology, First Edition. Edited by Carlo Di Mario, George D. Dangas, Peter Barlis.
© 2010 Blackwell Publishing Ltd. Published 2010 by Blackwell Publishing Ltd.

cerebrovascular events before clinical syndromes develop. Bearing that aim in mind, this chapter will focus on cellular and molecular mechanisms affecting plaque progression and serum markers correlated to plaque inflammation.

The Vulnerable Plaque

Atherosclerotic lesions, according to the classification of the American Heart Association modified recently by Virmani *et al.* [9], are divided in two groups: (a) non-atherosclerotic intimal lesions and (b) progressive atherosclerotic lesions which include stable, vulnerable and thrombotic plaques.

The different pathologic characterization of atherosclerotic lesions largely depends on the thickness of the fibrous cap and its grade of inflammatory infiltrate which is in turn largely constituted by macrophages and activated T lymphocytes. Typically, the accumulating plaque burden is initially accommodated by an adaptive positive remodelling with expansion of the vessel external elastic lamina and minimal changes in lumen size [15]. The plaque contains monocyte-derived macrophages, smooth muscle cells, and T lymphocytes. Interaction between these cells types and the connective tissue appears to determine the development and progression of the plaque itself, including important complications, such as thrombosis and rupture.

The lesions classified as vulnerable or thin cap fibrous atheroma (TCFA) identify a plaque prone to rupture and thrombosis characterized by a large necrotic core containing numerous cholesterol clefts. The overlying cap is thin and rich in inflammatory cells, macrophages and T lymphocytes with few smooth muscle cells [9,11,16]. Burke *et al.* identified a cut-off value for cap thickness of 65 microns to define a vulnerable coronary plaque [17]. With regard to carotid plaque vulnerability, our observations identified a thickness of 165 microns for differentiating stable from unstable carotid lesions (*pers. comm.*).

Despite the predominant hypothesis focusing on the responsibility of a specific vulnerable atherosclerotic plaque rupture [4,6] for acute coronary syndromes, some pathophysiologic, clinical and angiographic observations seem to suggest the possibility that the principal cause of coronary

instability is not to be found in the vulnerability of a single atherosclerotic plaque, but in the presence of multiple vulnerable plaques in the entire coronary tree, correlated with the presence of a diffuse inflammatory process [12,13,18,19].

Within this context, recent angiographic studies have demonstrated the presence of multiple vulnerable atheromatous plaques in patients with unstable angina [20] and in those affected by transmural myocardial infarction [19]. Recently by means of flow cytometry we have demonstrated the presence of an activated and multicentric inflammatory infiltrate in the coronary vessels of individuals who died of acute myocardial infarction [13]. Similar results have been obtained by Buffon *et al.*, who, through the determination of the neutrophil myeloperoxidase activity, have proved the presence of a diffuse inflammation in the coronary vessels in individuals affected by unstable angina [18]. These results have been confirmed by a morphological study of our group which demonstrated the presence of a high inflammatory infiltrate constituted by macrophagic cells and T lymphocytes activated in the whole coronary tree, also present in the stable plaques of individuals who died of acute myocardial infarction. These plaques showed a two- to four-fold higher inflammatory infiltrate than aged-matched individuals dying from noncardiac causes with chronic stable angina (SA) or without clinical cardiac history (CTRL), respectively [12]. Moreover, we have recently demonstrated that activated T lymphocytes infiltrate the myocardium both in the peri-infarctual area and in remote unaffected myocardial regions in patients who died of a first myocardial infarction [21]. The simultaneous occurrence of diffuse coronary and myocardial inflammation in these patients further supports the concept that both coronary and myocardial vulnerabilities concur in the pathogenesis of fatal AMI.

Acute myocardial infarction—at least associated with unfavorable prognosis—is therefore likely to be the consequence of a diffuse "active" chronic inflammatory process which determines the destabilization of both the entire coronary tree and the whole myocardium, not only the part of it affected by infarction. The causes of the diffuse inflammation associated with myocardial infarction are scarcely known. The presence of activated T lymphocytes suggests the "in-situ" presence of an antigenic stimulus which triggers adaptive immunity.

Role of Inflammation in the Natural History of Atherosclerosis

Inception of the Plaque

Endothelium injury has been proposed to be an early and clinically relevant pathophysiologic event in the atherosclerotic process [3,8]. Patients with endothelial dysfunction have an increased risk for future cardiovascular events including stroke [22]. Endothelial dysfunction was described as the ignition step in atherogenesis. From this point on, an inflammatory response leads to the development of the plaque.

Endothelial damage can be caused by physical and chemical forces, by infective agents or by oxidized LDL (ox-LDL). Dysfunctional endothelium expresses P-selectin (stimulation by agonists such as trombin) E-selectin (induced by IL-1 or TNF-α. Expression of intercellular adhesion molecule-1 (ICAM-1) both by macrophages and endothelium and vascular adhesion molecule-1 (VCAM-1) by endothelial cells is induced by inflammatory cytokines such as IL-1, TNFα and IFNγ.

Monocytes recalled in the subintimal space ingest lipoproteins and morph into macrophages. These generate reactive oxygen species (ROS), which convert ox-LDL into highly oxidized LDL. Macrophages upload ox-LDL via scavenger receptors until form foam cells. Foam cells with leukocytes migrate at the site of damage and generate the fatty streak. The loss of biologic activity of endothelium determines nitric oxide (NO) reduction together with increased expression of prothrombotic factors, proinflammatory adhesion molecules cytokines and chemotactic factors. Cytokines may decrease NO bioavailability increasing the production of reactive oxygen species (ROS). ROS reduces NO activity both directly, reacting with endothelial cells, and indirectly via oxidative modification of eNOS or guanylyl cyclase [23]. Low NO bioavailability can up-regulate vascular adhesion molecule-1 (VCAM-1) in the endothelial cell layer, that binds monocytes and lymphocytes in the first step of invasion of the vascular wall, via induction of

NFkB expression [24]. In addition, NO inhibits leukocyte adhesion [25] and NO reduction results in induction of monocyte chemotactic protein-1 (MCP-1) expression which recruits monocytes [26]. NO is in a sensitive balance with endothelin1 (ET-1) regulating vascular tone [27]. Plasma ET-1 concentrations are increased in patients with advanced atherosclerosis and correlate with the severity of the disease [28,29]. In addition to its vasoconstrictor activity, ET-1 also promotes leukocyte adhesion [30] and thrombous formation [31]. Dysfunctional endothelium expresses P-selectin (stimulation by agonists such as trombin) and E-selectin (induced by IL-1 or TNF-α [32]. The expression of both intercellular adhesion molecule1 (ICAM-1) by macrophages and endothelium, and VCAM-1 by endothelial cells is induced by inflammatory cytokines such as IL-1, TNFα, IFNγ. Endothelial cells also produce MCP-1, monocyte colony-stimulating factor and IL-6 which further amplify the inflammatory cascade [33]. IL-6 production by smooth muscle cells represents the main stimulus for C-reactive protein (CRP) production [2]. Recent evidence suggests that CRP may contribute to the proinflammatory state of the plaque both mediating monocytes recruitment and stimulating monocytes to release IL-1, IL-6, TNFα [34]. The damaged endothelium allows the passage of lipids into the subendothelial space. Fatty streaks represent the first step in the atherosclerotic process.

Evolving Fibro-atheromatous Plaque

The atheroma evolution is modulated by innate and adaptive immune responses [2,35,36]. The most important receptors for innate immunity in atherothrombosis are the scavenger receptors and the toll-like receptors (TLRs) [37]. Adaptive immunity is much more specific than innate immunity but may take several days or even weeks to be fully mobilized. It involves an organized immune response leading to generation of T and B cell receptors and immunoglobulins, which can recognize foreign antigens [38].

Stable Plaque

Macrophages take up lipid deposited in the intima via a number of receptors, including scavenger receptor-A, and CD36. Deregulated uptake of modified LDL through scavanger receptors leads to cholesterol accumulation and "foam cells" formation. The lipid laden macrophages (foam cells) forming the fatty streak secrete pro-inflammatory cytokines that amplify the local inflammatory response in the lesion, matrix metalloproteinases (MMPs), tissue factor into the local matrix, as well as growth factors, that stimulate the smooth muscle replication responsible for lesion growth. Macrophages colony stimulating factor (M-CSF) acts as the main stimulator in this process, next to granulocyte-macrophage stimulating factor (MG-CSF) and IL-2 for lymphocytes [39]. Lymphocytes enter the intima by binding adhesion molecules (VCAM-1, P-selectin, ICAM-1 MCP-1(CCL2), IL-8 (CxCL8) [33]. Such infiltrate constituted mainly by CD4+ T lymphocytes recognize antigens bound to MHC class II molecules involved in antigen presentation to T lymphocytes thus provoking an immune response [1]. The histocompatibility complex molecules (MHC II) are expressed by endothelial cells, macrophages and vascular smooth muscle cells in proximity to activated T lymphocytes in the atherosclerotic plaque. Pro-inflammatory cytokines manage a central transcriptional control point mainly mediated by nuclear factor-kB (NFkB). Macrophage/foam cells produce cytokines that activate neighbouring smooth-muscle cells, resulting in extracellular matrix production [1].

Repeated inflammatory stimuli induce foam cells to secrete growth factors that induce SMCs proliferation and migration into the intima. The continuous influx of cells in the subintimal space convert the fatty streak in a more complex and advanced lesion in which inflammatory cells (monocytes/macrophages, lymphocytes), SMCs, necrotic debris mainly due to cell death, oxLDL elicit a chronic inflammatory response by adoptive immune system. SMCs form a thick fibrous cap that cover the necrotic core and avoid the exposition of thrombogenic material to the bloodstream. The volume of lesion grows up and protrudes into the arterial lumen causing variable degree of lumen stenosis. These lesions are advanced complicated "stable" atherosclerotic lesions, asymptomatic and often unrecognized [40,41].

Vulnerable Plaque: A Shift Toward Th1 Pattern

Early phases of the plaque development are characterized by an acute innate immune response against exogenous (infectious) and endogenous non-infectious noxae. Specific antigens activate adaptive immune system leading to proliferation of T and B cells. A first burst of activation might occur in regional lymph nodes by dendritic cells (DCs) trafficking from the plaque to lymph node. Subsequent cycle of activation can be sustained by interaction of activated /memory T cells re-entering in the plaque by selective binding to endothelial cell surface adhesion molecules with plaque macrophages expressing MHC class II molecules. In this phase of the atherogenic process the selective recruitment of a specific subtype of CD4+ cells play a major role determining the future development of the lesion. Two subtypes of CD4+ cells have juxtaposed role Th1 and Th2 cells [42].

Th1 cells secreting proinflammatory cytokines, such as IFNγ promote macrophage activation, inflammation, and atherosclerosis, whereas Th2 cells (cytokine pattern IL-4, IL-5 and IL-10) mediate antibody production and generally have anti-inflammatory and antiatherogenic effects [22]. Therefore the switch to a selective recruitment of Th1 lymphocyte represents a key point toward plaque vulnerability/disruption. T cells in the plaque may encounter antigens such as oxLDL. Moreover T cell response can be triggered by heat shock proteins of endogenous or microbial origins [43]. It is still unknown why the initial inflammatory response becomes a chronic inflammatory condition. However, when the plaque microenvironment triggers the selective recruitment and activation of Th1 cells they in turn determine a potent inflammatory cascade.

The combination of IFNγ and TNFα upregulates the expression of fractalkine (CX3CL1) [44]. Interleukin 1 and TNFα-activated endothelium express also fractalkine (membrane bound form) that directly mediates the capture and adhesion of CX3CR1 expressing leukocytes providing a further pathway for leukocyte activation [45]. This cytokine network promotes the development of the Th-1 pathway which is strongly proinflammatory and induces macrophage activation, superoxide production and protease activity.

Role of Inflammation as Vulnerability Factor

Homeostasis of plaque "microenvironment", i.e. the balance between cell migration and cell proliferation, extracellular matrix production and degradation, macrophages and lymphocytes interplay, appears strictly related to the transition of a stable plaque into a vulnerable one.

A limited number of T cells, following the Th1 pathway, initiates the production of large amount of molecules downstream in the cytokine cascade orchestrating in the transition from the stable to unstable plaque [35,46].

Within the plaque, inflammatory cells such as foam cells and monocyte-derived macrophages are induced to produce matrix-degrading enzymes, cytokines and growth factors strictly implicated in extracellular matrix homeostasis. In particular, cytokines such as INF γ suppress collagen synthesis a major component of the fibrous cap [33]. Moreover infiltration of mononuclear cells results in release of proteases which causes plaque disruption [47]. The production of ROS within the atherosclerotic plaque has important implications for its structural integrity [23]. Deregulated oxidant production has the potential to promote the elaboration and activation of matrix degrading enzymes in the fibrous cap of the plaque. Moreover impaired NO function coupled with oxidative excess may activate MMPs [48], namely MMP-2 and MMP-9 which weaken the fibrous cap. Another mechanism which may determine the thinning of the fibrous cap is the apoptosis of smooth muscle cells. There is, in fact, evidence for extensive apoptosis of smooth muscle cells within the cap of advanced atherosclerosis, as well as those cultured from plaques [8,49].

A very important role, not yet well studied, is that of dendritic cells, namely cells specialized in antigen presentation with a key role in the induction of primary immune response and in the regulation of T lymphocytes differentiation, as well as in mechanisms of central and peripheral tolerance

aiming at the elimination of T lymphocytes that are potentially self-reactive toward self-antigens [50,51]. A characteristic of dendritic cells is also the ability to polarize T cell responses toward a T helper phenotype (Th1) in response to bacterial antigens. Molecules expressed by activated T lymphocytes, like CD40L, OX40, stimulate the release from dendritic cells of chemokines (fractalkines) able to attract other lymphocytes toward the inflammation site, amplifying the immune response [52].

Patients with ACS are characterized by the expansion of an unusual subset of T-cells, CD4+CD28null T-cells, with functional activities that predispose for vascular injury [53,54]. CD4+CD28null T-cells are a population of lymphocytes rarely found in healthy individuals. Disease-associated expansions of these cells have been reported in inflammatory disorders such as rheumatoid arthritis. CD4+CD28null T-cells are characterized by their ability to produce high amounts of IFN-γ [54]. Equally important, CD4+CD28null T cells have been distinguished from classical T helper cells by virtue of their ability to function as cytotoxic effector cells. Possible targets in the plaque are smooth muscle cells and endothelial cells, as recently shown [55]. In-vivo, CD4+CD28null cells have a tendency to proliferate with the frequent emergence of oligoclonality, raising the possibility of continuous antigenic stimulation, as it is the case in certain autoimmune disorders and in chronic infections. The demonstration of oligoclonality within the CD4+CD28null T-cell subsets and sharing of T-cell receptor sequences in expanded T-cell clones of patients with ACS strongly support the notion that these cells have expanded and are activated in response to a common antigenic challenge [56]. CD4+CD28null T-cells are long-lived cells. Clonality and longevity of these cells are associated with defects in apoptotic pathways [57]. Moreover, CD28 is relevant for the expansion of naïve T-cells, thus the absence of this molecule contributes to the senescence of lymphocytes. The excessive expansion of a pool of senescent T-lymphocytes might compromise the efficacy of the immune responses direct against exogeneous antigens as well as determinate autoimmune responses.

Recently, a sub-population of T CD4+ cells, expressing IL-2 receptor, CD25 membrane marker, has been pointed out. Such lymphocytes represent 7–10% of T CD4+ cells and their homeostasis is due to some co-stimulatory molecules, such as CD28 receptor expressed by T cells and B7 molecules expressed by dendritic cells [58]. The current knowledge of the role of this specific subset of T cells in human atherogenesis is still incomplete, even though a very recent study carried out on mice has demonstrated an anti-atherogenic effect of T CD4+CD25+ cells [59].

T helper 1 cells and T regulatory 1 cells have been demonstrated to play opposite roles in rupture of atherosclerotic lesion. The role of novel subset of T regulatory cells, known as CD4+CD25+Foxp3+ T cells, has been recently studied on coronary artery disease (CAD). Han et al. [60] found that the reduction of CD4+CD25+Foxp3+ T lymphocytes was consistent with the expansion of Th1 cells in patients with unstable CAD. The reversed development between CD4+CD25+ Tregs and Th1 cells might contribute to plaque destabilization.

Serum Markers Correlated to Plaque Inflammation

In recent years, a number of studies have correlated different serologic biomarkers with cardiovascular disease [3, 61] leading to a rapid increase in the number of biomarkers available (Table 2.1). These biomarkers are useful in that they can identify a population at risk of an acute ischemic event and detect the presence of so called vulnerable plaques and/or vulnerable patients [62,63]. Ideally, a biomarker must have certain characteristics to be a potential predictor of incident or prevalent vascular disease. Measurements have to be reproducible in multiple independent samples, the method for determination should be standardized, variability controlled, and the sensitivity and specificity should be good. In addition, the biomarker should be independent from other established risk markers, substantively improve the prediction of risk with established risk factors, be associated with cardiovascular events in multiple population cohorts and clinical trials, and the cost of the assays has to be acceptable. Finally, to be clinically useful a biomarker should correctly reflect the underlying biological process associated with plaque burden and progression.

Traditional biomarkers for cardiovascular risk include low-density lipoprotein (LDL) cholesterol and glucose. However, 50% of heart attacks and strokes occur in individuals that have normal LDL cholesterol, and 20% of major adverse events occur in patients with no accepted risk factors [64]. Therefore, in light of changing atherosclerotic models, vulnerable blood may be better described as blood that has an increased level of activity of plasma determinants of plaque progression and rupture.

In this context, proposed biomarkers fall into nine general categories: inflammatory markers, markers for oxidative stress, markers of plaque erosion and thrombosis, lipid-associated markers, markers of endothelial dysfunction, metabolic markers, markers of neovascularization, and genetic markers. The last six biomarker categories are not treated in the presented chapter but only listed in Table 2.1. As mentioned earlier, some of these markers may indeed reflect the natural history of atherosclerotic plaque growth and may not be directly related to an increased risk of cardiovascular events. On the contrary, other markers are more related to complex plaque morphological features and may reflect an active process within the plaque which is in turn related to the onset of local complications and onset of acute clinical events.

However, it is important to emphasize that in any individual patient, it is not yet clear how these biomarkers relate to quantitative risk of major adverse cardiovascular events. The best outcomes may be achieved by a panel of markers that will capture all of the different processes involved in plaque progression and plaque rupture, and that will enable clinicians to quantify an individual patient's true cardiovascular risk. In all likelihood, a combination of genetic (representing heredity) and serum markers (representing the net interaction between heredity and environment) will ultimately be the ones that should be utilized in primary prevention. Finally, different non-invasive and invasive imaging techniques may be coupled with biomarkers detection to increase the specificity, sensitivity

Table 2.1. Serologic markers of vulnerable plaque/patient.

Reflecting Metabolic and Immune Disorders	Reflecting Hypercoagulability	Reflecting Complex Atherosclerotic Plaque
• Abnormal lipoprotein profile (i.e. high LDL, low HDL, lipoprotein [a], etc.) • Non specific markers of inflammation (hs-CRP, CD40L, ICAM-1, VCAM, leukocytosis and other immuno-related serologic markers which may not be specific for atherosclerosis and plaque inflammation • Serum markers of metabolic syndrome (diabetes or hypertriglyceridemia) • Specific markers of immune activation (i.e. anti-LDL antibody, anti heat shock protein (HSP) antibody • Markers of lipid peroxidation (i.e. ox-LDL and ox-HDL) • Homocysteine • PAPP-A • Circulating apoptosis markers (i.e. Fas/Fas ligand) • ADMA/DDAH (i.e. asymmetric dimethylarginine/ dimethylarginine dimethylaminohydrolase) • Circulating NEFA (nonesterified fatty acids)	• Markers of blood hypercoagulability (i.e. fibrinogen, D-dimer, factor V of Leiden) • Increased platelet activation and aggregation (i.e. gene polymorphism of platelet glycoproteins IIb/IIIa, Ia/IIa, and Ib/IX) • Increased coagulation factors (i.e. clotting of factors V, VII, VIII, XIII, von Willebrand factor) • Decreased anticoagulation factors (i.e. protein S and C, thrombomodulin, antithrombin III) • Decreased endogeneous fibrinolysis activity (i.e. reduced tissue plasminogen activator, increased type I plasminogen activator (PAI), PAI polymorphisms) • Prothrombin mutation (i.e. G20210A) • Thrombogenic factors (i.e. anticardiolipin antibodies, thrombocytosis, sickle cell disease, diabetes, hypercholesterolemia) • Transient hypercoagulability (i.e. smoking, dehydratation, infection)	• *Morphology/Structure* Cap thickness Lipid core size Percentage stenosis Remodelling (positive vs. negative) Color (yellow, red) Collagen content vs. lipid content Calcification burden and pattern Shear stress • *Activity/function* Plaque inflammation (macrophage density, rate of monocyte and activated T cells infiltration) Endothelial denudation or dysfunction (local nitric oxide production, anti/procoauglation properties of the endothelium) Plaque oxidative stress Superficial platelet aggregation and fibrin deposition Rate of apoptosis (apoptosis protein markers, microsatellite) Angiogenesis, leaking vasa vasorum, intraplaque hemorrage Matrix metalloproteinases (MMP-2, -3, -9) Microbial antigens (Chlamydia pneumoniae) Temperature • *Pan Arterial* Transcoronary gradient of vulnerability biomarkers Total calcium burden Total coronary vasoreactivity Total arterial plaque burden (intima media thickness)

and overall predictive value of each potential diagnostic technique.

Markers of Inflammation

Markers of inflammation include C-reactive protein (CRP), inflammatory cytokines soluble CD40L (sCD40L), soluble vascular adhesion molecules (sVCAM), and tumour necrosis factor (TNF).

C-reactive protein is a circulating pentraxin that plays a major role in the human innate immune response [65] and provides a stable plasma biomarker for low-grade systemic inflammation. C-reactive protein is produced predominantly in the liver as part of the acute phase response. However, CRP is also expressed in smooth muscle cells within diseased atherosclerotic arteries [66] and has been implicated in multiple aspects of atherogenesis and plaque vulnerability, including expression of adhesion molecules, induction of nitric oxide, altered complement function, and inhibition of intrinsic fibrinolysis [67]. CRP is considered to be an independent predictor of unfavorable cardiovascular events in patients with atherosclerotic disease. Beyond CRP's ability to predict risk among both primary and secondary prevention patients, interest in it has increased with the recognition that statin-induced reduction of CRP is associated with less progression in adverse cardiovascular events that is independent of the lipid-associated changes [68] and that the efficacy of statin therapy may be related to the underlying level of vascular inflammation as detected by hs-CRP. Among patients with stable angina and established CAD, plasma levels of hs-CRP have consistently been shown associated with recurrent risk of cardiovascular events [69, 70]. Similarly, during acute coronary ischemia, levels of hs-CRP are predictive of high vascular risk even if troponin levels are non-detectable, suggesting that inflammation is associated with plaque vulnerability even in the absence of detectable myocardial necrosis [71,72]. Despite these data, the most relevant use of hs-CRP remains in the setting of primary prevention. To date, over two dozen large-scale prospective studies have shown baseline levels of hs-CRP to independently predict future myocardial infarction, stroke, cardiovascular death, and incident peripheral arterial disease [73,74]. Moreover, eight major prospective studies have had adequate power to evaluate hs-CRP after adjustment for all Framingham covariates, and all have confirmed the independence of hs-CRP [75]. Despite the evidence described above, it is important to recognize that there remain no firm data to date that lowering CRP levels *per se* will lower vascular risk. Further, as with other biomarkers of inflammation, it remains controversial whether CRP plays a direct causal role in atherogenesis [76], and ongoing work with targeted CRP-lowering agents will be required to fully test this hypothesis. However, the clinical utility of hs-CRP has been well established, and on the basis of data available through 2002, the Centers for Disease Control and Prevention and the American Heart Association endorsed the use of hs-CRP as an adjunct to global risk prediction, particularly among those at "intermediate risk" [77]. Data available since 2002 strongly reinforce these recommendations and suggest expansion to lower-risk groups, as well as

those taking statin therapy. Perhaps most importantly, data for hs-CRP provides evidence that biomarkers beyond those traditionally used for vascular risk detection and monitoring can play important clinical roles in prevention and treatment.

Cellular adhesion molecules can be considered potential markers of vulnerability since such molecules are activated by inflammatory cytokines and then released by the endothelium [78]. These molecules represent the one available marker to assess endothelial activation and vascular inflammation. The Physicians' Health Study evaluated more than 14,000 healthy subjects and demonstrated ICAM-1 expression positive correlation with cardiovascular risk and showed that subjects in the higher quartile of ICAM-1 expression showed 1.8 times higher risk compared to subjects in the lower quartile [79]. Furthermore, soluble ICAM-1 and VCAM-1 levels showed a positive correlation with atherosclerosis disease burden [80]. IL-6 is expressed during the early phases of inflammation and it is the principle stimuli for CRP liver production. In addition, CD 40 ligand, a molecule expressed on cellular membrane, is a TNF-α homologue which stimulates activated macrophages proteolytic substances production [81]. CD40 and CD40L have been found on platelets and several other cell types in functional-bound and soluble (sCD40L) forms. Although many platelet-derived factors have been identified, recent evidence suggests that CD40L is actively involved in the pathogenesis of acute coronary syndrome (ACS). CD40L drives the inflammatory response through the interaction between CD40L on activated platelets and the CD40 receptor on endothelial cells. Such interactions facilitate increased expression of adhesion molecules on the surface of endothelial cells and release of various stimulatory chemokines. These events, in turn, facilitate activation of circulating monocytes as a trigger of atherosclerosis. Beyond known proinflammatory and thrombotic properties of CD40L, experimental evidence suggests that CD40L-induced platelet activation leads to the production of reactive oxygen and nitrogen species, which are able to prevent endothelial cell migration and angiogenesis [82]. As a consequence of inhibiting endothelial cell recovery, the risk of subsequent coronary events may be greater. Clinical studies have supported the involvement of CD40L in ACS and the prognostic value in ACS populations. Levels of sCD40L have been shown to be an independent predictor of adverse cardiovascular events after ACS [83] with increased levels portending a worse prognosis [84]. Importantly, specific therapeutic strategies have shown to be beneficial in reducing risk associated with sCD40L [85]. IL-18 is a pro-inflammatory cytokine mostly produced by monocytes and macrophages, and it acts synergistically with IL-12 [63]. Both these interleukines are expressed in the atherosclerotic plaque and they stimulate IFN-γ induction which, on its turn, inhibits collagen synthesis, preventing a thick fibrous cap formation and facilitating plaque destabilization. Mallat *et al.* [86] examined 40 stable and unstable atherosclerotic plaques obtained from patients undergoing carotid endarterectomy and they highlighted how IL-18 expression was higher in macrophages and endothelial cells extracted from unstable rather than stable lesions and it correlated with clinical (symptomatic plaques) and pathological (ulceration) signs of vulnerability (Figures 2.1 and 2.2).

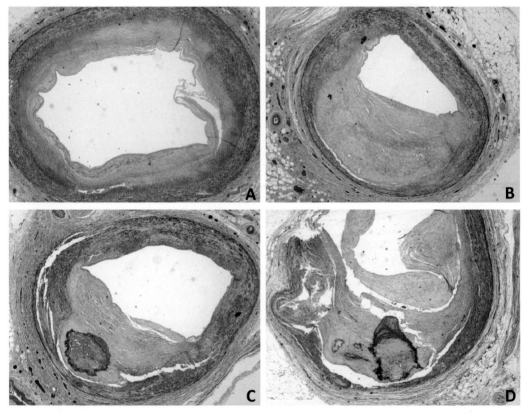

Figure 2.1. Stable atherosclerotic plaques characterized by the presence of a low inflammatory infiltrate:
A: "*Pathological intimal thickning*": this type of plaque is constituted by an intimal thickening associated to some deep lipid deposition without an evident true necrosis. The area overlying the lipid is rich on smooth muscle cells and proteoglycans and may contain a variable number of macrophages and T lymphocytes (Movat, 2x).
B: "*Fibroatheromata*": this type of lesion is constituted by a large lipidic-necrotic core constituted by extracellular lipid, cholesterol crystals and necrotic debris, covered by a thick fibrous cap consisting principally of smooth muscle cells in a collagenous-proteoglycan matrix, with varying degrees of infiltration by macrophages and T lymphocytes (Movat, 2x).
C: "*Fibrocalcific plaque*", characterized by a thick fibrous cap overlying extensive accumulations of calcium in the intima close to the media with a small lipid-laden necrotic and few inflammatory cells (Movat, 2x).
D: "*Healed lesion*": this type of lesion is constituted by distinct layers of dense collagen, suggestive of previous episodes of thrombosis. The necrotic core and inflammation are usually absent (Movat 2x).

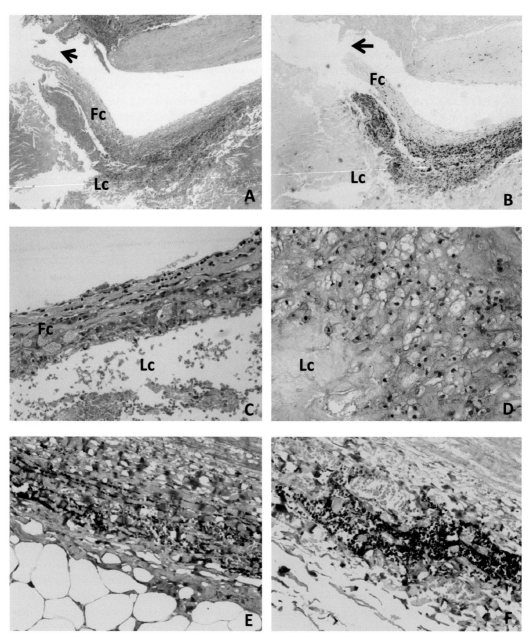

Figure 2.2. Unstable atherosclerotic plaques characterized by the presence of a high inflammatory infiltrate: A,B: "*Ruptured plaque*": An high power field of the site of the rupture (arrow) of the thin cap, associated with an acute thrombus (panel A, Movat, x4) showing many CD68 positive macrophagic cells (panel B, immunostaining anti-CD68, x4).

C,D: "*Vulnerable plaque*", characterized by a large lipidic-necrotic core associated with a thin fibrous cap, rich in inflammatory macrophagic foam cells cells and T lymphocytes (panel C, Movat x20). Numerous macrofagic foam cells area also observed in the shoulder of the plaque, near the lipidc necrotic core (panel D, Movat x20).

E,F: *Adventitial inflammation*: an abundant inflammatory infiltrate is frequently observed in unstable plaques, constituted mainly of T and B cells (Panel E, immunostaining anti-CD3, x20; Panel F: immunostaining anti-CD20, x20).

(Fc = fibrous cap; Lc = lipidic core)

Pregnancy Associated Plasma Protein- A (PAPP-A), is a high-molecular-weight, zinc-binding metalloproteinase, typically measured in women blood during pregnancy and later found in macrophages and smooth muscle cells inside unstable coronary atherosclerotic plaques. This protease cleaves the bond between Insulin Like Growth Factor-1 (IGF-1) and its specific inhibitor (IGFBP-4 e IGFBP-5), increasing free IGF-1 levels [87]. IGF-1 is important for monocytes-macrophages chemotaxis and activation in the atherosclerotic lesion, with consequent pro-inflammatory cytokine and proteolytic enzyme release, and stimulates endothelial cell migration and organizational behavior with consequent neo-angiogenesis. Hence IGF-1 represents one of the most important mediators in the transformation of a stable lesion into an unstable one [87]. Bayes-Genis *et al.* [88] demonstrated that PAPP-A is more expressed in the serum of patients with acute coronary syndromes (unstable angina, myocardial infarction), compared to subjects presenting with stable angina. In particular, PAPP-A serum levels > 10 mIU/l recognize patient vulnerability with a specificity of 78% and a sensibility of 89%. Recently we demonstrated that PAPP-A histological expression is higher in complex, vulnerable/ruptured carotid plaques compared to stable lesions [89]. Since PAPP-A serum levels can be easily measured today by means of ELISA, this protease could represent an easily quantifiable marker of vulnerability, with a reproducible method, allowing the identification of a patient subgroup with a high cerebrovascular risk, before its clinical event manifestation.

Jaffer *et al.* have recently published a detailed review on different techniques for detection of vulnerable plaque based on several biomarkers that have been implemented in recent years [90]. In this context, plaques with active inflammation may be identified directly by extensive macrophage accumulation [91]. Possible intravascular diagnostic techniques [92] based on inflammatory infiltration determination within the plaque include thermography [93], contrast-enhanced MRI [94], fluorodeoxyglucose positron emission tomography [95] and immunoscintigraphy [96]. In addition, non invasive techniques include MRI with superparamagnetic iron oxide [97,98] and gadolinium fluorine compounds [99,100].

Oxidative Stress Markers

Oxidative stress plays a very important role in atherogenesis [23]. Evidence shows that activation of vascular oxidative enzymes leads to lipid oxidation, foam cells formation, expression of vascular adhesion molecules and chemokines, and ultimately atherogenesis. Myeloperoxidase (MPO) is a heme peroxidase that is present in and secreted by activated phagocytes at sites of inflammation. Myeloperoxidase can generate several reactive, oxidatively derived intermediates, all mediated through a reaction with hydrogen peroxide, to induce oxidative damage to cells and tissues [101]. Oxidation products from MPO are found at significantly increased rates (up to 100-fold higher compared to circulating LDL) on LDL isolated from atherosclerotic lesions [102] and lead to accelerated foam-cell formation through nitrated apoB-100 on LDL and uptake by scavenger receptors [103]. Accumulating evidence suggests that MPO may play a causal role in plaque vulnerability [104]. Sugiyama *et al.* showed that advanced ruptured human atherosclerotic plaques, derived from patients with sudden cardiac death, strongly expressed MPO at sites of plaque rupture, in superficial erosions and in the lipid core, whereas fatty streaks exhibited little MPO expression. In addition, MPO macrophage expression and HOCl were highly co-localized immunochemically in culprit lesions of these patients. Several inflammatory triggers, such as cholesterol crystals, and CD40 ligand, induced release of MPO and HOCl production from MPO-positive macrophages in vitro [105]. Consistent with MPO's potential role in the atherosclerotic process, genetic polymorphisms resulting in MPO deficiency or diminished activity are associated with lower cardiovascular risk, although the generalizability of these findings is uncertain [106]. In parallel with MPO's effects on nitric oxide, LDL oxidation, and presence within ruptured plaques, several recent clinical studies have suggested that MPO levels may provide diagnostic and prognostic data in endothelial function, angiographically determined CAD, and ACSs. In a case control study of 175 patients with angiographically determined CAD, Zhang *et al.* [107] showed that the highest quartiles of both blood and leukocyte MPO levels were associated with ORs of 11.9 and 20.4, respectively, for the presence of CAD compared to the lowest quartiles. Brennan *et al.* [108] obtained MPO levels in the emergency department in 604 patients presenting with chest pain but no initial evidence of myocardial infarction, and showed that MPO levels predicted the in-hospital development of myocardial infarction, independent of other markers of inflammation, such as CRP. In addition, they showed that MPO levels were strong predictors of death, myocardial infarction, and revascularization six months after the initial event. The current data suggest that MPO may serve as both a marker of disease, providing independent information on diagnosis and prognosis of patients with chest pain, and also as a potential marker for assessment of plaque progression and destabilization at the time of acute ischemia.

Future Challenges in the Treatment of Vulnerable Plaques

With the concept of "vulnerable" plaque not nearly as straightforward as once thought, there are challenges to creating a therapeutic strategy for assessing the risk of rupture of vulnerable plaques in asymptomatic patients.

First, there must be an ability to identify the vulnerable plaque with non-invasive or invasive techniques. It has been demonstrated that coronary plaque composition can be predicted via invasive and non-invasive imaging techniques, allowing real-time analysis and in-vivo plaque characterization but clear identification of thin cap fibroatheroma (TCFA) is not possible yet and moreover the severity of the inflammatory infiltration of the cap, which certainly plays a major role in plaque disruption, cannot be evaluated as yet. Moreover, dynamic plaque changes, such as abrupt intraplaque haemorrhages from vasa-vasorum which may be fundamental in predicting the potentiality of a plaque to rupture, will be extremely difficult to identify with real-time imaging techniques.

A second challenge is that a lesion-specific approach requires that the number of vulnerable plaques in each patient needs to be known and the number of such lesions need to be limited. That's not the case, however. Several pathological studies indicate the presence of multiple "lipid-rich" vulnerable plaques in patients dying after ACS or with sudden coronary death [12,19]. Further complicat-

ing the issue: coronary occlusion and myocardial infarction usually evolve from mild to moderate stenosis—68% of the time, according to an analysis of data from different studies.

The third and fourth challenge is that the natural history of the vulnerable plaque (with respect to incidence of acute events) has to be documented in patients treated with patient-specific systemic therapy; and the approach has to be proven to significantly reduce the incidence of future events relative to its natural history. At this time, neither is documented nor proved.

Fifth, we believe that at the current stage it is not possible to know which vulnerable plaques will never rupture. Although we suspect it is the vast majority of them, we may have to shift to a more appropriate therapeutic target. In addition, targeting not only the vulnerable plaque but also the vulnerable blood (prone to thrombosis) and/or vulnerable myocardium (prone to life-threatening arrhythmia) may be also important to reduce the risk of fatal events.

Conclusions

Atherosclerosis is now recognized as a diffuse, and chronic inflammatory disorder involving vascular, metabolic and immune system with various local and systemic manifestations, A composite vulnerability index score comprising the total burden of atherosclerosis and vulnerable plaques in the coronary, carotid, aorta and femoral arteries, together with blood vulnerability factors, should be the ideal method of risk stratification. Obviously, such index is hard to achieve with today's tools. A future challenge is to identify patients at high risk of acute vascular events before clinical syndromes develop. At present, aside from imaging modalities such as IVUS- virtual histology, magnetic resonance, and local Raman spectroscopy that could help to identify vulnerable plaques, highly sensitive inflammatory circulating markers such as hsCRP, cytokines, pregnancy-associated plasma protein-A, pentraxin-3, LpPLA2 are currently the best candidates for diffuse active plaque detection. In order to achieve this aim a coordinate effort is needed to promote the application of the most promising tools and to develop new screening and diagnostic techniques to identify the vulnerable patient.

Questions

1. **What is the most important contributor to the enlargement of necrotic core?**
   A Smooth muscle cell necrosis
   B T lymphocytes infiltration
   C Intraplaque hemorrhage
   D Platelet aggregation

2. **What is the order of the frequency of underlying plaque morphology in patients dying with acute coronary thrombosis?**
   A Plaque rupture > Plaque erosion > Calcified nodule
   B Plaque rupture > Calcified nodule > Plaque erosion
   C Plaque erosion > Plaque rupture > Calcified nodule
   D Calcified nodule > Plaque rupture > Plaque erosion

3. **Plaque rupture occurs most commonly at:**
   A The junction between calcified and noncalcified atheroma
   B Sites of adventitial neovascularization
   C The necrotic core
   D The shoulder of the thin fibrous cap
   E The junction between the lipid pool and the adventitia

4. **After PCI, reendothelialization occurs in 4–6 weeks. What is the source of endothelial cells?**
   A Media
   B Intima
   C Adventitia
   D Adjunct endothelium
   E Circulating blood and adjunct endothelium

References

1. Libby P. Inflammation in atherosclerosis. Nature 2002; **420**(6917): 868–874.

2. Hansson GK, Libby P, Schonbeck U, et al. Innate and adaptive immunity in the pathogenesis of atherosclerosis. Circ Res 2002; **91**(4): 281–291.

3. Ross R. Atherosclerosis: an inflammatory disease. N Engl J Med 1999; **340**: 115–126.

4. Fuster V, Badimon L, Badimon JJ, et al. The pathogenesis of coronary artery disease and the acute coronary syndromes (1). N Engl J Med 1992; **326**(4): 242–250.

5. Falk E, Shah PK, Fuster V. Coronary plaque disruption. Circulation 1995; **92**: 657–671.

6. Davies MJ. Stability and instability: two faces of coronary atherosclerosis. The Paul Dudley White Lecture 1995. Circulation 1996; **94**(8): 2013–2020.

7. Ambrose JA, Tannenbaum MA, Alexopoulos D, et al. Angiographic progression of coronary artery disease and the development of myocardial infarction. J Am Coll Cardiol 1988; **12**(1): 56–62.

8. Long-term effectiveness and safety of pravastatin in 9014 patients with coronary heart disease and average cholesterol concentrations: the LIPID trial follow-up. Lancet 2002; **359**(9315): 1379–1387.

9. Virmani R, Kolodgie FD, Burke AP, et al. Lessons from sudden coronary death: a comprehensive morphological classification scheme for atherosclerotic lesions. Arterioscler Thromb Vasc Biol 2000; **20**(5): 1262–1275.

10. Spagnoli LG, Mauriello A, Sangiorgi G, et al. Extracranial thrombotically active carotid plaque as a risk factor for ischemic stroke. JAMA 2004; **292**(15): 1845–1852.

11. Virmani R, Burke AP, Farb A, Kolodgie FD. Pathology of the vulnerable plaque. J Am Coll Cardiol 2006; 47(8 Suppl): C13–18.

12. Mauriello A, Sangiorgi G, Fratoni S, et al. Diffuse and active inflammation occurs in both vulnerable and stable plaques of the entire coronary tree a histopathologic study of patients dying of acute myocardial infarction. J Am Coll Cardiol 2005; **45**(10): 1585–1593.

13. Spagnoli LG, Bonanno E, Mauriello A, et al. Multicentric inflammation in epicardial coronary arteries of patients dying after acute myocardial infarction. J Am Coll Cardiol 2002; **40**: 1579-8814.

14. Galis ZS, Sukhova GK, Lark MW, et al. Increased expression of matrix metalloproteinases and matrix degrading activity in vulnerable regions of human atherosclerotic plaques. J Clin Invest 1994; **94**(6): 2493–2503.

15. Schwartz RS, Topol EJ, Serruys PW, et al. Artery size, neointima, and remodeling: time for some standards. J Am Coll Cardiol 1998; **32**(7): 2087–2094.

16. Virmani R, Kolodgie FD, Burke AP, et al. Atherosclerotic plaque progression and vulnerability to rupture: angiogenesis as a source of intraplaque hemorrhage. Arterioscler Thromb Vasc Biol 2005; **25**(10): 2054–2061.

17. Burke AP, Farb A, Malcom GT, et al. Coronary risk factors and plaque morphology in men with coronary disease who died suddenly [see comments]. N Engl J Med 1997; **336**(18): 1276–1282.

18. Buffon A, Biasucci LM, Liuzzo G, et al. Widespread coronary inflammation in unstable angina. N Engl J Med 2002; **347**(1): 5–12.

19. Goldstein JA, Demetriou D, Grines CL, *et al.* Multiple complex coronary plaques in patient with acute myocardial infarction. N Engl J Med 2000; **343**: 915–922.

20. Garcia-Moll X, Cocolo F, Cole D, *et al.* Serum neopterin and complex stenosis morphology in patients with unstable angina. J Am Coll Cardiol 2000; **35**: 956–962.

21. Abbate A, Bonanno E, Mauriello A, *et al.* Widespread myocardial inflammation and infarct-related artery patency. Circulation 2004; **110**(1): 46–50.

22. Widlansky ME, Gokce N, Keaney JF, Jr., *et al.* The clinical implications of endothelial dysfunction. J Am Coll Cardiol 2003; **42**(7): 1149–1160.

23. Stocker R, Keaney JF, Jr. Role of oxidative modifications in atherosclerosis. Physiol Rev 2004; **84**(4): 1381–1478.

24. Khan BV, Harrison DG, Olbrych MT, *et al.* Nitric oxide regulates vascular cell adhesion molecule 1 gene expression and redox-sensitive transcriptional events in human vascular endothelial cells. Proc Natl Acad Sci USA 1996; **93**(17): 9114–9119.

25. Kubes P, Suzuki M, Granger DN. Nitric oxide: an endogenous modulator of leukocyte adhesion. Proc Natl Acad Sci USA 1991; **88**(11): 4651–4655.

26. Zeiher AM, Fisslthaler B, Schray-Utz B, *et al.* Nitric oxide modulates the expression of monocyte chemoattractant protein 1 in cultured human endothelial cells. Circ Res 1995; **76**(6): 980–986.

27. Teplyakov AI. Endothelin-1 involved in systemic cytokine network inflammatory response at atherosclerosis. J Cardiovasc Pharmacol 2004; **44** Suppl 1: S274–275.

28. Lerman A, Edwards BS, Hallett JW, *et al.* Circulating and tissue endothelin immunoreactivity in advanced atherosclerosis. N Engl J Med 1991; **325**(14): 997–1001.

29. Dang A, Wang B, Li W, *et al.* Plasma endothelin-1 levels and circulating endothelial cells in patients with aortoarteritis. Hypertens Res 2000; **23**(5): 541–544.

30. McCarron RM, Wang L, Stanimirovic DB, *et al.* Endothelin induction of adhesion molecule expression on human brain microvascular endothelial cells. Neurosci Lett 1993; **156**(1–2): 31–34.

31. Halim A, Kanayama N, el Maradny E, *et al.* Coagulation in vivo microcirculation and in vitro caused by endothelin-1. Thromb Res 1993; **72**(3): 203–209.

32. Feletou M, Vanhoutte PM. Endothelial dysfunction: a multifaceted disorder (The Wiggers Award Lecture). Am J Physiol Heart Circ Physiol September 2006; **291**(3): H985–1002.

33. Hansson GK, Libby P. The immune response in atherosclerosis: a double-edged sword. Nat Rev Immunol 2006; **6**(7): 508–519.

34. Verma S, Devaraj S, Jialal I. Is C-reactive protein an innocent bystander or proatherogenic culprit? C-reactive protein promotes atherothrombosis. Circulation 2006; **113**(17): 2135–2150; discussion 2150.

35. Hansson GK. Inflammation, atherosclerosis, and coronary artery disease. N Engl J Med 2005; **352**(16): 1685–1695.

36. Binder CJ, Chang MK, Shaw PX, *et al.* Innate and acquired immunity in atherogenesis. Nat Med 2002; **8**(11): 1218–1226.

37. Cook DN, Pisetsky DS, Schwartz DA. Toll-like receptors in the pathogenesis of human disease. Nat Immunol 2004; **5**(10): 975–979.

38. Nilsson J, Hansson GK, Shah PK. Immunomodulation of atherosclerosis: implications for vaccine development. Arterioscler Thromb Vasc Biol 2005; **25**(1): 18–28.

39. Clinton SK, Underwood R, Hayes L, *et al.* Macrophage colony-stimulating factor gene expression in vascular cells and in experimental and human atherosclerosis. Am J Pathol 1992; **140**(2): 301–316.

40. Fuster V, Lewis A. Connor memorial lecture: mechanism leading to myocardial infarction: insights from studies of vascular biology. Circulation 1994; **90**: 2126–2146.

41. Libby P. Coronary artery injury and the biology of atherosclerosis: inflammation, thrombosis, and stabilization. Am J Cardiol 2000; **86**(8B): 3J–8J; discussion 8J–9J.

42. Constant SL, Bottomly K. Induction of Th1 and Th2 CD4+ T cell responses: the alternative approaches. Annu Rev Immunol 1997; **15**: 297–322.

43. Benagiano M, D'Elios MM, Amedei A, *et al.* Human 60-kDa Heat Shock Protein Is a Target Autoantigen of T Cells Derived from Atherosclerotic Plaques. J Immunol 2005; **174**(10): 6509–6517.

44. Ludwig A, Berkhout T, Moores K, *et al.* Fractalkine is expressed by smooth muscle cells in response to IFN-gamma and TNF-alpha and is modulated by metalloproteinase activity. J Immunol 2002; **168**(2): 604–612.

45. Fong AM, Robinson LA, Steeber DA, *et al.* Fractalkine and CX3CR1 mediate a novel mechanism of leukocyte capture, firm adhesion, and activation under physiologic flow. J Exp Med 1998; **188**(8): 1413–1419.

46. Benagiano M, Azzurri A, Ciervo A, *et al.* T helper type 1 lymphocytes drive inflammation in human atherosclerotic lesions. Proc Natl Acad Sci USA 2003; **100**(11): 6658–6663.

47. Garcia-Touchard A, Henry TD, Sangiorgi G, *et al.* Extracellular proteases in atherosclerosis and restenosis. Arterioscler Thromb Vasc Biol 2005; **25**(6): 1119–1127.

48. Uemura S, Matsushita H, Li W, *et al.* Diabetes mellitus enhances vascular matrix metalloproteinase activity: role of oxidative stress. Circ Res June 22, 2001; **88**(12): 1291–1298.

49. Geng YJ, Wu Q, Muszynski M, *et al.* Apoptosis of vascular smooth muscle cells induced by in vitro stimulation with interferon-gamma, tumor necrosis factor-alpha, and interleukin-1 beta. Arterioscler Thromb Vasc Biol 1996; **16**(1): 19–27.

50. Adams S, O'Neill DW, Bhardwaj N. Recent advances in dendritic cell biology. J Clin Immunol 2005; **25**(2): 87–98.

51. Lanzavecchia A, Sallusto F. Regulation of T cell immunity by dendritic cells. Cell 2001; **106**(3): 263–266.

52. Kanazawa N, Nakamura T, Tashiro K, *et al.* Fractalkine and macrophage-derived chemokine: T cell-attracting chemokines expressed in T cell area dendritic cells. Eur J Immunol 1999; **29**(6): 1925–1932.

53. Liuzzo G, Kopecky SL, Frye RL, *et al.* Perturbation of the T-cell repertoire in patients with unstable angina. Circulation 1999; **100**: 2135–2139.

54. Liuzzo G, Vallejo AN, Kopecky SL, *et al.* Molecular fingerprint of interferon-gamma signaling in unstable angina. Circulation 2001; **103**(11): 1509–1514.

55. Nakajima T, Schulte S, Warrington KJ, *et al.* T-cell-mediated lysis of endothelial cells in acute coronary syndromes. Circulation 2002; **105**(5): 570–575.

56. Liuzzo G, Goronzy JJ, Yang H, *et al.* Monoclonal T-cell proliferation and plaque instability in acute coronary syndromes. Circulation 2000; **101**(25): 2883–2888.

57. Vallejo AN, Schirmer M, Weyand CM, *et al.* Clonality and longevity of CD4+CD28null T cells are associated with defects in apoptotic pathways. J Immunol 2000; **165**(11): 6301–6307.

58. Shimizu J, Yamazaki S, Takahashi T, *et al.* Stimulation of CD25(+)CD4(+) regulatory T cells through GITR breaks immunological self-tolerance. Nat Immunol 2002; **3**(2): 135–142.

59. Ait-Oufella H, Salomon BL, Potteaux S, *et al.* Natural regulatory T cells control the development of atherosclerosis in mice. Nat Med 2006; **12**(2): 178–180.

60. Han SF, Liu P, Zhang W, *et al.* The opposite-direction modulation of CD4+CD25+ Tregs and T helper 1 cells in acute coronary syndromes. Clin Immunol 2007; **124**(1): 90–97.

61. Naghavi M, Libby P, Falk E, *et al.* From vulnerable plaque to vulnerable patient: a call for new definitions and risk assessment strategies: Part II. Circulation 2003; **108**(15): 1772–1778.

62. Fuster V, Fayad ZA, Moreno PR, *et al.* Atherothrombosis and high-risk plaque: Part II: approaches by noninvasive computed tomographic/magnetic resonance imaging. J Am Coll Cardiol 2005; **46**(7): 1209–1218.

63. Fuster V, Moreno PR, Fayad ZA, *et al.* Atherothrombosis and high-risk plaque: part I: evolving concepts. J Am Coll Cardiol 2005; **46**(6): 937–954.

64. Tsimikas S, Willerson JT, Ridker PM. C-reactive protein and other emerging blood biomarkers to optimize risk stratification of vulnerable patients. J Am Coll Cardiol 2006; **47**(8 Suppl): C19–31.

65. Du Clos TW. Function of C reactive protein. Ann Med 2000; **32**: 274–278.

66. Calabro P, Willerson JT, Yeh ET. Inflammatory cytokines stimulated C-reactive protein production by human coronary artery smooth muscle cells. Circulation 2003; **108**: 1930–1932.

67. Verma S, Wang CH, Li SH, *et al.* A self-fulfilling prophecy:C-reactive protein attenuates nitric oxide production and inhibits angiogenesis. Circulation 2002; **106**: 913–919.

68. Ridker PM, Cushman M, Stampfer MJ, *et al.* Inflammation, aspirin, and the risk of cardiovascular disease in apparently healty men. N Engl J Med 1997; **336**: 973–979.

69. Ridker PM, Rifai N, Pfeffer MA, *et al.* Inflammation, pravastatin, and the risk of coronary events after myocardial infarction in patients with average cholesterol. Circulation 1998; **98**: 839–844.

70. Haverkate F, Thompson SG, Pyke SD, *et al.* Production of C-reactive protein and risk of coronary events in stable and unstable angina. European Concerted Action on Thrombosis and Disabilities Angina Pectoris Study Group. Lancet 1997; **349**: 462–466.

71. Liuzzo G, Biasucci LM, Gallimore JR, *et al.* The prognostic value of C-reactive protein and serum amyloid a protein in severe unstable angina. N Engl J Med 1994; **331**(7): 417–424.

72. Lindahl B, Toss H, Siegbahn A, *et al.* Markers of myocardial damage and inflammation in relation to long-term mortality in unstable coronary artery disease. FRISC Study Group. Fragmin during Instability in Coronary Artery Disease. N Engl J Med 2000; **343**(16): 1139–1147.

73. Ridker PM, Stampfer MJ, Rifai N. Novel risk factors for systemic atherosclerosis: a comparison of C-reactive protein, fibrinogen, homocysteine, lipoprotein(a), and standard cholesterol screening as predictors of peripheral arterial disease. JAMA 2001; **285**: 2481–2485.

74. Ridker PM, Rifai N, Rose L, *et al.* Comparison of C-reactive protein and low-density lipoprotein cholesterol levels in the prediction of first cardiovascular events. N Engl J Med 2002; **347**: 1557–1565.

75. Pai JK, Pischon T, Ma J, *et al.* Inflammatory markers and the risk of coronary heart disease in men and women. N Engl J Med 2004; **351**: 2599–2610.

76. Hirschfield GM, Gallimore JR, Kahan MC, *et al.* Transgenic human C-reactive protein is not proatherogenic in apolipoprotein E-deficient mice. Proc Natl Acad Sci USA 2005; **102**: 8309–8314.

77. Pearson TA, Mensah GA, Alexander RW, *et al.* Markers of inflammation and cardiovascular disease: application to clinical and public health practice: a statement for healthcare professionals from the Centers for Disease Control and Prevention and the American Heart Association. Circulation 2003; **107**: 499–511.

78. Davies MJ, Gordon JL, Gearing AJ. The expression of the adhesion molecules ICAM-1, VCAM-1, PECAM, and E-selectin in human atherosclerosis. J Pathol 1993; **171**: 223–229.

79. Ridker PM, Rifai N, Stampfer MJ, *et al.* Plasma concentration of interleukin-6 and the risk of future myocardial infarction among apparently healthy men. Circulation 2000; **101**(15): 1767–1772.

80. Peter K, Nawroth P, Conradt C, *et al.* Circulating vascular cell adhesion molecule-1 correlates with the extent of human atherosclerosis in contrast to circulating intercellular adhesion molecule-1, E-selectin, P-selectin, and thrombomodulin. Arterioscler Thromb Vasc Biol 1997; **17**(3): 505–512.

81. Libby P, Aikawa M. New insights into plaque stabilisation by lipid lowering. Drugs 1998; **56**: 9–13.

82. Urbich C, Dernbach E, Aicher A, *et al.* CD40 ligand inhibits endothelial cell migration by increasing production of endothelial reactive oxygen species. Circulation 2002; **106**: 981–986.

83. Varo N, de Lemos JA, Libby P, *et al.* Soluble CD40L: Risk prediction after acute coronary syndromes. Circulation 2003; **108**: 1049–1052.

84. Heeschen C, Dimmeler S, Hamm CW, *et al.* Soluble CD40 ligand in acute coronary syndromes. N Engl J Med 2003; **348**: 1104–1111.

85. Semb AG, van Wissen S, Ueland T, *et al.* Raised serum levels of soluble CD40 ligand in patients with familial hypercholesterolemia: downregulatory effect of statin therapy. J Am Coll Cardiol 2003; **41**: 275–279.

86. Mallat Z, Corbaz A, Scoazec A, *et al.* Expression of interleukin-18 in human atherosclerotic plaques and relation to plaque instability. Circulation 2001; **104**(14): 1598–1603.

87. Bayes-Genis A, Conover CA, Schwartz RS. The insulin-like growth factor axis: A review of atherosclerosis and restenosis. Circ Res 2000; **86**(2): 125–130.

88. Bayes-Genis A, Conover CA, Overgaard MT, *et al.* Pregnancy-associated plasma protein A as a marker of acute coronary syndromes. N Engl J Med 2001; **345**(14): 1022–1029.

89. Sangiorgi G, Mauriello A, Bonanno E, *et al.* Pregnancy-associated plasma protein-a is markedly expressed by monocyte-macrophage cells in vulnerable and ruptured carotid atherosclerotic plaques: a link between inflammation and cerebrovascular events. J Am Coll Cardiol 2006; **47**(11): 2201–2211.

90. Jaffer FA, Libby P, Weissleder R. Molecular and cellular imaging of atherosclerosis. J Am Coll Cardiol 2006; **47**: 1328–1338.

91. Constantinides P. Cause of thrombosis in human atherosclerotic arteries. Am J Cardiol 1990; **66**(16): 37G–40G.

92. Fayad ZA, Fuster V. Clinical imaging of the high-risk of vulnerable atherosclertic plaque. Circ Res 2001; **89**: 305–316.

93. Stefanidis C, Toutouzas K, Tsiamis E, *et al.* Thermal etherogeneity in stable human coronary atherosclerotic plaques is underestimated in vivo: the "cooling effect" of blood flow. J Am Coll Cardiol 2003; **41**: 403–408.

94. Ruehm SG, Corot C, Vogt P, *et al.* Magnetic resonance imaging of atherosclerotic plaque with ultrasmall superparamagnetic particles of iron oxide in hyperlipidemic rabbits. Circulation 2001; **103**(3): 415–422.

95. Lederman RJ, Raylmann RR, Fisher SJ, *et al.* Detection of atherosclerosis using a novel positron-sensitive probe and 18-fluorodeoxyglugose (FDG). Nucl Med Commun 2001; **22**: 747–753.

96. Ciavolella M, Tavolaro R, Taurino M, *et al.* Immunoscintigraphy of atherosclerotic uncomplicated lesions in vivo with a monoclonal antibody against D-dimers of insoluble fibrin. Atherosclerosis 1999; **143**(1): 171–175.

97. Schmitz SA, Coupland SE, Gust R, *et al.* Superparamagnetic iron oxide-enhanced MRI of atherosclerotic plaques in Watanabe hereditable hyperlipidemic rabbits. Invest Radiol 2000; **35**(8): 460–471.

98. Schmitz SA, Taupitz M, Wagner S, *et al.* Iron-oxide-enhanced magnetic resonance imaging of atherosclerotic plaques: postmortem analysis of accuracy, inter-observer agreement, and pitfalls. Invest Radiol 2002; **37**(7): 405–411.

99. Yuan C, Kerwin WS. MRI of atherosclerosis. J Magn Reson Imaging 2004; **19**(6): 710–719.

100. Yuan C, Kerwin WS, Ferguson MS, *et al.* Contrast-enhanced high resolution MRI for atherosclerotic carotid artery tissue characterization. J Magn Reson Imaging 2002; **15**(1): 62–67.

101. Vasilyev N, Williams T, Brennan ML, *et al.* Myeloperoxidase-generated oxidants modulate left

ventricular remodeling but not infarct size after myocardial infarction. Circulation 2005; **112**: 2812–2820.

102. Hazen SL, Heinecke JW. 3-Chlorotyrosine, a specific marker of myeloperoxidase-catalyzed oxidation, is markedly elevated in low density lipoprotein isolated from human atherosclerotic intima. J Clin Invest Radiol 1997; **99**: 2075–2081.

103. Podrez EA, Febbraio M, Sheibani N, *et al.* Macrophage scavenger receptor CD36 is the major receptor for LDL modified by monocyte-generated reactive nitrogen species. J Clin Invest 2000; **105**(8): 1095–1108.

104. Hazen SL. Myeloperoxidase and plaque vulnerability. Arterioscler Thromb Vasc Biol 2004; **24**: 1143–1146.

105. Sugiyama S, Okada Y, Sukhova GK, *et al.* Macrophage myeloperoxidase regulation by granulocyte macro-

phage colony-stimulating factor in human atherosclerosis and implications in acute coronary syndromes. Am J Pathol 2001; **158**: 879–891.

106. Asselbergs FW, Tervaert JW, Tio RA. Prognostic value of myeloperoxidase in patients with chest pain. N Engl J Med 2004; **350**: 516–518.

107. Zhang R, Brennan ML, Fu X, *et al.* Association between myeloperoxidase levels and risk of coronary artery disease. JAMA 2001; **286**(17): 2136–2142.

108. Brennan ML, Penn MS, Van Lente F, *et al.* Prognostic value of myeloperoxidase in patients with chest pain. N Engl J Med 2003; **349**(17): 1595–1604.

Answers

1. C
2. A
3. D
4. E—Circulating blood and adjunct endothelium—there are no endothelial cells in the media or adventitia; the sources of new endothelial cells are both the adjunct segments and circulating endothelial cells. (Kipshidze N, et al. Endoluminal reconstruction of the arterial wall with endothelial cell/glue matrix reduces restenosis in an atherosclerotic rabbit J Am Coll Cardiol 2000 36:1396–403)

CHAPTER 3

The Essentials of Vascular Access and Closure

Ted Feldman, & Gerald Yong
Evanston Hospital, Evanston, IL, USA

Introduction

Whilst we are often preoccupied with the coronary and cardiac complications of catheterization and intervention, it is femoral access complications that occur more frequently, and which are certainly more recognized and remembered by our patients. The incidence of local vascular complications that are considered major, as defined by the need for prolonged hospitalization, transfusion, or vascular surgery ranges between 1% and 1.5% in diagnostic catheterization procedures, and typically between 3% and 5% in interventional procedures. More recently, refinements in techniques and anti-thrombotic regimes have reduced femoral vascular complications in interventional procedures to 2%–3%, but they still remain frequent adverse events [1–3]. Risks of complications include advanced age, female gender, low BSA, aggressive anti-thrombin or anti-platelet agent use (e.g. GP IIb/IIIa inhibitors), emergent procedures, vascular disease, vessel size and puncture location [1,4]. The subjects of femoral access and management of femoral puncture after sheath removal are of vital importance in cardiac catheterizations and interventions, especially in patients with high risk of complications.

Interventional Cardiology, First Edition. Edited by
Carlo Di Mario, George D. Dangas, Peter Barlis.
© 2010 Blackwell Publishing Ltd. Published 2010 by
Blackwell Publishing Ltd.

Femoral Access

Anatomy

A good understanding of some key features of the local anatomy is essential for both optimal access and ideal management of the puncture site. Careful attention to access and careful evaluation of the access site are fundamental to both reduce sheath insertion trauma and ultimately to lead to uncomplicated sheath removal and the safe use of vascular closure devices.

It is important to puncture at the level of the common femoral artery. This allows compression of the vessel against the femoral head at the time of sheath removal. Punctures which are below the common femoral arterial bifurcation (hence in the profunda femoris or the superficial femoral artery) are over soft tissue and are difficult to compress (Figures 3.1, 3.2). Such punctures have been shown to be associated with increased risk of pseudoaneurysms and arteriovenous fistula formation [5,6]. Punctures which are above the inguinal ligament (hence in the external iliac artery) are in the retroperitoneal space which also represents an incompressible space. Such high punctures are associated with increased risk of retroperitoneal bleeding [6–8].

Landmarks on fluoroscopy are useful for identifying the position of the common femoral artery. Around 75%–80% of the common femoral bifurcation is at or below the inferior border of the femoral head and 95% is at or below the mid-

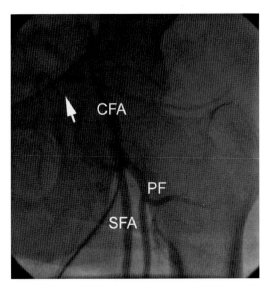

Figure 3.1. Femoral artery angiogram taken after sheath insertion. The sheath has been inserted into the superficial femoral artery (SFA). The profunda femoris or deep femoral artery is labeled PF. The sheath terminates in the common femoral artery (CFA). The arrow denotes the lower margin of the curve of the deep circumflex iliac artery. This lower border of the curve courses along the inguinal ligament. Punctures above this landmark are usually adjacent to the retroperitoneal space and poses a high risk for bleeding complications.

femoral head [5,9]. Whilst the inguinal ligament is not visualized under fluoroscopy, the deep circumflex iliac artery is commonly used as a surrogate marker of the upper border of the common femoral artery because it is the last arterial branch of the external iliac artery before the external iliac courses under the inguinal ligament and becomes the common femoral artery (Figure 3.1). The deep circumflex iliac artery arises from the lateral aspect of the external iliac artery nearly opposite the origin of the inferior epigastric artery. It ascends obliquely laterally behind the inguinal ligament, contained in a fibrous sheath formed by the junction of the transversalis fascia and iliac fascia, to the anterior superior iliac spine. Puncture above the most inferior border of the course of the deep circumflex iliac artery has been associated with increased risk of retroperitoneal hemorrhage. This landmark is above the most superior border of the acetabulum in most patients [6].

Puncture Technique

The basic technique of arterial access has changed very little since it was initially introduced by Seldinger [10]. Puncture of the common femoral

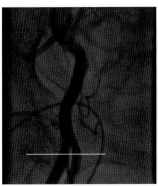
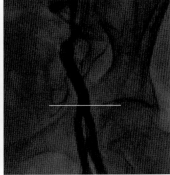
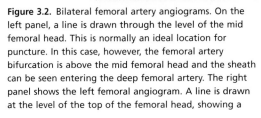

Figure 3.2. Bilateral femoral artery angiograms. On the left panel, a line is drawn through the level of the mid femoral head. This is normally an ideal location for puncture. In this case, however, the femoral artery bifurcation is above the mid femoral head and the sheath can be seen entering the deep femoral artery. The right panel shows the left femoral angiogram. A line is drawn at the level of the top of the femoral head, showing a remarkably high bifurcation in this patient. Even though the sheath insertion on this side is just below the top of the femoral head, it is also in the deep femoral artery. Although this puncture is compressible over the femoral head, the branch is relatively smaller than the common femoral artery and less well suited for use of closure devices.

artery is basically unchanged, save that the original concept used a through and through puncture and withdrawal of needle into the arterial lumen, whilst our current approach ideally punctures only the anterior surface of the femoral artery.

The technique, however, can be substantially improved by using fluoroscopy of bony landmarks to identify the likely course of the common femoral artery followed by confirmation with femoral angiography after sheath insertion [11]. A point of entry into the common femoral artery at the mid femoral head or slightly above is ideal. The femoral skin crease, which is a very commonly used landmark for puncture, is distal to the common femoral bifurcation in 72% of cases [12]. Generally speaking, younger patients have a mid femoral head location relatively close or slightly above the femoral crease, and older patients have a femoral head significantly above the femoral crease, since with age the crease tends to sag. Obese patients may have two or sometimes even three femoral creases.

The technique of puncture requires multiple small steps to be optimized. Before local anesthesia

is given, a clamp or needle can be laid at the point where the pulse is most easily felt, just above the femoral crease. Fluoroscopy can be used to locate the position of the needle relative to the center of the femoral head (Figure 3.3). Local anesthesia can thus be given accordingly. After local anesthesia is given, the needle is advanced to a point just above the arterial wall, using palpation as a guide. At this point, it is useful to fluoroscope the location of the needle once again. This is the last chance to adjust the puncture to enter the common femoral artery in the ideal landing zone. This method is not often adhered to, but in the long run is very worthwhile and justifies the few seconds of extra time at the beginning of the procedure.

Once the sheath has been inserted, a sheath angiogram should be taken. Usually a 20° ipsilateral angulation of the image intensifier will expose the entry point of the sheath, as well as the femoral bifurcation [6]. It can thus be determined whether the common femoral artery has in fact been entered, and whether or not there is atherosclerosis, calcification, or angulation of the puncture site. It is our practice to obtain the sheath angiogram at

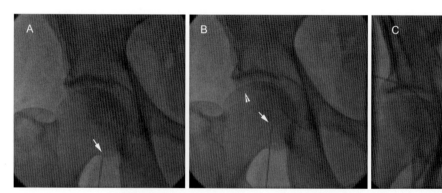

Figure 3.3. Panel A shows a fluoroscopic image recorded prior to puncture. The 18g thin wall needle has been laid on the skin at the point of anticipated femoral puncture based on palpation. The arrow shows the tip of the needle. Fluoroscopy demonstrates that the needle is at the lower border of the femoral head. This is an ideal location for skin entry since the needle will puncture the femoral artery superior to this point.

Panel B shows the needle advanced until the pulsation of the femoral artery is felt to be transmitted through the needle. The arrow shows the position of the needle. This is just below the mid femoral head and is an ideal "landing zone" for puncture. The majority of patients'

femoral artery bifurcation will be below this point and the probability of common femoral artery entry is high. The arrowhead pointing upward shows the location of the skin crease.

In Panel C, sheath angiography demonstrates that the entry point is in the common femoral artery above the line of the mid femoral head. This is higher than ideal but represents a good entry point for the sheath. Just above the sheath entry site, the U shaped branch of the external iliac artery denotes the location of the inguinal ligament and the division between the common femoral artery and the retroperitoneal iliac vessel. This branch is the deep circumflex iliac artery.

the beginning of the procedure, so that decisions about closure and sometimes anticoagulation can be made before the procedure is performed. If the sheath has been inserted into the branch vessels below the bifurcation, this will often have an impact on ultimate sheath size, e.g. in the setting of bifurcation or chronic total occlusion intervention, and may impact the choice of anticoagulation. When the puncture is above the most inferior border of the deep circumflex iliac artery, it is likely that the retroperitoneal space has been entered with the sheath. In this instance, an option is to defer intervention until a later time. Full anti-coagulation with the sheath in this location greatly increases the risk of retroperitoneal bleeding, which is one of the worst and more difficult local complications to manage.

Femoral Access Closure

Manual Compression

Manual compression has been the standard for sheath removal for decades. Classically after diagnostic catheterizations the technique involves sheath removal after normalization of the activated clotting time (ACT) to <160–180 seconds and direct digital pressures with fingers positioned over the arterial puncture site and more proximally. The manual pressure should be applied with enough force to allow for a faint palpable distal pulse. Pressure is held for 10–15 minutes, during which hemostasis should be achieved, after which the patient is kept under bed rest for 4–6 hours.

The use of larger arterial sheaths, more intensive anti-coagulation and anti-platelet regimes associated with coronary and cardiac interventions have led to the need for more prolonged direct pressure to achieve hemostasis and more prolonged bed rest prior to ambulation. A variety of mechanical manual compression aids, such as the Femostop (Radi Medical System, Sweden) and Compressar C-clamp (Advanced Vascular Dynamics, Portland, OR), have been developed to relieve the requirement for staff to physically apply prolonged direct digital pressure. A number of studies have compared such devices to direct manual pressure, with most studies finding lower vascular complications with mechanical compression devices [13–15]

although one recent small study (90 subjects) had found better results with direct manual pressure [16].

Clamp devices provide compression without the need to have someone using direct manual pressure. Whilst clamps may be less demanding on personnel, they do not obviate the need for careful supervision of the compression process. If clamps are applied with too much pressure or left in place for too long, they may result in arterial or venous thrombosis. If applied without adequate pressure, bleeding may result. The Femostop (RADI Medical) uses an inflatable bubble to apply pressure to the puncture site. This is our preferred device for compression in fully anti-coagulated patients with failed suture closure or large caliber arterial or venous sheaths. The bubble is clear, so the puncture site can be observed directly. The pressure is regulated with a blood pressure cuff bulb. Near systolic pressure can be applied for 15–30 minutes, and then the pressure can be decreased 10–15 mmHg every 10–20 minutes.

Even with interventional procedures, there have been some remarkable experiences with ambulation as early as two hours after simple manual compression. With the use of bivalirudin, in one study of 100 patients, after a mean manual compression time of 13 minutes, patients were able to ambulate at a mean of 2 hours and 23 minutes after sheath removal [17]. Even using heparin, there are various studies suggesting ability to ambulate early after two hours. Using a regime of a standard heparin dose of 5000U and 6Fr guiding catheters, two studies involving 359 and 907 patients were able to have sheaths removed immediately, with a mean compression time of around ten minutes and successful early ambulation within two hours with no significant excess in puncture site complications [18,19]. A study with more aggressive anti-coagulation (ACT to 300 seconds) and subsequent sheath removal when ACT is less than 150 seconds showed no difference in site complications between patients ambulating at two hours compared to four or six hours. In this latter study, there are also similar results in a subgroup of patients who received GP IIb/IIIa inhibitors [20]. Thus, manual compression is clearly an acceptable form of puncture site management in all patients.

Vascular Closure Devices

A variety of vascular closure devices have been developed to enhance vascular closure without need for prolonged compression. They are deployed at the conclusion of the cardiac catheterization procedure and may be used despite an elevated ACT. Table 3.1 shows the major categories of closure devices. Sutures, plugs, glues, and topical patches are all available. The current FDA-approved devices in most common use in the United States are the AngioSeal (Datascope Inc), Perclose, and StarClose (Abbott Vascular, Redwood City CA). Hemostatic patches are also approved for use in the United States (Figure 3.4).

AngioSeal

The AngioSeal device consists of a rectangular absorbable copolymeric anchor deployed intra-

Table 3.1. Types of closure devices.*

	Manufacturer	CE Mark	US Approval	Status
Plugs:				
VasoSeal	Datascope	+	+	Discontinued
AngioSeal	St Jude	+	+	
ExoSeal	J&J	+		US Trial ongoing
Suture Devices:				
Perclose	Abbott	+	+	
Superstich	Sutura	+	+	
X-Press	Datascope	+	+	
Staples/Clips:				
StarClose	Abbott	+	+	
Angiolink	Medtronic	+	+	Not yet launched
Liquid/Gel:				
Duett	Vascular Solutions	+	+	
Mynx	Access Closure	+	+	
Energy Based:				
Therus ultrasound	Therus			Investigational
Modified Guidewire:				
Boomerang	Cardiva	+	+	
EpiClose balloon	CardioDex			Investigational
Patches:				
Chito-Seal	Abbott		+	
V+	InterV	+	+	
Syvek	Marine Polymer	+	+	
Clo-Sur	Scion	+	+	
SafeSeal	Possis	+	+	
D-Stat	Vascular Solutions	+	+	
Neptune	TZ Medical	+	+	
Compression Devices:				
Femostop	Radi Medical	+	+	
Safeguard	Datascope	+	+	
QuickKlamp	TZ Medical	+		
EZ Hold	TZ Medical	+		

*List compiled December 2007.

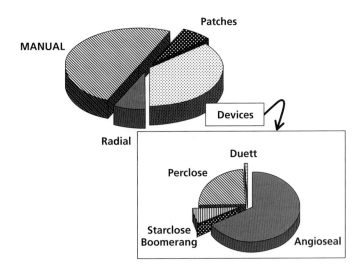

Figure 3.4. Use of vascular closure approaches in the United States.

vascularly against the arterial wall which is attached by an absorbable Dexon traction suture to an extravascular collagen plug applied to the outside of the arterial wall. The AngioSeal assembly consists of a carrier system with the anchor, collagen plug and traction suture compacted at the distal end. There is a delivery sheath with a modified locator dilator which identifies when the sheath is intravascular. After cardiac catheterization, the working sheath is changed over to the AngioSeal delivery sheath. Once the delivery sheath is intravascular as indicated by pulsatile flow in the arteriotomy locator system of the dilator, the dilator and wire are removed. The carrier is then advanced into the sheath, and locks in place with the sheath, and then the entire assembly withdrawn until resistance is felt. This indicates apposition of the anchor on the luminal arterial wall. Further withdrawal releases the collagen plug on the external surface of the artery, followed by a tamper tube. The tamper tube is used to compress the plug over the wire, followed by removal of the tamper tube and cutting of the suture which are external to the patient. Currently the AngioSeal is available in two sizes: 6Fr and 8Fr. Deployment success rates ranged from 92% to 98%, and hemostasis success ranged from 84% to 97% [21].

Perclose

The Perclose device is a suture mediated system which has undergone a steady evolution which included the Techstar device, Closer S 6Fr and the current Proglide 6Fr system. It incorporates two needles in the proximal compartment of the device and a catheter that houses the suture (Figure 3.5). The working sheath is exchanged over a wire for the Perclose device. The device is advanced until return of pulsatile blood in the locator, indicating appropriate intravascular placement. A lever is pulled to open the "feet," and the device is withdrawn until resistance is felt, indicating apposition of the foot processes and suture catch plates against the inner vessel wall. A plunger is depressed forcing the needles through the outer vessel wall into the suture catch plates. The catch plates are attached to the ends of the suture. Retraction of the plunger withdraws the needles and the attached sutures through the skin. With the current Proglide system, the device incorporates a non-absorbable polypropylene monofilament with pre-tied knot which is tightened and the vascular access site closed using a pusher device. With the Perclose system it is possible to reinsert a guidewire before withdrawing the device, so that vascular access can be preserved after deployment, as a wire can be reintroduced via the device after the needle and suture deployment, and the wire removed after confirmation of adequate hemostasis. This feature is unique among the closure approaches. In most series, the device is successfully deployed in 89%–100%, with hemostasis success seen in 86%–99%. The Prostar device is a Perclose-based suture mediated device which

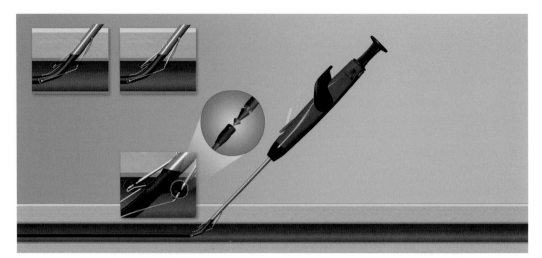

Figure 3.5. The Perclose Proglide device is used to deliver sutures through the puncture to close the arteriotomy site. The small insets of the upper left of the figure show feet that are opened inside the artery, and the mechanism by which needles are driven from the handle of the device into the feet to capture the sutures. The sutures are then withdrawn using the needles, and a pre-tied knot is pushed through the skin to the top of the arteriotomy site on the outside of the artery.

allows for closure of larger arteriotomy. It comes in 8Fr or 10Fr and may incorporate one or two sutures (associated with two or four needles respectively).

StarClose

StarClose device is a more recent entrant which applies a 4 mm low profile nitinol clip entirely on the external surface of the artery with no permanent intra-vascular component (Figures 3.6, 3.7). The tines of the clip grasp the arterial tissue and close the arteriotomy in a purse string fashion. The device consists of the clip applier and a proprietary 6Fr sheath. After conclusion of cardiac catheterization, the working sheath is changed over a wire to the proprietary sheath, with further blunt dissection during the process to ease subsequent advancement of the 12Fr clip applier through the skin and subcutaneous tissue. The clip applier has a vessel locator which is inserted into the sheath, until the clip applier snaps into the sheath. A button is depressed which deploys small flexible nitinol wings at the end of the vessel locator, inside the artery. The entire assembly is withdrawn until resistance is felt, indicating apposition of the wings against the inner vessel wall. The sliding element with the attached clip is then depressed splitting the sheath and applies the clip to the arterial wall at the end of the assembly. The procedure is completed by release of the clip using a button "trigger." In the CLIP trial, which compared the StarClose to manual compression, device success was 87% with no difference in complications between the groups [22].

Hemostatic Patches

Hemostatic patches were originally designed for military purposes to achieve temporary arterial hemostasis in the battlefield. The mechanisms of action include causing vasoconstriction, creation of a positively charged environment which attracts negatively charged red blood cells and platelets, or direct promotion of rapid coagulation [23–25]. Available patches (Table 3.1) include: Syvek Patch using poly-N-glucosamine (Marine Polymer Technologies, Danvers, MA), Neptune pad using calcium alginate (Biotronik, Bulach, Switzerland), Closure PAD (Medtronic, Santa Rosa, CA), Chito-Seal using chitosan gel (Abbott Vascular, Redwood, CA), SafeSeal using a microporous polysaccharide (Possis Medical, Minneapolis MN, formerly Stasys Patch, St Jude Medical, St Paul, MN), and D-Stat Dry using thrombin (Vascular Solutions, Minneapolis, MN) [23].

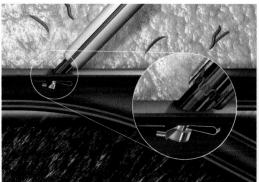 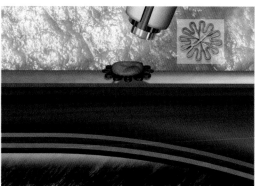

Figure 3.6. The Starclose device is delivered through a special sheath provided with the device. After the device is loaded into the artery, nitinol wings are opened within the artery and pulled back to capture the inner arterial wall. The clip device, shown on the left part of the figure, is then advanced to the outside surface of the artery. When a clip is fired, it inverts and the tines of the clip capture the arteriotomy and force it closed. This device is unique in that what is left behind is entirely extra-arterial.

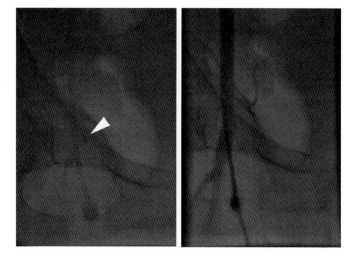

Figure 3.7. Femoral angiogram one year after closure with the Starclose device. The arrowhead on the left shows the device, and on the right contrast injection demonstrates the insertion site of the re-puncture. The device is entirely extravascular.

Hemostatic patches allows sheath removal in anti-coagulated patients, with ACT as high as 300 [24]. Studies on hemostatic patches have generally demonstrated shorter time to hemostasis and ambulation. However, a period of manual compression is generally required and may be longer than the recommended compression times from manufacturers [25–27]. It is likely a combination of both hemostatic properties of the patch and manual compression that leads to hemostasis. There are no consistent data demonstrating reduction in vascular complications with the use of hemostatic patches over manual compression. Neither the Syvek patch nor Chito-Seal have been shown to reduce vascular complications over manual compression in a review of cases registered with the ACC-NCDR [28]. D-Stat Dry used after diagnostic procedures has reduced vascular complications compared to manual compression a series utilizing a historical control [25], but no direct comparisons have been performed. Since the complication rate from vascular puncture in general appears to be declining with time, direct comparisons are necessary to clearly demonstrate decreased complication rates using these patches [29].

Evidence Based Issues for Vascular Closure Devices

The design goals of active vascular closure devices (as replacement of manual compression for management of femoral arterial sheath removal) would include reduction in hemostasis and ambulation times with associated improved patient comfort and reduction in hemorrhagic vascular complications. As experience with this family of devices has grown it is clear that hemostasis and ambulation times can be decreased, but the reduction of vascular complications has not been as well shown. There are real concerns for the potential to increase rare but serious complications such as infections, arterial occlusions, distal embolizations, and arterial wall injury with pseudoaneurysm. In addition, bleeding complications, should they occur, could potentially be more severe than seen with manual compression because manual compression requires normalization of ACT prior to sheath removal whilst vascular closure devices can be deployed at elevated ACT [4]. In a review of case series of AngioSeal and Perclose, the reported incidence of such complications include: infection 0.6%, pseudoaneurysm or arteriovenous fistula 0.6%–1%, occlusion or embolism 0.2%–0.4% [21]. In a review of four years of cardiac catheterizations and interventions at the Mayo clinic between 2000 and 2003, during which vascular closure devices were used in 1662 patients, the incidence of device-related infection was 0.24%.

There are numerous randomized and non-randomized comparisons of vascular closure devices and manual compression. There is significant heterogeneity between the trials in inclusion criteria and definitions of outcomes. Three recent meta-analyses have reviewed the studies involving collagen plug devices (AngioSeal and VasoSeal) and suture devices (Perclose) [28,30]. Use of vascular closure devices is associated with significant reductions in time to hemostasis (by 17 minutes), time to ambulation (by up to 11 hours) and time to discharge (by 0.6 days) [31]. However, in these analyses in both diagnostic and interventional settings, there are no substantial difference (benefits or harms) in vascular complications by the vascular closure devices, except for the VasoSeal device which has been associated with increased vascular complications in two of the meta-analyses [30–

32]. There are a number of limitations to assessing the relative rates of complications with manual compression and vascular closure devices. First, some trials have required femoral angiography, and higher risk patients may be eliminated from the trials, due to small caliber femoral vessels, atherosclerosis of the puncture site, or calcification. In addition, many of the trials have rigorous protocol specifications for the manner in which the closure devices are used, but generally give no guidance regarding manual compression methods. Manual compression methods are highly variable. In some institutions, there are sheath removal teams who become quite expert at sheath removal, manual compression, and puncture site management. It is difficult to make comparisons between these kinds of programs and lower volume programs or programs where new trainees are relegated to the task of sheath removal and manual compression.

The largest registry study of femoral hemostasis comes from the American College of Cardiology—National Cardiovascular Data Registry (ACC-NCDR) [33]. From this registry, the outcomes of 166,680 patients who underwent diagnostic and interventional cardiac catheterizations in 2001 were evaluated, with suture devices used in 25,495 cases, collagen-plug devices used in 28,160 cases, whilst the rest underwent manual compression. In the overall multivariate analysis, use of collagen plug devices was associated with reduced bleeding in diagnostic catheterization (odds ratio 0.68) and both types of closure devices were associated with reduced risk of pseudoaneurysm formation in diagnostic and interventional procedures (odds ratio 0.46–0.52). It is possible that among individual operators who develop special expertise with a particular closure device, there is potential to achieve improved success rates with lower complications [34].

What then are the advantages of vascular closure devices? Unquestionably, the complete avoidance of compression with immediate hemostasis and early ambulation improves patient satisfaction [35]. This alone may justify the use of these devices in many cases. However, with no clear difference in complication rates, possibly the strongest benefit may be an early (same-day) discharge of PCI patients that could result from early ambulation

[4,36]. Over the past five years, major vascular complications have decreased among patients undergoing percutaneous coronary intervention in the Northern New England Cardiovascular Disease Study Group. In their database, with 36,631 patients undergoing PCI, arterial complications decreased from 3.37% in 2002 to 1.98% in 2006 [30]. Whether this reflects more careful attention to needle puncture and sheath insertion, improved management of anti-coagulation, better manual compression, or optimized use of closure devices cannot be ascertained without a randomized trial. Such a trial would require such a large population that is not likely ever to be performed.

Preclosure for Large Arterial Sheaths

Large bore arterial sheaths up (12Fr–14Fr) may be required for certain interventions such as retrograde balloon aortic valvuloplasty, or more recently retrograde percutaneous aortic valve replacement (18Fr–24Fr). Such large bore arterial sheaths are commonly associated with need for prolonged compression to achieve hemostasis, prolonged bed rest prior to mobilization (up to 12–24 hours in certain cases), and high risk of recurrent bleeding and need for transfusion. Transfusions rates after manual compression following balloon aortic valvuloplasty have been in the range of 25%. Preclosure is a technique using the Perclose or Prostar device to "preload" the suture around the puncture site prior to access with the large bore sheath to allow for subsequent suture closure at removal of the large arterial sheath. After puncture, a standard 6Fr–8Fr sheath is inserted and subsequently exchanged over the wire to introduce a Perclose or Prostar device. Deployment of the needle is performed with the standard manner to preload the suture around the arteriotomy. The suture is not tightened. A wire is reintroduced into the device over which an exchange is made with the subsequent large bore arterial sheath. At completion of the procedure requiring the large bore sheath, the sheath is removed and closure performed by tightening of the pre-loaded sutures. With this technique, a 6Fr Perclose system had been successful in closing 12Fr arteriotomies and 10Fr Prostar system had been successful in closing 14Fr arteriotomies. In a non-randomized comparison, this technique had been successful in significantly reducing length of hospital stay and almost eliminating the need for blood transfusions after retrograde arterial balloon aortic valvuloplasty [37,38]

Conclusion

Proper management of femoral access is vital in reducing the femoral vascular adverse events which are the most common complications in cardiac catheterizations and interventions. Refinements in anti-thrombotic and anti-platelet regimes, and reductions in access size, have reduced ambulation times and reduced the risks of complications. Vascular closure devices have further significantly improved hemostasis and ambulation times, and current data suggest they are mostly safe. However, there is no unequivocal evidence to suggest they reduce vascular complications in either diagnostic or interventional subgroups. Experience and expertise with whichever techniques for femoral access site management one chooses are the best ways to minimize complications.

Just as important as management of vascular closure, careful attention to obtaining vascular access is important. Careful assessment of bony landmarks by fluoroscopy prior to femoral access will maximize the chance of sheath insertion into the common femoral artery with reductions in complications. Similarly, routine femoral angiography after femoral access to confirm sheath position is useful not only for assessing suitability of applications of vascular closure device but also for assessing the risks of bleeding with use of anti-thrombotics which may affect interventional decision making.

Questions

1. **The following can be said of radial artery access compared with femoral artery access:**
   A The complication rate is higher
   B The success rate is lower
   C The learning curve is less steep
   D The technique is associated with less discomfort

2. **Closure devices are associated with each of the following, except:**
   A Groin infection
   B Retroperitoneal hemorrhage
   C Lower complication rate than manual compression
   D Earlier ambulation than manual compression

3. **Compared to the femoral approach, the brachial approach to coronary intervention is associated with all of the following, except:**
   A More difficult catheter manipulation
   B Less radiation exposure
   C Easier superselective coronary intubation
   D Less local bleeding
   E Increased loss of pulse

4. **Which of the following statements about retroperitoneal hemorrhage is true**
   A The most common cause is vascular access of the femoral artery proximal to the inguinal ligament in a segment of vessel that dips posteriorly into the pelvic cavity
   B The classic description of discoloration over the flank or the abdomen (Grey Turner sign) occurs in 50% of cases
   C Ultrasound and CT scanning are equally sensitive and specific methods of establishing the diagnosis
   D Surgical exploration is often required
   E All of the above

References

1. Piper WD, Malenka DJ, Ryan TJ, Jr., *et al.* Predicting vascular complications in percutaneous coronary interventions. Am Heart J 2003; **145**: 1022–1029.
2. Lincoff AM, Bittl JA, Harrington RA, *et al.* Bivalirudin and provisional glycoprotein IIb/IIIa blockade compared with heparin and planned glycoprotein IIb/IIIa blockade during percutaneous coronary intervention: REPLACE-2 randomized trial. JAMA 2003; **289**: 853–863.
3. Waksman R, King SB, 3rd, Douglas JS, *et al.* Predictors of groin complications after balloon and new-device coronary intervention. Am J Cardiol 1995; **75**: 886–889.
4. Dauerman HL, Applegate RJ, Cohen DJ. Vascular Closure Devices: The Second Decade. J Am Coll Cardiol 2007; **50**:1617–1626.
5. Kim D, Orron DE, Skillman JJ, *et al.* Role of superficial femoral artery puncture in the development of pseudoaneurysm and arteriovenous fistula complicating percutaneous transfemoral cardiac catheterization. Cathet Cardiovasc Diagn 1992; **25**: 91–97.
6. Sherev DA, Shaw RE, Brent BN. Angiographic predictors of femoral access site complications: implication for planned percutaneous coronary intervention. Catheter Cardiovasc Interv 2005; **65**: 196–202.
7. Ellis SG, Bhatt D, Kapadia S, Lee D, Yen M, Whitlow PL. Correlates and outcomes of retroperitoneal hemorrhage complicating percutaneous coronary intervention. Catheter Cardiovasc Interv 2006; **67**: 541–545.
8. Farouque HM, Tremmel JA, Raissi Shabari F, *et al.* Risk factors for the development of retroperitoneal hematoma after percutaneous coronary intervention in the era of glycoprotein IIb/IIIa inhibitors and vascular closure devices. J Am Coll Cardiol 2005; **45**: 363–368.
9. Schnyder G, Sawhney N, Whisenant B, Tsimikas S, Turi ZG. Common femoral artery anatomy is influenced by demographics and comorbidity: implications for cardiac and peripheral invasive studies. Catheter Cardiovasc Interv 2001; **53**: 289–295.
10. Seldinger SI. Catheter replacement of the needle in percutaneous arteriography: a new technique. Acta radiol 1953; **39**: 368–376.
11. Turi ZG. Optimizing vascular access: routine femoral angiography keeps the vascular complication away. Catheter Cardiovasc Interv 2005; **65**: 203–204.
12. Grier D, Hartnell G. Percutaneous femoral artery puncture: practice and anatomy. Br J Radiol 1990; **63**: 602–604.
13. Pracyk JB, Wall TC, Longabaugh JP, *et al.* A randomized trial of vascular hemostasis techniques to reduce femoral vascular complications after coronary intervention. Am J Cardiol 1998; **81**: 970–976.
14. Semler HJ. Transfemoral catheterization: mechanical versus manual control of bleeding. Radiology 1985; **154**: 234–235.
15. Bogart MA. Time to hemostasis: a comparison of manual versus mechanical compression of the femoral artery. Am J Crit Care 1995; **4**:149–156.
16. Benson LM, Wunderly D, Perry B, *et al.* Determining best practice: comparison of three methods of femoral

sheath removal after cardiac interventional procedures. Heart Lung 2005; **34**: 115–121.

17. Ormiston JA, Shaw BL, Panther MJ, *et al*. Percutaneous coronary intervention with bivalirudin anticoagulation, immediate sheath removal, and early ambulation: a feasibility study with implications for day–stay procedures. Catheter Cardiovasc Interv 2002; **55**: 289–293.

18. Koch KT, Piek JJ, de Winter RJ, *et al*. Two hour ambulation after coronary angioplasty and stenting with 6 F guiding catheters and low dose heparin. Heart 1999; **81**: 53–56.

19. Koch KT, Piek JJ, de Winter RJ, Mulder K, David GK, Lie KI. Early ambulation after coronary angioplasty and stenting with six French guiding catheters and low-dose heparin. Am J Cardiol 1997; **80**: 1084–1086.

20. Vlasic W, Almond D, Massel D. Reducing bedrest following arterial puncture for coronary interventional procedures—impact on vascular complications: the BAC Trial. J Invasive Cardiol 2001; **13**: 788–792.

21. Hoffer EK, Bloch RD. Percutaneous arterial closure devices. J Vasc Interv Radiol 2003; **14**: 865–885.

22. Hermiller JB, Simonton C, Hinohara T, *et al*. The StarClose Vascular Closure System: interventional results from the CLIP study. Catheter Cardiovasc Interv 2006; **68**: 677–683.

23. Van Den Berg JC. A close look at closure devices. J Cardiovasc Surg (Torino) 2006; **47**: 285–295.

24. Nader RG, Garcia JC, Drushal K, Pesek T. Clinical evaluation of SyvekPatch in patients undergoing interventional, EPS and diagnostic cardiac catheterization procedures. J Invasive Cardiol 2002; **14**: 305–307.

25. Applegate RJ, Sacrinty MT, Kutcher MA, *et al*. Propensity score analysis of vascular complications after diagnostic cardiac catheterization and percutaneous coronary intervention using thrombin hemostatic patch-facilitated manual compression. J Invasive Cardiol 2007; **19**: 164–170.

26. Najjar SF, Healey NA, Healey CM, *et al*. Evaluation of poly-N-acetyl glucosamine as a hemostatic agent in patients undergoing cardiac catheterization: a double-blind, randomized study. J Trauma 2004; **57**: S38–41.

27. Palmer BL, Gantt DS, Lawrence ME, Rajab MH, Dehmer GJ. Effectiveness and safety of manual hemostasis facilitated by the SyvekPatch with one hour of bedrest after coronary angiography using six-French catheters. Am J Cardiol 2004; **93**: 96–97.

28. Tavris DR, Dey S, Albrecht-Gallauresi B, *et al*. Risk of local adverse events following cardiac catheterization by

hemostasis device use—phase II. J Invasive Cardiol 2005; **17**: 644–650.

29. Harold L. Dauerman, Robert J. Applegate, and David J. Cohen. Vascular Closure Devices: The Second Decade. J Am Coll Cardiol 2007; **50**: 1617–1626.

30. Koreny M, Riedmuller E, Nikfardjam M, Siostrzonek P, Mullner M. Arterial puncture closing devices compared with standard manual compression after cardiac catheterization: systematic review and meta-analysis. JAMA 2004; **291**: 350–357.

31. Nikolsky E, Mehran R, Halkin A, *et al*. Vascular complications associated with arteriotomy closure devices in patients undergoing percutaneous coronary procedures: a meta-analysis. J Am Coll Cardiol 2004; **44**: 1200–1209.

32. Vaitkus PT. A meta-analysis of percutaneous vascular closure devices after diagnostic catheterization and percutaneous coronary intervention. J Invasive Cardiol 2004; **16**: 243–46.

33. Tavris DR, Gallauresi BA, Lin B, *et al*. Risk of local adverse events following cardiac catheterization by hemostasis device use and gender. J Invasive Cardiol 2004; **16**: 459–464.

34. Warren BS, Warren SG, Miller SD. Predictors of complications and learning curve using the Angio-Seal closure device following interventional and diagnostic catheterization. Catheter Cardiovasc Interv 1999; **48**: 162–166.

35. Duffin DC, Muhlestein JB, Allisson SB, *et al*. Femoral arterial puncture management after percutaneous coronary procedures: a comparison of clinical outcomes and patient satisfaction between manual compression and two different vascular closure devices. J Invasive Cardiol 2001; **13**: 354–362.

36. Rickli H, Unterweger M, Sutsch G, *et al*. Comparison of costs and safety of a suture-mediated closure device with conventional manual compression after coronary artery interventions. Catheter Cardiovasc Interv 2002; **57**: 297–302.

37. Feldman T. Percutaneous Suture Closure for Management of Large French Size Arterial and Venous Puncture. J Interven Cardiol 2000; **13**: 237–241.

38. Solomon LW, Fusman B, Jolly N, Kim A, Feldman T. Percutaneous suture closure for management of large French size arterial puncture in aortic valvuloplasty. J Invasive Cardiol 2001; **13**: 592–596.

Answers

1. B. There have been a number of comparisons between the two approaches. In general, the success rate is somewhat lower with radial access but the complication rate is lower as well. Once through a somewhat steeper learning curve, most operators who perform radial access routinely have a success rate in the mid to high 90's. While a number of techniques limit discomfort associated with the radial approach, it can be painful.

2. C. Groin infection, although uncommon, is a potentially devastating complication, with a 4% associated mortality (Soheil, Mayo Proceedings, 2005). Retroperitoneal hemorrhage is statistically more likely with high sticks *and* vascular closure devices. Although this has only been demonstrated for Angio-Seal (Ellis, CCI, 2005) it is likely a class effect common to all devices. Closure devices do allow earlier ambulation. Lower complication rate has not been convincingly demonstrated – where claimed there is a high likelihood of selection bias. Some studies have suggested a higher complication rate, and the meta-analyses suggest parity at best.

3. B.

4. A.

CHAPTER 4

Optimal Angiographic Views for Coronary Angioplasty

Carl Schultz[1], & Carlo Di Mario[2]
[1] Thoraxcenter, Erasmus Medical Center, Rotterdam, The Netherlands
[2] Royal Brompton Hospital, London, UK

Introduction

The method for diagnostic coronary angiography was developed in an era when the only option for revascularization was coronary bypass surgery (CABG). Operators took multiple views focusing on distal target vessels and run-off. There was no need to be parsimonious with contrast because no further angiographic procedures were being planned. Angiography with a view to coronary angioplasty requires a different approach. In addition to clearly demonstrating the entire length of all epicardial arteries, the focus is to clearly delineate each significant coronary lesion from beginning to end without overlap or foreshortening. At the same time the number of views and contrast use is restricted to the minimum required, in anticipation of further contrast requirement during intervention. Percutaneous coronary angioplasty (PTCA) has supplanted CABG as the most frequently performed revascularization method. In many centres angiography is performed with a view to proceeding to PTCA in the same sitting. Yet many diagnostic angiographic procedures are performed without giving thought to which views that would be meaningful for planning PTCA. In the PTCA dominated era the operator needs to consider angiographic

Interventional Cardiology, First Edition. Edited by
Carlo Di Mario, George D. Dangas, Peter Barlis.
© 2010 Blackwell Publishing Ltd. Published 2010 by
Blackwell Publishing Ltd.

information as it is gained, from the first angiographic image, with a view to selecting subsequent views accordingly.

Catheter Selection

During the era of the predominant brachial approach when multipurpose catheters were in routine use, 7Fr catheters were the norm due to the requirement for torqueability. Contemporary diagnostic catheters are pre-shaped to facilitate intubation of the coronary ostia, in most cases with only minimal catheter manipulation. Less torqueable 5F and 6F catheters are used routinely and good quality images can also be obtained in a substantial proportion of patients using 4F catheters. The smaller size catheters have the advantage of being less likely to cause vessel trauma because they have very flexible tips.

Left Coronary

Judkins curve catheters are used most widely. A JL4 would suit the anatomy of most patients although a JL 3.5 may be required in patients with a smaller diameter aorta, e.g. women. If the aortic root is dilated a JL 4.5, JL5 or even JL6 with longer secondary curves may be required. Selective intubation may be encountered when there is a short left main stem or separate origin of the left anterior descending (LAD) and circumflex (Cx) arteries, which may necessitate selecting a catheter with an upwards pointing tip, e.g. JL3.5 for intubation of the LAD and a more horizontal tip, e.g. a JL4 for intubation of the Cx.

Right Coronary

The take off of the right coronary artery (RCA) varies more than the left. A JR4 curve is most often used successfully. High anterior origin of the RCA may necessitate the use of an Amplatz right or left curve if a JR is unsuccessful.

Radial Approach

The same catheter curves can be used via the radial approach as when using transfemoral arterial access (e.g. JL4, JR) although it may be necessary to downsize the left curve (e.g. to JL3.5 if a JL4 would have been suitable from the femoral approach). A Barbeau or a Tiger catheter suitable for both the left and right coronaries may also be used from the right radial approach [1].

Coronary Intubation

The left anterior oblique (LAO) view is most useful for intubation of the left and right coronary arteries, because the left and right coronary sinuses are maximally separated and there is minimal overlap between the ostia and the coronary sinuses (Figure 4.1). For intubation of the left system the J-wire is advanced up to just above the aortic leaflets. The catheter is advanced over the wire and when the tip nears the aortic sinuses the J-wire is withdrawn to allow it to approach close to or intubate the coronary ostium. Slow J-wire withdrawal is recommended to avoid the catheter tip flicking into the ostium which may cause dissection, plaque dislodgement or spasm and also to avoid sucking air into the proximal catheter hub. The right coronary is intubated by advancing the JR catheter over the J-wire until the tip is just above the aortic leaflets. The wire is then withdrawn into the distal catheter to facilitate manipulation. Gentle counter clockwise rotation aiming the catheter tip toward the left with concomitant withdrawal is usually required. Gentle movements are emphasized to avoid sudden or deep intubation which may precipitate spasm. Before proceeding to inject dye the pressure trace is checked. The pressure trace may be damped or ventricularized indicating the possibility of ostial right or left main stem disease, spasm, complete occlusion of a non-dominant RCA or that the catheter tip is abutting the vessel wall. Forceful contrast injection during any of these scenarios could result in dissection or plaque dislodgement. Contrast injection with an occlusive catheter with contrast remaining at the end of the injection, for instance holding up into the conus branch should also be avoided because this may precipitate ventricular fibrillation. Spasm may be reversed with intra-coronary nitrate e.g. isosorbide dinitrate (ISDN) 100 to 200 µg. Rapid but gentle catheter withdrawal is indicated until the coronary ostium is extubated or the pressure trace normalizes. A small dose of intra-coronary nitrate may be required to counteract any coronary vasospasm (e.g. ISDN 100 µg to 500 µg depending on the blood pressure). On occasion smaller e.g. 5F or 4F catheters may be required to avoid damping due to spasm in hyper-reactive arteries or when there is ostial plaque.

Diagnostic Angiography

Left Sided Views

The first view is chosen to identify left main stem disease. Either a post-anterior (PA) view with minimal angulation to the right to project the

Figure 4.1. The 3-dimensional reconstruction of a 64 slice CT coronary angiogram demonstrates clearly that in the post-anterior (PA) view the coronary ostia are superimposed on the aortic sinuses whereas there is maximal separation in the ~40° left anterior oblique (LAO) view.

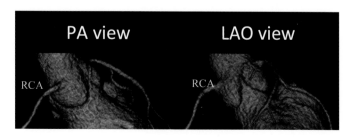

catheter tip off the spine or a LAO caudal (spider) view, are used most often. At least three to four perpendicular views are required to visualize the left coronary tree. Popular combinations of views are shown in Table 4.1. In many patients these views would suffice potentially even when proceeding immediately to angioplasty. However, due to variations in patient anatomy e.g. increased overlap caused by prominent tortuosity, displacement or rotation of the heart axis in the chest, e.g. when there is normal anatomical variation, chest wall deformity, previous cardiothoracic surgery or lung pathology, modification of views or additional views may be required. When a lesion is identified additional views may be indicated depending on how well the affected coronary segment has been visualized.

Right Sided Views

Two perpendicular views are advocated for the RCA, usually LAO and right anterior oblique (RAO). However, it is frequently impossible to exclude disease at or beyond the crux without an additional view with cranial angulation (e.g. PA cranial or LAO cranial).

Lesion Specific Approach

Optimal Views for Each Coronary Segment

Views that reliably demonstrate the full length of each coronary segment while minimizing foreshortening and overlap for the left coronary arteries are shown in Figures 4.2 and 4.3a. Due to the spectacular degree of variation in human anatomy there are no views that will in all cases demonstrate clearly a lesion in a particular coronary segment. An example of a patient where the lesion was only clearly demonstrated after further adjustment of the gantry to unusual angles is shown in Figure 4.4.

Left Main Stem (LMS)

Lesions in the ostium or mid segment of the left main stem are often best seen in the AP cranial view. The straight antero-posterior (AP) view with only slight rightward angulation to project the catheter tip off the spine is sometimes advocated but may not be optimal because the ostium of the LMS may be projected over the left coronary sinus.

Table 4.1. Popular view combinations for diagnostic angiography with benefits and limitations of each view.

View	Good for visualizing	Limitations
Combination 1		
AP (5-10° RAO)	Left main stem (ostium and main shaft)	Overlap on LMS bifurcation and sometimes LMS ostium with left coronary sinus
Lateral	Mid and distal LAD, mid Cx	Potentially high radiation dose to operator, Usually limited view of proximal LAD, patient arms need to be above head to visualize posterior arteries, often overlap Diagonals/LAD
RAO cranial	Proximal and mid LAD, distal Cx	Test injections may be required to adjust angulation to ensure diagonals are above LAD, overlap with dominant Cx, and position of the diaphragm
RAO caudal	Circumflex and distal LAD	
Combination 2		
LAO caudal	Left main stem bifurcation, proximal LAD and proximal circumflex	Potentially a higher radiation dose to the patient, poor quality images sometimes in large patients
LAO cranial	Mid LAD, origin of diagonals, proximal and mid Cx	Patient required to hold in inspiration during acquisition to elongate the proximal LAD
AP cranial	Proximal and mid LAD, distal Cx	Steep cranial angulation required can be a problem for patients with cervical spine fixation
RAO caudal	Circumflex and distal LAD, sometimes LAD ostium	

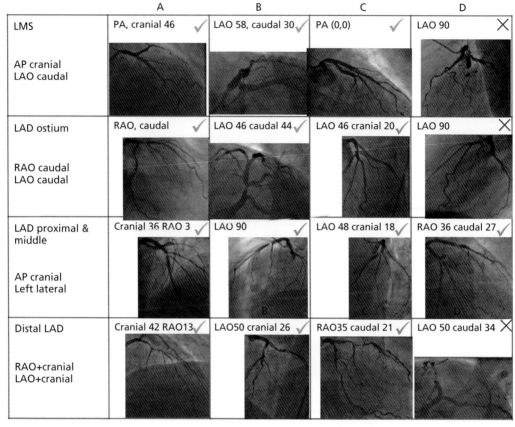

	A	B	C	D
LMS AP cranial LAO caudal	PA, cranial 46 ✓	LAO 58, caudal 30 ✓	PA (0,0) ✓	LAO 90 ✗
LAD ostium RAO caudal LAO caudal	RAO, caudal ✓	LAO 46 caudal 44 ✓	LAO 46 cranial 20 ✓	LAO 90 ✗
LAD proximal & middle AP cranial Left lateral	Cranial 36 RAO 3 ✓	LAO 90 ✓	LAO 48 cranial 18 ✓	RAO 36 caudal 27 ✓
Distal LAD RAO+cranial LAO+cranial	Cranial 42 RAO13 ✓	LAO50 cranial 26 ✓	RAO35 caudal 21 ✓	LAO 50 caudal 34 ✗

Figure 4.2. Optimal angiographic views for specific segments of the left anterior descending artery are indicated with a green tick mark. Some views that may be useful but are not generally recommended are indicated with a orange bracketed tick mark and inadequate views with a red cross.

The ostium of the LMS may also be seen clearly in an LAO caudal view (30 to 50° left; 25 to 40°caudal), which will also demonstrate the mid LMS and may sometimes be the only view to clearly separate the LMS bifurcation. In this view, also known as the "spider view", the picture may be grainy and poor quality particularly when angulation is steep and in obese patients. The image can be optimized by positioning the LMS in the centre of the field and reducing image contrast by blanking the field from 12 o'clock to 3 o'clock. A small test injection before acquisition is sensible because a more horizontal axis of the heart may require steeper caudal angulation and occasionally overlap at the LMS bifurcation may be separated by rotating more steeply to the left or toward AP caudal.

LAD
Separation of the bifurcation of the LMS in the LAO caudal view will also show the ostium of the LAD clearly as well as the proximal LAD and frequently also the origin of the first diagonal. For these reasons the LAO caudal view may be useful for wiring the proximal LAD or for stent positioning at the ostium of the LAD, but if possible it should be avoided as a working view because X-ray attenuation due to the highly angled projection through the spine results in higher x-ray doses. Working views for the LAD ostium include RAO caudal and RAO cranial although in the latter more than 30° degrees of rightward angulation may be required to move the circumflex off the region of interest.

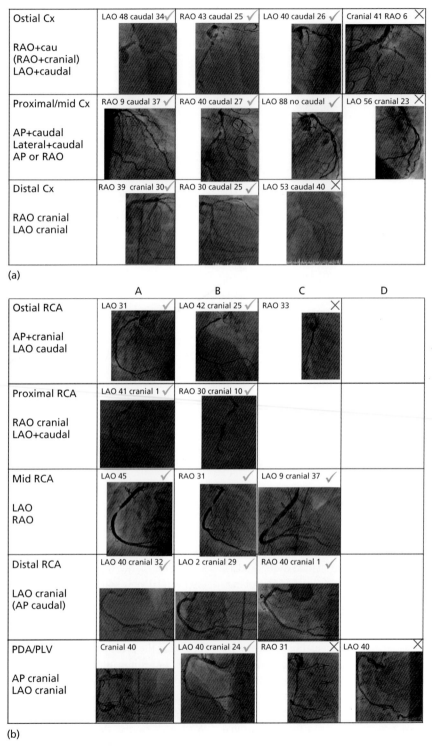

(a)

(b)

Figure 4.3a and 4.3b. Optimal angiographic views for specific segments in the circumflex and right coronary are indicated with a green tick mark. Some views that may be useful but are not generally recommended are indicated with a orange tick mark and inadequate views with a red cross.

Conventional views:

A) LAO 49 caudal 30

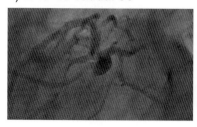

B) RAO38 caudal 27

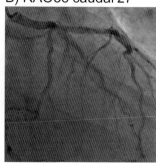

C) LAO 39 cranial 32

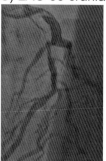

Modified views to demonstrate ostial LAD lesion:

D) LAO 60 caudal 50   E) LAO 90 cranial 15   F) After stenting

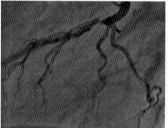

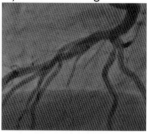

Figure 4.4. This male aged 47 with known coronary disease presented with deteriorating angina and reversible ischemia in the anterior territory on perfusion imaging. Conventional views (Panels A–C) raised suspicion of a lesion in the left anterior descending (LAD) ostium due to haziness (Panel A) but were limited by overlap at the ostium of the left anterior descending (LAD) due to unusual tortuosity (Panel A). Unusual modification including a steep spider view and a lateral view with cranial angulation were required to delineate the lesion (Panels D, E). The final angiographic result is shown after stenting (Panel F).

Although the RAO cranial view may clearly demonstrate lesions in the proximal and mid LAD this is not the ideal working view because steep ~40° rightward angulation may be required to eliminate ovelap with diagonals and wide diaphragmatic excursion during breathing causes highly variable contrast ratio in the field of view. Simply moving the gantry from AP to AP cranial elongates the proximal LAD and separates the diagonals to the right of the screen. A rightward tilt of ~5° may be required to separate the proximal segment from the spine and the catheter in order to produce an excellent standard working view for the proximal and mid LAD unaffected by movement of the diaphragm. For diagnostic purposes the ostia of the diagonals may be better seen in the LAO cranial view. However, LAO cranial is seldom used as a working view because a deep breath hold is required to reduce foreshortening and reduce projection of the diaphragm over the proximal and mid LAD. The body habitus of some patients also requires steep leftward angulation to project the LAD off the spine. An alternative but much less frequently used working view for lesions in the proximal and mid LAD is the left lateral. If the only vessel of interest is the LAD it is not necessary to ask patients to remove their arms from the field of view by keeping them above their heads, as this requirement can often be uncomfortable or sometimes impossible for the elderly and patients with arthritis or old shoulder injuries.

Panning is usually required in the RAO cranial and LAO cranial views to demonstrate the distal LAD. Smooth slow panning allows the X-ray generator to adjust automatically to changes in x-ray attenuation. The lateral view is a good alternative for demonstrating the distal LAD around the apex but may also require controlled movement of the table during the acquisition toward the floor and/ or in the direction of the head. The RAO caudal view may include the distal LAD without the requirement for table movement or being affected by diaphragmatic movement.

Circumflex

The circumflex ostium may be clearly seen together with the LMS bifurcation in the LAO caudal view. Occasionally eccentric ostial lesions not clearly seen in other views may be delineated in the RAO cranial view although steep angulation may be required. The RAO caudal is the most useful diagnostic view for the circumflex and may clearly define lesions in the ostium, proximal and mid vessel as well as the bifurcations and obtuse marginals. To obtain a working view with improved image quality by eliminating overlap with the diaphragm and reduced x-ray attenuation the view can be modified to AP caudal with only 10° to 15° rightward angulation.

The proximal and mid circumflex territory may also be viewed in the left lateral. A drawback of this view is that the patient has to remove their arms from the field of view by elevation above their head. Even young patients without arthritis may find this difficult to maintain for prolonged periods. Additional caudal angulation may be required to reduce overlap with marginal vessels.

RAO or LAO with cranial angulation may be required to view lesions in the distal circumflex when the RAO caudal is suboptimal. If the circumflex is dominant the LAO cranial or AP cranial views may open up the distal bifurcation and elongate the posterior descending artery (PDA).

RCA

Views that reliably demonstrate the full length of each coronary segment while minimizing foreshortening and overlap for the right coronary artery are shown in Figure 4.3a and b. Usually the only two views required to demonstrate lesions in the proximal, mid and distal RCA are LAO and RAO, because of the absence of side branches in these segments. Ostial lesions in the RCA are often detected in LAO but can be significantly foreshortened in this view. If stent placement is being considered finding the least foreshortened segment may facilitate accurate positioning at ostium. The ostial segment and proximal RCA often lay perpendicular to the X-ray beam in the AP cranial and LAO caudal views, despite variation in the origin of the RCA toward anterior or posterior. The lateral view with cranial angulation may identify occasional highly eccentric ostial lesions not clearly seen in other views. The lateral view may also occasionally help to better delineate lesions in a highly tortuous mid RCA or when right ventricular branches overlap the main vessel.

The distal RCA, PDA and posterior left ventricular (PLV) branches lie posterior to the heart and require cranial angulation (in LAO) or caudal angulation (in RAO or AP) to be visualized without overlap. Many operators routinely include a third view, either AP cranial or LAO cranial, in addition to LAO and RAO as standard during diagnostic imaging.

Vein Grafts

An operative report describing graft number and insertions is imperative to reduce the chances of missing a graft as well as to reduce fluoroscopy dose and procedure time spent hunting for an unknown number of grafts. An aortogram can be helpful for graft localization, potentially saving time and contrast, but it is not a panacea, because grafts may sometimes opacify only if the pigtail catheter is positioned at the level of the graft origin, if at all, when the take off is vertical and/or flow is slow. The insertions of vein grafts may vary substantially in particular after redo bypass surgery. A rule of thumb is that the aorto-ostial insertions of vein grafts to the left coronary system tend to arise lower and more anterior for grafts to an anterior artery (e.g.LAD) and progressively more superior and leftward as the insertion site moves more toward left lateral e.g. diagonal, intermediate, obtuse marginal, AV circumflex. In the RAO view left sided grafts may be intubated by pointing the catheter toward the right of the screen. Right sided grafts may be found in LAO by dragging the catheter pointing to the left of the screen along the ascending aorta starting above the RCA ostium. A patent graft with slow flow may only partially opacify and thus appear occluded if intubated with a catheter tip that is angulated toward the wall of the graft e.g vertical origin of vein grafts to the RCA intubated with a JR catheter. In these instances a coaxially aligned catheter e.g. multipurpose or RCB catheter for a right sided graft and a multipurpose or LCB for left sided grafts should be used to clarify whether or not a graft is occluded. The views are selected according to the native coronary segment where the graft inserts. Two perpendicular views are required.

LIMA Grafts

The left internal mammary artery (LIMA) graft is usually prognostically the most important. Selective intubation of the LIMA with demonstration of the entire length of the graft and native vessel including any lesions and collateral supply is the standard. The origin of the left subclavian artery is usually engaged in the AP view. An 0.035 inch J-wire is used to lead before the catheter is advanced over it to reduce the risk of trauma to the vessels. If difficulty is encountered with an abnormal aortic arch, severe tortuosity or stenosis the following steps can be tried: intubation of the left subclavian may be easier in the LAO view; making use of non-selective contrast injections to delineate the anatomy; using a JR rather than an IMA catheter to engage the left subclavian and exchanging it via a 300cm J-wire for an IMA catheter if necessary once the catheter is beyond the origin of the LIMA; making use of a 0.035 inch steerable hydrophilic J-wire if extreme tortuosity is preventing passage of the standard J-wire. Once the catheter tip is near the ostium of the LIMA the AP view may be most useful for engagement. If the JR catheter tip appears too horizontal during gentle withdrawal or too short to engage the ostium of the LIMA an IMA catheter may be used or sometimes the even more acute hook of a Bartorelli catheter may be required. Before contrast injection including test injections it is important to remember to check that the pressure tracing does not indicate wedging of the catheter tip against the vessel wall. If selective intubation via the femoral route proves elusive despite multiple attempts the left radial route may offer a safer alternative. A drawback of the left radial route is that RIMA grafts cannot be engaged, although there are reports of successful intubation of the LIMA via the right

radial route [2]. The first angiographic view for the LIMA requires panning from origin to the distal LAD. The views that best show the insertions are RAO cranial and left lateral. Collateral filling of other vessels should also be documented. Intubation to the diaphragm of a pedicle RIMA graft follows the same principles as for the LIMA, but with even greater care in view of the close proximity of the right internal carotid artery.

Coronary Variants

Aberrant coronary anatomy occurs infrequently and the prevalence of ~1.3 % is remarkably consistent in different series of patients attending for angiography [3,4]. Some anomalies are easy to identify e.g. abnormal origin of RCA (Figure 4.5) but others can be more subtle e.g. anomalous non-dominant circumflex, Figure 4.6. The culprit lesion may be missed if the aberrant anatomy is not identified (Figures 4.5 and 4.6). Systematic review to identify areas of the myocardium for which a vascular supply has not been demonstrated is helpful in this respect and also for identifying occlusions, Figure 4.6. Once it is known which vessel is anomalous a review of the images may identify ghosting of the vessel. If there are no clues as to the origin a systematic search starting with the most common variant is required. The diagnostic catheter shape may need to be changed as required to reach the wall of the aortic root in the area of interest. The most common coronary anomaly is an absent left main stem. A slightly smaller curve catheter may be required to intubate the LAD selectively, e.g. a JL3.5 if a JL4 preferentially and exclusively intubates the Cx. The Cx arising from the right coronary sinus can often be cannulated using the JR4 catheter, but a steep take off may require a multipurpose catheter whereas a posterior or high anterior origin may require an AR or AL shape. If the RCA arises from the left side separately from the left main stem an AL1 or multipurpose catheter are most likely to be successful.

Once the anomalous coronary vessel has been intubated the standard views are often sufficient for the mid and distal vessel if the heart has a normal position and orientation (Figures 4.2 and 4.3), while the views for the proximal vessel and ostium may need to be modified depending on the origin and course.

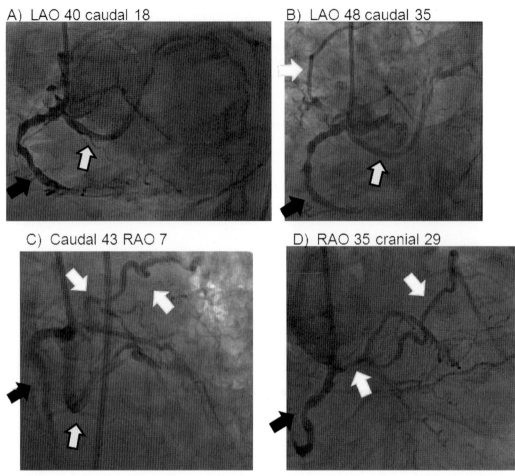

Figure 4.5. This obese female aged 80 years was admitted for angiography following a recent worsening of angina. She had a previous history of myocardial infarction. Preceding this presentation her angina symptoms had been stable for many years and were not previously investigated with angiography. A coronary ostium could not be engaged at the left aortic sinus. The left anterior descending (LAD), circumflex and right coronary arteries originated from a single right sided ostium. The right coronary artery (RCA) (black arrows) was occluded distally. The left anterior descending (LAD) (white arrows) was critically stenosed proximal to a large diagonal and the circumflex (grey arrows) was critically stenosed mid course. The catheter partially obscures the left anterior descending (LAD) in Panel A and the circumflex in Panel D.

Adding Information with CT-Angiography

Multidetector CT (MDCT) is becoming an established method for non-invasive coronary angiography and is discussed in more detail elsewhere. It can be a very useful diagnostic aid when information gained from invasive coronary angiography is incomplete due to technical or anatomical limitation, e.g. when a coronary graft or aberrant vessels cannot be selectively engaged (Figure 4.7). If significant coronary disease has been identified on MDCT and PCI is planned the optimal working view can easily be determined even when anatomy is challenging or unusual [5]. Information on the distribution of calcification and plaque can also be useful when planning complex angioplasty (e.g. bifurcations and chronic total occlusions) [6,7].

A) RAO 12   B) LAO 51 cranial 19 C) Lateral - early   D) Lateral - late

E) LAO 37   F) LAO 37   G) LAO 37

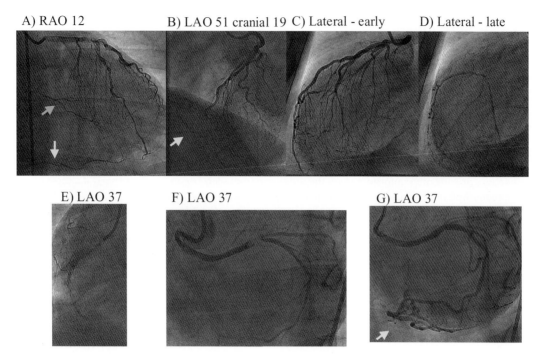

Figure 4.6. These views were taken during primary angioplasty performed in a male aged 41y who presented with an acute infero-lateral myocardial infarction. No antegrade perfusion was evident in the circumflex territory (Panels A to D), although retrograde collaterals to an obtuse marginal branch were seen in some views (green arrow, Panel A). The right coronary artery (RCA) was occluded and filled retrogradely via the left anterior descending (LAD) (yellow arrow, Panels A, B, D and E). The culprit lesion was in an aberrant circumflex arising from the right sinus (Panel F). Following aspiration thrombectomy and stent deployment it was evident that the aberrant circumflex provided the principle collateral supply to a chronically occluded dominant right coronary artery (RCA) (yellow arrow, Panel G).

Figure 4.7. Infrequently an anomalous right coronary may arise from the left aortic sinus. In this example the right coronary artery (RCA) could not be located with conventional angiography despite multiple attempts. 64-slice CT angiography demonstrates the origin anterior to the left main stem ostium, and at the same level rather than higher. Engaging the right coronary artery (RCA) in this position can be difficult and may require and AL1 curve catheter. A stent can be seen in the mid left anterior descending artery.

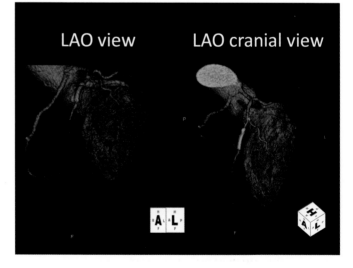

LAO view   LAO cranial view

Ventriculography

Knowledge of ventricular function is essential to interpreting the clinical relevance of coronary disease and planning appropriate treatment. Many patients may have a contemporary assessment of left ventricular function by non-invasive testing, which may include echocardiography, magnetic resonance imaging, nuclear imaging and MDCT, when attending for coronary angiography. These modalities provide more information on the function and morphology of the left ventricle that conventional ventriculography and may obviate the need for further assessment. Ventriculography should be performed in the catheter laboratory if LV function has not yet been assessed recently. The RAO view is standard although an additional LAO view could be considered if assessment of the postero-lateral wall, usually supplied by the circumflex, is likely to influence management.

Contrast Use

The number of angiographic views and volume of contrast used should be kept to the minimum required. However, contrast injections and acquisitions should last sufficiently long to demonstrate collateral filling and the length of occluded segments. Angiographic view should be set up so that the occluded segment will be demonstrated, e.g. in the LAO view to include an occluded RCA filling retrogradely, or in the RAO view to include the occluded LAD filling retrogradely from the RCA. If a complex chronic total occlusion is encountered the size and course of collaterals may also be important. Bilateral contrast injections may optimally demonstrate the length of an occluded segment and collaterals, but these are usually performed at the time of angioplasty rather than during diagnostic procedures to avoid an additional arterial puncture.

Questions

1. Which of the listed views is the best to visualize the mid segment of the LAD?

   A AP cranial

   B AP caudal

   C RAO caudal

   D LAO caudal

2. An elderly male smoker was referred for PCI of the LAD. Following introduction of an 8 French left Judkins guide catheter, the operator encountered difficulty in finding the way through the abdominal aorta apparently due to a large atherosclerotic burden. The catheter was subsequently advanced to the ascending aorta where it was flushed with saline. Chest pain, ST segment elevation and hypotension followed that resulted in a spiraling downhill clinical course in spite of intra-aortic balloon pumping. Which of the following is the most likely explanation of these events?

   A Left main coronary dissection

   B Air embolus

   C Atheroembolization

   D Aortic dissection

   E Left main coronary spasm

3. Considerable difficulty was encountered in finding a guide cathether which would selectively intubate a SVG to a posterior OM arising from a position high on the inner curvature of the ascending aorta. Which of the following is the best option?

   A Multipurpose

   B Left Judkins FL 4.0

   C Amplatz left 1.5

   D IMA

   E VODA

4. An obese 50-year-old female underwent coronary arteriography via the radial approach with 6-F catheters. Engagement of the left coronary artery was successful with difficulty using an Amplatz left catheter. After several pictures of the left coronary artery were taken, she developed sudden ST segment elevation and arrested. What is the most likely explanation?

   A Atheroembolic myocardial infarction

   B Aortic dissection

   C Pulmonary embolus

   D Left main coronary dissection

   E Air embolus

References

1. Ikari Y, Ochiai M, Hangaishi M, *et al.* Novel guide catheter for left coronary intervention via a right upper limb approach. Cathet Cardiovasc Diagn 1998; **44**(2): 244–247.

2. Cha KS, Kim MH. Feasibility and safety of concomitant left internal mammary arteriography at the setting of the right transradial coronary angiography. Catheter Cardiovasc Interv 2002; **56**(2): 188–195.

3. Yamanaka O, Hobbs RE. Coronary artery anomalies in 126,595 patients undergoing coronary arteriography. Cathet Cardiovasc Diagn 1990; **1**(1): 28–40.

4. Angelini P, Velasco JA, Flamm S. Coronary anomalies: incidence, pathophysiology, and clinical relevance. Circulation 2002; **105**(20): 2449–2454.

5. Otsuka M, Sugahara S, Nakamura M, *et al.* Optimal fluoroscopic view selection for percutaneous coronary intervention by multislice computed tomography. Int J Cardiol 2007; **118**(3): e94–96.

6. Van Mieghem CA, Thury A, Meijboom WB, *et al.* Detection and characterization of coronary bifurcation lesions with 64-slice computed tomography coronary angiography. Eur Heart J 2007; **28**(16): 1968–1976.

7. Mollet NR, Hoye A, Lemos PA, *et al.* Value of preprocedure multislice computed tomographic coronary angiography to predict the outcome of percutaneous recanalization of chronic total occlusions. Am J Cardiol 2005; **95**(2): 240–243.

Answers

1. A
2. C
3. D
4. D

CHAPTER 5

Material Selection

Carl Schultz,[1] Rohit Khurana,[2] & Carlo Di Mario[3]

[1] Thoraxcenter, Erasmus Medical Center, Rotterdam, The Netherlands

[2] Imperial College Health Trust, London, UK

[3] Royal Brompton Hospital and Imperial College, London, UK

Introduction

The legend tells that the first coronary angioplasty balloons were made by Andreas Gruentzig and his wife in a kitchen: they were very bulky, difficult to position as there was no guidewire lumen, and too compliant to safely expand resistant lesions in coronary arteries. These rudimentary instruments are light years away from the sophistication of the current material. Further understanding and developments in techniques and materials have reduced the profile of balloons, whilst increasing the robustness, deliverability, reliability and safety profile. Guidewires have reduced in size and seen improvements in torque and push transmission whilst becoming more robust with generally softer less traumatic but shapeable tips whereas specialty wires have been developed for the treatment of specific lesion types, e.g. chronic total occlusions. A wide range of guide catheters, guidewires and angioplasty balloons are now available, and continue to evolve to overcome variations in anatomy, changes in vascular access and evolution in technique. The appropriate selection and safe and optimal use of these devices can reduce procedural time whilst increasing success and safety and improve short and medium term outcomes

The fundamental principle of angioplasty pertaining to material selection and use are to know

Interventional Cardiology, First Edition. Edited by
Carlo Di Mario, George D. Dangas, Peter Barlis.
© 2010 Blackwell Publishing Ltd. Published 2010 by
Blackwell Publishing Ltd.

well advantages and limitations of each specific piece of equipment, be familiar with their characteristics and modalities of use, and be ready to have alternative strategies in case of failures or malfunction.

Guide Catheter Selection

Functional Design of Modern Guide Catheters

The functions of guide catheters are to allow safe intubation of the coronary ostia, accurate hemodynamic monitoring, and to provide a conduit for wires and balloons to be delivered and contrast to be injected. They are an important component to the system of support during equipment delivery to the coronary target. The clinical, anatomical and angiographic scenario must be considered when selecting the size, shape and length of a guiding catheter.

Modern catheters have a soft tip to reduce the risk of vessel trauma during intubation or manipulation. The wall consists of an outer layer that retains a predefined curve and increases shaft stiffness to provide backup support during angioplasty, a middle layer of wire braid to increase kink resistance, torque ability and shaft radiopacity, and a smooth lubricated inner layer to facilitate the transit of equipment. Guiding catheters have thinner walls than diagnostic catheters to increase inner lumen size and may be easily kinked, weakened or ruined by repeated or injudicious spinning (Table 5.1). Maintaining the J-wire within the catheter, rotation during with-

Table 5.1. Guide catheter inner lumen size by manufacturer and outer lumen size.

Guide/Manufacturer	Inner Lumen (in)	Outer lumen size (French)			
		5	6	7	8
Launcher / Medtronic		0.058	0.071	0.081	0.090
Vista Brite Tip/Cordis		0.056	0.070	0.078	0.088
Mach1/Boston Scientific		NA	0.070	0.081	0.091
Viking/Guidant Abbott		NA	0.068	0.078	0.091
Wiseguide/Boston Scientific		NA	0.066	0.076	0.086

drawal or advancement and deep inspiration may facilitate coronary intubation. If there is no torque control the problem may often be solved by the use of a peripheral sheath long enough to straighten the most tortuous arterial segments. The optimal view for left and right coronary intubation is the left anterior oblique because in most patients it offers the least superimposition of the coronary ostia with the left and right aortic sinuses.

Size Requirements

The advantages and disadvantages of smaller and larger catheter sizes are listed in Table 5.2. Routine angioplasty using 5French (Fr) guiding catheters may be ideal when direct stenting is planned, but not all stents are deliverable through a 5 Fr guide and most bifurcation techniques are not applicable [1]. The general standard is a 6 Fr (2.00 mm external diameter) guide which permits radial access, allows active engagement ("deep-throat"), accomodates two modern rapid exchange balloons or a 1.50/1.75 mm Rotablator burr and uses less contrast than larger catheter diameters. 7 Fr (2.33 mm diameter) guides are required for bifurcation techniques requiring the simultaneous insertion of 2 stents (Crush, V stenting), are necessary for chronic total occlusion techniques that require two over the wire (OTW) catheters for a parallel wire approach, facilitate the insertion of 1.75 mm Rotablator burrs and are indispensable for larger burrs (2.0 mm). 8 Fr (2.66 mm diameter) guides are used for directional atherectomy (Flexicut), Rotablator burrs more than 2.0 mm and chronic total occlusion techniques requiring intravascular ultrasound and an OTW catheter for guided recanalization.

Table 5.2. The advantages and disadvantages of smaller versus larger catheter diameters have to be weighed when selecting catheter size.

Smaller diameter	Larger diameter
Advantages	
Smaller puncture	Increased torque
Small vessel access	Increased support
Less traumatic radial access	Improved visualization
Allows deeper engagement without significant damping	Allows two balloon/stent strategy
Disadvantages	
Less torque	Larger puncture: increased access site trauma / recovery time
Reduced visualization	Pressure damping
Less support	Increased contrast use
Difficult or impossible to use two balloon/stent strategy	

Shape Selection

Shape selection to allow positioning of the catheter coaxially with the proximal segment of the artery is important to reduce the risk of catheter induced vessel trauma and optimize support during intervention. When selecting the shape of the catheter, the following factors may be considered: the curve and fit of the diagnostic catheter, size of the aortic root, origin and take off of the artery, location and complexity of the lesion and devices likely to be utilized during intervention.

Shape Selection for the Left Coronary System

Shapes for commonly used guide catheters for the left coronary system are shown in Figure 5.1. The

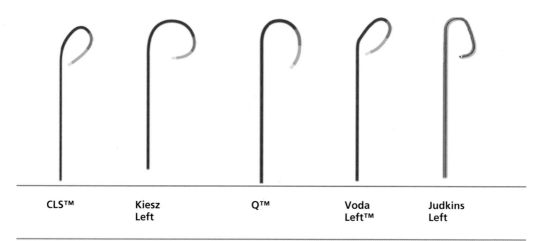

| CLS™ | Kiesz Left | Q™ | Voda Left™ | Judkins Left |

Figure 5.1. Shapes of a selection of guide catheters for the left coronary system.

Table 5.3. Comparability of curve sizes for different shapes of left sided guide catheters.

	AL (Amplatz) Curve	CLS or XB Curve	JL (Judkins Left) Curve	Q Curve	VL (Voda Left) Curve
Normal	AL 1	XB 4.0 or 3.5	JL 4	Q 4	VL 4
Dilated	AL 2	XB 4.0 or 4.5	JL 4.5	Q 4.5	VL 5
Narrow	AL 0.75	XB 3.0 or 3.5	JL 3.5	Q 3.5	VL 3

curve sizes of different shapes have been largely standardized and the comparable curve sizes that may be used most commonly are shown in Table 5.3.

For the left coronary artery, catheters with a smaller curve will point upward and selectively engage to LAD and a larger curve will selectively engage and provide better support for the circumflex. The tip of AL guides tend to point downward and is useful to selectively engage the circumflex when there is a short or absent left main.

The shape of the guide catheter is an important component of the backup or support system that allows delivery of devices to the target segment. Changing the guide catheter to improve support in the middle of a procedure can be problematic, e.g. if a stent cannot be delivered and predilation has caused coronary dissection or plaque disruption. It is also important to appreciate that by selection of a guide with optimal backup it is less likely that additional or stiffer wires or balloons would be required to provide backup, with a corresponding reduction in cost and procedure time.

Although JL curves are commonly used the support is less than for EBU- or Q-type curves. Because of the secondary curve on the JL, the tip moves suddenly downward when resistance is encountered. Q/Voda/XB/EBU or similar curves provide comparatively more support without an increased risk of damage to the coronary ostia. AL curves are required in certain situations, but should only be used by experienced operators in view of the increased risk of iatrogenic dissection. Techiques to obtain support other than the passive support allowed by the guide catheter shape are discussed in the final section of this chapter.

Shape Selection for the Right Coronary System

Shapes and sizes of commonly used guide catheters for the right coronary system are shown in Figure 5.2. The take off of the right coronary artery tends to vary more than the take off of the left coronary. If the take off is transverse the most commonly used guide would probably be a Judkins right (JR) 4.0. With a superiorly directed take off a JR, Hockeystick, EBU-R or Amplatz R or L are more suitable. Inferiorly directed take offs can be cannulated with a multipurpose or SLS catheter. Although the JR shape does not provide much passive support the guide can often be actively engaged more deeply to augment support if required.

Length

The standard length of a guide catheter is 100 cm. Occasionally shorter lengths (85 or 90 cm) may be required to reach for distal lesions (LIMA, sequential SVGs, retrograde approach to CTO). Longer lengths (110 to 115 cm) may be required for unusually tall patients or severely tortuous aorto-iliac vessels. The use of a long sheath and of longer balloon catheters (>145 cm) has partially overcome the problem but still there are no stent delivery catheters longer than 135 cm.

Side Holes or Not?

Side holes help to maintain coronary perfusion when there is the likelihood of damping, e.g. 7–8 Fr guides, ostial plaque, non-coaxial orientation and small caliber arteries at origin as is often found in women or Asian patients. Side holes may reduce contrast opacification of the arteries with a consequent reduction in image quality. Contrast consumption may also increase substantially, which is not desirable in patients at risk of contrast nephropathy. The persistence of aortic pressure morphology can mask severe damping which is of importance for measuring fractional flow reserve [2].

Variation in Access Site

The same guide catheters can be used via the transradial as would be for the transfemoral route. Dedicated transradial guide catheters include the Barbeau and brachial/radial curves. Both curves can be used for access to either the left or right coronary system and provide support against the opposite wall of the aorta (Figure 5.3).

Vein Grafts

Both right and left sided vein grafts with a transverse origin can often be cannulated with a JR4 guide catheter. If the vein graft points downwards

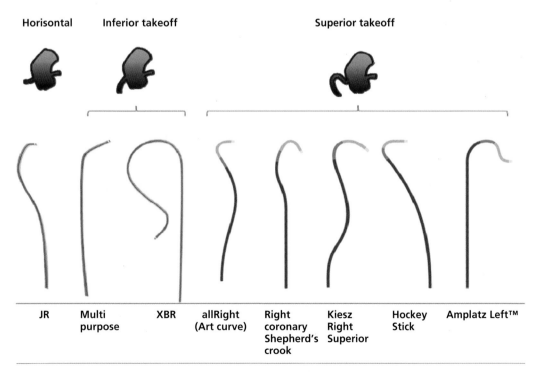

Figure 5.2. Shapes of commonly used guide catheters for the right coronary system.

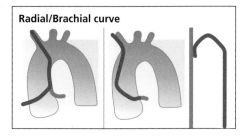 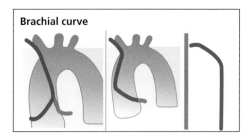

Figure 5.3. The Barbeau and Radial/Brachial curve catheters can be used via the radial route and have a "one size fits all" design for intervention to either the left or right coronary systems. (Diagram courtesy of Cordis International.)

(inferior or vertical such as often for RCA grafts), Opacification may be very poor using a JR catheter, in particular if the graft is ectatic and the flow slow. It is imperative to use a selectively engaged and coaxially aligned catheter before deciding that a graft may be blocked or to exclude disease at the anastomosis or downstream. A multipurpose or RCB guide is usually coaxially aligned when the takeoff is inferior and would also offer good support if required. Left sided vein grafts lesions can also often be attempted with a JR4 guide or, if more support is needed, with an Amplatz or Hockeystick guiding catheter. If the ascending aorta is large or dilated a guide with more pronounced secondary curve is required, e.g. LCB or an Amplatz shape.

Left and Right Internal Mammary Arteries

Although the left internal mammary can often be reached with a JR guide, the more acute primary angle and longer tip of an IMA guide may be required. Short tip hook shaped IMA catheters can occasionally be required to intubate a very steep takeoff angle. Sometimes, e.g. due to subclavian stenosis or extreme tortuousity, the IMA can only be selectively cannulated via the left radial approach.

Gastro-epiploic Artery Grafts

In an attempt to simulate the longevity of IMA grafts and overcome the problem of reaching the distal RCA the gastro-epiploic artery (GEA) is sometimes used as an in situ graft to the posterior or inferior surface of the heart (RCA, PDA, PLV) [3]. The GEA can be cannulated using catheters

designed for abdominal vascular intervention, e.g. a Cobra catheter [4]. The coeliac trunk is accessed from the abdominal aorta in the direction of the common hepatic artery (the other branch being the splenic artery) (Figure 5.4). The gastroduodenal artery arises in an inferior direction and gives off the pancreatico-duodenal branch beyond which it becomes the gastroepiploic artery, which passes through the diaphragm to reach the inferior wall of the heart (Figure 5.4). Insertional stenoses may require percutaneous treatment [5].

Guidewire Selection

Guidewires are required to cross the target lesion and to provide support for the delivery of balloons, stents and other devices whilst at the same time minimizing the risk of vessel trauma. A guidewire needs to be steerable, visible, flexible, lubricious and supportive. There is not a single wire that has the perfect combination of these characteristics for all situations. Variation in guidewire components have produced a wide range of wires. Wire selection depends on which characteristics are thought to optimally facilitate angioplasty for a given clinical and angiographic scenario.

Guidewires consist of a central core of steel or nitinol that makes up the proximal section of the wire, approximately 145 cm long, and which tapers toward a distal tip, a distal section measuring 35 to 40 cm has a further outer covering of either a fine coil spring consisting of tungsten, platinum or stainless steel, or a polymer coating loaded with a material such as tungsten to improve radiopacity, and the tip often has a lubricious coating that is

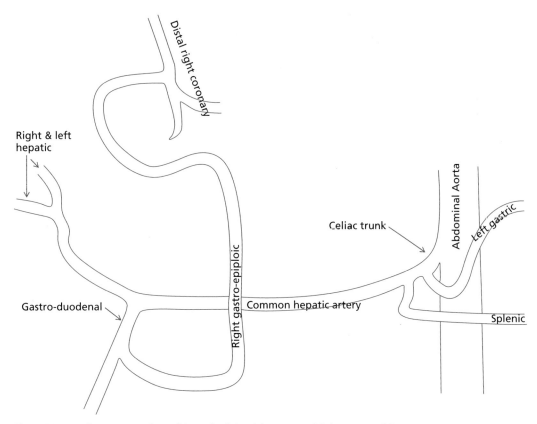

Figure 5.4. Vascular anatomy of a pedicle graft of the right gastro-epiploic artery to right coronary artery.

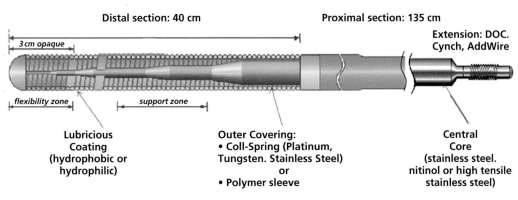

Figure 5.5. Components of guidewire design.

either hydrophobic or hydrophilic e.g. silicone or PTFE (Figure 5.5). Using steel as core material improves the steerability and torque control, but steel wires can be deformed by tortuosity and cannot be reshaped. A nitinol core also offers excellent torque control, but the wire will retain its shape much better and can be reshaped if deformed. Increasing the core diameter increases shaft

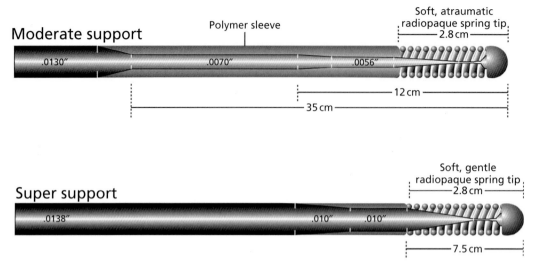

Figure 5.6. Support can be increased by increasing core diameter.

support (Figure 5.6). There is often a short transition zone between the tapered distal segment whereas some wires have a very gradually tapering central core, which tends to track better around tortuosities and prolapse less when there is extreme angulation (Figure 5.6). Features of the functional design of guidewires are listed in Table 5.4. Guidewires can be classified into general purpose and dedicated wires (Table 5.5).

Workhorse wires all have soft and gentle tips but the amount of shaft support may vary (Table 5.6). The guidewire may be exchanged for one with greater shaft support if required, or more frequently a buddy wire may be used because access to the true lumen is always maintained and the buddy wire can facilitate equipment passage by acting as an additional "rail".

Although some wires have preshaped tips the tip stiffness may be increased by heating during the preshaping process and the angle may not match the anatomy. As a result preshaping rarely offers an advantage except perhaps for polymer coated wires, which can be difficult to shape. When shaping the tip of a wire the primary curve should match the greatest angle to be negotiated, whereas the secondary curve is chosen to match the size of the vessel (Figure 5.7).

Hydrophilic wires are not recommended as a first choice for general purpose use, because the highly lubricious tip can easily slip beneath plaque and create a dissection during insertion, have a higher tendency to migrate distally and increase the risk of perforation, give less tactile feedback and have lower visibility. Highly tortuous vessels may require a flexible lubricious wire in the first instance (e.g. BMW, WhisperMS, Choice floppy), which can then be exchanged via an over the wire (OTW) balloon for a more supportive wire (e.g. Galeo HS, Choice extra support, Mailman, Ironman, Grand Slam, Platinum Plus).

The handling characteristics of different wires vary substantially and even the same wire may have a very different "feel" under different circumstances, e.g. diffuse disease with heavy calcification or angulation, etc. Inexperienced first operators may progress more confidently by becoming familiar with one workhorse wire used for most cases. It does not matter which method is used to shape the wire tip (curling over the side of the introducer needle or bending out of introducer needle tip), provided that it is done without damaging the wire. Nitinol wires are more forgiving and can be reshaped. An important principle is never to push when the wire bends, but rather to withdraw and rotate before gently readvancing it. Learning how to exchange a wire using OTW balloons/microcatheters is an essential skill before tackling complex lesions. More complex angioplasty will

Table 5.4. The selection of a guidewire depends on the characteristics required to deal with lesion complexity or particular vessel characteristics. The characteristics of guidewires can be altered by modifying specific components during the production process.

Flexibility	Flexible wires may better negotiate severe tortuosity or angulation without deformation	Shaft core material (nitinol offers greater flexibility and shape retention), core thickness (thinner core = more flexible)
Support	Improved equipment delivery when hampered by angulation, tortuosity, lesion severity, calcification	Shaft core material, core thickness
Steerability is a function of		
– torque transmission	1:1 transmission of torque to the tip is the ideal	Core materials are chosen for having good torque transmission, which is also improved by a thicker core with more gradual distal taper
—tip shape ability	Importance increases as lesion complexity increases	Nitinol is more difficult to shape, but can be reshaped; steel is easier to shape but can be ruined by being deformed
Lubricity	can ease wire passage in tight, calcified, severely tortuous lesions	tip or distal segment coating with silicon, hydrophilic coating or polymer coating: So called "plastic jacketed" wires are the most lubricious but also the most dangerous; when combined with a stiff tip long dissections can be inadvertently created —hydrophilic requires water for activation —hydrophobic does not require water for activation- allows feed-back from distal tip so that excessive friction when creating a subintimal dissection or going below stent struts can be detected
Tendency to prolapse	Can be important when negotiating angles >75 degrees	A gradually tapering core with a smooth transition towards the tip improves support and tracking around bends; abrupt tapers and floppy cores are more likely to prolapse
Visibility	The level of visibility becomes more important in obese patients or when angled working views are required	Lubricious polymer coated nitinol wires can be difficult to see, platinum, steel or tungsten markers at distal tip.
Tactile Feedback	Provides the operator with essential non-visual information, allows "palpation" of the lesion at the distal wire tip	hydrophylic wires provide poor tactile feedback, hydrophobic wires provide more feedback
Tip stiffness	A soft gentle tip is essential for all "workhorse" wires; to reduce the risk of vessel trauma, stiffer tips are required for dedicated CTO wires	More gradual distal taper, distal core material e.g. high tensile steel

Table 5.5. A classification of guidewires.

Workhorse	Dedicated	
	Problem	Proposed Solution
High Torque Floppy ACS	Tortuosity/calcification:	Polymer coated e.g. Faßdasher
Runthrough Terumo	Tortuousity (stent delivery	High support e.g. Grand Slam
ATW Cordis	after crossing)	
BMW Universal Guidant/Abbott	CTO	Stiffer tip: Cross-It, Persuader, Miracle,
		Confianza (Conquest), CrossWire, Shinobi
Prowater (Renato) Asahi/Abbott		Active Steer (Steer-It)
Galeo Flex Biotronik	Angulation	Highly flexible wires: Whisper
		RotaWire (0.09″, uncoated)
	Calcific/resistant lesions	Pressure wire (Radi, Certus)
	Functional assessment required	Optical coherence tomography wire
	Coronary imaging	Laser wire
	Resistant lesion	Filter wire (Angioguard)
	Distal protection	

Table 5.6. Hierarchies of increasing shaft support and tip stiffness.

Shaft support	Tip stiffness
Faßdasher (0.010″)	Soft
Choice PT	Intermediate
ATW Cordis	Standard
Pilot	Pilot 50
Prowater (Renato)	Crossit/Pilot 100
Runthrough	Crossit/Pilot 200
BMW Universal	Crossit 400
BMW	Miracle 3
Choice PT Support	Miracle 4.5
Galeo MJ	Miracle 6.0
Ironman	Miracle 12
Mailman	
Platinum Plus	
"Grand Slam" Asahi	

also provide an opportunity to gain familiarity with an expanded range of wires.

Dedicated wires for treating chronic total occlusions have stiffer tips. Tip stiffness is measured in grams of forward pressure required to flex the tip. Specialty wires are listed in Table 5.5 and Table 5.6 and will be discussed in other chapters.

Balloon Catheters

Balloon catheters were the key element once lumen enlargement was only achieved with balloon dilatation. At that time a correct choice of balloon diameter and length, compliance, pressure and duration of inflation were the key ingredients of a successful PCI and reflected the experience and quality of individual operators. The paradigm of today's PCI is a quick and easy direct stent deployment with no pre- or post-dilatation and a good result immediately achieved [6]. Unfortunately, this approach is applicable and successful only in a minority of cases and balloons are still used for predilation, stent delivery and postdilation. They also have additional useful applications, not directly concerning dilatation at the site of the lesion such as estimation of lesion size and length for the selection of stents, exchange after wire crossing (OTW), holding of the guiding in place when greater support is required (anchor balloon in side-branches or proximal-distal to the lesion in the main vessel). A balloon catheter consists from proximal to distal of a hub, a proximal shaft, a distal shaft. It has a cylindrical body with proximal and distal conical tapers and a distal tip (Figure 5.8). Balloon catheters are dual lumen with separate ports for the guidewire and balloon inflation.

Monorail or OTW?: The development of Monorail balloons by Tassilo Bonzel has followed and simplified the introduction from John Simpson of balloons with movable wires, a revolution from the first fixed wire balloons used by Gruentzig in the early days of angioplasty [7]. Fixed wire balloons remained used for some time because the absence of a second lumen for the guidewire

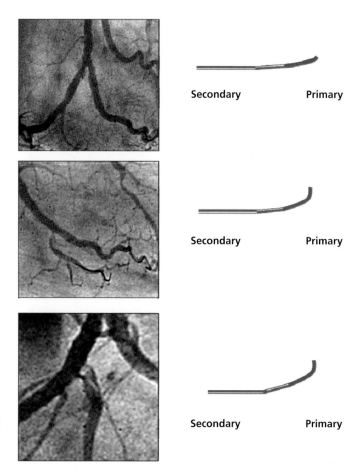

Figure 5.7. The primary curve is shaped to fit the tightest angle to be wired and the secondary curve to reflect vessel size.

allowed smaller profiles and smooth transition between wire and balloon. The principle of the Monorail technique is that the wire lumen is limited to a short segment (20 to 30 cm) at the distal tip which allows the rapid exchange of balloons with no need of long wires or wire extensions. The shaft of the catheter only contains a lumen for balloon inflation and deflation, i.e. can be thinner and often consists of a reinforced hollow metal tube providing great pushability. Over the wire (OTW) balloons have a lumen for the guidewire extending along the length of the catheter, a feature very useful and sometimes essential for procedures requiring wire exchange without re-wiring a vessel e.g. treatment of chronic total occlusions, crossing of very tortuous lesions, advancement of poorly steerable wires (Rotawire).

The parameters considered first when selecting a balloon are balloon diameter, length and compli-ance, although occasionally the shaft diameter, shaft length and crossing profile are also important considerations (e.g. bifurcations techniques using 6 Fr guides, retrograde recanalization of CTO, very tall patients, extreme tortuosity in peripheral vessels).

Balloon diameter is normally selected to match the vessel size. For long tapering lesions (typically the mid-LAD loosing caliber as multiple septal and diagonal branches leave the vessel), the diam-eter of the vessel at the distal end of the segment to be dilated must be selected. Vessel size can be measured using quantitative coronary angiogra-phy (QCA) but this method may grossly underes-timate the true vessel size. Aiming for a balloon to reference vessel ratio of 0.9 to 1.1 is a good rule of thumb. Imaging techniques such as intravas-cular ultrasound (IVUS) can very accurately measure the lumen diameter as well as the vessel

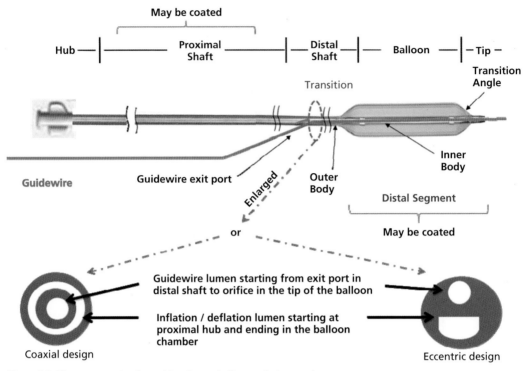

Figure 5.8. The components of a rapid exchange balloon catheter are shown.

diameter, which represents the maximum diameter which can be safely selected without risk of rupture. Especially in vessels with diffuse disease and gross positive remodeling the difference between balloon size chosen with angiography and IVUS can be as large as 1.0–1.5 mm. An appropriately sized balloon for postdilation is a critical step to achieve better expansion and apposition when the initial balloon deployment fails, despite the high pressures allowed by modern stent delivery balloons, to fully expand the stent.

Balloon length is selected depending on lesion and stent length. Especially after the introduction of drug eluting stents when the principle is to avoid injuring segments which will not be covered by stents, a situation known as geographical miss, smaller balloons tend to be used for predilation, just aiming to create a passage for stent insertion and exclude the presence of truly undilatable lesions [8]. Postdilatation balloons should be shorter than the stent and short balloons are recommended for postdilating resistant lesions.

The first angioplasty balloons were made of flexible PVC (polyvinyl chloride), a material characterized by great compliance. The following generations were made of cross-linked polyethylene, polyethylene terephthalate (PET), nylon, Pebax and polyurethane. Most modern balloons allow controlled limited expansion, burst resistance up to high pressure and have a low crossing profile. The tip style (tapering, length, flexibility) may vary substantially among different balloons, and is one of the factors contributing to a successful crossing (Figure 5.9). Compliant balloons show a linear increase in diameter with increasing inflation pressure whereas the diameter increase tends to plateau in semi- or non-compliant balloons until the rated burst pressure. More compliant balloons have a limited pressure range whereas non-compliant balloons have a limited diameter range and are useful for treating resistant lesions requiring high pressure inflation or post dilation. Semi-compliant balloons fall between these two extremes and tend to be multipurpose "workhorse" balloons. Familiarity with the compliance charts of

3.0 x 20 mm Test Length	Balloon Junction (prox. seal OD)	Proximal Shoulder (2/3)	Distal Profile (1 mm)	Tip seal (xing profile)	Tip Entry Profile	Tip I.D.
CrossSail	0.037″	0.031″	0.031″	0.024″	0.019″	0.0155″
Maverick	0.038″	0.034″	0.033″	0.026″	0.018″	0.0156″

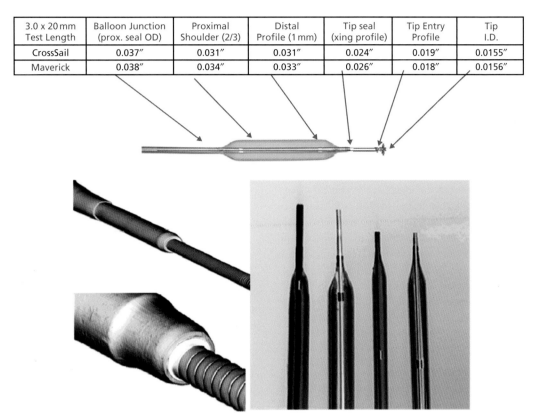

Figure 5.9. Distal tip styles and components contributing to the crossing profile of balloon catheters.

balloons is necessary to reduce the risk of trauma to the healthy vessel or of exceeding the vessel elasticity and induce dramatic vessel ruptures. Terms encountered on these charts include the following: Nominal, i.e. the pressure at which the balloon reaches its nominal diameter (diameter on the label); Rated burst pressure, i.e. the pressure below which in vitro testing has shown that 99.9% of the balloons will not burst with 95% confidence; Mean burst pressure, i.e. the mathematical mean pressure at which a balloon bursts. Wall stress within a cylindrical balloon can be represented by the following equations:

$$\sigma_{radial} = pd/2t$$

$$\sigma_{axial} = pd/4t$$

where σ_{radial} = radial stress, σ_{axial} = axial or longitudinal stress, p = pressure, d = diameter, t = wall thickness. It can be seen that wall stress is linearly proportional to diameter which means that higher

dilation pressure is possible with smaller diameter balloons. Furthermore axial stress is half of radial stress which means that balloon rupture is usually longitudinal rather than circumferential and therefore less likely to result in vessel trauma.

Specialty balloons include cutting balloons for treatment of instent restenosis and calcific lesions. The Angiosculpt in a non-compliant balloon with three nitinol wires or elements spiraling from the tip to the shaft transition. The function and application is similar to a cutting balloon.

Balloons have proximal and distal radiopaque markers to allow positioning (one central marker for some small diameter balloons). Rewrap refers to the ability of the balloon to regain its original folded state following deflation. Deflation and rewrapping can take time when large and long balloons are used. Rewrapping is essential to allow safe withdrawal of the balloon into the catheter. Stent deployment balloons tend to rewrap less well, have more variable expansion characteristics and should ideally not be used for postdilation. Balloon catheters may also be used to augment support when treating complex lesions.

Support

A detailed knowledge of the angioplasty equipment allows it to be used innovatively on occasions when required to complete a case successfully, often in order to increase support sufficiently to allow device delivery to the target in the context of tortuousity, calcification and or diffuse disease. The components of the support or backup system usually are the guide catheter, guidewire(s) and balloon(s) in the target artery. The components may be changed individually or in combination as demanded by the difficulties that are encountered. Hybrid strategies using more complex wire and or balloon based techniques may be required to overcome more challenging anatomy.

Guide Catheter Support

The role of shape selection is discussed in the relevant section. Guide catheter support may be either passive i.e. provided by a large diameter catheter positioned optimally in the coronary ostium or active i.e. provided by judiciously advancing a small diameter catheter to deeply intubate an epicardial artery.

Passive Support

Although 6 Fr guide catheters are successfully used for most cases of angioplasty, larger catheters may be required when complex lesions are tackled e.g. bifurcation stenting or when a parallel wire technique is required during CTO disobliteration (see section on guide catheter selection) [9] (Figure 5.10).

Active Support

Small ≤6 Fr guide catheters can be advanced over the guidewire and balloon catheter shaft to subselectively engage the proximal or mid segment of the artery (Figure 5.10). This technique is also referred to active engagement or "deep throating" of the guide catheter. The risk of damage to the artery may be minimized by ensuring that the catheter is advanced coaxially to a balloon already inside the vessel. Stabilization of the system whilst advancing the guide may sometimes be required and may be achieved by inflating a balloon within the artery. When considering the use of active support it is important to bear in mind that deep engagement of large arteries may cause profound ischemia. The use of side holes may not prevent and may even delay detection of catheter induced ischemia. A further risk is that of air embolism following aspiration through the Y-connector whilst the back pressure in the guide catheter is reduced due to damping inside the artery. Despite

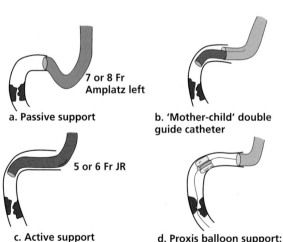

a. Passive support

b. 'Mother-child' double guide catheter

c. Active support

d. **Proxis balloon support:** Proximal balloon inflation arrests antegrade flow. The central lumen facilitates passage of guidewire and stent balloon to treat the target lesion

Figure 5.10. Approaches to increase guide catheter support for treating complex lesions.

these risks, for a skilled operator capable of rapid work active support offers an efficient solution in the majority of cases.

Hybrid Support

Several additional strategies have now been described based on the concept of inserting an additional device, wire, balloon or other catheter specifically to augment support when active and or passive support of the guide catheter proves insufficient (Figure 5.11).

Wire Support

The buddy wire technique, i.e. passage of a second or third wire distal to the lesion is a commonly used strategy for crossing difficult lesions with a balloon or a stent [10, 11]. The additional wire provides a rail that facilitates advancement across calcification, tortuosity or recently deployed stents. It facilitates active engagement of the guide catheter and may straighten tortuosity when a supportive wire is used. This technique is also the first essential step for the distal "anchor balloon" technique.

Although it may at first appear to be counterintuitive, advancing an additional wire into a branch that lies proximal to the target lesion may increase support only slightly, but sufficiently to allow passage of a balloon, stent or additional wire along the first wire into the tortuous distal vessel [12] (Figure 5.11). The risks of deep engagement or the delays and potential difficulties of upgrading the guide catheter may then be avoided. A floppy steerable wire may advance easily and may be exchanged using an OTW catheter for a wire with a supportive shaft but soft flexible tip. There is a risk of perforation of small branches but this usually occurs when a stiff hydrophilic wire is used. The techniques for support discussed to far will provide enough support for the majority of cases. Occasionally if support from the guide and an additional wire still proves insufficient an anchor balloon may be considered either proximal or distal to the target lesion.

Anchor Balloon Technique

Inflation of an adequately sized balloon at low pressure (3–6 atmospheres) in a proximal branch may tremendously augment support by anchoring the guide catheter to the branch [13] (Figure 5.11). Low inflation pressures are essential to reduce the

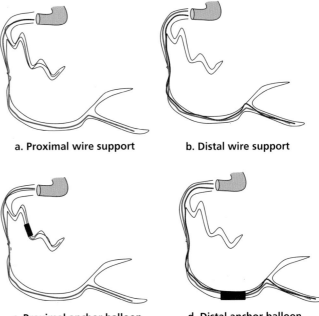

a. Proximal wire support   **b. Distal wire support**

c. Proximal anchor balloon support   **d. Distal anchor balloon support**

Figure 5.11. "Intraluminal" hybrid support techniques that may be used to substantially augment guide catheter support when treating complex lesions.

risk of dissection or damage to a small right ventricular branch or diagonal/marginal branch. In these branches, ischemia due to prolonged inflation is well tolerated. The technique is mostly used in treating CTO and requires a large guide catheter. Anticipation of potential damage or dislodgement of the stent caused by over-enthusiastic pushing may allow a timely change to a different strategy.

Another strategy that can be tried when a buddy wire does not resolve problems in tracking a stent to a target lesion due to turtuosity or calcification of the proximal segment, is to advance over the buddy wire a balloon optimally sized to match the diameter of the distal vessel (Figure 5.11). The balloon is positioned distal to the lesion and inflated at low pressure allowing enough space for the stent to be fully advanced across the target stenosis,. It is imperative to remember that the distal anchoring balloon must be deflated and removed before the stent is deployed. In addition to providing extra support, the shaft of the distal balloon also acts as a rail that may facilitate stent advancement. The operator needs to be experienced enough to anticipate when the force required may detach the stent from the balloon. Additional strategies can then be considered such as the need for better lesion preparation or the insertion of a sub-selectively engaged guiding catheter around the most tortuous segment, using the guide already in place or a 5 in 6/7 strategy as outlined in the next section (Figure 5.10).

Adjunctive Techniques
Double Coaxial Guiding Catheter Technique (Also Known as Mother-Child)

By placing one guide catheter inside another the advantages of the passive support provided by the large guide catheter are combined with the ability to actively engage the smaller catheter into the target vessel [14] (Figure 5.10).

Compatibility of different guide catheter lengths and diameter is a limiting factor. Mainly a 6 French 110 cm long "child" GC is combined within an 85/90 cm 7/8 French "mother" GC. A greater difference between the lengths of the "mother" and "child" GC, however, enables more flexibility because it permits further advancement of the daughter catheter into the artery.

The "mother" GC shape is selected to cannulate the ostium of the target vessel and is inserted first. In contrast, a straight "child" GC and with a soft atraumatic tip is desirable. If an unusual shape is required for the "mother" catheter that is not available in a short length, the solution is to cut the distal end of a 100 cm guiding catheter of the selected shape and insert within it a smaller valved sheath. Leakage due to an insufficiently tight seal may affect the quality of contrast injections. A further risk is the potential for air trapping within the sheath and subsequent inadvertent intracoronary air embolism.

This as an advanced technique that has been used for treating CTO, but may very occasionally also be useful in other situations where a very high level of backup may be required, e.g. extreme coronary tortuosity often combined with calcification. It may also be useful for example when a 7 or 8 French guide is too large to engage ostial disease or a critically diseased vessel and other situations where deep engagement of the guide is undesirable. The smaller guide can then be engaged into the vessel ostium, whereas the larger guide adds passive backup to the system. Relative adjustments of the positions of the two guide tips may help to achieve optimal orientation of the tip of the "daughter" catheter. When using this technique care has to be taken not to damage the proximal arterial segment.

Conclusion

A good operator will have a thorough knowledge of the advantages and limitations of each specific piece of equipment, familiarity with their specific characteristics and modalities of use, and a preparedness to change to an alternative strategy or alternative strategies if required.

References

1. Hamon M, Sabatier R, Zhao Q, *et al.* Mini-invasive strategy in acute coronary syndromes: direct coronary stenting using 5 Fr guiding catheters and transradial approach. Catheter Cardiovasc Interv 2002; **55**(3): 340–343.

2. De Bruyne B, Stockbroeckx J, Demoor D, *et al.* Role of side holes in guide catheters: observations on coronary pressure and flow. Cathet Cardiovasc Diagn 1994; **33**(2): 145–152.

3. Pym J, Brown P, Pearson M, *et al.* Right gastroepiploic-to-coronary artery bypass. The first decade of use. Circulation 1995; **92**(9 Suppl): II45–49.

4. Isshiki T, Yamaguchi T, Nakamura M, *et al.* Postoperative angiographic evaluation of gastroepiploic artery grafts: technical considerations and short-term patency. Cathet Cardiovasc Diagn 1990; **21**(4): 233–238.

5. Alam M, Safi AM, Mandawat MK, *et al.* Successful percutaneous stenting of a right gastroepiploic coronary bypass graft using monorail delivery system: a case report. Catheter Cardiovasc Interv 2000; **49**(2): 197–199.

6. Martinez-Elbal L, Ruiz-Nodar JM, Zueco J, *et al.* Direct coronary stenting versus stenting with balloon predilation: immediate and follow-up results of a multicentre, prospective, randomized study. The DISCO trial. DIrect Stenting of Coronary Arteries. Eur Heart J 2002; **23**(8): 633–640.

7. Bonzel T, Wollschläger H, Kasper W, *et al.*, The sliding rail system (monorail): description of a new technique for intravascular instrumentation and its application to coronary angioplasty. Z Kardiol 1987; **76 Suppl 6**: 119–122.

8. Blackman DJ, Porto I, Shirodaria C, *et al.* Usefulness of high-pressure post-dilatation to optimize deployment of drug-eluting stents for the treatment of diffuse in-stent coronary restenosis. Am J Cardiol 2004; **94**(7): 922–925.

9. Colombo A, Mikhail GW, Michev I, *et al.* Treating chronic total occlusions using subintimal tracking and reentry: the STAR technique. Catheter Cardiovasc Interv 2005; **64**(4): 407–411; discussion 412.

10. Burzotta F, Trani C, Mazzari MA, *et al.* Use of a second buddy wire during percutaneous coronary interventions: a simple solution for some challenging situations. J Invasive Cardiol 2005; **17**(3): 171–174.

11. Jafary FH. When one won't do it, use two-double "buddy" wiring to facilitate stent advancement across a highly calcified artery. Catheter Cardiovasc Interv 2006; **67**(5): 721–723.

12. Hamood H, Makhoul N, Grenadir E, *et al.* Anchor wire technique improves device deliverability during PCI of CTOs and other complex subsets. Acute Card Care 2006; **8**(3): 139–142.

13. Fujita S, Tamai H, Kyo E, *et al.* New technique for superior guiding catheter support during advancement of a balloon in coronary angioplasty: the anchor technique. Catheter Cardiovasc Interv 2003; **59**(4): 482–488.

14. Takahashi S, Saito S, Tanaka S, *et al.* New method to increase a backup support of a 6 French guiding coronary catheter. Catheter Cardiovasc Interv 2004; **63**(4): 452–456.

CHAPTER 6

Physiologic Assessment in the Cardiac Catheterization Laboratory

Narbeh Melikian[1], & Martyn R. Thomas[2]

[1] King's College London School of Medicine and King's College Hospital Foundation Trust, London, UK
[2] St Thomas' Hospital, London, UK

Coronary physiological parameters form an integral part of the clinical decision making process in the cardiac catheterization laboratory. Over the past two decades our understanding of the relationship between coronary arterial pressure and flow has paved the way for the validation of a number of physiological indices such as fractional flow reserve (FFR), coronary flow reserve (CFR) and the index of myocardial resistance (IMR), which have important clinical as well as research applications [1–3].

Arguably the most important clinical contribution of coronary physiology is its role in determining the physiological significance of epicardial coronary artery disease (CAD). Although, selective coronary angiography is accepted as the gold standard for determining the presence and extent of epicardial CAD, it has well recognized limitations. These included the inability to simultaneously combine anatomical and physiological data and a mismatch between angiographic two-dimensional images and actual levels of coronary stenosis.

Physiological indices (such as CFR and IMR) can also be used to assess coronary microvascular function. There is increasing evidence to suggest

Interventional Cardiology, First Edition. Edited by
Carlo Di Mario, George D. Dangas, Peter Barlis.
© 2010 Blackwell Publishing Ltd. Published 2010 by
Blackwell Publishing Ltd.

that assessment of coronary microvascular function may provide important information on diagnosis, risk stratification and prognosis of cardiac patients [4]. Furthermore, the ability to determine and monitor changes in the state of the coronary microcirculation has important research applications in investigating the cardiac influence of novel pharmacological agents and cardiovascular (CV) risk factors.

This chapter reviews the basic principles of coronary physiology and their clinical application in the cardiac catheterization laboratory.

Fundamentals of Coronary Pressure and Flow

Our understanding of the principles that govern the association between pressure and flow in the coronary circulation provides the basis from which clinically applicable coronary physiological indices have developed.

Epicardial vessel stenosis is known to increase conduit vessel resistance, which in turn reduces myocardial blood flow. In order to compensate for changes in myocardial blood flow, microvascular resistance vessels dilate to maintain regional basal blood flow at a level appropriate for concurrent myocardial oxygen demand. Under these conditions any increase in myocardial oxygen demand and/or a hyperemic stimulus will produce a smaller than expected incremental increase in post-stenotic coronary flow as compared to the coronary flow that would in theory be elicited in the same artery (or another myocardial region) without a stenosis (a diminished coronary flow velocity reserve; CVR) [2]. This principle is often exploited in the catheterization laboratory to assess CFR and relative CFR (rCFR).

In addition, an epicardial stenosis may also lead to a fall in distal artery pressure. This occurs in response to loss of kinetic (flow) energy to viscous friction, turbulence and flow separation across the epicardial stenosis. The reduction in distal arterial pressure results in a pressure differential/gradient between the driving aortic pressure and the post-stenotic coronary pressure [2]. As demonstrated in Figure 6.1, there is a curvilinear relationship between the loss of distal arterial pressure and flow rate [2]. Changes in coronary pressure gradient are used to assess FFR.

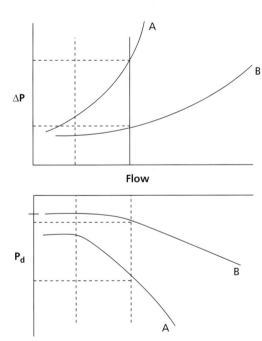

Figure 6.1. The relationship between coronary pressure and flow for two stenosis of the same angiographic severity (A and B). The top panel represents pressure gradient (ΔP) versus coronary flow and the bottom panel absolute distal coronary pressure (Pd) versus coronary flow. Increasing flow produces a marked reduction of Pd and an increase in ΔP. Loss of Pd can lead to myocardial ischemia. Reproduced from Kern [2].

Indices to Assess Hemodynamic Significance of Epicardial Vessel Stenosis

CFR and FFR are the two main indices available for routine assessment of epicardial vessel stenosis.

CFR and Relative CFR

At rest, myocardial blood flow remains normal until coronary artery stenosis exceeds 85% of the epicardial vessel cross sectional area. In contrast under conditions of maximal hyperemia myocardial blood falls with significantly lower levels of stenosis (around 50%) [5]. On the basis of these observations Gould *et al.* introduced the concept of CFR as an index to determine changes in the level of myocardial blood flow in the context of an epicardial stenosis [5]. *CFR is derived from the ratio of steady state maximal hyperemic flow to resting flow in a given artery* [1,2,6]. A comparison of CFR values with non-invasive functional imaging techniques has shown that a CFR <2.0 in a given artery correlates strongly with ischemia in the myocardial territory supplied by that artery [6,7].

However, clinical application of CFR in order to examine the physiological significance of an epicardial vessel stenosis has multiple limitations. As outlined, CFR is derived from the ratio of hyperemic to baseline myocardial blood flow. Myocardial blood flow can be influenced by changes in epicardial vessel stenosis, microvascular (resistance vessel) function or a combination of both [1–3]. The inability to differentiate between the relative contribution of the epicardial and microvascular compartments to myocardial blood flow is a major limitation of CFR as a clinical tool for interrogation of an epicardial stenosis.

To overcome the two-compartment limitation of CFR, the concept of relative CFR (rCFR) has been developed. rCFR attempts to reduce the influence of confounders on the CFR value by indexing the flow reserve of the interrogated vessel to an adjacent reference "normal"/unobstructed vessel [6]. *Relative CFR (rCFR) is defined as the ratio of maximal flow in an artery with a stenosis to flow in an adjacent "normal"/unobstructed artery.* The proposed normal range for rCFR is between 0.65 to 1.0 [3,6].

Despite the conceptual advantages of rCFR for assessment of epicardial vessel stenosis, there remain two major limitations. To assess rCFR, each patient must have at least one normal epicardial vessel. As a result rCFR cannot be used in patients with 3-vessel CAD who have no suitable reference vessel. In addition the concept of rCFR is based on the assumption that microvascular function is uniformly distributed throughout the myocardium.

In view of their multiple limitations, CFR and rCFR are rarely used for routine clinical assessment of epicardial vessel stenosis. However, as outlined later, CFR may have clinical applications for assessment of microvascular function in the context of "normal"/unobstructed coronary vessels.

Clinical Technique for Assessment of CFR/rCFR

A commercially available intra-coronary Doppler wire is commonly used to estimate coronary blood flow and hence derive CFR/rCFR. This method is based on the principle that in a vessel with a constant surface area flow is known to be directly proportional to velocity. Therefore, CFR is derived from the ratio of hyperemic to baseline coronary blood flow velocity.

A Doppler guidewire is introduced into the study artery under fluoroscopic guidance through a standard guiding catheter. Blood velocity is measured through a microscopic Doppler crystal at the tip of the Doppler guidewire, which is positioned distal to the epicardial vessel stenosis. Depending on the local set up the guide wire interfaces with either its dedicated interface and/or the hemodynamic monitoring equipment in the cardiac catheterization laboratory to produce real-time continuous Doppler traces. CFR is derived from the ratio of the average peak (blood flow) velocity (APV, calculated on line from continuous spectral traces) at baseline and maximal hyperemia (Figure 6.2) [6,8]. Although, this method for assessing CFR/rCFR is widely adopted it may at times be technically challenging to obtain high quality and readily reproducible spectral traces.

Induction of Maximal Hyperemia

A non-specific agonist such as adenosine or papaverine is often used to induce maximal hyper-

emia (see assessment of microvascular function). Adenosine can be administered either as an intra-coronary bolus or as a weight adjusted infusion of via a central vein. Papaverine is administered as a single intra-coronary bolus [9].

FFR

FFR is defined as the maximum myocardial blood flow in the presence of an epicardial stenosis divided by the theoretical maximum flow in the absence of a stenosis (maximum flow when the vessel is normal) in given artery [1–3,10]. In the cardiac catheterization laboratory, FFR is calculated from the ratio of distal (post-stenotic pressure) (Pd) to proximal (Pa) coronary pressure at maximal hyperemia. The derivation of FFR from Pd:Pa ratio is summarized in Figure 6.3 [1,2]. Currently FFR is the gold standard for investigating the hemodynamic significance of an epicardial vessel stenosis.

A cut-off FFR value of <0.75 across an epicardial stenosis is accepted to be indicative of myocardial ischemia [1,2]. Multiple clinical studies have demonstrated a close correlation between FFR <0.75 and different non-invasive indices of reversible myocardial ischemia [6,10,11]. Pijls *et al.* compared FFR with quantitative coronary angiography (QCA) and three different functional tests of myocardial ischemia (bicycle exercise test, thallium scintigraphy and dobutamine stress echocardiography) in patients with chest discomfort and moderate epicardial vessel stenosis (Figure 6.4) [11]. In this study the sensitivity of FFR to identify reversible ischemia was 88%, the specificity 100%, positive predictive value 100% and negative predictive value 88%. FFR is now routinely used as part of the diagnostic angiographic work-up of patients with chest pain and angiographically mild/moderate coronary stenosis to determine the need for revascularization.

As an index for assessment of epicardial vessel stenosis, FFR has multiple advantages in comparison to CFR. Unlike CFR, which cannot discriminate between epicardial disease, microvascular disease or a combination of both, FFR is a specific index for epicardial stenosis [1,6,10]. Therefore, it provides practical and clinically applicable information as regards to myocardial ischemia and the clinical need for coronary revascularization. In addition FFR has an unequivocal normal value of

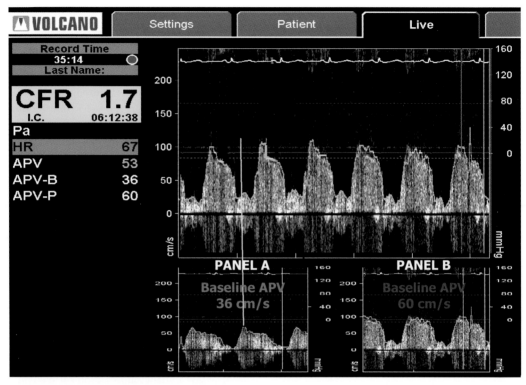

Figure 6.2. Intra-coronary Doppler spectral traces at baseline (PANEL A) and at maximal steady state hyperemia (PANEL B). Maximal steady state hyperemia was achieved by central infusion of adenosine (140 µg/kg/min). Considering in a vessel with a constant surface area flow is directly proportional to velocity, CFR is derived from the ratio of average peak velocity (APV) at maximal hyperemia to baseline (CFR = APV at maximal hyperemia: APV at baseline = 60:36 = 1.6).

Figure 6.3. Schematic illustration of the coronary artery and its dependent myocardial vascular bed. Myocardial blood flow equals the perfusion pressure across the myocardium, divided by myocardial resistance. Because at maximum arteriolar vasodilatation resistance is minimal and constant (R_{min}), maximum flow in the stenotic situation as a ratio to normal maximum flow equals the ratio of the myocardial perfusion pressure in the presence of the stenosis ($P_d - P_v$) to normal myocardial perfusion pressure ($P_a - P_v$), both measured after administration of a maximal hyperemic stimulus. In other words, FFR = ($P_d - P_v$)/($P_a - P_v$). Considering under most circumstances P_v is close to or equal to 0, FFR can therefore be assumed to be very close to P_d/P_a. In this example, FFR equals 0.70. (Reproduced from Pijls and De Bruyne [10].)

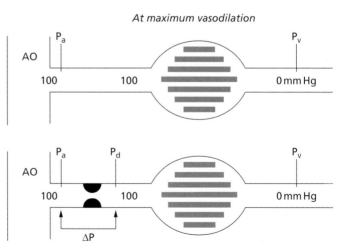

At maximum vasodilation

P_a = Proximal coronary driving pressure as measured in the aorta
P_d = Distal coronary pressure as measured from the distal pressure wire sensor
P_v = Myocardial venous pressure which is often near to or equal to 0 mmHg
AO = Aorta

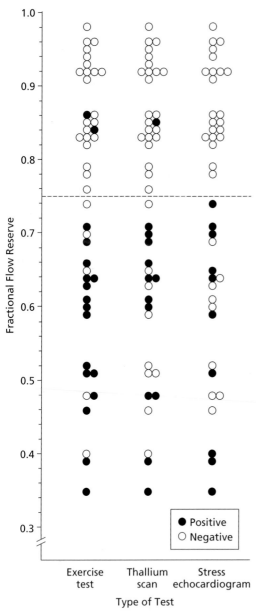

Figure 6.4. Relation between FFR and three different non-invasive functional tests of myocardial ischemia. Reproduced from Pijls and De Bruyne [11].

1.0 in every patient and coronary artery. FFR is also entirely independent of haemodynamic parameters (such as heart rate, blood pressure and contractility) and in comparison to CFR is highly reproducible. Furthermore, as there is no need for a normal reference artery, FFR can be applied in the context of multivessel disease [1,6,10].

The clinical utility of FFR as a robust decision making tool for revascularization in patients with intermediate angiographic stenosis has been validated. Bech *et al.* examined the 24-month outcome (DEFER Study) in three groups of patients with angiographic intermediate coronary stenosis undergoing percutaneous coronary intervention (PCI) [12]. FFR was measured in all stenosis. Patients with FFR was <0.75, underwent PCI as planned (reference group) and patients with FFR >0.75 were randomly assigned to medical therapy (deferral group) or PCI (performance group). At 12- and 24-month follow-up both event free survival and recurrent angina were similar in the deferral and performance groups (Figure 6.5) [12]. The low event rate in the deferral group was maintained at 5 year follow-up [13]. In addition, FFR value post-PCI also provides prognostic information. Adverse event rates at both 6 and 12 months after PCI correlate inversely with post-procedure FFR values (Figure 6.6) [14]. Clinical trials such as FAME (*F*ractional *F*low *R*eserve *V*ersus *A*ngiography for *M*ulti-vessel *E*valuation) have provided valuable information on the comparison of FFR- versus angiographic-guided PCI in patients with multi-vessel CAD, showing that limiting stent implantation only to functionally significant stenoses reduces immediate adverse events and cost with persistent improvement of outcome up to 2 years [15].

Clinical Technique for Assessment of FFR

A commercially available pressure/temperature sensor-tipped angioplasty guidewire (pressure wire) is used to asses FFR [6,10]. The pressure wire is introduced through a standard guiding catheter and positioned distal to the coronary stenosis being investigated under fluoroscopic guidance. Post-stenotic Pd is measured through a pressure sensor near the tip of the guidewire and Pa is measured through the tip of the guiding catheter. As for an intra-coronary Doppler wire, the pressure wire also interfaces with either its dedicated interface and/or the monitoring equipment in the catheterization laboratory. Pd and Pa traces and the corresponding FFR value are displayed continuously allowing live access to FFR during diagnostic and/or interventional procedures (Figure 6.7). FFR can be measured across a single stenosis by maintain-

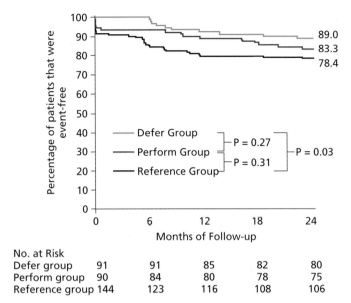

Figure 6.5. Kaplan-Meier survival curves for freedom from adverse cardiac events during 24 months of follow-up for three groups in the DEFER study. Reproduced from Bech, De Bruyne, Pijls *et al.* [12].

No. at Risk				
Defer group	91	91	85	82	80
Perform group	90	84	80	78	75
Reference group	144	123	116	108	106

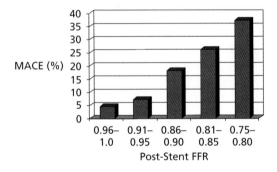

Figure 6.6. Clinical outcome of PCI and relationship to post-PCI FFR. A strong inverse correlation was present between FFR post-PCI and event rate at six months follow-up. Reproduced from Pijls, Klauss, Siebert *et al.* [14].

ing the position of the pressure wire. In addition by applying a gentle "pull back" on the pressure wire from a distal to proximal position in a given artery FFR values can be monitored along the entire length of a vessel. This will allow identification of hemodynamically significant stenosis in diffusely diseased epicardial vessel (Figure 6.8).

Induction of Maximal Hyperemia

As for assessment of CFR, adenosine or papaverine can be used to induce hyperemia. An intra-coronary bolus injection of adenosine is suitable for assessing FFR across a single discrete stenosis. However, when assessing FFR across a length of

vessel hyperemia needs to be maintained for longer than a few seconds and thus a weight adjusted central infusion of adenosine is required. An intra-coronary bolus of papaverine is suitable for assessment of both a discrete stenosis as well as coronary "pull back" (papaverine has a longer half-life in comparison to adenosine).

Assessment of Coronary Microvascular Function

There is increasing evidence that the functional state of the coronary microcirculation (resistance vessels) may play an important role in determining cardiac prognosis [4]. Therefore, apart from research applications clinical assessment of coronary microvascular function has an emerging role in diagnosis and risk stratification of patients.

Currently there is no technique which allows direct visualization and/or functional assessment of coronary microvascular function *in vivo* in humans. Vascular tone in resistance vessels determines coronary blood flow. In the catheterization laboratory this principle forms the basis for assessment of microvascular function where changes in epicardial vessel blood flow in response to a specific agonist are taken as an indirect marker of microvascular response. Comprehensive assessment of the coronary microcirculation requires specific interrogation of both the endothelium-

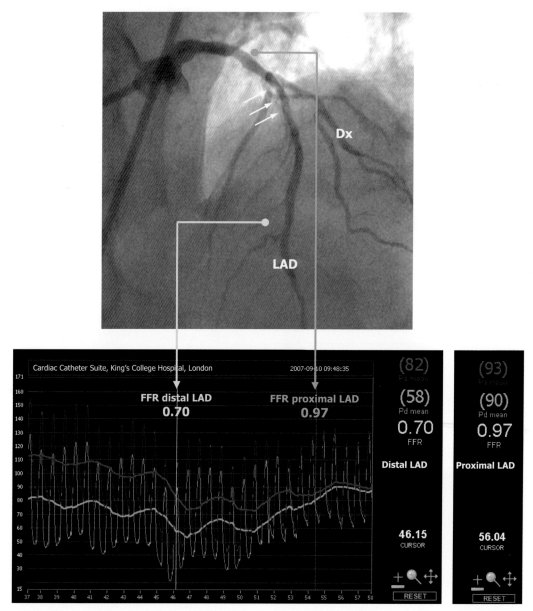

Figure 6.7. FFR to assess the physiological significance of an angiographic mild to moderate mid-LAD stenosis (white arrows) in a patient with stable angina. FFR distal to the stenosis is 0.70, indicating that the mid-LAD stenosis is hemodynamically significant and the patient would benefit from revascularization of the LAD (yellow arrow). Pullback of the wire through to the proximal LAD demonstrates an improvement in FFR (0.97) across the stenosis (green arrow). The red trace represents the continuous estimate of the mean proximal pressure and the green trace the continuous estimate of the distal pressure. The ratio between the two (FFR) can be calculated at any point. (LAD = left anterior descending artery, Dx = diagonal artery.)

PANEL A

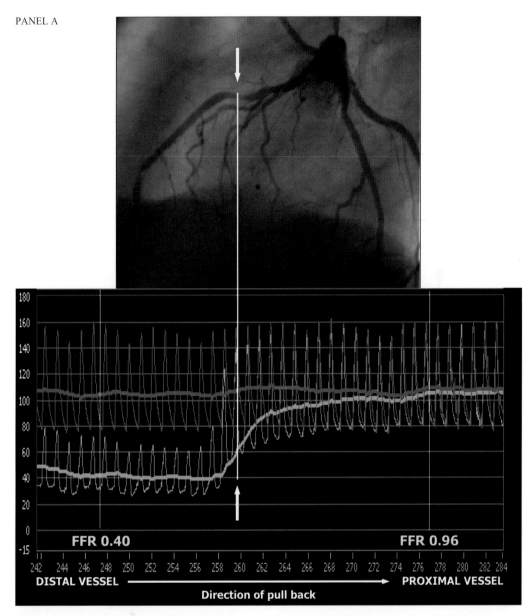

Figure 6.8. Proximal (in red) and distal (in green) pressure traces as derived from an intra-coronary pressure wire and changes in the pressures traces with "pull back" of the pressure wire along the length of two diffusely diseased LAD arteries in different patients with stable angina. In PANEL A there is a clear step-up in FFR value from 0.40 to 0.96 in the mid-LAD (white arrow) indicating the presence of a hemodynamically significant stenosis not detected in the angiographic image. In PANEL B there is a gradual change in pressure traces and no step-up in FFR indicating diffuse atherosclerotic changes in the LAD, which corresponds to the angiographic appearance of diffuse disease present in the vessel. FFR = fractional flow reserve, LAD = left anterior descending artery

PANEL B

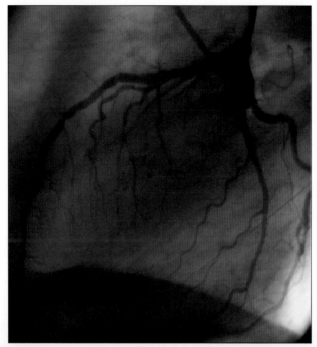

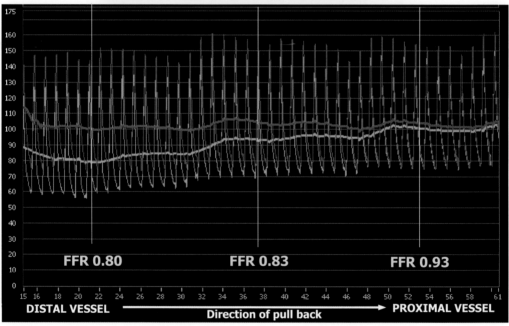

Figure 6.8. *Continued*

dependent (using agonists such as substance-P, acetylcholine, bradykinin) and -independent (using agonists such as nitrate, nitroprusside) microvascular responses [4,16]. The level of change in coronary blood flow in response to a given agonist is taken as marker of microvascular function and is inversely proportional to the functional state of the microcirculation.

Clinical Technique for Assessment of Coronary Microvascular Function

In a given vessel flow can be derived from the product of the cross sectional area of the vessel and the average velocity of the fluid within [flow = $(\pi D^2/4) \times (0.5 \times APV)$, where D is the diameter of the vessel and APV is the average peak velocity]. This principle forms the basis for measuring coronary flow when assessing coronary microvascular function in the catheterization laboratory. Quantitative coronary angiography (QCA)

is used to measure diameter of the study vessel (and hence derive coronary cross sectional area) and an intra-coronary Doppler guidewire to measure blood flow velocity.

An intra-coronary Doppler guidewire (as used for assessment of CFR) is introduced through a guiding catheter and positioned in the study vessel. Baseline AVP is recorded from continuous Doppler spectral traces. This is followed by a baseline selective coronary angiogram of the study vessel to measure vessel diameter using QCA. QCA is performed in a 2.5–5 mm length segment approximately 2.5 mm distal to the tip of the Doppler wire. Velocity and vessel diameter measurements are repeated a second time immediately after administration of an agonist (Figure 6.9). Coronary flow is calculated as outlined above at baseline and maximal flow and the percentage change in flow derived from these figures. Agonists are either given as a continuous infusion through a guiding

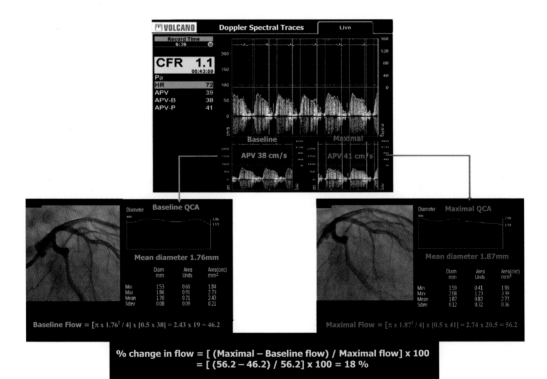

Figure 6.9. Intra-coronary Doppler spectral traces and corresponding QCA at baseline (Baseline) and at maximal blood flow (Maximal) after a 2 minute intra-coronary infusion of substance P to assess endothelium-dependent coronary microvascular function. Absolute coronary blood flow is calculated from the APV values and QCA-derived coronary artery diameter at baseline and maximal flow [coronary blood flow = $(\pi \times$ diameter^2/4$) \times (0.5 \times$ APV$)$]. The % change in coronary blood flow was obtained from baseline and maximal blood flow values.

catheter and/or infusion catheter using a high-speed infusion pump (such as substance P and acetylcholine) or as an intra-coronary bolus injection (such as nitrates).

However, detailed assessment of coronary microvascular function as outlined above is cumbersome and time consuming and thus is rarely undertaken outside research protocols. Instead in clinical practice two simple clinical indices, namely thermodilution CFR and IMR, are commonly used to assess coronary microvascular function.

Clinical Technique for Assessment of Thermodilution CFR

The transit time of an intra-coronary injectate, derived from a thermodilution curve, is inversely proportional to flow [2]. On this basis of this principle CFR can be derived from the ratio of the of mean transit time of an intra-coronary injectate at baseline and maximal hyperemia.

A commercially available combined pressure/temperature angioplasty guidewire, as used for assessment of FFR, is used to measure the transit time of a hand held 3–4 ml intra-coronary injectate of room temperature saline [17–19]. The shaft of this wire, on which the temperature-dependent electrical resistance is monitored, acts as a proximal thermistor. The distal pressure sensor also allows simultaneous high-fidelity temperature measurements. Software within the dedicated interface to which the pressure wire is attached formulates thermodilution curves and their corresponding transit times (in seconds) from changes in proximal and distal temperature profile within the pressure wire (Figure 6.10). Thermodilution curves are produced in triplicate at baseline and at maximal steady state hyperemia and mean transit times used to derive CFR. Hyperemia is induced by a weight adjusted infusion of adenosine or a bolus of intra-coronary papaverine. In addition the pressure wire concurrently displays Pd:Pa allowing simultaneous FFR measurements in conjunction with CFR (Figure 6.10). Assessment of CFR using thermodilution is technically less challenging and more reproducible in comparison to Doppler-derived CFR.

IMR

The two compartment nature of the CFR value and its exposure to influence by haemodynamic factors are two major limitations of this index. IMR is a novel specific index of microvascular function, which unlike CFR is independent of the influences of the epicardial vessel and/or haemodynamic parameters [20,21]. *IMR measures the resistance of coronary microvascular vessels and is derived from the ratio of Pd and flow at maximal hyperemia* [20]. Unlike CFR, there is currently no accepted cut-off value to distinguish between normal and abnormal IMR. As for the assessment of FFR and thermodilution-CFR a commercially available, combined, pressure/temperature guide wire is used to assess IMR [20,21]. The ability to derive all three indices simultaneously with a single coronary instrumentation using the pressure wire is important as it provides a simple, quick and reproducible method to comprehensively assess the functional status of the epicardial and microvascular compartments simultaneously.

Clinical Technique for Assessment of IMR

A combined intra-coronary pressure/temperature guidewire is once again used for assessment of IMR and positioned in the study vessel as for assessment of CFR/FFR. Pd is recorded from the pressure transducer near the tip of the wire and coronary flow is assessed using the principles of thermodilution (see above) in response to a hand-held, brisk, 3 ml injection of room temperature saline. Both measurements are recorded at maximal steady state hyperemia and displayed on a dedicated interface. IMR as outlined is derived from the ratio of the Pd and distal coronary flow (which is inversely proportional to the mean transit time of the intra-coronary injectate and saline) (Figure 6.11). As for thermodilution-CFR measurements are performed in triplicate. A weight adjusted intra-coronary in fusion of adenosine and/or bolus intra-coronary injection of papaverine is used to induce maximal steady state hyperemia.

Numerous alternative techniques for the assessment of coronary microvascular function based on direct volumetric coronary blood flow measurements [22] and invasive arterial wave analysis [23] have also been proposed. However, the clinical applicability of these techniques remains unclear.

Non-specific agents such as adenosine and papaverine are commonly used to induce maximal

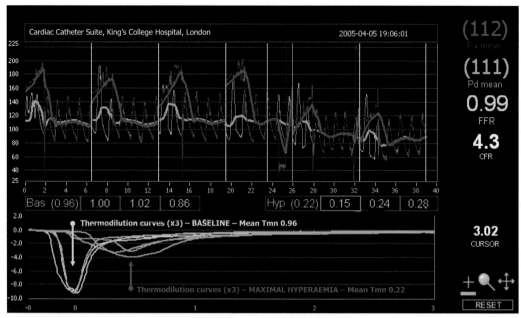

Bas = mean baseline Tmn, Hyp = mean hyperaemic Tmn

Figure 6.10. Thermodilution curves and corresponding transit times (Tmn) (in triplicate) of a hand held brisk intra-coronary injection of 3 ml room temperature saline as measured by a commercially available combined pressure/temperature guide wire. CFR is calculated from the ratio of mean baseline Tmn to mean steady state hyperemic Tmn [CFR = Tmn baseline/Tmn hyperemia = 0.96/0.22 = 4.5]. Pa (in red) and Pd (in green) are also displayed continuously at baseline and maximal hyperemia. FFR is calculated from the ratio of mean Pd to Pa [FFR = Pd/Pa = 111/112 = 0.99].

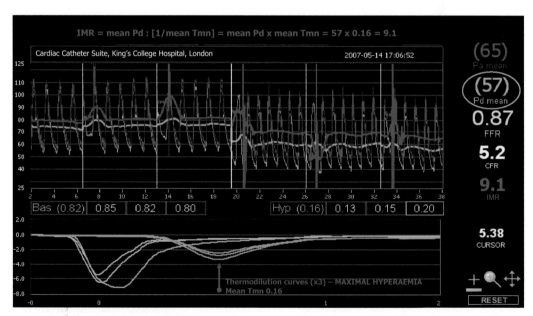

Figure 6.11. A combined pressure/temperature guide wire is used to obtain mean Pd and mean distal coronary blood flow (based on the principles of thermodilution in response to a 3 ml hand held intra-coronary injection of room temperature saline). IMR is derived from the ratio of mean Pd (green circle) and mean distal coronary flow at maximal hyperemia. Distal coronary flow is inversely proportional to the mean transit time (Tmn) of the injectate. Therefore IMR = Pd : 1/Tmn = Pd × Tmn.

hyperemia for assessment of indices such as CFR, FFR and IMR. It is assumed that non-specific agents are capable of interrogating both the endothelium-dependent and the endothelium-independent components of the microcirculation, thus inducing maximal change in coronary blood flow as well as providing a comprehensive overview of microvascular function. Maximal hyperemia is believed to occur in two stages. Both agents primarily achieve maximal hyperemia through their vasodilator action on microvascular smooth muscle cells (an endothelium-independent response). The resultant increase in blood flow is thought to stimulate shear stress-induced endothelial nitric oxide release, which promotes further vasodilatation of the microcirculation (flow-mediated dilatation) and increase in blood flow (an endothelium-dependent response).

Conclusion and Future Directions

Increasingly physiological data play an important role in the management of patients passing through the cardiac catheterization laboratory. In particular, information generated is used to determine the need for coronary revascularization, especially in the context of angiographically intermediate stenosis. In addition, data on the functional state of the microcirculation has emerging implications in risk stratification and determination of CV prognosis. Increasing acquisition of simultaneous physiological data and traditional imaging of coronary vessels has been shown to streamline evidence based patient care in a cost-effective manner.

Questions

1. **All of the following are true regarding the use of intravenous (IV) adenosine compared to intracoronary (IC) adenosine bolus for measuring FFR, except:**

   A IV adenosine is associated with less dyspnea and chest pain.

   B IV adenosine allows a slow pullback of the pressure wire to assess serial lesions or diffuse disease.

   C IV adenosine may provide slightly greater hyperemia in a subset of patients.

   D IV adenosine should be used to assess left main lesions.

2. **A 60 year old diabetic woman presents with classic stable chest pain and your colleague performs a coronary angiogram. It shows a tortuous, occluded RCA, a moderate 50% distal left main lesion and mild proximal LAD disease with collaterals to the RCA. After multiple cineangiograms in different projections, he decides to perform IVUS and finds an MLA in the left main of 6.2 mm2. He then performs FFR and with IV adenosine and the sensor in the mid-distal LAD the FFR is 0.70. Once the sensor is in the ostial LAD the ratio of is 0.80. Your colleague asks for your advice:**

   You tell him:

   A Both the IVUS and the FFR suggest that the left main lesion is not significant.

   B The FFR in the LAD is significant only because the LAD is supplying collaterals to the RCA and he should open the RCA CTO.

   C The combination of the left main and proximal LAD disease is causing ischemia and revascularization should be performed.

   D He should perform a stress imaging study and base his decision on that result.

3. **A 49-year old male with typical angina and a reversible perfusion defect in the inferior wall at MIBI-Spect, has a moderate (50%) stenosis in the proximal part of the large dominant RCA and a severe (90%) stenosis just before the crux.**

   FFR, measured by the pressure wire (located in the posterior descending branch) at maximum hyperemia, equals 0.39.

   The hyperemic pressure pull-back recording shows a pressure gradient of 51 mmHg at the level of the distal stenosis and a gradient of 12 mmHg at the level of the proximal stenosis.

   Which of the following statements is correct?

   A Only the distal stenosis should be stented.

   B Both lesions should be stented anyway.

   C It is very likely that the pressure gradient across the proximal stenosis will increase after stenting the distal one.

   D It is unlikely that the pressure gradient across the proximal stenosis will increase after stenting the distal one.

4. **A 60-year-old male, six weeks after transmural anterior wall infarction, and having akinesia of the anterolateral and apical wall segments on the echocardiogram, has an 80% residual stenosis in the mid LAD. FFR equals 0.92 and IVUS cross-sectional area equals 2.9 mm2.**

   Most likely:

   A This stenosis is functionally significant and should be dilated.

   B FFR is false negative.

   C IVUS is true positive.

   D There is extensive necrosis and little viable tissue and dilating the stenosis does not make much sense.

References

1. Melikian N, MacCarthy PA. Pressure and flow measurements in PCI. In Banning AP and Di Mario C, eds. *The Year in Interventional Cardiology 2004.* Clinical Publishing, Oxford, Volume 3: 37–59.

2. Kern MJ. Coronary physiology revisited: Practical insights from the cardiac catheterisation laboratory. Circulation 2000; **101**: 1344–1351.

3. Kern MJ, De Bruyne B, Pijls NHJ. From research to clinical practice: Current role of intracoronary physiology based decision making in the cardiac catheterisation laboratory. J Am Coll Cardiol 1997; **30**: 631–620.

4. Camici PG, Crea F. Coronary microvascular dysfunction. N Eng J Med 2007; **356**: 830–840.

5. Gould KL, Lipscomb K, Hamilton GW. Physiologic basis for assessing critical coronary stenosis: instantaneous flow response and regional distribution during coronary hyperemia as measures of coronary flow reserve. Am J Cardiol 1974; **33**: 87–94.

6. Bishop AH, Samady H. Fractional flow reserve: Critical review of an important physiologic adjunct to angiography. Am J Cardiol. 2004; **147**: 792–802.

7. Miller DD, Donohue TJ, Younis LT, *et al.* Correlation of 99mTc-sestamibi myocardial perfusion imaging with post-stenotic coronary flow reserve in patients with angiographically intermediate coronary artery stenosis. Circulation 1994; **89**: 2150–2160.

8. Gould KL, Kirkeeide RL, Buchi M. Coronary flow reserve as a physiologic measure of stenosis severity. J Am Coll Cardiol 1990; **15**: 459–474.

9. De Bruyne B, Pijls NH, Barbato E, *et al.* Intracoronary and intravenous adenosine 5′-triphosphate, adenosine, papaverine, and contrast medium to assess fractional flow reserve in humans. Circulation 2003; **107**: 1877–1883.

10. Pijls NHJ, De Bruyne B. Coronary pressure measurement and fractional flow reserve. Heart 1998; **80**: 539–542.

11. Pijls NH, De Bruyne B, Peels K, *et al.* Measurement of fractional flow reserve to assess the functiona; severity of coronary-artery stenosis. N Eng J Med 1996; **334**: 1703–1708.

12. Bech GJW, De Bruyne B, Pijls NHJ, *et al.* Fractional flow reserve to determine the appropriateness of angioplasty in moderate coronary stenosis: A randomised trial. Circulation 2001; **103**: 2928–2934.

13. Pijls NH, van Schaardenburgh P, Manoharan G, *et al.* Percutaneous coronary intervention of functionally non-significant stenosis: 5 year follow-up of the DEFER Study. J Am Coll Cardiol 2007; **49**: 2105–2111.

14. Pijls NHJ, Klauss V, Siebert U, *et al.* Fractional Flow Reserve (FFR) Post-Stent Registry Investigators: Coronary pressure measurement after stenting predicts adverse events at follow-up. A multicenter registry. Circulation 2002; **105**: 2950–2954.

15. Tonino PA, De Bruyne B, Pijls NH, *et al.* FAME Study Investigators. Fractional flow reserve vs angiography for guiding percutaneous coronary interventions. N Engl J Med 2009; **360**: 213–24.

16. Melikian N, Kearney MT, Thomas MR, *et al.* A simple thermodilution technique to assess coronary endothelium-dependent microvascular function in humans: Validation and comparison with coronary flow reserve. Eur Heart J 2007; **28**: 2188–2194.

17. De Bruyne B, Pijls NHJ, Smith L, *et al.* Coronary thermodilution to assess flow reserve: Experimental validation. Circulation 2001; **104**: 2003–2006.

18. Pijls NHJ, De Bruyne B, Smith L, *et al.* Coronary thermodilution to assess flow reserve: Validation in humans. Circulation. 2002; **105**: 2482–86.

19. Fearon WF, Farouque O, Balsam LB, *et al.* Comparison of coronary thermodilution and Doppler velocity for assessing coronary flow reserve. Circulation 2003; **108**: 2198–200.

20. Ng MKC, Yeung AC, Fearon WF. Invasive assessment of the coronary microcirculation: Superior reproducibility and less hemodynamic dependence of index of microcirculatory resistance compared with coronary flow reserve. Circulation 2006; **113**: 2054–2061.

21. Fearon WF, Aarnoudse W, Pijls NHJ, *et al.* Microvascular resistance in not influenced by epicardial coronary artery stenosis severity: Experimental validation. Circulation 2004; **109**: 2269–2272.

22. Aarnoudse W, van't Veer M, Pijls NHJ, *et al.* Direct volumetric blood flow measurement in coronary arteries by thermodilution. J Am Coll Cardiol 2007; **50**: 2294–2304.

23. Davies JE, Whinnett ZI, Francis DP, *et al.* Evidence of a dominant backward-propagating "suction" wave responsible for diastolic coronary filling in humans, attenuated in left ventricular hypertrophy. Circulation. 2006; **113**: 1768–1778.

Answers

1. A
2. C
3. C
4. D

CHAPTER 7

Quantitative Coronary and Vascular Angiography

Joan C. Tuinenburg, Gerhard Koning, & Johan H.C. Reiber
Leiden University Medical Center, Leiden, The Netherlands

Introduction

In the late 1970s, quantitative coronary arteriography (QCA) was developed to quantify vessel motion and the effects of pharmacological agents on the regression and progression of coronary artery disease in straight vessels [1]. So far, QCA has been the only technique that allows the accurate and reliable assessment of arterial dimensions within the entire coronary vasculature over time, despite its known limitations [2].

In interventional cardiology, QCA has been used for on-line vessel sizing, for the selection of the interventional devices and the assessment of the efficacy of the individual procedures, for the on-line selection of patients to be included or excluded in clinical trials (e.g. small vessel disease), and for training purposes.

But, in particular, QCA has been applied worldwide in core laboratories and clinical research sites to study the efficacy of the procedures and devices in smaller and larger patient populations in off-line situations.

Basic Principles of Automated Contour Detection

The general principles and characteristics of a modern QCA/QVA (for both coronary and vascu-

Interventional Cardiology, First Edition. Edited by
Carlo Di Mario, George D. Dangas, Peter Barlis.

lar analysis) software package are illustrated by the QAngio® XA (Medis medical imaging systems bv, Leiden, the Netherlands) algorithms developed in our laboratory [3–5].

The contour detection procedure is carried out in two iterations relative to a model. In the first iteration, the pathline, found by the wavefront propagation principle ("the wavepath approach" [6–7]), is used as the model (Figure 7.1a). To detect the contours, scanlines are defined perpendicular to the model (Figure 7.1b). For each point or pixel along such a scanline, the corresponding edge-strength value (local change in brightness level) is computed. The resulting edge-strength values are input to the so-called minimal cost analysis (MCA) contour detection algorithm, which searches for an optimal contour path along the entire segment (Figure 7.1c). The individual left and right vessel contours, detected in the first iteration, now serve as models for the MCA contour detection procedure in the second iteration, resulting in the initially detected arterial contours (Figure 7.1d).

If the operator does not agree with one or more parts of the initially detected contours, these can be edited/corrected in various ways. For example, the MCA approach works very well as long as the vessel outlines are relatively smooth in shape. However, in its design, the MCA technique is hampered when tracing very irregular and complex boundaries, which may occur before (e.g. complex lesions) or after the coronary intervention (e.g. dissections or radiopaque stents). To circumvent this limitation, a more complex algorithm, the

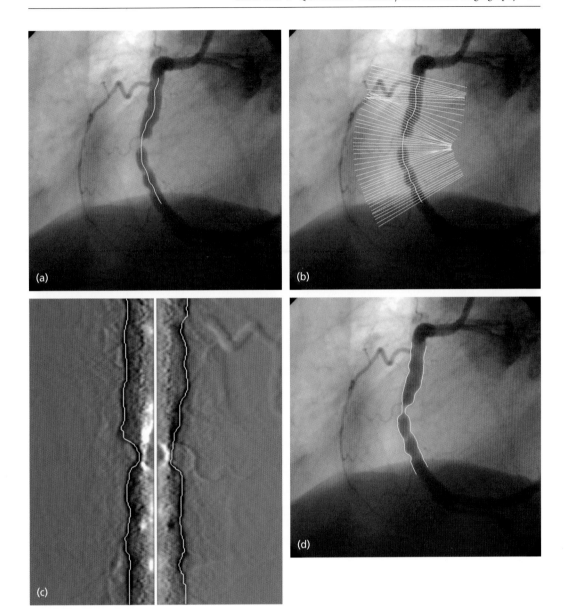

Figure 7.1. Basic principles of the minimum cost analysis (MCA) contour detection algorithm. (a) Initial segment with pathline, (b) scanlines defined, (c) straightened for analysis; contours calculated, (d) contours returned to initial image; diameter measurements performed.

gradient field transform (GFT®) was developed [8], which can follow much more abrupt changes in morphology, and which is carried out as a next iteration of the contour detection. An illustrative example of the GFT is given in Figure 7.2.

Another approach of automatic contour correction is the option to add an attraction point at the improperly detected vessel part. In the subsequent MCA iteration, the contour is forced through the vicinity of this attraction point. In this way the attraction point pulls the arterial contour automatically toward another and better (user indicated) vessel edge.

Finally, if these semi-automated correction methods fail and do not result in the correct

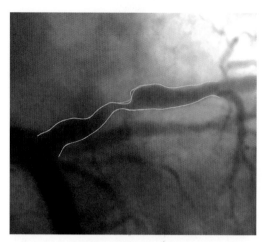

Figure 7.2. Example of outcome of gradient field transform (GFT) analysis on a vessel segment with very severe complex stenosis. Conventional approaches with the minimal cost analysis (MCA) algorithm are not able to follow automatically the abrupt changes in morphology. The light blue contour is minimal cost analysis (MCA), and the yellow contour is gradient field transform (GFT).

contour, the user can re-draw the arterial contour manually.

Calibration Procedure

The calibration procedure is one of the most important steps in any QCA/QVA analysis procedure. The goal of the calibration procedure is to assess the size of each picture element or pixel in the image as expressed in mm/pixel based on the calibration device with known dimensions. Therefore, any error in the calibration will directly translate into an error in the absolute measures of the arterial segment.

A potential problem with calibration in general is the out-of-plane magnification, which occurs when the calibration object and the vessel segment of analysis are positioned at different distances with respect to the image intensifier. Another big problem may be the variable image quality of the displayed calibration devices. For that reason, extra attention to the quality of the outcome of the calibration is really mandatory.

For the coronary application the contrast catheter (preferably of size 6 French or bigger) is used as calibration device. A frame is chosen in which the contrast-filled catheter is in a "stable" posi-

tion, i.e. minimal motion with respect to neighboring frames to prevent motion blur. This will result in an image in which the image contrast of the catheter and the sharpness of the edges are maximal. The calibration is performed on a non-tapering portion of the catheter, using the MCA edge detection procedure similar to that applied to the arterial segment. In this case, however, additional information is used in the edge detection process because this part of the catheter is known to be characterized by parallel boundaries.

For peripheral applications, other devices might be used for calibration as well: the marker catheter or -guidewire, the cm-grid or ruler, or the sphere or coin of known dimension (see Figure 7.3a, b and c). The advantage of each of these devices is that the distance over which the calibration is carried out is larger than in the catheter diameter measurements in the coronary applications, leading to more accurate calibration factors. A typical advantage of the marker catheter is that it is inside and very close to the arterial segment of interest, thereby avoiding any out-of-plane errors. The disadvantage is that it is more expensive.

Vessel Segment Analysis

From the lefthand and righthand contours of the arterial segment, a diameter function is determined (Figure 7.4a) [9]. To calculate the arterial diameter function (the width of a vessel segment along its trajectory from proximal to distal), the exact centerline of the vessel is derived from the arterial contours, followed subsequently by the assessment of the width values at every pixel distance along the centerline and measured perpendicular to this centerline.

The most widely used parameter to describe the severity of an obstruction is the percentage diameter stenosis. Calculation of this parameter requires that a reference diameter value is computed, for which two options are available: (1) a user-defined reference diameter as positioned by the user at a so-called "normal" portion of the vessel, and (2) the automated or interpolated reference diameter value. In practice, this last approach is preferred because it requires no user interaction and takes care of any tapering of the vessel. For that

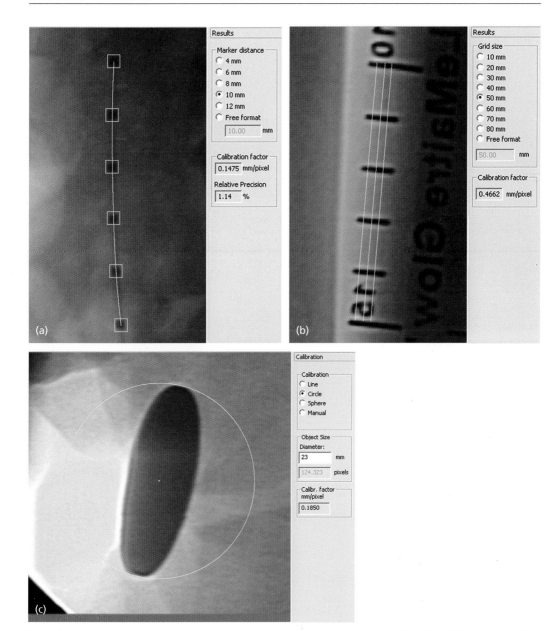

Figure 7.3 Some examples of calibration objects: (a) Marker catheter; the true marker distance in mm is divided by the average distance between the automatically detected markers calculated in pixels, (b) cm-ruler; the true (displayed) length in mm is divided by the average length of manually indicated lines calculated in pixels, and (c) coin; the true diameter of the coin in mm is divided by the diameter of the manually indicated circle calculated in pixels. All calibration measurements lead to a calibration factor in mm/pixel.

purpose, a reference diameter function is calculated by an iterative regression technique (excluding the influence of any obstructive area) and displayed in the diameter function as a (slightly tapering) horizontal straight line, which represents the best approximation of the vessel size before the occurrence of a focal narrowing.

Now that the reference diameter function is known, reference contours can be reconstructed around the actual vessel segment, representing the

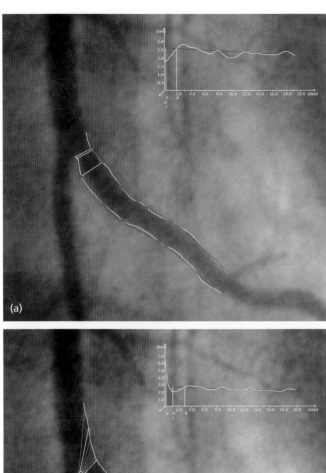

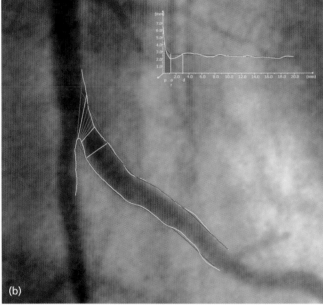

Figure 7.4. The diameter function:
(a) The contours and the diameter
function of a straight analysis,
and (b) the contours and the diameter
function of an ostial analysis.

original size and shape of the vessel before any disease occurred.

The value of the reference diameter function at the location of the obstruction diameter equals the reference diameter, so that neither overestimation nor underestimation occurs. Finally, from the reference diameter and the obstruction diameter, the percentage diameter stenosis is calculated.

The Flagging Procedure

In the large majority of vessel analyses, the calculation of the reference diameter function and the reconstruction of the reference contours provide a reliable representation of the vessel segment. However, overdilated stents, vessels with large lesions or ectatic areas, overlap of vessel segments, and so forth, may negatively influence the calculation of the reference diameter function. This is illustrated in Figure 7.5a. The ectatic area distal to the obstruction results in a significant tapering of the reference diameter function, so that the normal vessel size would not be measured correctly. Therefore, an option called the "flagging" procedure has been developed. The user can "flag" the abnormal portion of the vessel segment (in Figure 7.5b, the ectatic area), and the corresponding arterial diameter values are excluded from the subsequent calculation of the reference diameter function. The correctly calculated reference diameter function and reconstructed reference contours are presented in Figure 7.5b, which is more in line with what one would expect.

Ostial Analysis

For the analysis of a true ostial lesion, whether in a coronary or peripheral vessel, the ostial analysis option was developed. Particular advantage of this option is that the contours of the arterial segment are properly detected at the ostium, which is not possible with the conventional straight analysis approach (see Figure 7.4a and b).

An example of an ostial analysis on a renal artery is given in Figure 7.6. The user indicates three points to define the arterial segment: two start points in the main segment at either side of the side branch, and one end point in the side branch. Subsequently, two pathlines are determined (Figure 7.6a) and the corresponding arterial contours detected. From these contours, the ostial diameter function is calculated. In this case, the arterial diameter function needs to include the proximal part at the ostium (which can be strongly curved). Therefore, firstly the exact location where the side branch separates from the main vessel and the direction of the side branch at that location are determined. Secondly, the position where a straight analysis would start in this case is calculated. This information is then used to interpolate the diameter values near the ostium (pink lines), which results in a complete arterial diameter function (Figure 7.6b). At the position near the ostium, the direction of the reference diameters changes in order to match the direction of the main vessel.

Therefore, the reference diameter function is adjusted according to a model that takes into account the angle between the side branch and the main vessel. Because of the increasing arterial diameter function at the ostium, this part is flagged by default (pink lines) in order to obtain a suitable reference diameter function, leading to a proper assessment of the percentage diameter stenosis (Figure 7.6b).

Bifurcation Analysis

For the quantification of true bifurcating arterial segments (e.g. carotid arteries) and with the increasing interest for a bifurcation application in the coronary arteries (as a result of the increased use of bifurcation stenting in clinical studies [10]), it became clear that a special bifurcation analysis option had to be developed. The first approach that we developed is the so-called three-section analysis model. The particular advantage of this model is that it combines the proximal and two distal artery segments with the central fragment of the bifurcation, resulting in three separate analyses each with its own set of parameters, all derived in one analysis procedure.

An example of a bifurcation analysis on a coronary artery is given in Figure 7.7. The user indicates three points to define the arterial bifurcation segment: one start point in the proximal segment and an end point in each of the two distal segments. Subsequently, two pathlines are detected (see Figure 7.7a) and the corresponding arterial contours determined. Next, the central fragment of the bifurcation is defined by three automatically determined delimiters; one distally in the proximal segment and two proximally in each distal segment (see Figure 7.7b).

From the section contours, three bifurcation diameter functions are calculated. In our three-section bifurcation analysis the reference diameter function should only be based upon the arterial diameters outside the central fragment, since the normally increasing arterial diameters in the central fragment are not representative for the fragments outside the central fragment. Therefore, the central fragment arterial diameters are all flagged by default in all three sections (see Figure 7.7c).

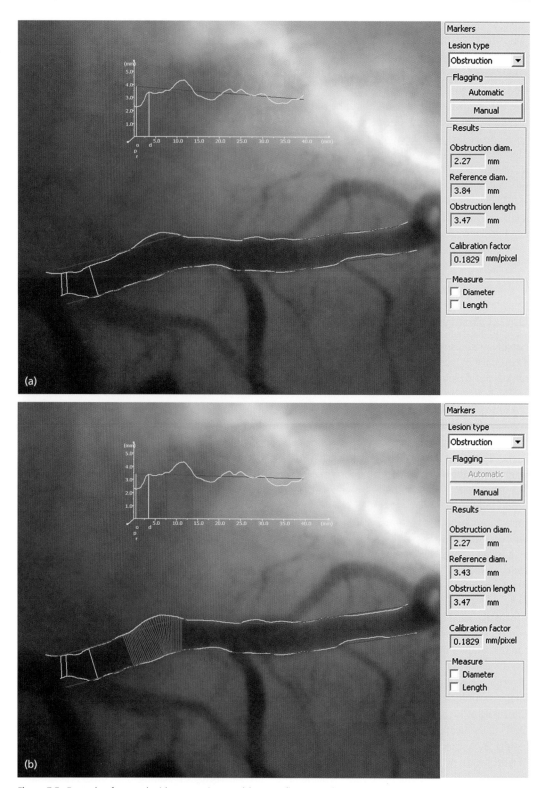

Figure 7.5. Example of a vessel with an ectatic area: (a) The initial (interpolated) reference diameter function significantly tapers, which would lead to arbitrary, erroneous parameter results. In this case, a stenosis of 41% would be measured (obstruction diameter of 2.27 mm, reference diameter of 3.84 mm). (b) By "flagging" the ectatic area (pink lines), a proper tapering of the reference diameter function is obtained. The reference diameter changes from 3.84 mm before flagging to 3.43 mm after flagging. For this case, this leads to a less severe narrowing of 34% (obstruction diameter of 2.27 mm).

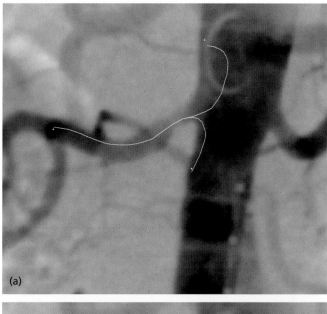

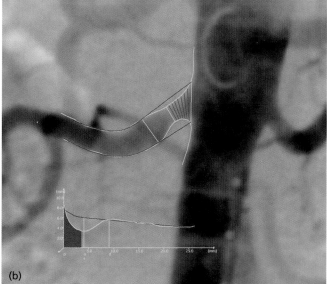

Figure 7.6. Example of an ostial analysis on a renal artery. (a) The two pathlines of the ostial analysis, (b) the contours and the diameter function of an ostial analysis.

Guidelines for QCA Acquisition Procedures

The primary objective of QCA measurements in clinical trials is to allow more precise and reliable analyses of the real changes after interventions, namely, acute lumen gain, late lumen loss, and net lumen gain, expressed in millimeters. This is best achieved when exactly the same setting is applied during the procedure at baseline, post-interven-

tion and at the follow-up studies, that is, replication of the same angiographic X-ray views, same doses of intra-arterial nitroglycerin, same contrast agent, same catheter type or material, and, if feasible, same catheterization room. Further details can be found in [11, 12]. The best and most reproducible results are obtained, if proper standard operating procedures (SOPs) are in place and used in the core lab [13].

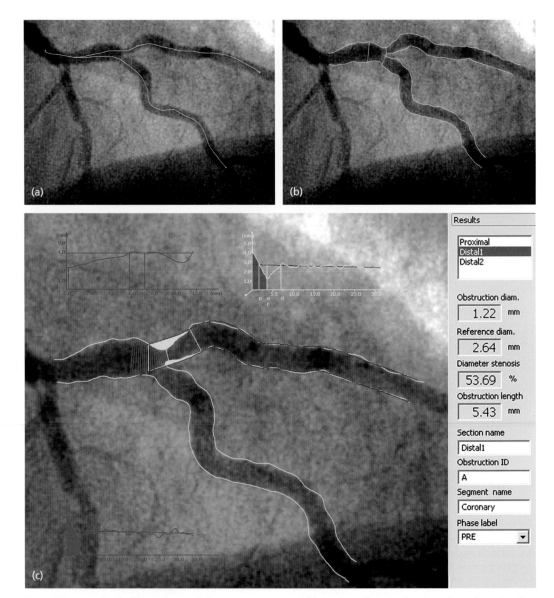

Figure 7.7. Example of a bifurcation analysis on coronary artery. (a) The two pathlines of the bifurcation analysis, (b) the three delimiters of the bifurcation analysis, and (c) the three diameter functions for each section. In this case, the distal 1 section is selected and the corresponding main parameter results are displayed.

Conclusion

Semi-automated segmentation techniques are able to trace the luminal boundaries of coronary arteries from two-dimensional digital X-ray arteriograms after minimal user interaction. Quantitative coronary arteriography or QCA allows the derivation of such luminal dimensions and derived indices with small systematic and random errors as demonstrated by a range of validation studies. QCA can be used in an off-line mode for clinical research studies and in an on-line mode during the interventional procedure to support the clinical decision making process. New options have become available for more extensive analyses in both coronary and peripheral vessels, such as the brachytherapy- and drug eluting stent analyses, the ostial and bifurcation analyses, and the quantification of both obstructive and/or aneurysmal lesions.

References

1. Brown BG, Bolson E, Frimer M, *et al.* Quantitative coronary arteriography: estimation of dimensions, hemodynamic resistance, and atheroma mass of coronary artery lesions using the arteriogram and digital computation. Circulation 1977; **55**(2); 329–337.

2. De Feyter PJ, Vos J, Reiber JHC, *et al.* Value and limitations of quantitative coronary angiography to assess progression and regression. In: Reiber JHC and Serruys PW, eds. *Advances in Quantitative Coronary Arteriography.* Kluwer Academic Publishers, Dordrecht, 1993, pp. 255–271.

3. Reiber JHC, Serruys PW, Kooijman CJ, *et al.* Assessment of short-, medium-, and long-term variations in arterial dimensions from computer-assisted quantitation of coronary cineangiograms. Circulation 1985; **71**(2); 280–288.

4. Reiber JHC, van der Zwet PM, Koning G, *et al.* Accuracy and precision of quantitative digital coronary arteriography: observer-, short-, and medium-term variabilities. Cathet Cardiovasc Diagn 1993; **28**(3); 187–198.

5. Reiber JHC, Koning G, Dijkstra J, *et al.* Angiography and intravascular ultrasound. In: Sonka M & Fitzpatrick JM (eds) *Handbook of Medical Imaging—Volume 2: Medical Image Processing and Analysis.* SPIE Press, Belligham WA, 2001, pp. 711–808.

6. Janssen JP, Koning G, de Koning PJ, *et al.* A novel approach for the detection of pathlines in X-ray angiograms: the wavefront propagation algorithm. Int J Cardiovasc Imaging 2002; Oct **18**(5); 317–324.

7. Janssen JP, Koning G, de Koning PJ, *et al.* Validation of a new method for the detection of pathlines in vascular x-ray images. Invest Radiol 2004 September; **39**(9); 524–530.

8. Van der Zwet PM, Reiber JHC. A new approach for the quantification of complex lesion morphology: The gradient field transform; basic principles and validation results. J Am Coll Cardiol 1994; **24**(1); 216–224.

9. Reiber JHC, Schiemanck L, van der Zwet PM, Goedhart B, Koning G, Lammertsma M, *et al.* State of the art in quantitative coronary arteriography as of 1996. In: Reiber JHC and van der Wall EE, eds. *Cardiovascular Imaging.* Kluwer Academic Publishers, Dordrecht, 1996, pp. 39–56.

10. Lefevre T, Louvard Y, Morice MC, *et al.* Stenting of bifurcation lesions: a rational approach. J Interv Cardiol 2001; **14**(6); 573–585.

11. Reiber JHC, Jukema JW, Koning G, Bruschke AVG. Quality control in quantitative coronary arteriography. In: Bruschke AVG, Reiber JHC, Lie KI and Wellens HJJ (eds.) *Lipid lowering therapy and progression of coronary artherosclerosis.* Kluwer Academic Publishers, Dordrecht, 1996, pp. 45–63.

Reiber JHC, Tuinenburg JC, Koning G, *et al.* Quantitative coronary arteriography. In: Oudkerk M, Reiser MF, eds. *Coronary Radiology*, 2nd edn. Springer-Verlag, Berlin, 2009, pp. 41–65.

13. Tuinenburg JC, Koning G, Hekking E, *et al.* One core lab at two international sites, is that feasible? An intercore lab and intra-observer variability study. Cath Cardiovasc Int 2002 July: **56**(3); 333–340.

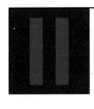

PART II
Interventional Pharmacology

CHAPTER 8

Oral Antiplatelet Agents in PCI

Annunziata Nusca, & Germano Di Sciascio
Campus Bio-Medico University of Rome, Rome, Italy

Optimization of antiplatelet therapy is crucial for the prevention of peri-procedural acute ischemic complications in patients undergoing percutaneous coronary interventions (PCI) and dual antiplatelet therapy with aspirin and clopidogrel is the regimen of choice. The thienopyridine clopidogrel is a prodrug that needs to be metabolized to an active compound that targets the platelet ADP P2Y12 receptor, affecting intracellular signalling events that modulate the ADP-induced platelet activation.

We will discuss several "hot issues" in contemporary interventional pharmacology regarding oral antiplatelet therapy, in particular:
- What is the optimal clopidogrel loading dose (300 mg vs. 600 mg vs. 900 mg)?
- How much anti-aggregation is really needed to improve clinical outcome?
- Glycoprotein IIb/IIIa antagonists: do they provide additional benefit when a 600 mg clopidogrel loading dose is used?
- What is the optimal loading dose for patients already receiving clopidogrel?
- Can clopidogrel be given less than two hours before percutaneous coronary intervention (i.e. after coronary angiography and immediately before PCI)?

- What is the role of early clopidogrel loading dose in acute coronary syndromes, including acute myocardial infarction?
- What is beyond clopidogrel?

Search for the Optimal Clopidogrel Loading Dose

Clopidogrel has become a mainstay of the pharmacological therapy for patients undergoing PCI and drug dosing is critically important. "Double, double, dose in trouble" is the subtitle of an editorial by David O. Williams [1] published on *Circulation* in April 2005 commenting on the results of the ARMYDA-2 trial, which demonstrated in a randomized design the superiority of a 600 mg pre-PCI clopidogrel loading dose in improving outcome compared with a 300 mg loading dose [2].

Indeed, previous pharmacokynetic studies had already indicated that a higher and faster suppression of platelet function evaluated with ADP-induced aggregation can be achieved with a 600 mg loading dose of clopidogrel vs. 300 mg loading or ticlopidine within two hours after drug administration [3] and that increasing doses (75 mg to 675 mg) provide a progressive decrease of platelet function with a dose-dependent effect [4].

Moreover, a 600 mg loading dose of clopidogrel given to patients not previously treated with this drug achieves a platelet inhibition similar to that observed with chronic therapy of 75 mg/die and the same loading dose in patients already receiving

Interventional Cardiology, First Edition. Edited by Carlo Di Mario, George D. Dangas, Peter Barlis.
© 2010 Blackwell Publishing Ltd. Published 2010 by Blackwell Publishing Ltd.

clopidogrel can provide a further degree platelet suppression [5].

A 600 mg loading dose has been used across the board as antiplatelet therapy pre-PCI in the ISAR-REACT trial [6], which investigated the usefulness of abciximab in patients at low-to-moderate risk for early ischemic complications after elective PCI, thus the conventional 300 mg loading dose was not even tested against 600 mg, the latter being instead considered optimal by the investigators. In fact, whilst in the CREDO trial [7] clinical benefit with 300 mg loading vs. placebo started being evident only with pre-treatment duration longer than 15 hours, the Munich group demonstrated that 600 mg loading was somewhat of an "equalizer" in terms of pre-treatment times, i.e. increasing the pre-treatment interval beyond two to three hours was not associated with a measurable clinical benefit (death, myocardial infarction—MI, target vessel revascularization—TVR) [6]. This observation is in agreement with data from a non-randomized PCI cohort reporting no difference in inhibition of platelet aggregation whether treatment with clopidogrel pre-intervention was administered two hours before or longer (up to six hours) [8].

With this background, the ARMYDA-2 trial [2] was the first randomized trial to evaluate the impact of a 600 mg loading dose of clopidogrel versus the "standard" 300 mg in patients undergoing coronary interventions. In this study, 329 patients with stable angina or NSTE-acute coronary syndromes were randomized to 300 mg or 600 mg of clopidogrel 4–8 hours before cardiac catheterization. After coronary angiography 44 patents were excluded for indication to medical therapy and 30 patients for indication to surgery; 255 remaining patients (129 in 300 mg arm; 126 in 600 mg arm) underwent coronary angioplasty. The primary composite endpoint of death, MI and TVR at 30 days was 4% in the 600 mg group and 12% in the 300 mg group (p = 0.041) (Figure 8.1). A 600 mg dose was also superior in preventing peri-procedural myocardial damage, measured by any elevation of troponin I above upper normal limit (ULN) and CK-MB (above one, two and three times ULN). The beneficial effect of a higher loading dose was not associated with increase in bleeding complications; no patient

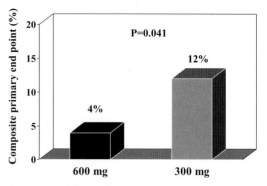

Figure 8.1. Incidence of composite primary endpoint (30 days occurrence of death, MI and TVR) in patients pre-treated with high loading dose of clopidogrel (600 mg) vs. standard dose of 300 mg in the ARMYDA 2 study.

had major bleeding and a similar incidence of minor bleeding was observed in the two groups. Multivariable analysis identified pre-treatment with 600 mg loading dose as an independent predictor of decreased risk of peri-procedural MI (OR 0.48, 95% CI 0.15–0.97; p = 0.044); an additive reduction in the risk of MI was found in the patients randomized to 600 mg who were taking statins before PCI (OR 0.20, 95% CI 0.10–0.74; p = 0.017). Thus, the results of the ARMYDA-2 trial indicate that use of 600 mg loading dose before planned PCI improves clinical outcome compared to 300 mg. On the basis of the above, the latest guidelines of the European Society of Cardiology for Percutaneous Coronary Intervention [9] state: "*To ensure full antiplatelet activity, clopidogrel should be initiated at least 6 hours prior to the procedure with a loading dose of 300 mg, ideally administered the day before a planned PCI. If this is not possible, a loading dose of 600 mg should be administered at least 2 hours before PCI.*"

Different mechanisms can explain the greater efficacy of a high clopidogrel loading dose. Gurbel *et al.* [10] demonstrated that a 600 mg loading dose of clopidogrel is associated with a significant reduction of non-responsive patients compared to a 300 mg administration (8% vs. 32%; p < 0.001) (Figure 8.2). Clopidogrel seems to have important anti-inflammatory effects, enhanced by a higher dose administration. Reduced C-reactive protein (CRP) and soluble P-selectin levels were

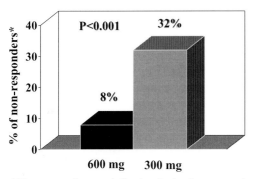

*Non-responsiveness defined as Δ platelet aggregation
<10% (at the time of PCI – 24 hrs/5days post)*

Figure 8.2. Influence of 600 mg loading dose in individual response vs. 300 mg standard dose.

found in patients treated with loading dose of 600 mg compared with a standard dose of 300 mg [11,12]. Seminal observations by Angiolillo *et al.* showed a significant "rebound" increase in markers of inflammation and platelet activation (CRP and P-selectin) after one month following clopidogrel withdrawal in diabetic patients on long-term (12 months) dual antiplatelet therapy [13].

How Much Antiaggregation is Necessary?

A large individual variability in response to clopidogrel has been identified and multiple mechanisms may be involved: differences in individual drug absorption, variations in the biotransformation rate into active metabolite or P2Y12 receptor polymorphisms affecting receptor number and activity; response to clopidogrel is also reduced in presence of high pre-treatment platelet reactivity, as observed in patients with diabetes mellitus and acute coronary syndromes, and may be also due to accelerated platelet turnover and up-regulation of P2Y-dependent or P2Y-independent pathways induced by coagulation agonists (collagen, epinephrine, thromboxane A_2, thrombin) [14]. Reported prevalence of impaired clopidogrel responsiveness varies from 4% to 30%, depending on assays used, empirically applied definitions and presence of potential confounders. In several studies using optical aggregometry, a low degree of platelet

response to clopidogrel has been prospectively associated with a poorer outcome after PCI, due to an increased incidence of short and mid-term periprocedural myocardial injury and cardiovascular events [15].

Potential additional benefit of a loading dose of clopidogrel >600 mg in improving procedural outcome has been investigated, but, to date, no studies with a clinical or platelet function endpoint have demonstrated a favourable evidence. The Albion study, enrolling patients with non-STE ACS randomized to receive a 300 mg, 600 mg, or 900 mg clopidogrel loading dose, observed that a 900 mg does not provide a higher inhibition of platelet aggregation evaluated by optical aggregometry (5 μmol ADP stimulation) compared with a 600 mg dose [16]. These results were confirmed by Von Beckerath *et al.* in the ISAR-CHOICE study, also demonstrating that the administration of 900 mg was not associated with further increase in plasma concentration of the active thiol metabolite of clopidogrel when compared with administration of 600 mg (p = 0.38) [17].

In addition to preloading issues, duration and intensity of chronic clopidogrel therapy after stenting requires careful investigation. Kastrati *et al.* observed at one month after PCI a lower ADP-induced aggregation in patients receiving a 150 mg/day chronic dose of clopidogrel compared to patients receiving the standard 75 mg/die chronic dose. This mechanistic improvement has translated into a clinical benefit at 30 days in the recent CURRENT-OASIS 7 trial, suggesting that a higher loading dose and initial dose in the first days postprocedure is highly recommended if clopidogrel is used [18].

Glycoprotein IIb/IIIa Antagonists: Do They Provide Additional Benefit When a 600 mg Clopidogrel Loading Dose Is Used?

Efficacy of Glycoprotein IIb/IIIa antagonists after a pre-treatment with a 600 mg clopidogrel loading dose is strongly related to patients' clinical features and risk profiles.

In the first ISAR-REACT trial (Intracoronary Stenting and Antithrombotic Regimen: Rapid early Action for Coronary Treatment) abciximab was not found to provide additional benefit when given in addition to adequate pre-treatment with clopidogrel in patients with low-to-moderate risk. However, this study excluded patients with acute coronary syndromes, a group of patients that may potentially derive the greatest benefit from adjunctive therapy with GP IIb/IIIa antagonists [19]. ISAR-REACT 2 solved this concern, enrolling patients with ACS and demonstrating that there was no difference in the incidence of ischemic events (death, MI, TVR at 30 days) between the abciximab and the placebo groups among patients without elevated troponin levels (p = 0.98); conversely, in patients with an elevated troponin levels the incidence of ischemic events was significantly lower in the abciximab group (p = 0.02) [20].

In addition, Gurbel *et al.* demonstrated with the CLEAR-PLATELETS study that administration of eptifibatide with either a standard or high loading dose of clopidogrel provides the most sustained platelet inhibition evaluated by optical aggregometry and this is associated with the lowest incidence of myocardial necrosis markers release [21].

What is the Optimal Loading Dose for Patients Receiving Clopidogrel?

As mentioned above, Kastrati *et al.* observed that in patients chronically treated with clopidogrel a further loading dose of 600 mg results in a significant additional inhibition of ADP induced platelet aggregation [5]. In order to verify if this more intense antiaggregation leads to clinical improvement, the ARMYDA study group is conducting the ARMYDA-4 trial [22], a multicenter, randomized, controlled study to evaluate whether a 600 mg loading dose of clopidogrel given before PCI in patients receiving chronic treatment with the drug influences clinical outcome. Patients with indication to PCI and on chronic treatment (>1 month) with clopidogrel (75 mg/day) were randomized to receive a further 600 mg loading dose of clopidogrel 4–8 hours before planned coronary angioplasty or the standard 75 mg daily dose.

Can Clopidogel be Given Less Than Two Hours Before Percutaneous Coronary Intervention (After Coronary Angiography and Immediately Before PCI)?

The administration of a loading dose of clopidogrel after coronary angiography, immediately before PCI, when the coronary anatomy is known and revascularization indications are more clear, could be an advantage especially in patients in need of coronary bypass surgery.

The ARMYDA study group has designed the ARMYDA-5 trial, a prospective, randomized trial evaluating the influence on outcome of 600 mg of clopidogrel given 4–8 hours before angiography compared to 600 mg loading dose administered in the catheterization laboratory at the time of PCI. Preliminary results, utilizing point of care aggregometry determinations, suggest better antiaggregation in the pre-load group, without, however, an evident advantage in clinical benefits. To be noted, unlike the PRAGUE-8 study, the ARMYDA-5 trial did not show an increased rate of bleeding complications in the latter patients.

What is the Role of Early Clopidogrel Loading Dose in Acute Coronary Syndromes?

An ARMYDA-2 substudy, the ARMYDA-HIGH RISK, evaluating patients with high risk features (69% of total population) of which the most severe was NSTE-ACS, together with age >70 years, diabetes, multivessel intervention, demonstrated a maintained benefit of 600 mg loading dose of clopidogrel versus 300 mg with a significant reduction peri-procedural CK-MB and troponin-I levels [2]. On the other end, the ISAR-REACT-2 had already shown the advantage of the 600 mg protocol in clinically more complex patients, with or without the association with IIb-IIIa antagonists according to the troponin status.

Therefore, even if future studies are needed to resolve this concern, 600 mg of clopidogrel is recommended also in high risk patients with acute coronary syndromes.

STEMI and attendant acute reperfusion modalities represent a more complex clinical setting, in which clopidogrel loading at the first medical contact may prove to be beneficial on top of other established recanalization attempts (lysis and/or PCI): this also deserves careful consideration in future studies.

What is Beyond Clopidogrel?

Novel antiplatelet agents with a more rapid onset of action and a higher efficacy would provide a valuable tool in the treatment of patients undergoing PCI. A number of such agents are currently being developed, and include an oral, irreversible thienopyridine agent (prasugrel), and two reversible non-thienopyridine agents: one oral (AZD6140, ticagrelor) and the other intravenous (cangrelor). These agents act upon the same platelet receptor as clopidogrel (P2Y12), but are distinguished by their routes of administration, reversibility, and pharmacodynamic properties.

Prasugrel is an orally administered agent that provides faster, higher, and more consistent inhibition of platelet aggregation than clopidogrel. Current data suggest that the effects of this drug on clinical outcome compare favorably with those of clopidogrel. In the Joint Utilization of Medications to Block Platelets Optimally (JUMBO)—Thrombolysis In Myocardial Infarction (TIMI) 26 trial (Phase 2 trial), prasugrel was associated with lower incidence of major adverse cardiac events at 30 days without difference in bleeding complications [23]. The recently published phase 3 TRITON (TRial to assess Improvement in Therapeutic Outcomes by optimizing platelet inhibitioN with prasugrel)—TIMI 38 trial, enrolling more than 13.000 patients, compared the efficacy and safety of prasugrel (60 mg loading dose, 10 mg daily maintenance dose) and clopidogrel (300 mg loading dose, 75 mg daily maintenance dose) in patients with ACS scheduled for PCI [24]. The incidence of primary efficacy end-point (a composite of death from cardiovascular causes, non-fatal MI or non-fatal stroke) was significantly decreased in patients receiving prasugrel (9.9% vs. 12.1%; p < 0.001) (Figure 8.3); this difference was largely due to a reduction in the

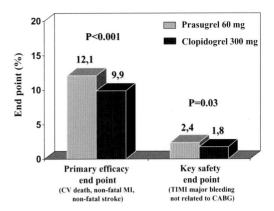

Figure 8.3. Incidence of the primary efficacy end point (death from cardiovascular causes, non-fatal MI or non-fatal stroke) and the key safety end point (TIMI major bleeding not related to CABG) in patients received 60 mg of prasugrel vs. 300 mg of clopidogrel in the TRITON-TIMI 38 Trial.

occurrence of non-fatal MI. However, TIMI major bleeding not related to coronary artery bypass grafting (CABG) occurred in 2.4% of patients treated with prasugrel vs. 1.8% of patients in the clopidogrel group (p = 0.03) (Figure 8.3), with a higher incidence of life-threatening and fatal bleedings in the first group, an excess not previously reported with clopidogrel. Thus, the greater antiplatelet inhibition and the consequent more effective prevention of ischemic events associated with prasugrel needs to be weighed against a significant increase in bleeding. Therefore, subgroups of patients who would benefit or be jeopardised by prasugrel therapy need to be identified and treatment will eventually have to be individualized.

One of the concerns about the TRITON-TIMI 38 study was the fact that this trial did not use the optimal loading dose of 600 mg of clopidogrel, as several studies have suggested. A recently completed laboratory study (PRasugrel IN Comparison to Clopidogrel for Inhibition of Platelet Activation and AggrEgation—PRINCIPLE-TIMI 44) has evaluated the antiplatelet effects of the prasugrel 60 mg loading dose versus a 600 mg loading dose of clopidogrel in patients undergoing elective PCI. Preliminary data show higher levels of platelet inhibition with prasugrel after 30 minutes vs. clopidogrel 600 mg even after 6 hours [25].

AZD6140 is another orally administered platelet inhibitor but, unlike prasugrel, has a rapid and reversible action. The Dose-finding Investigative Study to assess the Pharmacodynamic Effects of AZD6140 in atherosclerotic disease (DISPERSE) 2 trial had suggested that at a twice daily dose of 180 mg, AZD6140 may be more effective than clopidogrel 75 mg/day in preventing thrombotic events in patients with ACS [26]. These results were recently confirmed by the PLATO study, showing in 18624 patients that at 12 months, death from vascular causes, myocardial infarction, or stroke had occurred in 9.8% of patients receiving ticagrelor as compared with 11.7% of those receiving clopidogrel (hazard ratio, 0.84; 95% confidence interval [CI], 0.77 to 0.92; $P < 0.001$). The difference was significant also for mortality alone and was not associated with a significant increase in bleeding events [27].

Cangrelor is an intravenously administered, reversible, short-acting agent with a rapid onset of activity. Unfortunately, the results of a large trial comparing Cangrelor to Clopidogrel in subjects with acute coronary syndromes requiring PCI (CHAMPION-PCI) has not fulfilled the promise that faster, higher, and more consistent inhibition of platelet aggregation demonstrated in mechanistic studies of platelet function translates into an improved clinical outcome.

Learning Points

- Optimal dose of clopidogrel, (i.e. influencing clinical outcome) appears to be 600 mg across a variety of clinical syndromes and risk profiles, including ACS.
- A loading dose higher than 600 mg has not been proven to have additional clinical benefit after coronary stenting.
- A 150 mg/die chronic dose in the first week after PCI is more effective in preventing ischemic/thrombotic complications.
- Glycoprotein IIb/IIIa antagonists use in addition to 600 mg clopidogrel loading dose should be administered in patients with troponin-I-positive ACS, but does not provide a clinical benefit in patients with low-to-moderate risk profile.
- A 600 mg loading dose confers a measurable additional clinical benefit in patients already receiving chronic antiplatelet therapy including clopidogrel.
- In patients undergoing PCI, statins may provide additional benefit to clopidogrel through anti-inflammatory and microvascular protective effects.
- Prasugrel may represent an effective choice in certain subgroups of patients with a higher risk of ischemic events, and when mnimisation of the interval between loading dose administration and start of the pharmacological effect is mandatory such in primary PCI for AMI.

Ticagrelor has the potential to revolutionise the antiplatelet treatment because of a combination of greater efficacy and maintained safety.

References

1. Williams DO. Clopidogrel pre-treatment for percutaneous coronary intervention: Double, double, dose in trouble. Circulation 2005; **111**: 2019–2021.
2. Patti G, Colonna G, Pasceri V, et al. A randomized controlled trial if high dose of clopidogrel for reduction of peri-procedural myocardial infarction in patients undergoing coronary intervention. Results from the ARMYDA 2 (Antiplatelet therapy for Reduction of Myocardial Damage during Angioplasty) Study. Circulation 2005; **111**: 2099–2106.
3. Muller I, Seyfarth M, Rudiger S, et al. Effect of high loading dose of clopidogrel on platelet function in patients undergoing coronary stent placement. Heart 2001; **85**: 92–93.
4. Leimbach ME, Peyrou V, Marzec UM, et al. Single dose clopidogrel inhibition of platelet adenosine receptor function in patients with atherosclerotic coronary artery disease (abstr). Circulation 1999; **100**: 1–681P.
5. Kastrati A, von Beckerath N, Joost A, et al. Loading with 600 mg of clopidogrel in patienst with coronary artery disease with and without chronic clopidogrel therapy. Circulation 2004; **110**: 1916–1919.
6. Kandzari DE, Berger PB, Kastrati A, et al. ISAR-REACT Study Investigators. Influence of treatment duration with a 600-mg dose of clopidogrel before percutaneous coronary revascularization. J Am Coll Cardiol 2004; **44**: 2133–2136.
7. Steinhubl SR, Darrah S, Brennan D, et al. Optimal duration of pre-treatment with clopidogrel prior to PCI: data from the CREDO trial. Circulation 2003; **108** Suppl I: I1742.
8. Hochholzer W, Trenk D, Frundi D, et al. Time dependence of platelet inhibition after a 600-mg loading dose of clopidogrel in a large, unselected cohort of candidates

for percutaneous coronary intervention. Circulation 2005; **111**: 2560–2564.

9. European Society of Cardiology Guidelines for Percutaneous Coronary Intervention. Eur Heart J 2005; **26**: 804.

10. Gurbel PA, Bliden KP, Hayes KM, *et al.* The relation of dosing to clopidogrel responsiveness and the incidence of high post-treatment platelet aggregation in patients undergoing coronary stenting. J Am Coll Cardiol 2005; **45**: 1392–1396.

11. Patti G, Colonna G, Pasceri V, *et al.* A randomized trial of high loading dose of clopidogrel for reduction of peri-procedural myocardial infarction in patients undergoing coronary intervention. Eur Heart J 2005; Abstract Suppl. P433.

12. Patti G, Chello M, Colonna D, *et al.* Clinical benefit of pre-treatment with high dose of clopidogrel before percutaneous coronary intervention is associated with lower procedural levels of P-selectin. Results from the ARMYDA-2 (Antiplatelet therapy for Reduction of MYocardial Damage during Angioplasty) SELECT substudy. J Am Coll Cardiol 2006; **47**(Suppl 2): 18 B.

13. Angiolillo DJ, Fernandez-Ortiz A, Bernardo E, *et al.* Clopidogrel withdrawal is associated with proinflammatory and prothrombotic effects in patients with diabetes and coronary artery disease. Diabetes 2006; **55**: 780–784.

14. Angiolillo DJ, Fernandez-Ortiz A, Bernardo E, *et al.* High clopidogrel loading dose during coronary stenting: effects on drug response and interindividual variability. Eur Heart J 2004; **25**: 1903–1910.

15. Geisler T, Langer H, Wydymus M, *et al.* Low response to clopidogrel is associated with cardiovascular outcome after coronary stent implantation Eur Heart J 2006; **27**: 2420–2425.

16. Montalescot G, Sideris G, Meuleman C, *et al.* A randomized comparison of high clopidogrel loading doses in patients with non-ST-segment elevation acute coronary syndromes: the ALBION (Assessment of the Best Loading Dose of Clopidogrel to Blunt Platelet Activation, Inflammation and Ongoing Necrosis) trial. J Am Coll Cardiol 2006; **48**: 931–938.

17. von Beckerath N, Taubert D, Pogatsa-Murray G, *et al.* Absorption, metabolization, and antiplatelet effects of 300-, 600-, and 900-mg loading doses of clopidogrel: results of the ISAR-CHOICE (Intracoronary Stenting and Antithrombotic Regimen: Choose Between 3 High Oral Doses for Immediate Clopidogrel Effect) Trial. Circulation 2005; **112**: 2946–2950.

18. Mehta SR, Bassand JP, Chrolavicus S, *et al.* Design and Rationale of CURRENT-OASIS 7: a randomized 2 × 2 factorial trial evaluating optimal doses of clopidogrel and aspirin in patients with ST and non-ST elevation acute coronary syndromes managed with an early invasive strategy. Am Heart J 2008; **156**: 1080–1088.

19. Kastrati A, Mehilli J, Schuhlen H, *et al.* A clinical trial of abciximab in elective percutaneous coronary intervention after pretreatment with clopidogrel. N Engl J Med 2004; **350**: 232–238.

20. Kastrati A, Mehilli J, Neumann FJ, *et al.* Abciximab in patients with acute coronary syndromes undergoing percutaneous coronary intervention after clopidogrel pretreatment: the ISAR-REACT 2 randomized trial. JAMA 2006; **295**: 1531–1538.

21. Gurbel PA, Bliden KP, Zaman KA, *et al.* Clopidogrel loading with eptifibatide to arrest the reactivity of platelets: results of the Clopidogrel Loading With Eptifibatide to Arrest the Reactivity of Platelets (CLEAR PLATELETS) study. Circulation 2005; **111**: 1153–1159.

22. Patti G, Pasceri V, Colonna G, *et al.* Role of an Additional Clopidogrel Loading Before Percutaneous Coronary Intervention in Patients on Chronic Therapy. Preliminary Results of the ARMYDA-4 (Antiplatelet therapy for Reduction of MYocardial Damage during Angioplasty) Randomized Trial. Eur Heart J 2007; Abstract Suppl. P2007.

23. Wiviott SD, Antman EM, Winters KJ, *et al.* Randomized comparison of prasugrel (CS-747, LY640315), a novel thienopyridine P2Y12 antagonist, with clopidogrel in percutaneous coronary intervention: results of the Joint Utilization of Medications to Block Platelets Optimally (JUMBO)-TIMI 26 trial. Circulation 2005; **111**: 3366–3373.

24. Wiviott SD, Braunwald E, McCabe CH, *et al.* Prasugrel versus Clopidogrel in patients with acute coronary syndromes. N Engl J Med 2007; **357**: 2001–2015.

25. Wiviott SD, Trenk D, Frelinger AL, *et al.* Prasugrel compared with high loading- and maintenance-dose clopidogrel in patients with planned percutaneous coronary intervention: The Prasugrel in Comparison to Clopidogrel for Inhibition of Platelet Activation and Aggregation-Thrombolysis in Myocardial Infarction 44 trial. Circulation 2007; **116**: 2923–2932.

26. Cannon C, Husted S, Storey R, *et al.*, for the DISPERSE 2 Investigators. The DISPERSE 2 Trial: safety, tolerability and preliminary efficacy of AZD6140, the first oral reversible ADP receptor antagonist, compared with clopidogrel in patients with non–STsegment elevation acute coronary syndrome. Circulation 2005; **112** Suppl II: 615.

27. Wallentin L, Becker RC, Budaj A, *et al.* Ticagrelor versus Clopidogrel in Patients with Acute Coronary Syndromes. N Engl J Med 2009; **361**.

CHAPTER 9

Heparin, LMWH, GIIb/IIIa, and Direct Thrombin Inhibitors

Eric Heller, & George D. Dangas
Columbia University Medical Center, New York, NY, USA

Introduction

Aspirin and unfractionated heparin have been the mainstay of anti-coagulation in ischemic coronary disease for over a quarter of a century. However, pharmacologic treatment options have expanded rapidly over the past decade with the advent of glycoprotein IIB/IIIA inhibitors, low molecular weight heparins, direct thrombin inhibitors and factor Xa inhibitors. Discrete bodies of evidence have emerged to support the use of each of these agents along the spectrum of urgent/elective percutaneous coronary intervention, acute coronary syndromes, and acute myocardial infarction. This chapter will examine the primary data which guides the use of each agent in these three scenarios and synthesize this data to make summary recommendations for best clinical practice.

Heparin

Structure and Function

Heparin was fortuitously isolated from a dog liver in 1916. Its structure was elucidated some twenty years later at approximately the same time it was introduced into clinical practice. Unfractionated

Interventional Cardiology, First Edition. Edited by Carlo Di Mario, George D. Dangas, Peter Barlis.
© 2010 Blackwell Publishing Ltd. Published 2010 by Blackwell Publishing Ltd.

heparin (UFH) is a sulfated glycosaminoglycan composed of alternating uronate and glucosamine units that contain straight chain mucopolysaccharides of highly variable length. This complex heterogeneous substance has a molecular weight ranging from 3–30 kDa with a mean of 15 kDa.

Heparin functions as an indirect thrombin inhibitor, exerting its effects through the endogenous serine protease antithrombin III (Figure 9.1). As AT complexes with heparin it undergoes a conformational change, accelerating its enzymatic activity by 1000X to 4000X. This results in the rapid inhibition of factor IIA (thrombin), factor Xa, and, to a lesser extent, factors IXa, XIa and Xa (Figure 9.2). Heparin requires a specific pentasaccharide motif for AT binding and polysaccharide chains of at least 18 units of length for thrombin inactivation (ternary complex formation with AT and thrombin) (Figure 9.3).

Clinically, heparin prevents the formation and propagation of thrombus in acute coronary syndromes (ACS), acute myocardial infractions (AMI), and percutaneous coronary interventions (PCI). In fact, despite the advent of new pharmacologic therapies and intracoronary interventions UFH remains the standard of care for anticoagulation in ischemic heart disease.

ACS

Several randomized trials constructed the foundation for heparin use in ACS. The heparin versus atenolol trial randomized 214 ACS patients to

Heparin	Enoxaparin	Direct Thrombin Inhibitors

• Indirect thrombin inhibitor
 	
• Non-specific binding to:
  •Serine proteases
  •Endothelial cells
 	
• Reduced effect in ACS
  •Inhibited by PF-4
  •Clot-bound thrombin
 	
• Causes platelet aggregation
 	
• Nonlinear pharmacokinetics
 	
• Risk of HIT
	• Indirect thrombin inhibitor
	
	• Less non-specific binding than UFH
	
	• Reduced effect in ACS
	  •Compared to UFH, markedly less inhibition by PF-4
	  •Clot-bound thrombin
	
	• Causes much less platelet aggregation than UFH
	
	• Predictable anticoagulation
	
	• Markedly reduced risk of HIT
		• Do not require a cofactor
		
		• Not inhibited by PF-4 or anti-heparin proteins
		
		• Effective against clot-bound thrombin
		
		• No platelet aggregation
		
		• Predictable anticoagulation
		
		• No thrombocytopenia

Figure 9.1. Comparison of different antithrombotic agents.

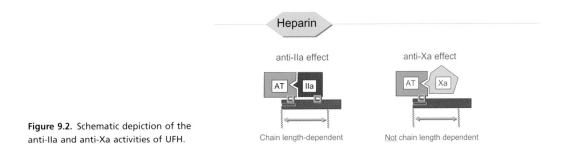

Figure 9.2. Schematic depiction of the anti-IIa and anti-Xa activities of UFH.

heparin, atenolol or placebo [1]. Heparin, but not atenolol, was associated with a significant reduction in transmural MI. The Canadian heparin-aspirin trial randomized 479 ACS patients to heparin, ASA or both [2]. Heparin (alone and in combination) was associated with a significant reduction in MI compared to aspirin alone. The ATACS trial randomized 214 patients to aspirin versus a combination of aspirin and heparin followed by warfarin [3]. ASA/heparin/warfarin therapy was associated with a significant reduction in the primary endpoint of 2 week recurrent death, MI or recurrent angina that persisted at 12 weeks. Bleeding was slightly increased with combination therapy. A meta-analysis of six randomized studies demonstrated a significant reduction in death or

MI with heparin/ASA combination therapy as opposed to aspirin alone [4]. These initial trials established the ischemic benefit of heparin, the routine use of heparin in ACS and optimized dosing and bolus plus continuous infusion as opposed to intermittent bolus therapy.

Discontinuation of heparin may result in rebound ischemia within 12 hours of discontinuation secondary to thrombin activation and clot formation. This is averted with concomitant administration of anti-platelet therapy (ASA, thienopyridine, GP IIB/IIIA inhibitor).

There is no evidence for a direct correlation between the degree of anticoagulation once heparin is therapeutic and ischemic clinical endpoints (bleeding is clearly increased). Therefore the optimal

Heparin Activities

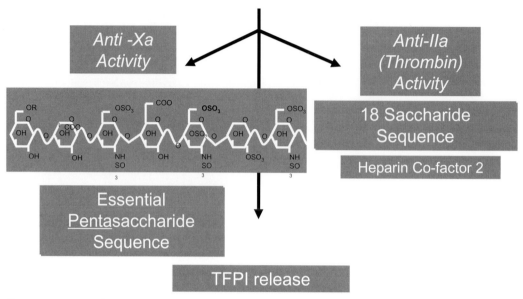

Figure 9.3. Structural depiction of the anti-IIa and anti-Xa activities of UFH.

therapeutic window had been set as 1.5–2X control activated partial thromboplastin time (PTT).

Despite limitations of the data (many studies underpowered for clinical outcomes) heparin remains the gold standard for anticoagulation in ACS and is an ACC/AHA class I indication for anticoagulation in ACS with either a conservative or invasive strategy (Figure 9.4) [5].

AMI

Thrombolysis

In AMI the greatest risk for recurrent thrombosis and MI occurs during the first 24 hours following thrombolysis. Thrombin activity increases along with that of other coagulation factors. The rationale behind heparin therapy is to prevent thrombus formation during this critical period. There is some data to suggest heparin favorably impacts ischemic clinical outcomes with the use of fibrin specific lytic agents such as alteplase, tenecteplase, and reteplase. However when using non-fibrin specific lytic therapy such as streptokinase or anistreplase, heparin does not appear to have any effect on infarct vessel patency or hard clinical

endpoints such as death or recurrent MI [6–9]. The ISIS-3 and GISSI-2/International trials showed that delayed subcutaneous heparin therapy (12,500 U SC twice daily starting 4 and 12 hours following thrombolysis respectively) does not have any mortality benefit compared to IV heparin therapy and results in more bleeding complications [10–12].

The most recent ACC/AHA guidelines recommend the routine use of heparin with fibrin specific thrombolytic therapy to continue for 48 hours following thrombolysis (Figure 9.4) [13]. Heparin is only recommended for use with streptokinase or anistreplase when the patient is at a high risk for systemic embolization (i.e. atrial fibrillation, left ventricular thrombus, poor LV function, large or anterior MI) (Figure 9.4).

Primary PCI

Heparin was initially used in the angioplasty era as adjunctive therapy to prevent abrupt vessel closure during primary PCI. The advent of stents, GP IIB/IIIA inhibitors and thienopyridines has significantly reduced this risk of abrupt closure. However,

ACC/AHA Guidelines for UFH in ACS
Class I Recommendations

Patients in whom an early invasive strategy is selected
Patients in whom a conservative strategy

ACC/AHA Guidelines for UFH in AMI
Class I Recommendations

Percutaneous or surgical revascularization
Reperfusion with fibrin-specific thrombolytics (alteplase, reteplase, tenecteplase)
Reperfusion with nonselective thrombolytics (streptokinase, urokinase, anistreplase) who are at high risk for systemic emboli (large or anterior MI, atrial fibrillation, LV thrombus, previous embolus)

Class II Recommendations

Anticoagulation with no reperfusion	IIA
Reperfusion with streptokinase in low to intermediate risk patients	IIB

Figure 9.4. ACC/AHA recommendations for UFH use in ACS, Circulation 2007; **116**(7): e148–304, ACC/AHA recommendations for UFH use in AMI. Circulation 2004; **110**: 588–636. (Source: *American Heart Association, Inc.*).

	Median molecular weight	Anti-Xa IU/mg	Anti-IIa IU/mg	Xa/IIa
Enoxaparin	4800	104	32	3.3
Dalteparin	5000	122	60	2.0
Nadroparin	4500	94	31	3.0
Tinzaparin	4500	90	50	1.8
Clivarine	3900	130	40	3.3

Figure 9.5. Comparison of Low Molecular Weight Heparins.

heparin remains the standard of care for antithrombotic therapy in this scenario (Figure 9.5) [13]. Heparin is often administered as a bolus prior to PCI, and is given intermittently to maintain an ACT between 250 and 300 seconds in the presence and >300 seconds in the absence of GP IIB/IIIA inhibitors. Heparin is discontinued at the end of PCI and sheath removal occurs when ACT reaches ≤150–180 seconds.

No Reperfusion

Heparin is often used in the absence of reperfusion therapy to prevent further thrombus formation

(Figure 9.6) [13]. There is little data to support its use in the presence of aspirin [14,15], especially in patients who are at a high risk of bleeding such as the elderly [16].

Special Considerations

Heparin should be continued and anticoagulation transitioned to warfarin for a duration of six months in patients who either have a large anterior MI or develop a left ventricular thrombus. If the patient has undergone PCI, heparin should not be restarted until 4–6 hours following sheath removal or vessel closure.

Elective/Urgent PCI

Heparin is used during urgent or elective PCI to prevent abrupt vessel closure. The parameters for dosing, stoppage and sheath removal are the same as those with *primary PCI*.

Dosing Guidelines

For ACS/AMI heparin is initiated with a bolus of 60 units/kg and a maintenance infusion of 12 units/kg/hr to achieve a goal PTT of 1.5–2X control (50–70 seconds). PTT should be checked every 4–6 hours. Heparin should be continued through the completion of cardiac catheterization/PCI with an

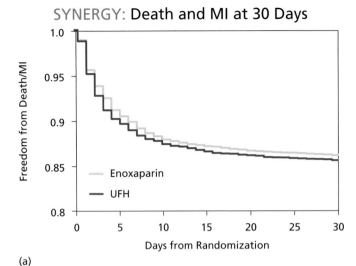

SYNERGY: **Death and MI at 30 Days**

SYNERGY: **Bleeding Events**

	Enoxaparin (n = 4993)	UFH (n = 4985)	P-value
GUSTO severe	2.9	2.4	0.106
TIMI major	9.1	7.6	0.008
CABG-related	6.8	5.9	0.081
Non-CABG-related	2.4	1.8	0.025
H/H drop – algorithm	15.2	12.5	0.001
Any RBC transfusion	17.0	16.0	0.155
ICH	< 0.1	< 0.1	NS

(b)

Figure 9.6. Synergy: (a) death and MI and (b) bleeding at 30 days JAMA: 2004; **292**: 45–54. Copyright © (2004) American Medical Association. All rights reserved.

early invasive strategy/primary PCI and for 48–72 hours with a conservative strategy. In the setting of AMI and thrombolysis dosing and target PTT are the same but heparin is continued for 48 hours. For PCI heparin bolus and maintenance infusion are administered to maintain an ACT of 250–300 in the absence and 200–250 in the presence of a GP IIB/IIIA inhibitor. Heparin is discontinued at the end of the procedure. Heparin has a half life of 1–2 hours.

Reversal

In the event of bleeding complications the ant-IIa effects of heparin may be reversed by the administration of protamine sulfate. Protamine should be given as a slow IV infusion administration of 1 mg of protamine/100 units of circulating heparin remaining results in full reversal. Intermittent readministration may be required in patients who have received large doses of subcutaneous heparin. Patients should not receive a protamine bolus of >25–50 mg and should not receive an infusion >20–50 mg/min over any 10 minute period. Excess protamine administration may lead to paradoxical anticoagulation. Those who have been previously exposed to protamine, including diabetics receiving NPH insulin, have a 1% risk of a hypersensitivity/anaphylactic reaction.

Limitations

The use of heparin has a number of limitations and can result in serious complications (Figure 9.4). Heparin is unable to bind clot-bound thrombin or factor Xa bound to platelets in the prothrombinase complex. It does bind non-specifically to platelets, macrophages and endothelial cells, and can activate platelet function, possibly through a GPIIB/IIIA receptor pathway. These phenomena theoretically reduce heparin's ischemic efficacy. Heparin may bind to osteoblasts, leading to the release of osteoclast activating factors. Prolonged use (>6 months) may cause osteoporosis. Heparin also binds plasma proteins; its interaction with platelet factor 4 may results in neoepitope formation and the production of antibodies that leads to heparin induced thrombocytopenia (HIT) type 2. All of this non-specific binding results in a variable dose–response relationship, a narrow therapeutic window. The XLM fraction [or "extra large" material (>8 kDa) heparin contains] may also contribute to an increased risk of hemorrhagic complications.

Heparin Induced Thrombocytopenia

As many as 20% of patients receiving UFH may experience thrombocytopenia or and/or >50% drop in their platelet count after 48 hours of initiation of therapy. This thrombocytopenia is often benign, usually normalized even with continued heparin therapy, and is often referred to as heparin induced thrombocytopenia (HIT) type 1. HIT-1 is thought to result as a byproduct of platelet.

In 0.2–0.3% of individuals receiving heparin, platelet counts will drop precipitously (thrombocytopenia with median count 60,000/μl, >50% drop in initial platelet count) after 4–10 days following initial administration and will not reverse. Thrombocytopenia is often associated with thrombotic and rarely with hemorrhagic complications (i.e. adrenal hemorrhage). This serious disorder is referred to as HIT type 2 (HIT-2). Early onset HIT-2 occurs <10.5 hours after the initiation of heparin and is seen in the setting of previous heparin exposure within 3–4 months' time. Delayed onset HIT-2 occurs after termination of heparin therapy.

HIT-2 results from IgG and IgM antibody formation to a neoepitope created by the heparin-PF4 complex. Antibody formation leads to platelet consumption and often thrombosis; antibodies may also mediate heparin induced skin necrosis. The heparin-PF4-antibody complex may bind platelet Fc-γ-RIIA, leading to platelet activation, PF4 release and further propagation of platelet activation. The same complex may bind microvascular endothelial cells leading to the release of platelet secretagogues and adhesion molecules. Furthermore, the heparin-PF4-antibody complex may interact with monocytes to cause the release of tissue factor.

Thrombosis occurs in up to 75–90% of patients with HIT-2 and is more commonly occurs in the venous (DVT/PE, gangrene, cerebral sinus thrombosis) as opposed to the arterial (MI, stroke, acute limb ischemia, mesenteric ischemia) circulation.

HIT-2 is a clinical diagnosis but may be aided by laboratory testing. Many hospitals use ELISA to detect antibodies to the heparin-PF4 complex. This test is highly sensitive (>90–95% sensitivity) but much less specific (75–85% specificity) for HIT-2. Serotonin release and heparin-induced platelet aggregation have also been utilized to aid in making a diagnosis.

The first step in the treatment of HIT-2 is the immediate cessation of all heparin therapy including subcutaneous heparin and heparin flushes. In the United States direct thrombin (argatroban and lepirudin are FDA approved) inhibitors are used to prevent primary or recurrent thrombosis (the heparin analogue danapranoid is used outside of the USA). Details of therapy are discussed below in the section on direct thrombin inhibitors. If a patient has thrombocytopenia but not thrombosis, a DTI is continued until the platelet count normalizes. Observation is reasonable if the patient is at high risk for bleeding but bear in mind that the patient is still at risk for thrombosis. If a patient requires ongoing anticoagulation for thrombosis or a comorbidity (AF, mechanical valve) then a DTI is continued and overlapped with warfarin therapy for at least five days. Warfarin should be continued for 2–3 months (INR 2–3) in the absence and 3–6 months in the presence of thrombosis. Heparin may be re-introduced for short periods of time in HIT-2 patients who are clear of antibodies because the assumption is it would take approximately three days tom mount an anamnestic response to repeated exposure. This may occur in the setting of surgery requiring cardiopulmonary bypass.

Low Molecular Weight Heparin

Structure and Function

Low molecular weight heparin (LMWH) is produced through the enzymatic or chemical (nitrous acid, alkaline) degradation of UFH. These processes result in smaller molecules containing shorter polysaccharide chains (Figure 9.5). The molecular weight of LMWH ranges from 2–9 kDa with an average of 4–5 kDa. LMWH has a few theoretical advantages over UFH. LMWH still acts through AT, but because many of its chains contain <18 monosaccharides they cannot form a ternary complex with AT and thrombin; therefore LMWH has preferential anti-Xa as opposed to anti-thrombin activity.

LMWH has complete bioavailability, greater than twice the half life of UFH (4.5–7 hours for enoxaparin) and a predictable dose response relationship. It can therefore be administered subcutaneously. LMWH incurs much less non-specific binding and therefore presents a lower risk of HIT-2 and results in less platelet activation than with UFH. LMWH is cleared predominantly by the kidneys but also by the reitculoendothelial system. This becomes important for dosing in renal failure. Enoxaparin is the best studied LMWH for ischemic prophylaxis in coronary artery disease (Figure 9.1).

ACS

Initial trials of LMWH in ACS focussed almost exclusively on its use in a conservative strategy. A meta-analysis of ESSENCE and TIMI 11B evaluated over 7000 ACS patients undergoing a conservative strategy were randomized to either UFH or enoxaparin. Enoxaparin was associated with a 20% reduction in death and major ischemic events (non-fatal MI, urgent revascularization) within the first few days of treatment that persisted through 43 days. Enoxaparin was associated with a significant increase in minor, but not major bleeding. To reduce this section, it is better to talk about the meta-analysis of these two trials that employed conservative (selective invasive strategy for ACS) enoxaparin therapy. FRISC randomized 1506 ACS patients to dalteparin versus placebo. Dalteparin was associated with a significant decrease in the primary endpoint of death and recurrent MI which persisted at 40 days. There was no difference in major or minor bleeding [17]. Phase A of the A to Z trial studied 3987 ACS patients who received tirofiban plus either enoxaparin or UFH for up to seven days [18]. Sixty percent of patients received an early invasive strategy. The study met non-inferiority criteria for enoxaparin with respect to the primary endpoint of death, MI or refractory ischemia at seven days. Subgroup analysis suggested the combination of tirofiban and enoxaparin was superior to tirofiban plus UFH in patients undergoing a conservative strategy. There was a significant increase in major bleeding with enoxaparin.

Since most patients with ACS in the USA undergo an early invasive strategy it was important to evaluate enoxaparin within this treatment framework. SYNERGY was the major study that accomplished this goal. In SYNERGY 10027 high risk ACS patients assigned to an early invasive strategy received either open-label enoxaparin (1 mg/kg) or UFH until anticoagulation was no longer required as judged by the patient's treating physician [19]. The majority of patients received contemporary pharmacologic therapy including ASA (95%)\, thienopyridines (66%) and GP IIB/IIIA inhibitors (57%). 92% of patients underwent coronary angiography (47% PCI, 19% CABG). For those undergoing PCI who were assigned to enoxaparin, if the last enoxaparin dose was given <8 hours prior to the procedure no additional drug was given. If the last enoxaparin dose was given >8 hours prior to PCI 0.3 mg/kg of enoxaparin was administered prior to any intervention. The enoxaparin group met non-inferiority criteria with respect to the primary efficacy composite endpoint of 30 day all-cause death or non-fatal MI (Figure 9.6a). No significant differences were observed for ischemic events during PCI including abrupt closure, threatened abrupt closure, unsuccessful PCI or emergency CABG. Seventy-five percent of trial patients received antithrombin therapy prior to randomization. Enoxaparin demonstrated a statistically significant reduction in the primary endpoint for those who received either no antithrombin therapy prior randomization or received the same pre- and post randomization therapy. There was a significant increase in bleeding complications

ACC/AHA Guidelines for Enoxaparin in ACS
Class I Recommendations

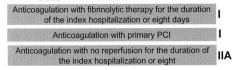

Patients undergoing an invasive strategy

Patients undergoing a conservative strategy

Class II Recommendations

Enoxaparin is preferable to UFH in patients undergoing a conservative strategy unless CABG is planned within 24 hours	IIA

ACC/AHA Guidelines for Enoxaparin in AMI
Class II Recommendations for LMWH

Anticoagulation with fibrinolytic therapy for the duration of the index hospitalization or eight days	I
Anticoagulation with primary PCI	I
Anticoagulation with no reperfusion for the duration of the index hospitalization or eight	IIA

Figure 9.7. ACC/AHA recommendations for LMWH use in ACS, Circulation 2007; **116**(7):e148–304, ACC/AHA recommendations for LMWH use in AMI, Circulation 2004; **110**: 588–636. (Source: *American Heart Association, Inc.*).

with enoxaparin, specifically TIMI major bleeding (Figure 9.6b).

Enoxaparin (dosed as 1mg/kg SQ BID) is certainly as efficacious as UFH for anticoagulant therapy in ACS. In fact, according to the 2007 ACC/AHA guidelines the overall weight of the evidence in ACS favors enoxaparin and provides a class 1 recommendation to this drug regardless of treatment strategy (Figure 9.7) [5]. Enoxaparin has been shown to be superior to UFH in a conservative strategy (ESSENCE, TIMI 11B, FRISC, A to Z), and, by subgroup analysis, in high risk patients (troponin positive, TIMI risk score ≥4). (TIMI 11B, FRISC). SYNERGY showed that enoxaparin has similar ischemic efficacy to UFH in an early invasive strategy but results in more major bleeding. Therefore, one must balance the advantages of LMWH (ease of administration, decreased incidence of HIT-2, lack of required laboratory monitoring) with the ischemic and bleeding risks of the individual patient.

Acute Myocardial Infarction

In CREATE 15570 patients from India and China presenting with ST-elevation MI or new left bundle branch block were randomly assigned to either placebo or the LMWH reviparin [20]. 73% of patients received thrombolysis (predominantly streptokinase). There was a significant reduction in of death, recurrent MI or stroke with the use of reviparin that was greater with early initiation of reviparin therapy. This benefit persisted over 30 days.

Three major trials compared UFH to LMWH in AMI. ASSENT-3 randomized 6095 AMI patients to full dose tenecteplase plus enoxaparin for ≤7 days, half-dose tenecteplase plus low dose UFH and abciximab for 12 hours or full dose tenecteplase plus UFH for 48 hours [21]. The primary endpoint of 30 day death, in-hospital reinfarction or in-hospital refractory ischemia was significantly reduced mortality in both the enoxaparin and abciximab arms compared to UFH alone. In addition there was a significant reduction in recurrent MI for the same two groups at 30 days. There was a significant increase in bleeding in patients over 75 for those who received enoxaparin [22].

ASSENT-3 PLUS randomized 1639 patients with AMI who received pre-hospital tenecteplase to enoxaparin or UFH [23] . There was no difference with regards to the primary endpoint of 30 day mortality or in-hospital reinfarction, but there was a trend toward increased mortality with enoxaparin and a significant increase in stroke and intracranial hemorrhage. Virtually all of the intracranial hemorrhages occurred in patients older than 75.

EXTRACT TIMI-25 randomized 20,506 patients with AMI receiving thrombolytic therapy to enoxaparin (30 mg IV bolus followed by 1mg/kg SC BID for a mean of seven days) or UFH (≥ 48 hours) [24]. Enoxaparin was associated with a significant reduction in the primary endpoint of 30 day death or MI (driven by a reduction in recurrent MI). There was also a significant reduction in urgent revascularization. Further analysis showed benefit in all subgroups, including those who received streptokinase (previous trials had not shown any significant benefit for LMWH as compared to UFH) and those who had PCI within 30 days of presentation. Enoxaparin was, however, associated with an increase in major bleeding.

LMWH is considered an AHA/ACC class I alternative to UFH as anticoagulant therapy with fibrinolysis in AMI for the duration of the index hospitalization or eight days (Figure 9.7) [13,25]. The best studied regimen is that from the EXTRACT-TIMI 25 trial and should ideally be used with full dose tenecteplase.

Primary PCI

Enoxaparin is an ACC/AHA class I alternative to UFH in primary PCI based upon data from CREATE and EXTRACT-TIMI 25 (Figure 9.7) [25].

No Reperfusion

In CREATE 3325/15570 patients randomized did not receive any reperfusion therapy. In this group treatment with reviparin resulted in a significant reduction in death, recurrent MI or stroke as compared with UFH. TETAMI randomized 1224 patients with AMI who did not receive any reperfusion therapy to enoxaparin or UFH and then to tirofiban or placebo [26]. There was no significant difference in the primary endpoint of death, reinfarction or recurrent angina with enoxaparin. It is reasonable to conclude there is sufficient evidence for LMWH as an alternative therapy to UFH for anticoagulation in AMI for patients who do not receive reperfusion therapy. Patients should receive LMWH for the duration of the index hoispitalization or eight days [13,25] (Figure 9.7).

PCI

SYNERGY evaluated the safety and efficacy of enoxaparin within the context of an early invasive strategy in 10,027 patients with high risk ACS. These results and the dosing protocol may be extrapolated for use in elective and urgent PCI, with the caveat of potentially increased bleeding with enoxaparin versus UFH. STEEPLE was an open-label trial that randomized 3528 patients undergoing elective PCI to either IV enoxaparin (0.5 ton 0.75 mg/kg) or UFH [27]. The primary endpoint of non-CABG bleeding over 48 hours was significantly reduced for the lower dose (0.5 mg/kg) but not the higher dose (0.75 mg/kg) group. Major bleeding was significantly reduced in both enoxaparin groups and with more predictable anticoagulation. A trial dedicated to ischemic efficacy and safety will be required before enoxaparin can be routinely recommended as alternative anticoagulant therapy in elective/urgent PCI.

Dosing Guidelines

Enoxaparin should be administered at a dose of 1 mg/kg SC BID in USA patients receiving a conservative strategy and AMI patients receiving thrombolytic or no reperfusion therapy. Pharmacotherapy should be continued for at least 48 hours. Enoxaparin should be administered per the SYNERGY protocol (1 mg/kg SC BID with a bolus of 0.3 mg/kg IV before PCI if the last dose was administered >8 hours prior to intervention) in ACS patients receiving an early invasive strategy.

Enoxaparin therapy should be reduced to 1 mg/kg daily in patients with a creatinine clearance<30 L/min and is contraindicated in dialysis. Caution should be used when treating the elderly and patients at both extremes of the weight spectrum for fear of an unreliable dose-response and an increased risk of bleeding.

A rough estimate of anticoagulation with LMWH may be contained my measuring antifactor Xa activity; however, anti-Xa activity does not correlate well with the risk of bleeding or thrombosis.

Protamine may reverse the anti-IIa effect of the higher molecular weight components of heparin but does not completely reverse the drug's anti-Xa activity. Protamine administered as 1 mg/100 units of circulating LMWH can reduce clinical bleeding. The dose should be reduced if LMWH was given >8 hours before the inciting bleeding event.

Limitations

LMWH can cause HIT-2, although the incidence is markedly decreased compared to UFH therapy. LMWH is also associated with bleeding complications without an ideal option for reversal. Enoxparin accumulates in the setting of renal failure and must be dosed accordingly to avoid bleeding complications. There is no viable reversal option for LMWH, although protamine may inhibit anti-IIA effects.

Glycoprotein IIB/IIIA Inhibitors

The IIB/IIIA integrin receptor on the surface of platelets binds preferentially to collagen and fibrinogen as well as fibronectin, vitronectin, and Von Willebrand's Factor. IIB/IIIA activation triggers the final common pathway of platelet aggregation: fibrinogen cross-linking of platelets. Activation of the receptor also fosters platelet adhesion to the vascular endothelial surface. GP IIB/IIIA inhibitors abrogate the effects of the IIB/IIIA receptor on

	Abciximab	Eptifibatide	Tirofiban
Type	Monoclonal antibody fragment	Small molecule (KGD sequence)	Small molecule (RGD sequence)
Platelet-Bound Half-life	Long (hours)	Short (secs)	Short (secs)
Plasma Half-life	Short (mins)	Long (2.5 hours)	Long (2 hours)
Drug-to-Receptor Ratio	1.5–2.0	250–2,500[*]	>250[†]
% of Dose in Bolus	~75%[‡]	<2–5%	<2–5%
Dosage Adjustment in Renal Insufficiency	None	Yes	Yes

*IMPACT-II and PURSUIT doses.
†RESTORE and PRISM-PLUS doses.
‡For any individual receiving a weight-adjusted, 12-hour infusion.

	Abciximab	Eptifibatide	Tirofiban
Specificity/Selectivity			
IIb/IIIa	xxx	xxx	xxx
$\alpha_v\beta_3$	xxx	x	
Mac-1	x		
Anticoagulant Properties			
↓Thrombin Generation	++	+	+
↑Activated Clotting Time[§]	+30 sec	+20 sec	0
Reversibility Without Platelets*	24 hours	~4 hours†	~4 hours†
Reversibility With Platelets	Yes	No	No

§ With high-dose heparin (100U/kg)
*50% return of platelet function with/without platelet transfusion.
†Assumes adequate renal function.

Figure 9.8. Characteristics of GP IIB/IIIA inhibitors.

platelet aggregation and adhesion through reversible or irreversible inhibition. There are three different GP IIB/IIIA inhibitors commercially available in the USA (Figure 9.8).

Abciximab

Abciximab is a chimeric murine-human monoclonal antibody that consists of the FAB fragment of a murine GP IIB/IIIA antibody fused the constant region of human IgG. Abciximab binds to platelets with high affinity and irreversibly. It is a long acting agent (>48 hours) whose effects are reversible with platelet transfusions. Abciximab is rapid in onset, has a half life of 30 minutes, and causes complete platelet inhibition within two hours of administration. Abciximab is eliminated by protease degradation. Patients may produce anti-chimeric antibodies; however hypersensitivity/anaphylactic reactions to abciximab are rare.

Eptifibatide

Eptifibatide is a non-immunogenic cyclic heptapeptide that reversibly inhibits the platelet IIB/IIIA receptor as a competitive inhibitor of the fibrinogen binding site. Eptifibatide contains an active pharmacophore derived from barbourin, the primary component of southeastern pigmy rattlesnake poison. This agent is short acting (2–4 hours) and its effects are not reversible platelet transfusions. Eptifibatide is rapid in onset, has a half life 2.5 hours and causes high level platelet inhibition within two hours prior to administration. Eptifibatide is cleared predominantly by the kidneys (75% renal, 25% hepatic clearance) and should be dosed with caution in patients with renal insufficiency.

Tirofiban

Tirofiban is a reversible non-peptide GP IIB/IIIA inhibitor that acts as a competitive inhibitor of the fibrinogen binding site. This agent is short acting (2–4 hours) and its effects are not reversible with platelet transfusions. Tirofiban is slower in onset than the other two GP IIB/IIIA inhibitors, has a half life of two hours, and causes high level platelet inhibition within two hours after administration. Caution should be used for dosing in renal insufficiency.

ACS

Abciximab has been well studied in ACS. EPIC evaluated 2099 patients with USA, NSTEMI, or high risk anatomy undergoing either PTCA or atherectomy [28]. Patients received ASA and heparin, and were randomized to either abciximab or placebo immediately prior to PCI. Abciximab was associated with a significant reduction in the primary composite endpoint of 30 day death, MI, or urgent repeat revascularization. This benefit was maintained out to three year follow-up. Subgroup analysis suggested that USA/NSTEMI patients derived the greatest benefit from abciximab.

CAPTURE randomized 1265 patients with refractory ACS to abciximab vs. placebo given 18–24 hours prior to PTCA [29]. Abciximab was associated with a significant reduction in the primary endpoint of 30 day death, MI or urgent revascularization. The benefit of abciximab was driven by a reduction MI. Subgroup analysis identified troponin positive patients as those most likely to benefit from abciximab therapy [30]. GUSTO 4-ACS randomized 7800 patients with ACS undergoing a conservative strategy to abciximab bolus plus 24 or 48 hour infusion versus placebo [31]. In contrast to other studies of GP IIB/IIIA inhibitors in ACS, there was no difference in the primary endpoint of 30 day death or MI and no difference in death or MI at one year [32].

ISAR-REACT 2 specifically addressed the issue of the use of GP IIB/IIIA inhibitors in combination with a thienopyridine for ACS; 2002 ACS patients undergoing an early invasive strategy who were pre-loaded with 600 mg of clopidogrel ≥2 hours prior to PCI were randomized to abciximab or placebo in the catheterization laboratory [33]. Abciximab was associated with a significant reduction in the primary endpoint of 30 day death, MI or urgent target vessel revascularization (Figure 9.9). Subgroup analysis suggests this benefit was confined to troponin positive patients.

Tirofiban is also well studied in ACS. RESTORE randomized 2139 patients with ACS undergoing PCI within 72 hours of presentation to tirofiban versus placebo [34]. Tirofiban was associated with a significant reduction in the primary endpoint of 30 day death, MI, PTCA failure requiring unplanned CABG or stenting or recurrent ischemia requiring repeat PTCA. PRISM randomized 3232 patients with ACS undergoing a conservative strategy to tirofiban or placebo [35]. Tirofiban was associated with a significant reduction in the primary endpoint of death, MI or refractory ischemia at 48 hours. Subgroup analysis suggested that high risk (troponin positive) patients derived particular benefit from tirofiban [36]. PRISM-PLUS randomized 1915 ACS patients to tirofiban, heparin, or a combination of both [37]. Catheterization after 48 hours was at the discretion of the treating physician. Tirofiban plus heparin was associated with a significant reduction in the primary endpoint of seven day death, MI or refractory ischemia (mortality) was increased with tirofiban alone). These differences persisted at 30

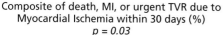

Composite of death, MI, or urgent TVR due to Myocardial Ischemia within 30 days (%)
$p = 0.03$

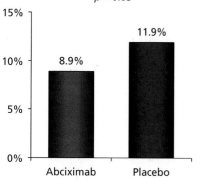

- The primary composite endpoint occurred less frequently in the abciximab group compared to placebo (8.9% vs 11.9%; relative risk [RR] 0.75 p = 0.03)

Figure 9.9. ISAR-REACT 2: primary endpoint, JAMA 2006; **295**: 1531–1538.

days and 6 months. Subgroup analysis showed that those treated conservatively and invasively both benefited from tirofiban, and that high risk patients derived particular benefit [38].

There is adequate data to support the use of eptifibatide in ACS. PURSUIT randomized just less than 11,000 ACS patients to either two different eptifibatide regimens or placebo for ≤3 days [38]. Eptifibatide was associated with a significant reduction in the primary endpoint of 30 day death or nonfatal MI. Subgroup analysis suggested that patients undergoing conservative and invasive strategies both benefited from eptifibatide therapy. IMPACT-II randomized 4010 patients undergoing PCI electively, urgently, or for ACS to low dose eptifibatide bolus and infusion, high dose eptifibatide or placebo 60 minutes prior to PCI [39]. Eptifibatide was associated with a significant reduction in the primary endpoint of 30 day death, MI, unplanned revascularization or stent placement for abrupt closure. Further analysis revealed that the low dose eptifibatide group derived particular ischemic benefit.

A meta-analysis of six randomized trials (31,400 patients) looked at the treatment of ACS with all three of the GP IIB/IIIa inhibitors for patients who received medical therapy for at least 48 hours (Figure 9.10) [40]. This meta-analysis showed a significant reduction in the primary endpoint of death or MI at five days for GP IIB/IIIA inhibitors. Significant reductions were seen for each of the two individual endpoints. Subgroup analysis suggests

this benefit was confined to patients who underwent PCI or CABG within 30 days of presentation and tom patients with positive troponin. GP II/IIIA inhibitors were associated with an increase in major bleeding.

Synthesizing this data, the following recommendation can be made regarding the use of GP IIB/IIIA inhibitors in ACS: (1) GP IIB/IIIA inhibitors should be administered to patients undergoing an early invasive strategy in the absence of clopidogrel; (2) GP IIB/IIIA inhibitors should be administered to troponin positive patients who have been pre-loaded with clopidogrel and are undergoing an early invasive strategy; (3) GP IIB/IIIA inhibitors should be administered to high risk patients (troponin positive, TIMI risk score ≥4) undergoing a conservative strategy; (4) GP IIB/IIIA inhibitors should be administered upstream at presentation; and (5) GP IIB/IIIA inhibitors should be used as bailout therapy in the setting of angiographic complications or a suboptimal angiographic result. These recommendations are in keeping with the current ACC/AHA guidelines (Figure 9.11) [5].

All of these recommendations are made in the setting of heparin therapy for anticoagulation. As described later on in more detail, bivalirudin therapy appears to be an adequate alternative in ACS to heparin plus GP IIB/IIIA inhibitors.

All three GP IIB/IIIA inhibitors have demonstrated efficacy in ACS but practical considerations dictate their individual use. Eptifibatide is often used with an early invasive strategy because it costs

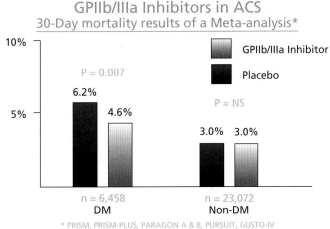

Figure 9.10. Meta-analysis of GP IIB/IIIA inhibitors in ACS. (Reproduced with permission from Platelet Glycoprotein IIb/IIIa Inhibitors Reduce Mortality in Diabetic Patients With Non-ST-Segment-Elevation Acute Coronary Syndromes, Marco Roffi, Circulation 2001; **104**: 2767–2771.)

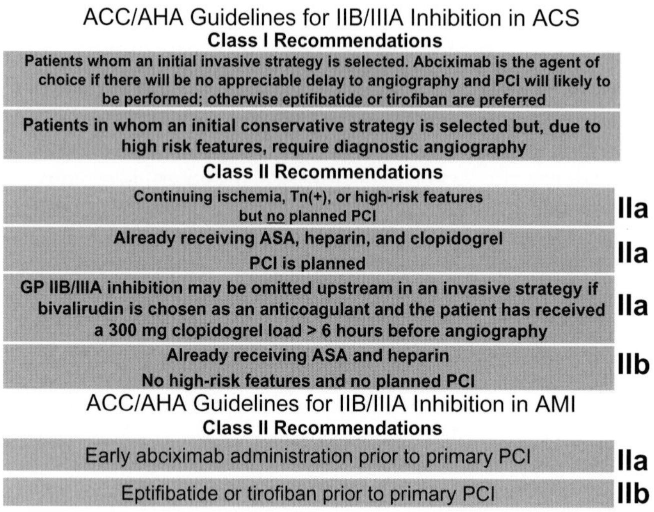

ACC/AHA Guidelines for IIB/IIIA Inhibition in ACS
Class I Recommendations

| Patients whom an initial invasive strategy is selected. Abciximab is the agent of choice if there will be no appreciable delay to angiography and PCI will likely to be performed; otherwise eptifibatide or tirofiban are preferred |
| Patients in whom an initial conservative strategy is selected but, due to high risk features, require diagnostic angiography |

Class II Recommendations

Continuing ischemia, Tn(+), or high-risk features but <u>no</u> planned PCI	IIa
Already receiving ASA, heparin, and clopidogrel PCI is planned	IIa
GP IIB/IIIA inhibition may be omitted upstream in an invasive strategy if bivalirudin is chosen as an anticoagulant and the patient has received a 300 mg clopidogrel load > 6 hours before angiography	IIa
Already receiving ASA and heparin No high-risk features and no planned PCI	IIb

ACC/AHA Guidelines for IIB/IIIA Inhibition in AMI
Class II Recommendations

| Early abciximab administration prior to primary PCI | IIa |
| Eptifibatide or tirofiban prior to primary PCI | IIb |

Figure 9.11. ACC/AHA recommendations for GP IIB/IIIA inhibition in ACS, Circulation 2007; **116**(7): e148–304, ACC/AHA recommendations for GP IIB/IIIA inhibition in AMI, Circulation 2004; **110**: 588–636. (Source: *American Heart Association, Inc.*).

less than abciximab and its standard dosing regimen has been better studied and better refined for rapid and complete platelet inhibition than that or tirofiban. Eptifibatide or Tirofiban may be administered to patients undergoing a conservative strategy.

AMI

Thrombolysis

Multiple lines of investigation have evaluated the use of half dose thrombolysis plus GP IIB/IIIA inhibitors in AMI. This regimen appears better restore coronary perfusion, accelerate ST segment resolution and reduce ischemic complications as compared to standard thrombolysis. However, large randomized trials such as GUSTO V and ASSENT 3 have found no ischemic benefit and increased bleeding for this proposed therapy [21,41,42]. There is currently no role for GP IIB/IIIA inhibitors in thrombolysis for AMI.

No Reperfusion

TETAMI randomized 1224 patients with MI who did not receive any reperfusion therapy to tirofiban or placebo. There was no difference in the primary endpoint of death, MI or recurrent angina. There is currently no role for GP IIB/IIIA inhibitors in patients with AMI who do not receive any reperfusion therapy.

Primary PCI

Abciximab is the most extensively studied GP IIB/IIIA inhibitor in primary PCI. RAPPORT randomized 483 AMI patients undergoing PTCA to abciximab versus placebo. Abciximab was associated with a significant reduction in the primary endpoint of 7 day death, MI or target vessel revascularization which persisted at 30 days [43]. There was also a reduction in the need for "bailout" stenting. The results were primarily driven by a reduction in urgent revascularization. CADILLAC randomized 2082 AMI patients to PTCA +/– abciximab or stenting +/– abciximab [44]. The composite primary endpoint of death, recurrent MI, disabling stroke or repeat ischemia-driven revascularization was significantly reduced by stenting as opposed to PTCA regardless of abciximab use.

ISAR-2 randomized 401 patients with AMI undergoing primary stenting to full dose heparin versus reduced-dose heparin plus abciximab [33]. Abciximab was associated with a significant reduction in the primary endpoint of 30 day death, recurrent MI or target lesion revascularization that did not persist one year. ADMIRAL randomized 300 patients with AMI undergoing primary PTCA or stenting to abciximab versus placebo [45]. Abciximab was associated with a significant reduction in the primary endpoint of 30 day death, recurrent MI or target vessel revascularization that persisted at six months. All-cause mortality was reduced at three years. Subgroup analysis revealed a benefit for patients who received abciximab upstream (pre-hospital, emergency room) as opposed to immediately prior to primary PCI. ACE randomized 400 patients with AMI receiving primary stenting to abciximab vs. placebo [46]. Abciximab was associated with a significant reduction in the primary endpoint of one month death, recurrent MI, target vessel revascularization or stroke. Stroke and reinfarction were both decreased with abciximab out to one year.

Tirofiban and eptifibatide have not been adequately studied as adjunctive therapy to primary PCI. A metavfbnalysis of the five randomized trials evaluating the use of abciximab in primary PCI showed that abciximab was associated with a significant reduction in mortality at 30 days and 6–12 months and a reduction in recurrent MI at 30 days [41]. There was no significant increase in bleeding.

Barring a contra-indication, patients undergoing primary PCI should receive abciximab as early as possible prior to primary PCI (Figure 9.11) [13].

Elective/Urgent PCI
EPISTENT randomized 2399 patients undergoing elective or emergent stenting to stenting alone, stenting plus abciximab or PTCA plus abciximab [47,48]. Abciximab was associated with a significant reduction in the primary endpoint of 30 day death, MI or urgent revascularization which persisted at six months. Subgroup analysis suggests that both ACS and stable angina patients benefited from abciximab therapy. Abciximab was also associated with mortality reduction at one and three years. EPILOG randomized 2792 patients undergoing elective or urgent PCI to abciximab plus standard dose heparin, abciximab plus low dose heparin or placebo plus standard dose heparin [49]. Abciximab was associated with a significant reduction in the primary endpoint of 30 day death which persisted at six months and one year. Subgroup analysis suggested abciximab reduced the primary endpoint in both low and high risk patients. ISAR-REACT randomized 2159 patients undergoing elective stenting who were pre-treated with 600 mg of clopidogrel to abciximab versus placebo [50]. There was no dif-

ference in the primary endpoint of 30 day death, MI or urgent target vessel revascularization. There was also no difference in major bleeding. ISAR-SWEET randomized 701 diabetic patients undergoing elective PCI and pre-treated with 600 mg of clopidogrel to abciximab versus placebo [51]. Although abciximab was associated with a significant reduction in angiographic restenosis at a mean of seven months, there was no difference in death or MI at one year. A study looking at patients from EPILOG and EPISTENT with complex lesions undergoing PCI found that abciximab significantly reduces one year death or MI but has no effect on target vessel revascularization [52].

As discussed above, the ADVANCE trial showed that tirofiban was associated with a reduction in death, MI, target vessel revascularization or bailout use of a GP IIB/IIIA inhibitor at 6 months; however subgroup analysis showed no difference with abciximab in patients with stable angina.

ESPRIT randomized 2064 patients undergoing elective stenting to eptifibatide versus placebo [53]. Eptifibatide was associated with a significant reduction in the primary endpoint of 48 hour death, MI, urgent target vessel revascularization, or use of a "bailout" GP IIB/IIIA inhibitor and the secondary endpoint of 30 day death, MI or urgent target vessel revascularization. Eptifibatide was also associated with a reductions in death or MI and death, MI or target vessel revascularization at one year. Subgroup analysis suggests high risk but not low risk patients benefited from eptifibatide at one year. There were no differences in angiographic complications.

Finally, TARGET randomized 4809 patients undergoing elective/urgent PCI to abciximab versus tirofiban [54]. Abciximab was associated with a significant reduction in the primary endpoint of 30 day death, MI or urgent revascularization. The primary endpoint was driven by a reduction in MI. Subgroup analysis suggested the benefit of abciximab was restricted to ACS patients and non-diabetics. There was no difference in the composite endpoint at six months. The benefit of eptifibatide over tirofiban may have been to less rapid and effective platelet inhibition with tirofiban dosing (10 μg/kg bolus and a 0.15 μg/kg/min infusion for 18–24 hours). A high dose tirofiban regimen (25 ug/kg bolus and a 0.15 µg/kg/min infusion for 18 hours) was more successful in the ADVANCE trial, likely due to more rapid and complete platelet inhibition.

The following recommendations can be made for the administration of GP IIB/IIIA inhibitors in elective or urgent PCI: (1) Either clopidogrel or a GP IIB/IIIA inhibitor should be used for ischemic prophylaxis of low–medium risk patients. (2) GP IIB/IIIA inhibitors should be considered for use in high risk patients regardless of concomitant adjunctive pharmacotherapy. (3) GP IIB/IIIA inhibitors should be used as bailout therapy in the setting of angiographic complications or a suboptimal angiographic result.

Eptifibatide is often the agent of choice in elective/urgent PCI because it costs less than abciximab and its standard dosing regimen has been better studied and better refined for rapid and complete platelet inhibition than that of tirofiban.

Dosing Guidelines

Eptifibatide should be dosed with a bolus of 180 mcg/kg over 1–2 minutes, a second bolus of 180 µg/kg 10 minutes later, and an infusion of 2 µg/kg./min to continue until hospital discharge or up to 18–24 hours. For ACS with a conservative strategy Eptifibatide should be dosed as a single bolus and infusion up to hospital discharge or CABG for up to 72 hours. Reduce the infusion by half in the setting of a creatinine clearance <50 ml/min.

Abciximab should be dosed in AMI and ACS with an early invasive strategy as a bolus of 0.25 µg/kg followed by an infusion of 10 µg/kg/min to continue for up to 18–24 hours and finish one hour after PCI. For patients at high risk for abrupt closure during PCI abciximab should be dosed with a 0.25 µg/kg bolus 10–60 minutes prior to PCI followed by a 0.125 µg/kg/min infusion to continue for 12 hours. There is no adjustment for renal insufficiency.

Tirofiban is dosed for ACS/PCI at 0.4 µg/kg/min for 30 minutes and continued at 0.1 µg/kg/min until 12–24 hours following PCI. For ACS with an early invasive strategy and elective/urgent PCI. The bolus and infusion should be reduced y 50% with a creatinine clearance <30 ml/min.

Limitations

The major concerns with GP IIB/IIIA inhibitor therapy are for bleeding complications and thrombocytopenia, especially with concomitant anticoagulation and anti-platelet therapy (Figure 9.18a–c). Bleeding is a particular concern following cardiac catheterization given the risk of renal failure secondary to contrast nephropathy. The effects of abciximab, but not tirofiban or eptifibatide, are readily reversed with platelet transfusions. For the latter two agents one must wait for approximately four hours for the effects to wear off.

Direct Thrombin Inhibitors

Direct thrombin inhibitors (DTI) are small molecules which can bind and inactivate both circulating and clot-bound thrombin (Figures 9.1, 9.12). DTI do not interact non-specifically with plasma proteins or cells; therefore DTI do not activate platelets and do not cause HIT. In fact, they are used for the treatment of HIT. DTI have a much more predictable dose response than UFH. The major differences in DTI are in their valency and reversibility. The three commercially available DTI in the USA are argatroban. L-hirudin (lepirudin) and bivalirudin (Figure 9.13).

Hirudin

Hirudin was initially isolated from *hirudo medicinalis*, the medicinal leech, and identified as an antithrombotic agent in 1884. Hirudin is a bivalent protein which binds irreversibly to thrombin. It is renally cleared and is relatively contraindicated in patients with renal insufficiency. Production of anti-hirudin antibodies is relatively common and may affect dosing, but there is only a 0.015% incidence of anaphylaxis with L-hirudin exposure and a 0.016% incidence with re-exposure.

Argatroban

Argatroban is a small, monovalent DTI which binds reversibly to thrombin. It has a half life of 50 minutes and is hepatically cleared. Argatroban is relatively contraindicated in patients with liver dysfunction. Argatroban is not immunogenic.

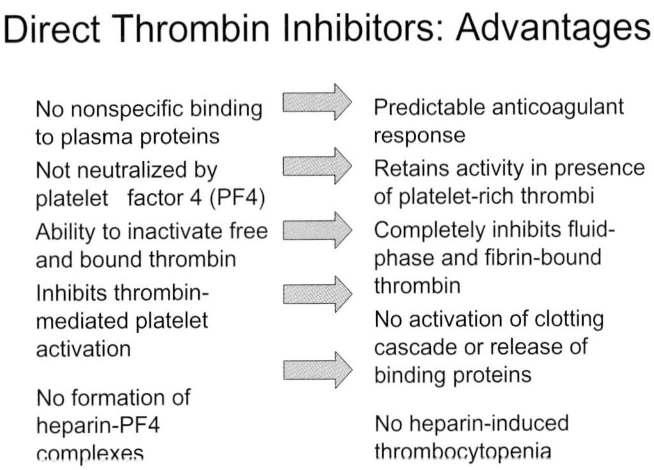

Direct Thrombin Inhibitors: Advantages

No nonspecific binding to plasma proteins ⟹ Predictable anticoagulant response

Not neutralized by platelet factor 4 (PF4) ⟹ Retains activity in presence of platelet-rich thrombi

Ability to inactivate free and bound thrombin ⟹ Completely inhibits fluid-phase and fibrin-bound thrombin

Inhibits thrombin-mediated platelet activation ⟹ No activation of clotting cascade or release of binding proteins

No formation of heparin-PF4 complexes ⟹ No heparin-induced thrombocytopenia

Figure 9.12. Advantages of direct thrombin inhibition.

	lepirudin	argatroban	bivalirudin
Bivalent	Yes	No	Yes
Reversible	No	Yes	Yes
Half-life	80 min	50 min	25 min
Excretion	Renal	Hepatic	Renal
Plasma metabolism with reversal of activity	No	No	Yes
Indication	HIT	HIT/ HIT-PCI	PCI, HIT-PCI

Figure 9.13. Comparison of direct thrombin inhibitors.

Bivalirudin

Bivalirudin is a bivalent 20 amino acid protein that reversibly inhibits thrombin. It has a half life of 25 minutes and is cleared predominantly through proteolytic cleavage by proteases and the reticuloendothelial system; therefore, it may be used safely in patients with hepatic and/or renal dysfunction. Bivalirudin is not immunogenic. Bivalirudin is the most extensively studied DTI in the treatment of ischemic heart disease.

Heparin Induced Thrombocytopenia

Lepirudin is effective for thrombotic prophylaxis in HIT-2 and is FDA approved for the treatment of this disorder in the absence of significant renal insufficiency. Lepirudin is dosed in HIT as a continuous infusion at 0.05–0.075 mg/kg/hr to a target PTT 1.5–2.5X control. Argatroban has also shown efficacy for HIT and is FDA approved for this

purpose in patients with significant hepatic dysfunction. Argatroban is dosed as a continuous infusion at 2 μg/kg/min with a goal PTT of 1.5–3X control. Although bivalirudin has been studied as a treatment for HIT, it is not currently FDA approved for this specific purpose.

PCI-HIT

ARG-216/310/311 was a prospective open label study that evaluated the use of argatroban (350 μg/kg bolus followed by a 25 μg/kg/min infusion adjusted to achieve an ACT of 3adjusted to achieve an ACT of 350 to 400 seconds) in 91 patients with HIT-2 undergoing PCI [55]. One hundred and twelve interventions were performed for AMI (38%), USA (25%) or stable angina. Ninety-four and a half percent of patients achieved procedural success (angiographic success), 97.8% achieved clinical success (angiographic success and no major acute complications) and 97.8% achieved adequate anticoagulation. For 7.7% of patients, death, MI or urgent revascularization occurred. Argatroban was used safely and successfully in repeat procedures and outcomes compared favorably with historical controls.

ATBAT was also a prospective open label study that evaluated the use of bivalirudin in 52 HIT-2 patients undergoing PCI [56]. Patients received either high dose (1 mg/kg bolus followed by a four hour infusion at 2.5 mg/kg/min) or low dose (0.75 mg/kg bolus followed by a four hour infusion at 1.75 mg/kg/min) bivalirudin five minutes prior to intervention. Ninety-six percent of patients achieved procedural success whilst 98% of patients achieved clinical success (no death, Q-wave MI, or emergency CABG). One patient in the high dose group had a major bleed. There was no significant thrombocytopenia.

Based upon this data the FDA has approved argatroban and bivalirudin for the use in HIT-2 patients undergoing elective, urgent or emergent PCI.

Urgent/Elective PCI

HELVETICA randomized 1141 patients undergoing PTCA to one of two hirudin regimens or UFH in an attempt to evaluate the use of this DTI to prevent restenosis [57]. There was no difference in the primary endpoint of seven month cardiac event free survival; however, hirudin was associated with a significant reduction in cardiac events at 96 hours with no difference in bleeding complications compared to UFH.

The Hirulog (bivalirudin) Angioplasty Study was the first large randomized trial to evaluate the safety and efficacy of bivalirudin during balloon angioplasty [58]. A total of 4,098 patients with unstable or post-infarction angina received either bivalirudin or UFH prior to PTCA. There was no difference in the primary endpoint of major adverse cardiac events. Subgroup analysis suggests that bivalirudin was associated with a significant reduction in both the primary ischemic endpoint and in bleeding complications in the post-infarction angina cohort. This benefit did not persist at six months. A re-analysis of HAT used an intention to treat analysis, redefined MI with respect to post-PTCA CPK-MB levels and evaluated contempo-

rary clinical outcomes [59]. Bivalirudin was associated with a significant reduction in the new primary endpoint of death, MI or urgent revascularization at 7, but not at 90 or 180 days. The same differences were present for bleeding complications and in the post-infarction angina population.

CACHET randomized 268 patients undergoing PCI to UFH plus abciximab, bivalirudin plus planned abciximab and two different regimens of bivalirudin plus provisional abciximab [60]. The pooled bivalirudin treatment arm was superior to UFH with respect to the composite endpoint of death, MI, repeat revascularization or major bleeding. The ADEST registry evaluated the use of bivalirudin in 1182 patients undergoing PCI with sirolimus eluting stents (SES) [61]. This "real world" study demonstrated low rates of bleeding, stent thrombosis, and major adverse coronary events.

REPLACE-1 randomized 1056 patients undergoing PCI to heparin vs. bivalirudin. Fifty-six percent of patients were pre-loaded with clopidogrel, 72% received a GP IIB/IIIA inhibitor and 85% received a bare metal stent (BMS) [62]. There was no difference in the primary endpoint of death, MI or urgent revascularization prior to hospital discharge. There was also no difference in major bleeding.

REPLACE-2 randomized 6010 low-moderate risk patients undergoing elective or urgent PCI to UFH plus planned GP IIB/IIIA inhibition vs. bivalirudin plus provisional GP IIB/IIIA inhibition [63]. Eighty-five percent of patients were pre-loaded with clopidogrel and 85% received a BMS. Bivalirudin plus provisional GP IIB/IIIA inhibition met non-inferiority with respect to the primary endpoint of 30 day death, MI, urgent repeat revascularization and in-hospital major bleeding and this result persisted at one year follow-up (Figure 9.14a, b). The bivalirudin arm also met non-inferiority criteria with respect to the secondary ischemic endpoint of death, MI or urgent revascularization. The bivalirudin arm was associated with a significant reduction both TIMI and REPLACE-2 major bleeding. An imputed comparison of bivalirudin to UFH alone showed that bivalirudin was superior with respect to both the primary and secondary endpoints. REPLACE-2 was a seminal

- Intent-to-treat population

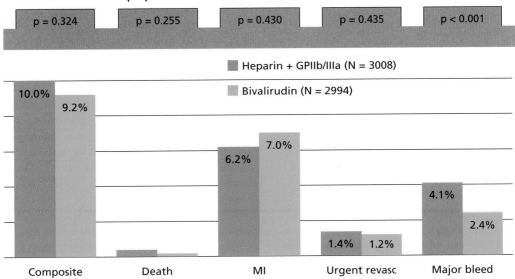

Non-inferiority confirmed for both the quadruple and triple ischemic endpoints

(a)

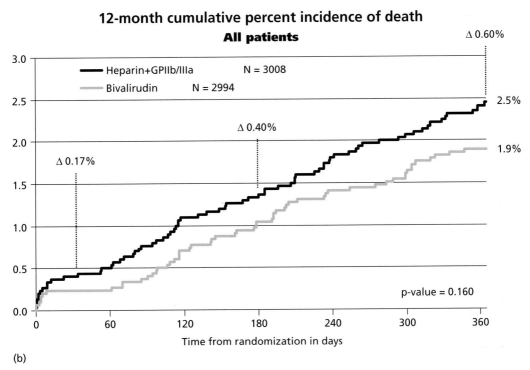

(b)

Figure 9.14. REPLACE-2: (a) primary endpoint; (b) one year mortality, JAMA 2004; **292**: 696–703. Copyright © (2004) American Medical Association. All rights reserved.

study which demonstrated that bivalirudin mono-therapy had similar ischemic efficacy as compared to UFH plus planned GP IIB/IIIA inhibition in contemporary PCI whilst incurring a lower bleeding risk.

Bivalirudin with provisional use of a GP IIB/IIIA inhibitor is an attractive alternative to UFH plus planned GP IIB/IIIA inhibition. The two strategies have similar ischemic efficacy whilst bivalirudin is associated with a significant reduction in major bleeding.

ACS

TIMI 8 was the initial dose-finding study that evaluated the safety and efficacy of bivalirudin in ACS [64]. This study randomized 133 ACS patients to bivalirudin vs. UFH fort ≥72 hours. There was no significant in either the primary endpoint of 14 day all cause mortality or recurrent MI or in bleeding complications. PROTECT (TIMI-30) randomized 857 moderate to high risk ACS patients undergoing an early invasive strategy to bivalirudin, eptifibatide plus reduced dose UFH or eptifibatide plus reduced dose enoxaparin [65]. Bivalirudin monotherapy was associated with a significant increase in the primary angiographic endpoint of coronary flow reserve; however, the eptifibatide arms were associated with a better myocardial perfusion grade and shorter post-PCI ischemic time. There was no difference in TIMI major bleeding, but bivalirudin was associated with a significant

decrease in TIMI minor bleeding and transfusion requirements.

ACUITY was the first and only large scale randomized trial to assess the use of bivalirudin as an alternative to UFH for anti-coagulation in the contemporary treatment of ACS [66]. It was found that 13,819 moderate to high risk ACS patients managed with contemporary pharmacotherapy and undergoing an early invasive strategy were randomized to UFH or enoxaparin plus planned GP IIB/IIIA inhibition, bivalirudin plus planned GP IIB/IIIA therapy or upstream (administered in the emergency room) bivalirudin monotherapy (Figure 9.15). GP IIB/IIIA inhibition was randomized to deferred (catheterization laboratory) or upstream administration. Ninety-nine percent of patients underwent angiography within 19.6 hours following admission. Pretreatment with clopidogrel was left to the discretion of the treating physician. Fifty-six percent of patients received PCI, 11% were taken to CABG, and 33% received medical therapy. Bivalirudin monotherapy met non-inferiority criteria with respect to the primary ischemic endpoint of 30 day death, MI or unplanned revascularization and was superior with respect to the primary safety endpoint of 30 day major bleeding (Figure 9.16a, b). Bivalirudin monotherapy was non-inferior with respect to the net clinical outcome (ischemic plus safety outcomes combined). Bivalirudin monotherapy was associated signifi-

ACUITY Study Design – First Randomization
Moderate-high risk unstable angina or NSTEMI
undergoing an invasive strategy (N = 13,800)

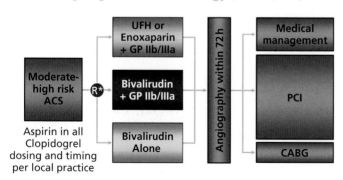

*Stratified by pre-angiography thienopyridine use or administration

Figure 9.15. ACUITY: study design. Reprinted with permission from the American Heart Journal 2004; **148**: 764–775.

Net Clinical Outcome Composite Endpoint
UFH/Enoxaparin + GPI vs. Bivalirudin + GPI vs. Bivalirudin Alone

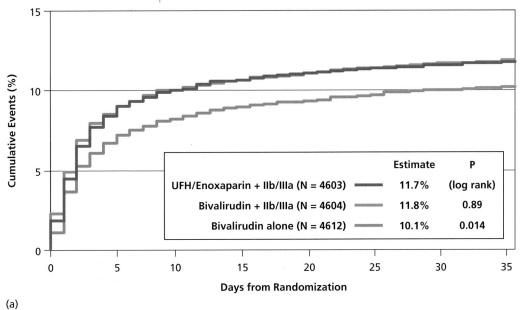

	Estimate	P
UFH/Enoxaparin + IIb/IIIa (N = 4603)	11.7%	(log rank)
Bivalirudin + IIb/IIIa (N = 4604)	11.8%	0.89
Bivalirudin alone (N = 4612)	10.1%	0.014

(a)

Major Bleeding Endpoint
UFH/Enoxaparin + GPI vs. Bivalirudin + GPI vs. Bivalirudin Alone

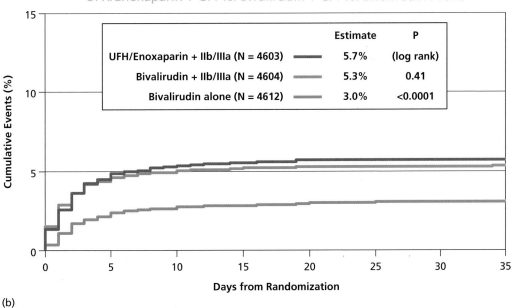

	Estimate	P
UFH/Enoxaparin + IIb/IIIa (N = 4603)	5.7%	(log rank)
Bivalirudin + IIb/IIIa (N = 4604)	5.3%	0.41
Bivalirudin alone (N = 4612)	3.0%	<0.0001

(b)

Figure 9.16. ACUITY: (a) net clinical outcome; (b) major bleeding, NEJM 2006; **355**: 2203–2216. Copyright © *[2006] Massachusetts Medical Society. All rights reserved.*

cant reductions in minor bleeding, TIMI major and minor bleeding and transfusion requirement. Subgroup analysis suggested that while lack of clopidogrel pre-treatment did not affect the ischemic outcome for the two groups receiving GP IIB/IIIA inhibition, it resulted in a significant increase in the ischemic endpoint for those receiving bivalirudin monotherapy.

A fastidious analysis of bleeding outcomes in ACUITY showed that major bleeding was an independent predictor of the primary ischemic endpoint, stent thrombosis and mortality at 30 days [67]. Ninety-eight percent of ACUITY patients received one year follow-up [68]. There continued to be no difference between the three treatment arms with respect to the composite ischemic endpoint. A landmark analysis revealed no differences in either early or late mortality. Remarkably, while one year mortality was highest in the setting of MI and major bleeding at 30 days, major bleeding was a better predictor of mortality and MI, underscoring its prognostic significance.

ACUITY PCI analyzed outcomes for the 7789 patients in the PCI subgroup (Figure 9.17a, b) [69]. Sixty percent of patients received DES and 37% received BMS. There was no difference in the primary ischemic endpoint or stent thrombosis but bivalirudin monotherapy was associated with a significant reduction in major bleeding, minor bleeding and transfusion requirements (Figure 9.17c). There was no difference in angiographic parameters. The ACUITY Timing Trial evaluated deferred vs. upstream GP IIB/IIIA inhibition [70]. There was a trend toward an increased risk of ischemic events with deferred use that was balanced by a reduction in bleeding complications (Figure 9.18 a, b).

Bivalirudin has been FDA approved for anticoagulation in ACS and has been given an ACC/AHA class I recommendation when used as part of an invasive strategy (Figure 9.19) [5]. Based upon the data one can recommend the following: (1) Careful thought is required regarding the ischemic and bleeding risks of each individual patient when deciding whether to use bivalirudin monotherapy vs. UFH plus planned IIB/IIIA inhibition. (2) Patients receiving bivalirudin monotherapy should be pre-loaded with a

thienopyridine prior to coronary angiography. (3) Bivalirudin monotherapy with provisional GP IIB/IIIA inhibition may be optimal pharmacotherapy to optimize ischemic benefit and bleeding risk.

AMI

Thrombolysis

The HERO pilot study randomized 268 AMI patients who received ASA and streptokinase to UFH, low dose bivalirudin or high dose bivalirudin [71]. Bivalirudin (composite of low and high dose arms) was associated with significant reductions in TIMI 3 flow and bleeding complications but there was no difference in ischemic clinical endpoint. HERO-2 randomized 17,073 AMI patients to the same three treatment arms [72]. Bivalirudin was associated with a significant reduction in reinfarction at 96 hours but there was no difference in mortality at 30 days. Bivalirudin was associated with a significant increase in mild and moderate bleeding with a trend towards increases in severe bleeding and intracranial hemorrhage. Use of the HERO-2 protocol with streptokinase is an ACC/AHA class IIa recommendation [13].

Primary PCI

HORIZONS AMI is a large multi-center open label trial which randomized 3602 AMI patients (93% primary PCI) to bivalirudin vs. heparin plus planned GP IIB/IIIA inhibition [73] (Figure 9.20). A secondary randomization was made to paclitaxel eluting vs. bare metal stents. A preliminary presentation of the data revealed bivalirudin was associated with a significant reduction in the primary composite endpoint of death, MI, ischemic target vessel revascularization, stroke or major bleeding (Figure 9.21a–b). Bivalirudin was also associated with a significant reduction in TIMI major or minor bleeding. There was no difference in major adverse coronary; however, cardiac death was significantly lower in the bivalirudin group. Bivalirudin was associated with an increased rate of acute stent thrombosis (≤24 hours) but no difference in stent thrombosis at 30 days (Figure 9.21c). These initial results show bivalirudin looks very promising as adjunctive anticoagulation therapy in primary PCI.

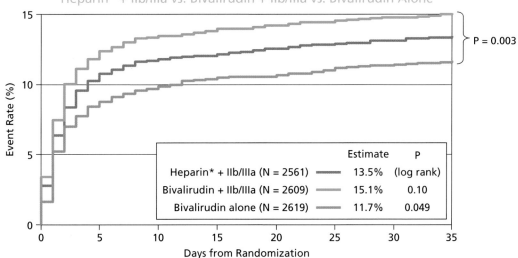

*Heparin=unfractionated or enoxaparin

(a)

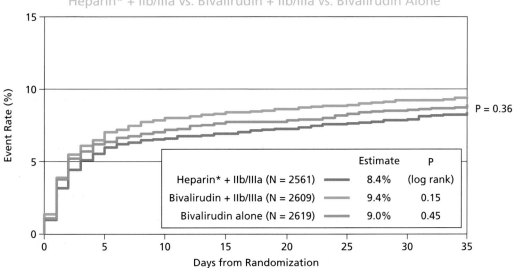

*Heparin=unfractionated or enoxaparin

(b)

Figure 9.17. ACUITY PCI: a) net clinical outcome b) composite ischemia c) adjudicated stent thrombosis. Reprinted with permission from the Lancet 2007; **369**: 907–919.

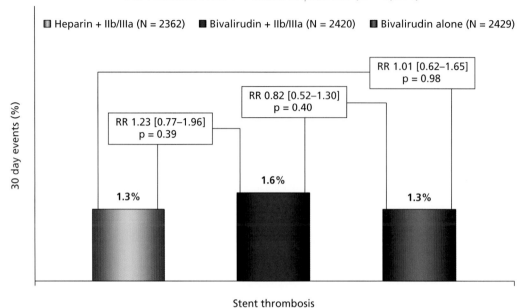

Adjudicated Stent Thrombosis
PCI Patients With ≥1 Stent Implanted (N = 7,211)

☐ Heparin + IIb/IIIa (N = 2362)   ■ Bivalirudin + IIb/IIIa (N = 2420)   ■ Bivalirudin alone (N = 2429)

RR 1.01 [0.62–1.65]
p = 0.98

RR 0.82 [0.52–1.30]
p = 0.40

RR 1.23 [0.77–1.96]
p = 0.39

1.6%

1.3%

1.3%

30 day events (%)

Stent thrombosis

(c)

Figure 9.17. *Continued*

No Reperfusion

Although bivalirudin monotherapy seems reasonable, there is no evidence that specifically addresses the use of bivalirudin in this scenario.

It is reasonable to conclude that bivalirudin may be considered an alternative to heparin as adjunctive therapy with streptokinase for AMI. Pending the results of HORIZONS there is no other indication for bivalirudin in AMI at this time.

Dosing Guidelines

In accordance with REPLACE-2 bivalirudin should be administered in elective or urgent PCI as a bolus of 0.75 mg/kg prior to intervention followed by an infusion of 1.75 mg/kg/hr to be stopped at the conclusion of the procedure. In accordance with ACUITY bivalirudin should be administered in the emergency room as a bolus of 0.1 mg/kg followed by a 0.25 mg/kg/hr infusion. If the patient requires PCI an additional IV bolus of 0.5 mg/kg should be given prior to intervention and the infusion should be increased to 1.75 mg/kg/hr and terminated at the end of the procedure.

In renal insufficiency the bolus of bivalirudin remains the same but the infusion is reduced to 1 mg/kg/hr for a creatinine clearance <30 ml/min and 0.25 mg/kg/hr in dialysis dependent patients.

An ACT need not be measured and ACT prolongation does not correlate with efficacy; however an ACT is often checked once to ensure adequate infusion. A sheath may be pulled safely two hours following discontinuation of bivalirudin.

There is currently no pharmacotherapy available to reverse anticoagulation with bivalirudin; therefore bivalirudin is relatively contraindicated in PCI with a high risk of dissection or perforation such as recanalization of a chronic total occlusion.

Factor Xa Inhibitors

Factor Xa inhibitors are the most refined and lowest molecular weight heparin. They contain a pentasaccharide sequence which specifically binds Xa. Fondaparinux, the most well studied and widely used of these agents, is a 1.7 KDa synthetic pentasaccharide that rapidly and reversibly binds AT, inducing a conformational change that

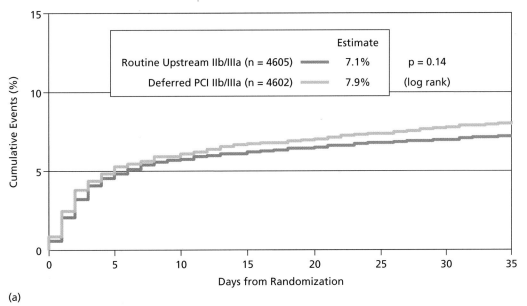

(a)

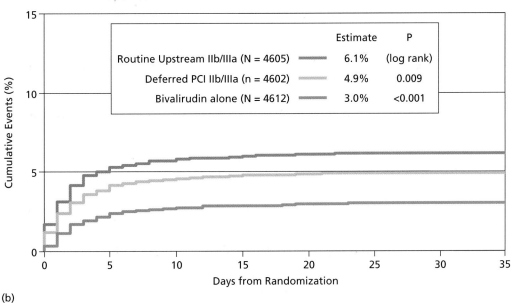

(b)

Figure 9.18. Acuity Timing: a) 30 day ischemic composite endpoint b) 30 day major bleeding. JAMA 2007; **297**: 591–602. Copyright © (2007) American Medical Association. All rights reserved.

accelerates AT-Xa interactions by >300 fold. Fondaparinux can be administered in a fixed dose (2.5 mg for creatinine clearance>30 L/minute) with no need for weight based adjustment or routine monitoring. This drug does not significantly interact with any cells or other plasma proteins, and therefore does not affect platelet function or cause HIT. Fondaparinux has been approved by the FDA for prophylaxis of venous thromboembolism in patients undergoing major orthopedic surgery on their lower limbs; however, it has recently been studied in ACS and AMI.

AMI

OASIS-6 randomized 12092 AMI patients presenting up to 12–24 hours following symptom onset to fondaparinux (2.5 mg SC daily) vs. matched subcutaneous placebo or UFH for up to eight days or hospital discharge [74]. The primary endpoint was death or reinfarction at 30 days with secondary assessments at nine days and final follow-up (3–6 months). Patients were stratified by the absence (stratum 1) or presence (stratum 2) of a standard indication for UFH. In stratum 1 fondaparinux was associated with a significant reduction in death or MI at all time points. Severe bleeding was reduced at 30 days. In stratum 2 fondaparinux was associated with a significant ischemic benefit at 30 days and final follow-up in those patients undergoing thrombolysis (30.9%) or reperfusion therapy (15.9%); however, there was no benefit in patients undergoing primary PCI (53.2%). In fact, there was a higher rate of catheter thrombosis and coronary complications (abrupt closure, dissection, perforation) for those receiving fondaparinux during coronary interventions with UFH vs. fondaparinux. There were no differences in bleeding in patients undergoing PCI. There is currently no role for fondaparinux in AMI.

Based upon data from OASIS-6 fondaparinnux has received a class I recommendation for anticoagulation in AMI with fibrinolytics or primary PCI (provided its is not used as the sole anticoagulant during PCI) (Figure 9.22) [25]. Fondaparinux is also an acceptable alternative for anticoagulation in AMI patients who receive no reperfusion (Figure 9.22) [25].

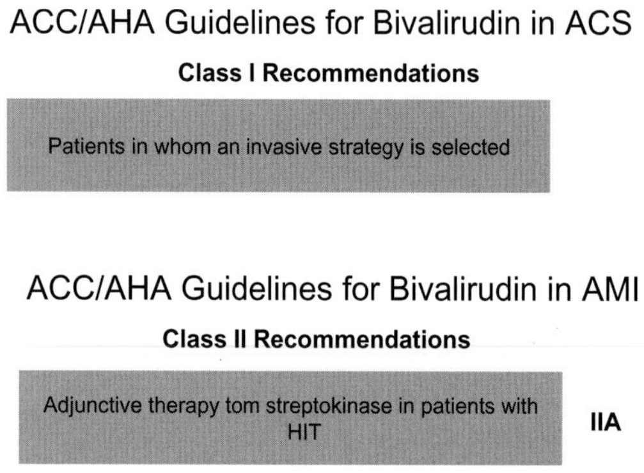

ACC/AHA Guidelines for Bivalirudin in ACS

Class I Recommendations

Patients in whom an invasive strategy is selected

ACC/AHA Guidelines for Bivalirudin in AMI

Class II Recommendations

| Adjunctive therapy tom streptokinase in patients with HIT | IIA |

Figure 9.19. ACC/AHA recommendations for bivalirudin use in ACS, Circulation 2007. **116**(7): e148–304, ACC/AHA recommendations for bivalirudin use in AMI, Circulation 2004; **110**: 588–636. (Source: *American Heart Association, Inc.*).

HORIZONS AMI Trial Design
n=3,400 randomized patients undergoing primary PCI

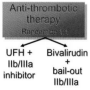

Anti-thrombotic therapy
Randomize 1:1

UFH + IIb/IIIa inhibitor

Bivalirudin + bail-out IIb/IIIa

Hypothesis: Use of bivalirudin + bail-out IIb/IIIa will reduce the composite rate of death, reinfarction, TVR, disabling stroke and major bleeding at 30-days

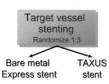

Target vessel stenting
Randomize 1:3

Bare metal Express stent

TAXUS stent

Hypothesis: Use of the polymer-based slow-release paclitaxel-eluting TAXUS stent will safely reduce the 1-year rate of ischemia-driven TVR

Figure 9.20. Horizons AMI: Study Design. Transcatheter Therapeutics (TCT), 2007.

Primary Outcome Measures

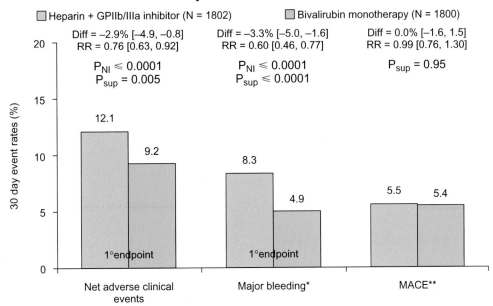

Not related to CABG
**MACE = All cause death, reinfarction, ischemic TVR or stroke

(a)

Primary PCI Cohort (N = 3,340; 92.7%)

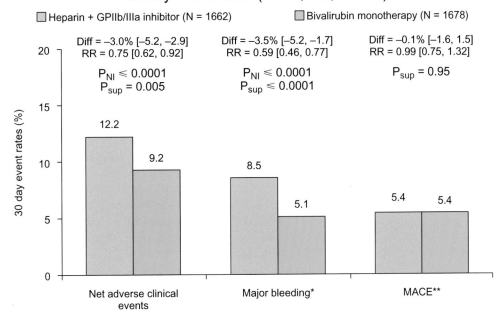

*Not related to CABG
**MACE = All cause death, reinfarction, ischemic TVR or stroke

(b)

Figure 9.21. HORIZONS AMI: (a) primary outcome; (b) primary outcome in patients undergoing primary PCI; (c) adjudicated 30 day stent thrombosis. Transcatheter Therapeutics (TCT), 2007.

30 Day Stent Thrombosis (N = 3,124)

	UFH + GP IIb/IIIa (N = 1553)	Bivalirudin (N = 1571)	P Value
ARC definite or probable*	1.9%	2.5%	0.30
- definite	1.4%	2.2%	0.09
- probable	0.5%	0.3%	0.24
- acute (≤24 hrs)	0.3%	1.3%	0.0007
- subacute (>24 hrs–30d)	1.7%	1.2%	0.28

*Protocol definition of stent thrombosis, CEC adjudicated

(c)

Figure 9.21. *Continued*

ACC/AHA Guidelines for Fondaparinux in ACS
Class I Recommendations

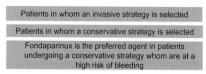

Patients in whom an invasive strategy is selected

Patients in whom a conservative strategy is selected

Fondaparinux is the preferred agent in patients undergoing a conservative strategy whom are at a high risk of bleeding

ACC/AHA Guidelines for Fondaparinux in AMI

Anticoagulation with fibrinolytic therapy for the duration of the index hospitalization or eight days. I

Anticoagulation with primary PCI I

Anticoagulation with no reperfusion for the duration of the index hospitalization or eight days. IIA

Fondaparinux should not be used as a sole anticoagulant with primary PCI III

Figure 9.22. ACC/AHA recommendations for fondaparinux in ACS, Circulation 2007; **116**(7): e148–304. (Source: *American Heart Association, Inc.*).

ACS

OASIS-5 randomized 20078 ACS patients to fondaparinux (2.5 SC daily) vs. enoxaparin (1 mg/kg twice daily) for a mean of six days [75]. The primary endpoints were death, MI or refractory ischemia at nine days, major bleeding, or a combination. Fondaparinux met non-inferiority criteria for the ischemic endpoint and was superior with respect to major bleeding and the net clinical endpoint. Fondaparinux was associated with a significant decrease in stroke at six months and a significant decrease in mortality at 30 days and 6 months. The most concerning portion of this study, especially considering the prevalence of an early invasive strategy in the USA, was a significant increase in the rate of guiding catheter thrombus with fondaparinux. This difference persisted despite an amendment to the study allowing centers to flush catheters with 200 IU of UFH. A subgroup analysis of those patients in OASIS-5 who underwent PCI also showed that fondaparinux had similar efficacy to enoxaparin while significantly reducing major bleeding [76]. Although fondaparinux was associated with an increased risk of catheter related thrombus, this was largely reduced by the addition of UFH without any significant increase in major bleeding. The current AHA/ACC guidelines give a class I recommendation for the use of fondaparinux with either a conservative or invasive strategy; fondaparinux is considered the agent of choice for anticoagulation in conservative therapy in patients at a high risk of bleeding (Figure 9.22) [5].

Questions

1. **Factors associated with an increased risk of bleeding complications in patients with acute coronary syndromes include:**
   A Advanced age
   B Female gender
   C Renal insufficiency
   D Use of glycoprotein inhibitors plus heparin
   E All of the above

2. **The SYNERGY Trial found which of the following for enoxaparin compared to unfractionated heparin in patients with acute coronary syndromes:**
   A Enoxaparin showed greater efficacy and caused less major bleeding
   B Enoxaparin showed greater efficacy but caused more major bleeding
   C Enoxaparin showed similar efficacy and caused less major bleeding
   D Enoxaparin showed similar efficacy but caused more major bleeding

3. **In a patient with suspected HIT with thrombosis syndrome, and serum creatinine value of 2.8 mg/dl, which agent can be used?**
   A Lepirudin
   B Argatroban
   C Enoxaparin
   D Bivalirudin
   E Unfractionated heparin with aPTT target of >3.5Xcontrol

4. **A 53 year old male presents with ACS and undergoes diagnostic catheterization and stenting of a proximal high grade LAD stenosis. The patient receives aspirin, clopidogrel, and heparin as well as eptifibatide during the procedure. You are called 2 hours later because of restlessness and a blood pressure of 70/30 mmHg. A stat hematocrit returns at 25% and ACT at 220 sec. In addition to volume resuscitation you should do all of the following except**
   A Give protamine
   B Discontinue eptifibatide
   C Request a platelet transfusion
   D Request a blood transfusion
   E None of the above

References

1. Telford AM, Wilson C. Trial of heparin versus atenolol in prevention of myocardial infarction in intermediate coronary syndrome. Lancet 1981; 1(8232): 1225–1228.

2. Theroux P, Ouimet H, McCans J, et al. Aspirin, heparin, or both to treat acute unstable angina. N Engl J Med 1988; 319(17): 1105–1111.

3. Cohen M, et al. Combination antithrombotic therapy in unstable rest angina and non-Q-wave infarction in non-prior aspirin users. Primary end points analysis from the ATACS trial. Antithrombotic Therapy in Acute Coronary Syndromes Research Group. Circulation 1994; 89(1): 81–88.

4. Oler A, Ouimet H, McCans J, et al. Adding heparin to aspirin reduces the incidence of myocardial infarction and death in patients with unstable angina. A meta-analysis. JAMA 1996; 276(10): 811–815.

5. Anderson JL, Adams CD, Antman EM, et al. ACC/AHA 2007 guidelines for the management of patients with unstable angina/non ST-elevation myocardial infarction: A report of the American College of Cardiology/American Heart Association Task Force on Practice Guidelines (Writing Committee to Revise the 2002 Guidelines for the Management of Patients With Unstable Angina/Non ST-Elevation Myocardial Infarction): Developed in collaboration with the American College of Emergency Physicians, the Society for Cardiovascular Angiography and Interventions, and the Society of Thoracic Surgeons: Endorsed by the American Association of Cardiovascular and Pulmonary Rehabilitation and the Society for Academic Emergency Medicine. Circulation 2007; 116(7): e148–304.

6. The effects of tissue plasminogen activator, streptokinase, or both on coronary-artery patency, ventricular function, and survival after acute myocardial infarction. The GUSTO Angiographic Investigators. N Engl J Med 1993; 329(22): 1615–1622.

7. de Bono DP, Simoons ML, Tijssen J, et al. Effect of early intravenous heparin on coronary patency, infarct size, and bleeding complications after alteplase thrombolysis: results of a randomised double blind European Cooperative Study Group trial. Br Heart J 1992; 67(2): 122–128.

8. Granger CB, Hirsch J, Califf RM, et al. Activated partial thromboplastin time and outcome after thrombolytic therapy for acute myocardial infarction: results from the GUSTO-I trial. Circulation 1996; 93(5): 870–878.

9. Nallamothu BK, Bates ER, Hochman JS, et al. Prognostic implication of activated partial thromboplastin time after reteplase or half-dose reteplase plus abciximab:

results from the GUSTO-V trial. Eur Heart J 2005; **26**(15): 1506–1512.

10. GISSI-2: A factorial randomised trial of alteplase versus streptokinase and heparin versus no heparin among 12,490 patients with acute myocardial infarction. Gruppo Italiano per lo Studio della Sopravvivenza nell'Infarto Miocardico. Lancet 1990; **336**(8707): 65–71.

11. In-hospital mortality and clinical course of 20,891 patients with suspected acute myocardial infarction randomised between alteplase and streptokinase with or without heparin. The International Study Group. Lancet 1990; **336**(8707): 71–75.

12. ISIS-3: A randomised comparison of streptokinase vs tissue plasminogen activator vs anistreplase and of aspirin plus heparin vs aspirin alone among 41,299 cases of suspected acute myocardial infarction. ISIS-3 (Third International Study of Infarct Survival) Collaborative Group. Lancet 1992; **339**(8796): 753–770.

13. Antman EM, Anbe DT, Armstrong PW, et al. ACC/AHA guidelines for the management of patients with ST-elevation myocardial infarction–executive summary: a report of the American College of Cardiology/American Heart Association Task Force on Practice Guidelines (Writing Committee to Revise the 1999 Guidelines for the Management of Patients With Acute Myocardial Infarction). Circulation 2004; **110**(5): 588–636.

14. Randomised trial of intravenous streptokinase, oral aspirin, both, or neither among 17,187 cases of suspected acute myocardial infarction: ISIS-2. ISIS-2 (Second International Study of Infarct Survival) Collaborative Group. Lancet 1988; **2**(8607): 349–360.

15. Late Assessment of Thrombolytic Efficacy (LATE) study with alteplase 6–24 hours after onset of acute myocardial infarction. Lancet 1993; **342**(8874): 759–766.

16. Krumholz HM, Hennen J, Ridker PM, et al. Use and effectiveness of intravenous heparin therapy for treatment of acute myocardial infarction in the elderly. J Am Coll Cardiol 1998; **31**(5): 973–979.

17. Low-molecular-weight heparin during instability in coronary artery disease, Fragmin during Instability in Coronary Artery Disease (FRISC) study group. Lancet 1996; **347**(9001): 561–568.

18. Blazing MA, de Lemos JA, White HD, et al. Safety and efficacy of enoxaparin vs unfractionated heparin in patients with non-ST-segment elevation acute coronary syndromes who receive tirofiban and aspirin: a randomized controlled trial. JAMA 2004; **292**(1): 55–64.

19. Ferguson JJ, Califf RM, Antman EM, et al. Enoxaparin vs unfractionated heparin in high-risk patients with non-ST-segment elevation acute coronary syndromes managed with an intended early invasive strategy:

primary results of the SYNERGY randomized trial. JAMA 2004; **292**(1): 45–54.

20. Yusuf S, Mehta SR, Xie C, et al. Effects of reviparin, a low-molecular-weight heparin, on mortality, reinfarction, and strokes in patients with acute myocardial infarction presenting with ST-segment elevation. JAMA 2005; **293**(4): 427–435.

21. Efficacy and safety of tenecteplase in combination with enoxaparin, abciximab, or unfractionated heparin: the ASSENT-3 randomised trial in acute myocardial infarction. Lancet 2001; **358**(9282): 605–613.

22. Van de Werf F. ASSENT-3: implications for future trial design and clinical practice. Eur Heart J 2002; **23**(12): 911–912.

23. Wallentin L, Goldstein P, Armstrong PW, et al. Efficacy and safety of tenecteplase in combination with the low-molecular-weight heparin enoxaparin or unfractionated heparin in the prehospital setting: the Assessment of the Safety and Efficacy of a New Thrombolytic Regimen (ASSENT)-3 PLUS randomized trial in acute myocardial infarction. Circulation 2003; **108**(2): 135–142.

24. Antman EM, Morrow DA, McCabe CH, et al. Enoxaparin versus unfractionated heparin with fibrinolysis for ST-elevation myocardial infarction. N Engl J Med 2006; **354**(14): 1477–1488.

25. Antman EM, Hand M, Armstrong PW, et al. 2007 Focused update of the ACC/AHA 2004 Guidelines for the Management of Patients With ST-Elevation Myocardial Infarction. A report of the American College of Cardiology/American Heart Association Task Force on Practice Guidelines. Circulation 2007.

26. Cohen M, Gensini GF, Maritz F ,et al. The safety and efficacy of subcutaneous enoxaparin versus intravenous unfractionated heparin and tirofiban versus placebo in the treatment of acute ST-segment elevation myocardial infarction patients ineligible for reperfusion (TETAMI): A randomized trial. J Am Coll Cardiol 2003; **42**(8): 1347–1356.

27. Montalescot G, White HD, Gallo R, et al. Enoxaparin versus unfractionated heparin in elective percutaneous coronary intervention. N Engl J Med 2006; **355**(10): 1006–1017.

28. Topol EJ, Califf RM, Weisman HF, et al. Randomised trial of coronary intervention with antibody against platelet IIb/IIIa integrin for reduction of clinical restenosis: results at six months. The EPIC Investigators. Lancet 1994; **343**(8902): 881–886.

29. Randomised placebo-controlled trial of abciximab before and during coronary intervention in refractory unstable angina: the CAPTURE Study. Lancet 1997; **349**(9063): 1429–1435.

30. Hamm CW, Heeschen C, Goldmann B, et al. Benefit of abciximab in patients with refractory unstable angina in

relation to serum troponin T levels. c7E3 Fab Antiplatelet Therapy in Unstable Refractory Angina (CAPTURE) Study Investigators. N Engl J Med 1999; **340**(21): 1623–1629.

31. Simoons ML. Effect of glycoprotein IIb/IIIa receptor blocker abciximab on outcome in patients with acute coronary syndromes without early coronary revascularisation: the GUSTO IV-ACS randomised trial. Lancet 2001; **357**(9272): 1915–1924.

32. Ottervanger JP, Armstrong P, Barnathan ES, et al. Long-term results after the glycoprotein IIb/IIIa inhibitor abciximab in unstable angina: one-year survival in the GUSTO IV-ACS (Global Use of Strategies To Open Occluded Coronary Arteries IV–Acute Coronary Syndrome) Trial. Circulation 2003; **107**(3): 437–442.

33. Neumann FJ, et al. Effect of glycoprotein IIb/IIIa receptor blockade with abciximab on clinical and angiographic restenosis rate after the placement of coronary stents following acute myocardial infarction. J Am Coll Cardiol 2000; **35**(4): 915–921.

34. Effects of platelet glycoprotein IIb/IIIa blockade with tirofiban on adverse cardiac events in patients with unstable angina or acute myocardial infarction undergoing coronary angioplasty. The RESTORE Investigators. Randomized Efficacy Study of Tirofiban for Outcomes and REstenosis. Circulation 1997; **96**(5): 1445–1453.

35. A comparison of aspirin plus tirofiban with aspirin plus heparin for unstable angina. Platelet Receptor Inhibition in Ischemic Syndrome Management (PRISM) Study Investigators. N Engl J Med 1998; **338**(21): 1498–1505.

36. Heeschen C, Hamm CW, Goldmann B, et al. Troponin concentrations for stratification of patients with acute coronary syndromes in relation to therapeutic efficacy of tirofiban. PRISM Study Investigators. Platelet Receptor Inhibition in Ischemic Syndrome Management. Lancet 1999; **354**(9192): 1757–1762.

37. Inhibition of the platelet glycoprotein IIb/IIIa receptor with tirofiban in unstable angina and non-Q-wave myocardial infarction. Platelet Receptor Inhibition in Ischemic Syndrome Management in Patients Limited by Unstable Signs and Symptoms (PRISM-PLUS) Study Investigators. N Engl J Med 1998; **338**(21): 1488–1497.

38. Inhibition of platelet glycoprotein IIb/IIIa with eptifibatide in patients with acute coronary syndromes. The PURSUIT Trial Investigators. Platelet Glycoprotein IIb/IIIa in Unstable Angina: Receptor Suppression Using Integrilin Therapy. N Engl J Med 1998; **339**(7): 436–443.

39. Randomised placebo-controlled trial of effect of eptifibatide on complications of percutaneous coronary intervention: IMPACT-II. Integrilin to Minimise Platelet Aggregation and Coronary Thrombosis-II. Lancet 1997; **349**(9063): 1422–1428.

40. Boersma E, et al. Platelet glycoprotein IIb/IIIa inhibitors in acute coronary syndromes: a meta-analysis of all major randomised clinical trials. Lancet 2002; **359**(9302): 189–198.

41. De Luca G, Suryapranata H, Stone GW, et al. Abciximab as adjunctive therapy to reperfusion in acute ST-segment elevation myocardial infarction: a meta-analysis of randomized trials. JAMA 2005; **293**(14): 1759–1765.

42. Topol EJ. Reperfusion therapy for acute myocardial infarction with fibrinolytic therapy or combination reduced fibrinolytic therapy and platelet glycoprotein IIb/IIIa inhibition: the GUSTO V randomised trial. Lancet 2001; **357**(9272): 1905–1914.

43. Brener SJ, Barr LA, Burchenal JE, et al. Randomized, placebo-controlled trial of platelet glycoprotein IIb/IIIa blockade with primary angioplasty for acute myocardial infarction. ReoPro and Primary PTCA Organization and Randomized Trial (RAPPORT) Investigators. Circulation 1998; **98**(8): 734–741.

44. Stone GW, Grines CL, Cox DA, et al. Comparison of angioplasty with stenting, with or without abciximab, in acute myocardial infarction. N Engl J Med 2002; **346**(13): 957–966.

45. Montalescot G, Barragan P, Wittenberg O, et al. Platelet glycoprotein IIb/IIIa inhibition with coronary stenting for acute myocardial infarction. N Engl J Med 2001; **344**(25): 1895–1903.

46. Antoniucci D, Rodriguez A, Hempel A, et al. A randomized trial comparing primary infarct artery stenting with or without abciximab in acute myocardial infarction. J Am Coll Cardiol 2003; **42**(11): 1879–1885.

47. Randomised placebo-controlled and balloon-angioplasty-controlled trial to assess safety of coronary stenting with use of platelet glycoprotein-IIb/IIIa blockade. Lancet 1998; **352**(9122): 87–92.

48. Lincoff AM, Califf RM, Moliterno DJ, et al. Complementary clinical benefits of coronary-artery stenting and blockade of platelet glycoprotein IIb/IIIa receptors. Evaluation of Platelet IIb/IIIa Inhibition in Stenting Investigators. N Engl J Med 1999; **341**(5): 319–327.

49. Platelet glycoprotein IIb/IIIa receptor blockade and low-dose heparin during percutaneous coronary revascularization. The EPILOG Investigators. N Engl J Med 1997; **336**(24): 1689–1696.

50. Kastrati A, Mehilli J, Schuhlen H, et al. A clinical trial of abciximab in elective percutaneous coronary intervention after pretreatment with clopidogrel. N Engl J Med 2004; **350**(3): 232–238.

51. Mehilli J, Kastrati A, Schuhlen H, et al. Randomized clinical trial of abciximab in diabetic patients undergoing elective percutaneous coronary interventions after

treatment with a high loading dose of clopidogrel. Circulation 2004; **110**(24): 3627–3635.

52. Cura FA, Bhatt DL, Lincoff AM, *et al.* Pronounced benefit of coronary stenting and adjunctive platelet glycoprotein IIb/IIIa inhibition in complex atherosclerotic lesions. Circulation 2000; **102**(1): 28–34.

53. Novel dosing regimen of eptifibatide in planned coronary stent implantation (ESPRIT): a randomised, placebo-controlled trial. Lancet 2000; **356**(9247): 2037–2044.

54. Topol EJ, Moliterno DJ, Herrmann HC, *et al.* Comparison of two platelet glycoprotein IIb/IIIa inhibitors, tirofiban and abciximab, for the prevention of ischemic events with percutaneous coronary revascularization. N Engl J Med 2001; **344**(25): 1888–1894.

55. Lewis BE, Matthai WH Jr, Cohen M, *et al.* Argatroban anticoagulation during percutaneous coronary intervention in patients with heparin-induced thrombocytopenia. Catheter Cardiovasc Interv 2002; **57**(2): 177–184.

56. Mahaffey KW, *et al.* The anticoagulant therapy with bivalirudin to assist in the performance of percutaneous coronary intervention in patients with heparin-induced thrombocytopenia (ATBAT) study: main results. J Invasive Cardiol 2003; **15**(11): 611–616.

57. Serruys PW, Herrman JP, Simon R, *et al.* A comparison of hirudin with heparin in the prevention of restenosis after coronary angioplasty. Helvetica Investigators. N Engl J Med 1995; **333**(12): 757–763.

58. Bittl JA, *et al.* Treatment with bivalirudin (Hirulog) as compared with heparin during coronary angioplasty for unstable or postinfarction angina. Hirulog Angioplasty Study Investigators. N Engl J Med 1995; **333**(12): 764–769.

59. Bittl JA, Chaitman BR, Feit F, *et al.* Bivalirudin versus heparin during coronary angioplasty for unstable or postinfarction angina: Final report reanalysis of the Bivalirudin Angioplasty Study. Am Heart J 2001; **142**(6): 952–959.

60. Lincoff AM, Kleiman NS, Kottke-Marchant K, *et al.* Bivalirudin with planned or provisional abciximab versus low-dose heparin and abciximab during percutaneous coronary revascularization: results of the Comparison of Abciximab Complications with Hirulog for Ischemic Events Trial (CACHET). Am Heart J 2002; **143**(5): 847–853.

61. Dangas G, Lasic Z, Mehran R, *et al.* Effectiveness of the concomitant use of bivalirudin and drug-eluting stents (from the prospective, multicenter BivAlirudin and Drug-Eluting STents [ADEST] study). Am J Cardiol 2005; **96**(5): 659–663.

62. Lincoff AM, Bittl JA, Kleiman NS, *et al.* Comparison of bivalirudin versus heparin during percutaneous coronary intervention (the Randomized Evaluation of PCI Linking Angiomax to Reduced Clinical Events [REPLACE]-1 trial). Am J Cardiol 2004; **93**(9): 1092–1096.

63. Lincoff AM, Bittl JA, Harrington RA, *et al.* Bivalirudin and provisional glycoprotein IIb/IIIa blockade compared with heparin and planned glycoprotein IIb/IIIa blockade during percutaneous coronary intervention: REPLACE-2 randomized trial. JAMA 2003; **289**(7): 853–863.

64. Antman EM, McCabe CH, Braunwald E. Bivalirudin as a replacement for unfractionated heparin in unstable angina/non-ST-elevation myocardial infarction: observations from the TIMI 8 trial. The Thrombolysis in Myocardial Infarction. Am Heart J 2002; **143**(2): 229–234.

65. Gibson CM, Morrow DA, Murphy SA, *et al.* A randomized trial to evaluate the relative protection against post-percutaneous coronary intervention microvascular dysfunction, ischemia, and inflammation among antiplatelet and antithrombotic agents: the PROTECT-TIMI-30 trial. J Am Coll Cardiol 2006; **47**(12): 2364–2373.

66. Stone GW, McLaurin BT, Cox DA, *et al.* Bivalirudin for patients with acute coronary syndromes. N Engl J Med 2006; **355**(21): 2203–2216.

67. Manoukian SV, Feit F, Mehran R, *et al.* Impact of major bleeding on 30-day mortality and clinical outcomes in patients with acute coronary syndromes: an analysis from the ACUITY Trial. J Am Coll Cardiol 2007; **49**(12): 1362–1368.

68. Stone GW A Prospective, Randomized Trial of Bivalirudin in Acute Coronary Syndromes: Final One Year Results from the ACUITY Trial. Presentation at the American College of Cardiology Meeting. New Orleans, LA, March 2007.

69. Stone GW, White HD, Ohman EM, *et al.* Bivalirudin in patients with acute coronary syndromes undergoing percutaneous coronary intervention: A subgroup analysis from the Acute Catheterization and Urgent Intervention Triage strategy (ACUITY) trial. Lancet 2007; **369**(9565): 907–919.

70. Stone GW, Bertrand ME, Mose JW, *et al.* Routine upstream initiation vs deferred selective use of glycoprotein IIb/IIIa inhibitors in acute coronary syndromes: the ACUITY Timing trial. JAMA 2007; **297**(6): 591–602.

71. White HD, *et al.* Randomized, double-blind comparison of hirulog versus heparin in patients receiving streptokinase and aspirin for acute myocardial infarction (HERO). Hirulog Early Reperfusion/Occlusion (HERO) Trial Investigators. Circulation 1997; **96**(7): 2155–2161.

72. White H. Thrombin-specific anticoagulation with biva-lirudin versus heparin in patients receiving fibrinolytic therapy for acute myocardial infarction: the HERO-2 randomised trial. Lancet 2001; **358**(9296): 1855–1863.

73. Ston, GW. Harmonizing Outcomes With Revasculari-zation and Stents in Acute Myocardial Infarction (HORIZONS AMI). Transcatheter Therapeutics (TCT) 2007, 2007.

74. Yusuf S, Mehta SR, Chrolavicius S, *et al.* Effects of fon-daparinux on mortality and reinfarction in patients with acute ST-segment elevation myocardial infarction: the OASIS-6 randomized trial. JAMA 2006; **295**(13): 1519–1530.

75. Yusuf S, Mehta SR, Chrolavicius S, *et al.* Comparison of fondaparinux and enoxaparin in acute coronary syn-dromes. N Engl J Med 2006; **354**(14): 1464–1476.

76. Mehta SR, *et al.* Efficacy and Safety of Fondaparinux Versus Enoxaparin in Patients With Acute Coronary Syndromes Undergoing Percutaneous Coronary Intervention: Results From the OASIS-5 Trial. J Am Coll Cardiol 2007; **50**(18): 1742–1751.

Answers

1. E
2. D
3. B
4. C

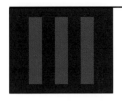

PART III

Complementary Imaging Techniques

CHAPTER 10

Intravascular Ultrasound: Principles, Image Interpretation, and Clinical Applications

Adriano Caixeta[1], Akiko Maehara[1], & Gary S. Mintz[2]

[1] Columbia University Medical Center and the Cardiovascular Research Foundation, New York, NY, USA

[2] Cardiovascular Research Foundation, New York, NY, USA

Medical uses of ultrasound came shortly after the end of World War II. However, real-time ultrasound imaging originated in the late 1960s and early 1970s when Bom *et al.* [1] pioneered the development of linear array transducers for use in the cardiovascular system. By the late 1980s, Yock *et al.* [2] had successfully miniaturized a single-transducer system that could be placed within coronary arteries. Ever since, intravascular ultrasound (IVUS) has become an increasingly important catheter-based imaging technology providing both practical guidance for percutaneous coronary interventions (PCI) as well as many different clinical and research insights [3–8]. For example, IVUS directly images the atheroma within the vessel wall, allowing measurement of plaque size, distribution, and to some extent its composition. Thus, IVUS has been established as the method of choice for the serial assessment of atherosclerotic plaque burden in progression-regression trials.

This chapter will review the rationale, technique, and interpretation of IVUS imaging in diagnostic and therapeutic applications.

Principles of IVUS Imaging

Ultrasound is acoustic energy with a frequency above human hearing. The highest frequency that

Interventional Cardiology, First Edition. Edited by Carlo Di Mario, George D. Dangas, Peter Barlis. © 2010 Blackwell Publishing Ltd. Published 2010 by Blackwell Publishing Ltd.

the human ear can detect is approximately 20 thousand cycles per second (20,000 Hz). This is where the sonic range ends and where the ultrasonic range begins. In medical imaging high-frequency acoustic energy is the range of millions of cycles per second (megahertz—MHz).

IVUS supplements angiography by providing a tomographic perspective of lumen geometry and vessel wall structure. The equipment required to perform intracoronary ultrasound consists of a catheter incorporating a miniaturized transducer and a console to reconstruct the images [9]. The IVUS transducer converts electrical energy into acoustical energy through a piezoelectric (pressure-electric) crystalline material that expands and contracts to produce sound waves when electrically excited (i.e. a series of pulse/echo sequences or vectors). After reflection from tissue part of the ultrasound energy returns to the transducer; the transducer then generates an electrical impulse that is converted into moving pictures [10]. All materials in the body reflect sound waves. Sound waves bounce back at various intervals depending on the type of material and the distance from the transducer. It is the variation in reflective sound waves that creates the ultrasound image on the console.

The intensity of reflected (or backscattered) ultrasound depends on a number of variables including the intensity of the transmitted signal, the attenuation of the signal by the tissue, the distance from the transducer to the target, the angle of the signal relative to the target, and the density of the tissue [3]. Several clinically relevant properties of the ultrasound image—such as the resolution, depth of penetration, and attenuation of the acoustic—are dependent on the geometric and frequency properties of the transducer. The higher the center frequency, the better the axial resolution, but the lower the depth of penetration. For coronary imaging because the transducer is close to the vessel wall, high ultrasound frequencies are used that are centered at 20 to 40 MHz [8]. The use of high ultrasound frequencies provides axial resolution between 80 and 120 μm and lateral resolution (dependent on imaging depth and beam shape) between 200 and 500 μm [3].

Equipment for IVUS Examination

Two different transducer designs are commonly used yielding comparable information: mechanically rotated and electronically activated phased-array. Mechanical probes use a drive cable to rotate a single-element transducer at the tip of the catheter at 1800 rpm. At approximately 1° increments, the transducer sends and receives ultrasound signals providing 256 individual radial scan lines for each image. The mechanical transducer has the advantage of a simple design, greater signal-to-noise ratio, and higher temporal and spatial resolution. In electronic systems, multiple tiny transducer elements in an annular array are activated sequentially to generate the cross-sectional image [3,10].

The IVUS console contains numerous imaging controls such as zoom, gain, TGC (time-gain-compensation), gamma curves, compression and reject, and others.

Imaging Artifacts

Artifacts often appear in images generated by contemporary IVUS devices and may interfere in imaging interpretation and measurements.

Ring-Down
Ring-Down artifacts usually appear as a series of parallel bands or halos of variables thickness surrounding the catheter obscuring near field imaging. Phased-array systems tend to have more ring-down artifacts (Figure 10.1).

Non-uniform Rotational Distortion (NURD)
NURD arises from frictional forces to the rotating elements in mechanical catheters. NURD creates stretched or compacted portions of the images. Because accurate reconstruction of IVUS two-dimensional images is dependent on uniform

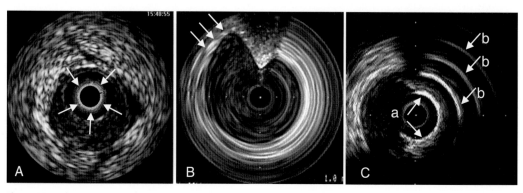

Figure 10.1. Three examples of artifacts. In Panel A, ring-down artifacts in an electronic-array system image, near-field bright halos (arrows) close to the face of the catheter may obscure the area immediately adjacent to the catheter. In Panel B, NURD—non-uniform rotation distortion—occurs only with mechanical systems. Part of the image is expanded causing deformation of the image in its circumferential view—the image appears elliptical (arrows). In Panel C, reverberations are repetitive echoes of the same structure. This is an example of reverberations from calcium. The arcs of calcium are indicated by the arrows a; and the false structures (reverberations) are indicated by arrows b.

rotation of the catheter, nonuniform rotation may create errors during IVUS measurements [11] (Figure 10.1). For practical propose the mean lumen area tends to increase as the degree of distortion increases [12]. NURD artifacts can also occur because of bends in the catheter drive-shaft or in the presence of acute bends in the artery.

Reverberations

Strong spatial tissue heterogeneity creates acoustic noise and pulse reverberations—multiple echoes reaching the transducer before the next pulse transmission to give rise to multiple copies of the anatomy (Figure 10.1). Reverberation artifacts are more common from strong echoreflectors such as stents, guidewires, guiding catheters, and calcium (especially after rotational atherectomy).

Other Artifacts

There are a few other artifacts that can also interfere in IVUS interpretation including *side lobes* and *ghost* artifacts also generated from strong echoreflectors such as calcium and stent metal [3]. In longitudinal or L-mode display, catheter motion artifacts during the pullback may results in a "saw tooth" appearance (Figure 10.2).

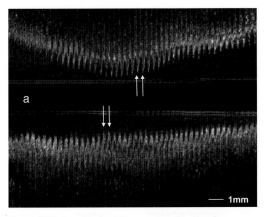

Figure 10.2. Longitudinal image reconstruction (or L-mode) is shown. There is excessive motion of the transducer (a) relative to the artery, causing zigzag or sawtooth appearance (white arrows). This artifact is more of a problem with the right and circumflex arteries, because of the wide atrioventricular groove movement between systole and diastole.

Catheter position also plays an important role in image quality. Off-axis position of the catheter may alter vessel geometry in an elliptical fashion to mislead the operator to overestimate the lumen and vessel area [13]. Axial (antegrade-retrograde) movement of the IVUS probe during the cardiac cycle scrambles consecutive image slices that may have implications for three-dimensional reconstruction and attempts to assess coronary artery compliance [14].

Image Acquisition and Presentation

Two important consensus documents have been published: Standards for the acquisition, measurement, and reporting of IVUS studies: a report of the American College of Cardiology Task Force on Clinical Expert Consensus Documents [10] and the Study Group on Intracoronary Imaging of the Working Group of Coronary Circulation and the Subgroup on Intravascular Ultrasound of the Working Group of Echocardiography of the European Society of Cardiology [15].

IVUS is displayed as a tomographic cross-sectional view. A longitudinal view (L-Mode or long-view) can be also displayed, but this should be done only when using motorized transducer pullback. Longitudinal representation of IVUS images is useful for lengths measurements, for interpolation of shadowed deep arterial structures (i.e. external elastic membrane behind calcium or stent metal) [10].

There are advantages and disadvantages using manual or motorized pullback; however, motorized pullback is usually preferable. Using motorized transducer pullback allows assessment of lesion length, volumetric measurements, consistent and systematic IVUS image acquisition among different operators, and uniform and reproducible image acquisition for multicenter and serial studies.

In standard image acquisition after anticoagulation and intracoronary nitroglycerin administration, the IVUS catheter should be placed distal to the segment of interest (at least 10 mm of distal reference); and a continuous pull-back to the aorta should be recorded. The preferred pullback speed is 0.5 mm/sec.

Normal Artery Morphology

The ultrasound appearance of normal human arteries in vitro and in vivo has been reported [16–19]. In the coronary artery there are three layers: intima, media, and adventitia. Normal intima thickness increases with age, from a single endothelial cell at birth to a mean of 60 μm at 5 years to 220–250 μm at 30–40 years of age [20]. The definition of abnormal intimal thickness by IVUS is still controversial; in general, the threshold of "normal intimal thickness" is <300 μm (0.3 mm). The innermost layer of the intima is relatively echogenic compared with the lumen and media and displayed on the screen as a single bright concentric echo. The lower ultrasound reflectance of the media is due to its homogeneous smooth muscle cells distribution and smaller amounts of collagen, elastic tissue, and proteoglycans. The thickness of media histologically averages 200 μm, but

medial thinning occurs in the presence of atherosclerosis [21]. The intima/media border is poorly defined because the intimal layer reflects ultrasound more strongly than the media. Conversely, the media/adventitia border, consistent with the location of the external elastic membrane (EEM), is accurately defined because a step-up in echo reflectivity occurs without *blooming*. The outermost layer, the adventitia, is composed of collagen and elastic tissue; it is 300–500 μm thick. The outer border of the adventitia is also indistinct due to echo reflectivity similar to the surrounding peri-adventitial tissues [13,21]. Therefore, the normal coronary artery is either (1) "mono-layered" in cases of intimal thickness <100 μm because of a 40 MHz IVUS catheter resolution is less than 100 μm or (2) "three-layered" to include a bright echo from the intima, a dark zone from the media, and bright surrounding echoes from the adventitia (Figure 10.3).

Three-layer

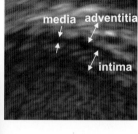

Mono-layer

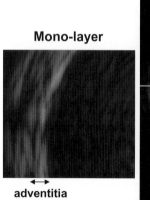

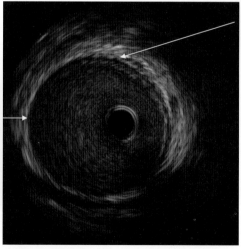

Figure 10.3. This is an example of normal coronary artery morphology in a cross-sectional view. In the magnified image in the right, the bright inner layer (intima), middle echolucent zone (media), and outer bright layer (adventitia) are representative of the "three-layered" appearance of IVUS. In the magnified image in the left, only the outer bright adventitial layer is representative of the "mono-layered" appearance.

Quantitative Analysis

In non-stented lesions there are two strong acoustic interfaces that are well visualized by ultrasound: the leading edge of the intima and the outer border of the media (or media/adventitia junction). Therefore, two cross-sectional area (CSA) measurements can be defined by IVUS: the lumen CSA and the media/adventitia CSA (or EEM CSA). The atheroma or plaque&media (P&M) complex is calculated as EEM minus lumen; the media cannot be measured as a distinct structure. Thus, complete quantification of a non-stented lesion is possible by tracing the EEM and lumen areas of the proximal reference, lesion, and distal reference; calculating derived measures (minimum and maximum EEM and lumen diameters, P&M area and thickness, and plaque burden [P&M divided by EEM]); and measuring lesion length (distance between the proximal and distal reference) (Figure 10.4).

In stented vessels the stent forms a third measurable structure (stent CSA). It appears as bright points along the circumference of the vessel. Complete quantification of a stented lesion is possible by tracing the EEM and lumen areas of the proximal and distal reference and the EEM, lumen, and stent areas of the stented lesion; calculating derived measures (minimum and maximum EEM, stent, and lumen diameters; peri-stent P&M area and thickness; and intra-stent intimal hyperplasia [IH, area and %IH]); and measuring stent length.

Qualitative Analysis

Greyscale IVUS has some ability to differentiate plaque composition based on different echoreflectivity of the tissue. Atherosclerotic plaques are rarely homogeneous and contain a mixture of plaque components with different impedance (density). A standard approach is to compare the echointensity or "brightness" of the plaque to the

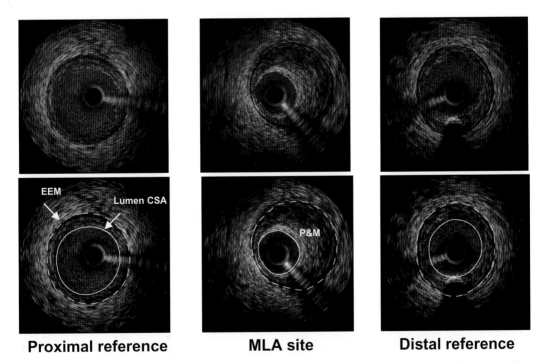

Proximal reference   **MLA site**   **Distal reference**

Figure 10.4. IVUS measurements pre-intervention in a non-stented artery. The proximal and distal reference and minimum lumen area (MLA) of the lesion are shown. The IVUS study is shown in duplicate: one unlabeled and one highlighted with lines to illustrate quantitative analysis. The dashed line highlights each external elastic membrane cross-sectional area (EEM CSA), and the solid line indicates each lumen interface (lumen CSA). The minimal lumen cross sectional area (lumen CSA) at the lesion site is 2.1 mm². Between the EEM CSA and lumen CSA, the atheroma or plaque&media (P&M) complex is calculated.

surrounding adventitia that is used as a reference. Three basic types of lesions are distinguished according to plaque echogenicity: (1) "soft" or hypoechoic plaque does not reflect much ultrasound and appears dark with less echointensity compared to the adventitia (Figure 10.5); (2) fibrous and (3) calcific plaques are characterized by equal or greater intensity than the adventitia. A plaque that is not so reflective as to cause shadowing is labeled "hard" or hyperechoic and is composed primarily of fibrous tissue (Figure 10.5). The presence of acoustic shadowing along with the brightest echoes and reverberations are characteristic of the presence of calcification (Figure 10.5).

Intimal hyperplasia due to in-stent restenosis often appears to have low echogenecity depending, in part, on age and adjunct therapies (i.e. brachytherapy) (Figure 10.6).

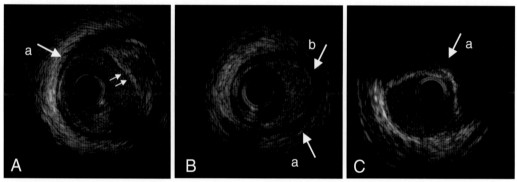

Figure 10.5 A pure soft or hypoechoic plaque is uncommon because atherosclerotic plaques are rarely homogeneous. Panel A shows an example of a predominantly soft plaque—a thin fibrous cap (small arrows) and lipid core underlying it; the plaque is less bright than the adventitia (a). In Panel B, fibrous plaque or hyperechoic plaque is shown. Hyperechoic plaque is as bright as or brighter than the adventitia (a) without shadowing. In this eccentric plaque, the thickness of the media behind the thickest part of the plaque (b) is an artifact caused by attenuation of the beam as it passes through the hyperechoic plaque. In reality, the media becomes thinner with increasing atherosclerosis. Note that the media behind the thinnest part of the plaque is also thinner—without artifacts. The Panel C shows superficial calcium—defined as calcium (a) that is closer to the intima than it is to the adventitia. Calcium shadows the deeper arterial structures; in this case, the arc of calcification is ~180°.

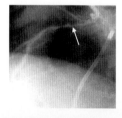

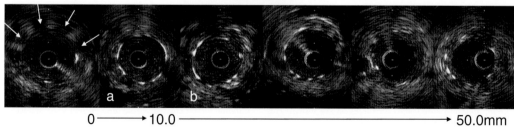

0 ——→ 10.0 ————————————————————————→ 50.0mm

Figure 10.6. This patient presented with diffuse in-stent restenosis (white arrow on angiogram). Neointimal tissue is packed around the IVUS catheter at a and b, where the maximum amount of intimal hyperplasia occurs. There is also stent malapposition proximally (white arrows). Reproduced from Mintz [3].

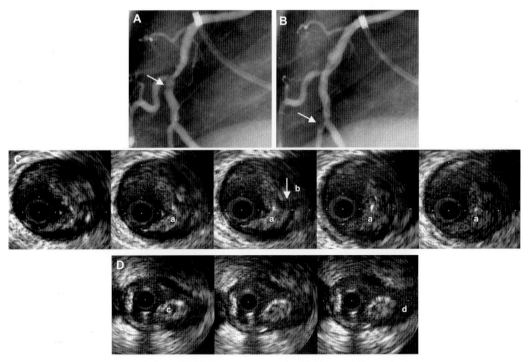

Figure 10.7. This example shows an unstable plaque before (white arrow in Panel A) and after balloon angioplasty (Panel B). A new, post-balloon angioplasty filling defect at the origin of the acute marginal branch is shown (white arrow in Panel B). Pre-intervention IVUS (Panel C) shows a lobulated and penduculated thrombus (a) and a distinct interface with the underlying vessel wall (b). Post-balloon angioplasty IVUS (Panel D) shows the thrombus (c) that has embolized into the acute marginal branch (d). Reproduced from Mintz [3].

The identification of thrombus is difficult by IVUS. It may appears as lobulated hypoechoic mass within the lumen, scintillating echoes, a distinct interface between the presumed thrombus imaging and underlying plaque, and blood flow through the thrombus (Figure 10.7) [3].

Comparison of IVUS and Angiography

Coronary angiography depicts the coronary anatomy as a longitudinal silhouette of the lumen. Conversely, IVUS with its tomographic perspective directly images the lumen, atheroma, and the vessel wall. Coronary angiography significantly underestimates the presence, severity, and extent of atherosclerosis compared to IVUS [22,23]. Furthermore, IVUS routinely shows significant atherosclerosis in angiographically 'normal' segments in patients undergoing PCI [24]. This phenomenon may be explained by three major factors: (1) coronary atherosclerosis is often diffusely distributed involving long segments of the vessel containing no truly normal reference segment for comparison, (2) complex atherosclerotic plaques are not appreciated by the two-dimensional 'silhouette,' and (3) most importantly, the presence of arterial wall remodeling [10]. In some circumstances diffuse, concentric, and symmetrical coronary disease can affect the entire length of the vessel resulting in an angiographic appearance of a small artery with minimal luminal narrowing.

Coronary Artery Remodeling

Arterial remodeling of the vessel wall at the site of coronary plaques was originally described from necropsy examinations by Glagov *et al.* [25] and later validated in vivo by IVUS imaging [26]. "Positive," "outward," or "expansive" remodeling

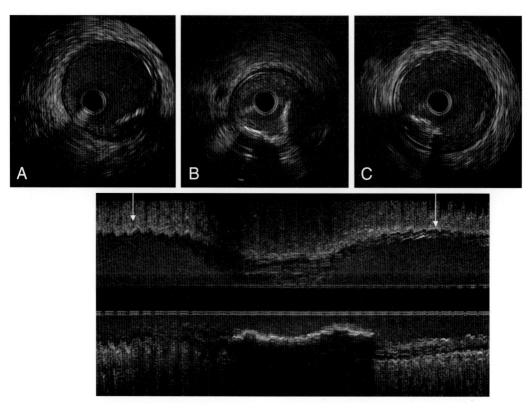

Figure 10.8. These illustrations show an eccentric, calcific, and small plaque accumulation leading to negative remodeling. Panels A and C refer to proximal and distal vessel references and their respective longitudinal views (white arrows). In Panel B, notice how the vessel cross-sectional area (or EEM) is smaller than both the proximal and distal vessels. The longitudinal view depicts clearly the artery shrinkage at the lesion site.

is defined as an increased in arterial dimensions; and "negative," "inward," or "constrictive" remodeling is defined as a smaller arterial dimension. Positive remodeling occurs as a compensatory increase in local vessel size in response to increasing plaque burden, especially during early stages of atherosclerosis [27]. An absolute reduction in lumen dimensions typically does not occur until the lesion occupies, on average, an estimated 40–50% of the area within the EEM (40–50% plaque burden) [25]. Conversely, negative remodeling has been implicated in the development of native significant stenosis in the absence of plaque accumulation (Figure 10.8) [28,29].

A number of definitions of remodeling have been proposed and published [10,26–32]. One definition compares the lesion EEM CSA to the average of the proximal+distal reference EEM CSA; positive remodeling is an index >1.0 and

negative remodeling <1.0. A second definition defines positive remodeling as a lesion EEM greater than the proximal reference EEM, intermediate remodeling as a lesion EEM between the proximal and distal reference EEM, and negative remodeling as a lesion EEM less than the distal reference EEM. Using a third definition, arterial remodeling has been calculated by a remodeling index (lesion/reference EEM); positive remodeling is an index >1.05, intermediate remodeling is an index of 0.95–1.05, and negative remodeling is an index <0.95. It is important to note that all of these remodeling definitions are based on a comparison of the reference EEM and lesion EEM. Accordingly, because both reference and lesion sites may have undergone quantitative changes in EEM during the atherosclerotic process, the evidence of remodeling derived from this index is relative and indirect [10]. It depends on the definition of the reference, and the classification of an individual lesion depends on the definition used.

Unstable Lesions

In patients with acute coronary syndromes, culprit lesions more frequently exhibit positive remodeling and a large plaque area; conversely, patients with a stable clinical presentation more frequently show negative remodeling and a smaller plaque area [30]. Echolucent plaques are also more common in unstable than in stable patients. In addition, unstable lesions have less calcium than stable lesions; and when present, calcific deposits in unstable lesions are small, focal, and deep [33]. Plaque ruptures can occur with varying clinical presentations although they are more often associated with acute coronary syndromes (Figure 10.9) [34]. Multiple ruptured plaques have been reported in patients with acute coronary syndromes; their prevalence, however, is the subject of controversy [35,36].

Intermediate Lesions

Coronary angiography underestimates stenosis severity most markedly in arteries with a 50–75% plaque burden and in patients with multivessel disease [37–39]. An IVUS measured minimum luminal area (MLA) of $\leq 4.0\,mm^2$ in a major (>3.0 mm) proximal epicardial artery excluding the LMCA has been a consensus criterion of a significant coronary artery stenosis since it correlates well with the findings of other methods for diagnosing myocardial ischemia including single-photon emission computed tomography [40], Doppler FloWire studies [41], and pressure wire measurements [42]. The clinical importance of this criterion has been confirmed by a study of 300 patients showing that deferral of revascularization is safe for patients with an MLA of $>4.0\,mm^2$ [43].

Left Main Coronary Artery (LMCA) Disease

LMCA atherosclerosis is often underestimated by coronary angiography. Several studies have showed that a very high percentage of patients with angiographically normal LMCA have disease by IVUS [44–47]. Others have shown that IVUS is helpful in assessing ambiguous LMCA disease (Figure 10.10) [48–50]. The main reasons for the discrepancy between angiography and IVUS are the following: (1) diffuse atherosclerotic plaque involvement may lead to a lack of a normal reference segment, (2) a short LMCA makes identification of a normal reference segment difficult, (3) the presence of arterial remodeling, (4) the correlation between angiography and necropsy or IVUS appears to be better in non-LMCA lesions possibly because of unique geometric issues in the LMCA [51,52], and (5) significant inter and intraobserver variability in the angiographic assessment of LMCA disease [53–55], especially in ostium location [56].

IVUS assessment of lumen dimensions has been shown to correlate with fractional flow reserve

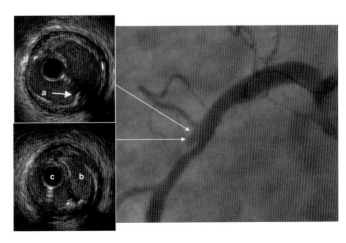

Figure 10.9. This patient presented with an acute coronary syndrome and a complex right coronary lesion (white arrows) and disrupted plaque by IVUS. The IVUS imaging run shows the residual fibrous cap (a), the evacuated plaque cavity (b), and the true lumen containing the catheter (c).

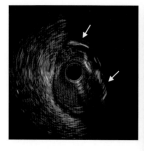
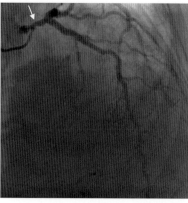

Figure 10.10. The figure illustrates a mildly diseased ostium in the left main by angiography (white arrow). The IVUS diagnostic study shows an eccentric stenotic plaque with a minimum lumen area of 4.4 mm². Notice the superficial and deep calcium with shadowing (arrows).

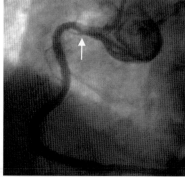

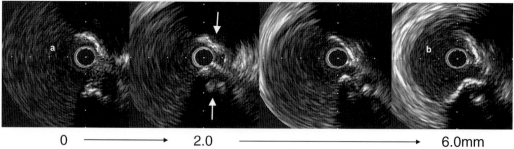

0 ⟶ 2.0 ⟶ 6.0mm

Figure 10.11. Diagnostic IVUS was performed to assess this angiographic filling defect at the proximal right coronary artery (white arrow in the angiogram). The IVUS imaging run begins at the ostium (a) of the right coronary artery to beyond the filling defect (b). Note the calcification (white arrow in the IVUS) without lumen compromise. Reproduced from Mintz [3].

[50], and both IVUS and fractional flow reserve predict clinical outcome in patients with LMCA disease [48,57]. In general an LMCA MLA <6.0 mm² has been used as a criteria of significant stenosis because it is the best predictor of FFR <0.75 and correlates with MLA >4.0 mm² in the LAD and LCX using Murray's Law [58].

Other Unusual Lesion Morphology

During coronary angiography it is common to encounter unusual appearing lesions that elude accurate characterization despite thorough examination using multiple radiographic projections. The use of IVUS allows accurate characterization of unusual morphology: filling defects, aneurysms,

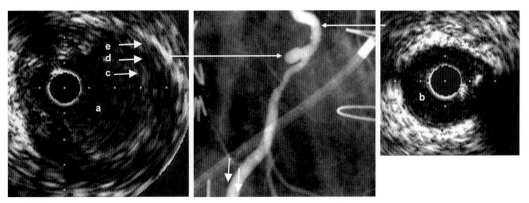

Figure 10.12. This patient presented with a true saccular aneurysm in the right coronary artery. IVUS imaging shows the aneurysm (a) and the proximal vessel (b). Note that the intima (c), the media (d), and the adventitia (e) are intact, making this a true aneurysm. Reproduced from Mintz [3].

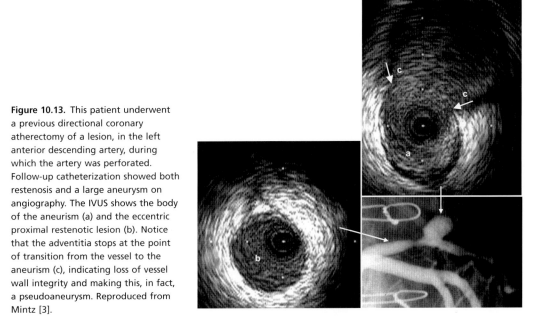

Figure 10.13. This patient underwent a previous directional coronary atherectomy of a lesion, in the left anterior descending artery, during which the artery was perforated. Follow-up catheterization showed both restenosis and a large aneurysm on angiography. The IVUS shows the body of the aneurism (a) and the eccentric proximal restenotic lesion (b). Notice that the adventitia stops at the point of transition from the vessel to the aneurism (c), indicating loss of vessel wall integrity and making this, in fact, a pseudoaneurysm. Reproduced from Mintz [3].

and spontaneous dissections. While most filling defects are true thrombi, a small percentage are highly calcified plaque (Figure 10.11) or even calcified nodules, an unusual form of vulnerable plaque.

In an IVUS analysis of 77 angiographically diagnosed aneurysms, 27% were true aneurysms (Figure 10.12), 4% were pseudoaneurysms (Figure 10.13), 16% were complex plaques, and 53% were normal arterial segments adjacent to stenoses [59].

By IVUS, a spontaneous dissection appears as a medial dissection with an intramural hematoma occupying some or all of the dissected false lumen without identifiable intimal tears and without a communication between the true and false lumens, typically in a non-atherosclerotic artery.

Guidance for Stent Implantation

Stent Sizing

Pre-interventional IVUS is performed to assess stenosis severity and plaque composition and distribution, measure reference vessel size, and measure lesion length. As a result stent size can be chosen more accurately than solely by angiography. There are a number of paradigms that can be used. Stent size can be selected by identifying the maximum reference *lumen* diameter (proximal or distal to the lesion); it results in stent upsizing without an increase in complications. At the other extreme, stents can be sized to the "true vessel," "media-to-media," or mid-wall dimensions to reflect the amount of angiographically silent disease and, in most cases, the extent of positive remodeling, not just vessel size. Typically, this measurement will be larger than reference *lumen* reference and, thus, should be used only by experienced operators who understand its limitations.

IVUS measures lesion length more accurately than angiography because IVUS eliminates foreshortening, vessel tortuosity, or bend points.

Stent Expansion and Malapposition

IVUS studies have shown that lumen enlargement after stent implantation is a combination of vessel expansion and plaque redistribution/embolization, not plaque compression [60–62]. Plaque reduction in patients with acute coronary syndromes is attributed to plaque or thrombus embolization. Intrusion or prolapse of plaque through the stent mesh into the lumen is more common in acute coronary syndromes and in saphenous vein graft lesions. Importantly, after stent implantation there is a significant residual plaque burden behind the stent struts that almost always measures 50–75% at the center of the lesion. Thus, the stent CSA always looks smaller than the EEM even when the stent is fully expanded.

Apposition refers to the contact between the stent struts to the arterial wall [10]. Incomplete stent apposition is defined as one or more struts clearly separated from vessel wall with evidence of blood speckles behind the strut (Figure 10.14). There is no conclusive evidence suggesting that isolated acute incomplete stent apposition (in the absence of concomitant underexpansion) is associated with adverse clinical outcomes.

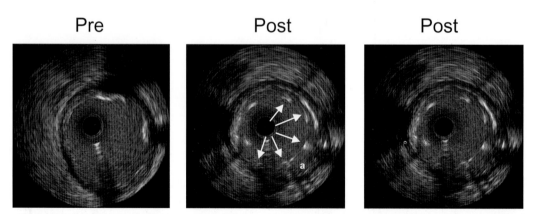

Figure 10.14. An example of acute stent malapposition is shown. Notice the space between the stent strut and the intima and the blood speckle behind the stent struts (a). Five stent struts are malapposed (white arrows). Because of stent malapposition, the stent area (9.4 mm²) is smaller than the lumen area (14.4 mm²). The post-stent implantation IVUS image is shown in duplicate.

IVUS-guided Stent Implantation and Predictors of Restenosis and Thrombosis

The two main uses of IVUS are to insure optimal stent expansion (stent CSA) and full coverage of the lesion (especially with DES implantation). In the majority of pre-drug-eluting stent (DES) studies, IVUS use optimized stent expansion; and the initially larger minimum stent area (MSA) achieved was associated with a lower restenosis rate [63–77].

At the introduction of DES, the importance of optimal stent deployment was initially underestimated. Suboptimal stent expansion with both BMS and DES was a risk factor for restenosis and target vessel revascularization, but also for stent thrombosis [78–80]. Recently, Roy *et al.* reported that IVUS guidance during DES implantation had the potential to reduce both DES thrombosis and the need for repeat revascularization [81]. In this study 884 patients undergoing IVUS-guided DES implantation were compared with 884 propensity-score matched patients undergoing DES implantation with angiographic guidance alone. At 30 days and at 12 months, a lower rate of definite stent thrombosis using the ARC definition was seen in the IVUS-guided group (0.5% vs. 1.4%; P = 0.046) and (0.7% vs. 2.0%; P = 0.014), respectively. At one year, target lesion revascularization was also lower in the IVUS-guided group (5.1% vs. 7.2%; P = 0.07). A multicenter Korean registry of 805 LMCA interventions showed that the 595 patients treated with IVUS-guided DES implantation had better three-year survival than the 210 patients in whom IVUS was not used to guide LMCA DES implantation (HR = 0.43, p = 0.019).

Complications

IVUS has a higher sensitivity than angiography in identifying complications that may occur during PCI. Angiography tends to underestimate the presence and extent of dissection. Stent edge dissections are common since the junction between stent metal and reference segment tissue is a site of compliance mismatch. Edge dissections may be more common when the stent ends in a reference segment that contains (1) both plaque and normal vessel wall or (2) both calcific (or hard) and soft plaque elements (Figure 10.15). Dissection may not be visible by IVUS if the true lumen is severely stenotic and the ultrasound catheter presses the flap against the arterial wall or if the dissection occurs behind a calcified plaque that prevents accurate morphological definition. In general, the treatment of coronary dissection with stent implantation depends on the combination of angiographic assessment, flow assessment, and signs or symptoms of ischemia, and residual IVUS MLA. Treatment of dissections should be based on IVUS findings when they show evidence (1) reduced lumen dimensions below the threshold for an optimum result, (2) impingement of the dissection flap on the IVUS catheter, (3) mobility, and (4) increased length. In general, minor edge dissections should not be treated unless they result in lumen compromise; the vast majority have healed when imaged at follow-up.

Intramural hematoma is a variant of dissection. Blood accumulates in the medial space; the EEM expands outward, and the internal elastic membrane is pushed inward to cause lumen compromise. Intramural hematomas are typically

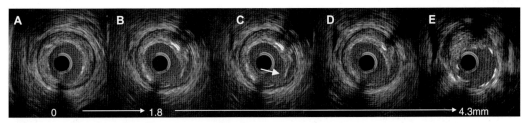

Figure 10.15. This patient presented with proximal edge dissection after coronary stenting. Panel A depicts the proximal reference segment, which contains mild plaque. Panel E shows the stent. Notice the tear into the lumen (arrow) and the dissection reaching the medial layer of the vessel (Panels B, C and D).

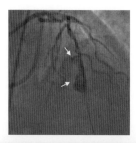

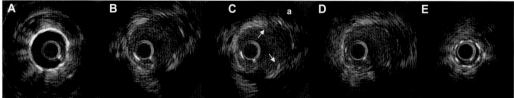

Figure 10.16. This patient presented with in-stent restenosis. After balloon dilation, coronary perforation with myocardial contrast extravasation occurred, as seen by angiography (arrows). On IVUS, notice the small vessel with stenting at a distal site (Panel E) and the medial and adventitial discontinuation at the site of perforation (Panel B, C and D, and arrows). Notice also an accumulation of blood outside the EEM (a). One stent graft was implanted prior to IVUS assessment (Panel A), followed by an additional stent graft after IVUS assessment.

hyperechoic and crescent shaped, with straightening of the internal elastic membrane [82]. In general, an intramural hematoma should be treated because of the propensity for propagation and lumen compromise.

Coronary perforation and rupture usually occurs with overaggressive and/or oversized balloon dilation although it can occur with a guidewire and stenting as well. In general, there are 3 distinct IVUS morphologic patterns indicating arterial rupture: (1) free blood speckle outside the EEM (Figure 10.16), (2) extramural hematoma—an accumulation of blood outside the EEM, and (3) less common, a new peri-adventitial echolucent interface representing contrast extravasation [3]. Acute management ranges from a conservative strategy of monitoring to prolonged balloon inflations, covered stents, and surgery.

Serial IVUS Studies of Restenosis

Restenosis
Serial IVUS studies have shown that the main mechanism of restenosis in non-stented arteries is negative arterial remodeling (decrease in EEM area), not intimal hyperplasia [29,83]. Conversely, in-stent restenosis is primarily due to neointimal proliferation, not chronic stent recoil. By IVUS, %IH (IH volume divided by stent volume) has been shown to be consistent for each stent type. DES reduce restenosis by reducing IH from an average of 30% in BMS [84] to 3 to 5% in sirolimus-eluting stents (SES) [85,86], to 6% in everolimus-eluting stents [87], to 8 to 13% in polymer-based paclitaxel-eluting stents [88], and to 16% in zotarolimus-eluting stents [89].

Serial IVUS analysis of the first-in-human ABSORB trial of the Bioabsorbable Vascular Solutions (BVS, Abbott Vascular) fully absorbable DES showed a significant reduction in stent CSA at follow-up (−11.8%), absence of vessel negative remodeling, and IH of 30%. Of concern, was the higher incidence of late-acquired incomplete stent apposition of 27% [90].

Stent underexpansion is a common finding in restenotic stents. It is the result of poor expansion at implantation, not chronic stent recoil. In an analysis of over 1000 patients with BMS restenosis, 15% had a MSA <4.5 mm²; and 25% had a MSA between 4.5 and 6.0 mm². In addition, in 4.5% there were technical and mechanical complications

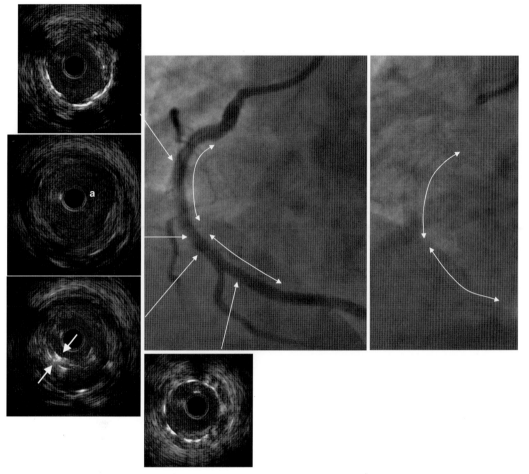

Figure 10.17. An example of stent crush at the right coronary artery detected at IVUS follow-up. Two stents have been implanted with a gap between them (a). The proximal edge of the second stent has been crushed as shown on IVUS (arrows) but not on angiography.

of stent implantation that contributed to the restenosis. Examples of mechanical complications have included (1) missing the lesion (e.g. an aorto-ostial stenosis), (2) stent "crush" (Figure 10.17), (3) having the stent stripped off the balloon during the implantation procedure, or (4) DES fracture (Figure 10.18) [91].

Acquired late stent malapposition

Late stent malapposition (LSM) is usually caused by regional vessel positive remodeling (Figure 10.19). LSM has been reported in 4–5% after BMS implantation [92–94]. Studies have suggested a higher incidence of LSM after DES (especially after SES) [95–97]. Hoffmann *et al.* studied the impact of LSM after SES implantation on four-year clinical events. This pooled IVUS analysis from three randomized trials comparing SES with BMS showed that LSM at follow-up was more common after SES than after BMS (25% vs. 8.3%; p = 0.001); however, major adverse cardiac event free survival at four years was identical for those with and without LSM (11.1% vs. 16.3%, p = 0.48), and LSM was not a predictor for target lesion revascularization, target vessel failure, or late stent thrombosis during the

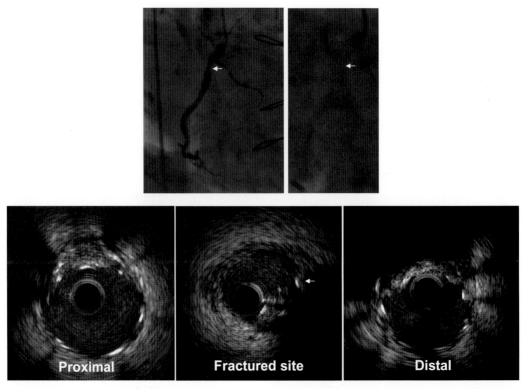

Figure 10.18. A patient presented with restenosis at follow-up after Cypher™ stent implantation in the right coronary artery (arrows on angiogram). Note the stent fracture with acquired transection on fluoroscopy. On IVUS, all stent struts have been seen at proximal and distal references, whereas at the fracture site, only one stent strut has been seen (arrow).

four-year follow-up period in either patient group [98].

Conversely, others have suggested that LSM can contribute to late stent thrombosis [99–101]. Cook *et al.* studied 13 patients presenting with very late stent thrombosis (>1 year) after DES implantation and compared them to 144 control patients who did not experience stent thrombosis. Compared with DES controls, patients with very late stent thrombosis had longer lesions and stents, more stents per lesion, and more stent overlap. Vessel cross-sectional area was significantly larger for the in-stent segment ($28.6 \pm 11.9\,mm^2$ vs. $20.1 \pm 6.7\,mm^2$; $P = 0.03$) in very late stent thrombosis patients compared with DES controls, denoting evidence of positive arterial remodeling. Although IVUS was not performed at stent implan-

tation in any patients of either group, incomplete stent apposition was more frequent (77% vs. 12%, $P < 0.001$) and maximal incomplete stent apposition area was larger ($8.3 \pm 7.5\,mm^2$ vs. $4.0 \pm 3.8\,mm^2$; $P = 0.03$) in patients with very late stent thrombosis compared with controls.

Based on these studies with conflicting data, it is still speculative as to how to treat patients with IVUS findings of LSM.

Conclusions

Greyscale IVUS provides (1) high-quality, tomographic imaging of the lumen, the atheroma, and the vessel wall, (2) incremental and more detailed qualitative and quantitative information than coronary angiography, (3) practical guidance for per-

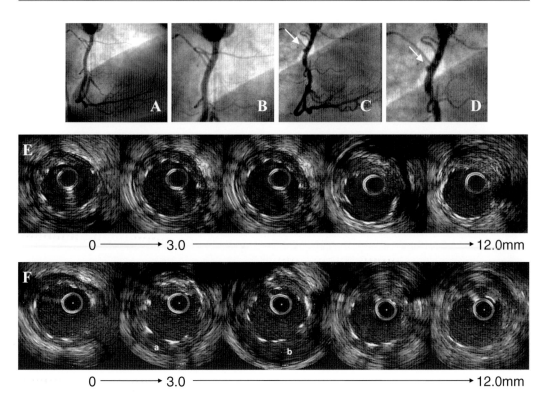

Figure 10.19. This patient underwent sirolimus-eluting stent (Cypher™) implantation in a right coronary stenosis. The final angiogram is shown in Panels A and B. At follow-up (Panels C and D), there was a proximal and focal angiographic aneurysm (white arrows). Final (post-stent implantation) IVUS image is shown in Panel E, and the follow-up IVUS image is shown in Panel F. Note the late stent malapposition (a and b). At the site of maximum stent malapposition (b), there has been an increase in EEM CSA from 17.8 mm² to 28.9 mm². The stent CSA (8.8 mm²) and the peri-stent P&M (8.9 mm²) have not changed. Reproduced from Mintz [102].

cutaneous coronary intervention, and (4) many different clinical and research insights. More recently, IVUS has become an indispensable part of all DES studies, representing the most effective way to understand the mechanisms, effects, and complications of this new stent technology.

Questions

1. **IVUS minimum lumen has been correlated with:**
   A Coronary flow reserve (measured by Doppler FloWire)
   B Stress perfusion imaging
   C Fractional Flow Reserve (measured by the pressure wire)
   D All of the above
   E None of the above

2. **A Meta-analysis of IVUS-guided PCI compared to Angiography-guided PCI using bare metal stents demonstrated:**
   A Decreased Death with IVUS guidance
   B Decreased MI with IVUS guidance
   C Decreased TVR with IVUS guidance
   D Decrease MACE with IVUS guidance
   E Both C and D

3. **Late stent malapposition**
   A Is more common after DES than bare metal stent implantation
   B Is the most common cause of DES restenosis
   C Is the most common cause of DES thrombosis
   D Should always be treated
   E None of the above is correct

4. **Which of the following best predicts IVUS or angiographic restenosis after DES implantation?**
   A Absolute minimum stent CSA
   B Stent CSA divided by mean reference lumen CSA
   C Stent CSA divided by distal reference lumen CSA
   D Stent CSA divided by lesion EEM CSA
   E Stent CSA divided by reference EEM CSA

5. **Which of the following formulas is correct?**
   A Plaque = Media minus lumen
   B Intimal hyperplasia = EEM minus stent
   C Remodeling = Lesion EEM divided by reference EEM
   D Plaque burden = Reference lumen CSA minus lesion lumen CSA divided by reference lumen CSA

References

1. Bom N, Lancee CT, Honkoop J, *et al.* Ultrasonic viewer for cross-sectional analyses of moving cardiac structures. Biomedical Eng 1971; **6**: 500–503, 505.

2. Yock PG, Johnson EL, DTL. Intravascular ultrasound: development and clinical potential. Am J Card Imaging 1988; **2**: 185–193.

3. Mintz G. Intracoronary Ultrasound. Abingdon, UK: Taylor & Francis; 2005.

4. Yock PG, Linker DT. Intravascular ultrasound. Looking below the surface of vascular disease. Circulation 1990; **81**(5): 1715–1718.

5. Tobis JM, Mallery J, Mahon D, *et al.* Intravascular ultrasound imaging of human coronary arteries in vivo. Analysis of tissue characterizations with comparison to in vitro histological specimens. Circulation 1991; **83**(3): 913–926.

6. Mintz GS, Potkin BN, Cooke RH, *et al.* Intravascular ultrasound imaging in a patient with unstable angina. Am Heart J 1992; **123**(6): 1692–1694.

7. Nissen SE, De Franco AC, Tuzcu EM, *et al.* Coronary intravascular ultrasound: diagnostic and interventional applications. Coron Artery Dis 1995; **6**(5): 355–367.

8. Honda Y, Fitzgerald PJ. Frontiers in Intravascular Imaging Technologies. Circulation 2008; **117**: 2024–2037.

9. Nissen S. Coronary angiography and intravascular ultrasound. Am J Cardiol 2001; **87**(4A): 15A–20A.

10. Mintz GS, Nissen SE, Anderson WD, *et al.* American College of Cardiology Clinical Expert Consensus Document on Standards for Acquisition, Measurement and Reporting of Intravascular Ultrasound Studies (IVUS). A report of the American College of Cardiology Task Force on Clinical Expert Consensus Documents. J Am Coll Cardiol 2001; **37**(5): 1478–1492.

11. Kimura BJ, Bhargava V, Palinski W, *et al.* Distortion of intravascular ultrasound images because of nonuniform angular velocity of mechanical-type transducers. Am Heart J 1996; **132**: 328–336.

12. Kearney PP, Ramo MP, Spencer T, *et al.* A study of the quantitative and qualitative impact of catheter shaft angulation in a mechanical intravascular ultrasound system. Ultrasound Med Biol 1997; **23**: 87–93.

13. Takahashi T, Honda Y, Russo RJ, *et al.* Intravascular ultrasound and quantitative coronary angiography. Catheter Cardiovasc Interv 2002; **55**(1): 118–128.

14. Arbab-Zadeh A, DeMaria AN, Penny WF, *et al.* Axial movement of the intravascular ultrasound probe during the cardiac cycle: implications for three-

dimensional reconstruction and measurements of coronary dimensions. Am Heart J 1999; **138**: 865–872.

15. Di Mario C, Gorge G, Peters R, *et al.* Clinical application and image interpretation in intracoronary ultrasound. Study Group on Intracoronary Imaging of the Working Group of Coronary Circulation and of the Subgroup on Intravascular Ultrasound of the Working Group of Echocardiography of the European Society of Cardiology. Eur Heart J 1998; **19**(2): 207–229.

16. Siegel R, Chae JS, Maurer G, *et al.* Histopathologic correlation of the three-layered intravascular ultrasound appearance of normal adult human muscular arteries. Am Heart J 1993; **126**: 872–878.

17. Nishimura RA, Edwards WD, Warnes CA, *et al.* Intravascular ultrasound imaging: in vitro validation and pathologic correlation. J Am Coll Cardiol 1990; **16**(1): 145–154.

18. Gussenhoven EJ, Essed CE, Lancee CT, *et al.* Arterial wall characteristics determined by intravascular ultrasound imaging: an in vitro study. J Am Coll Cardiol 1989; **14**(4): 947–952.

19. Yock PG, Linker DT, Angelsen BA. Two-dimensional intravascular ultrasound: technical development and initial clinical experience. J Am Soc Echocardiogr 1989; **2**(4): 296–304.

20. Velican D, Velican C. Comparative study on age-related changes and atherosclerotic involvement of the coronary arteries of male and female subjects up to 40 years of age. Atherosclerosis 1981; **38**(1–2): 39–50.

21. Isner JM, Donaldson RF, Fortin AH, *et al.* Attenuation of the media of coronary arteries in advanced atherosclerosis. Am J Cardiol 1986; **58**(10): 937–939.

22. Topol EJ, Nissen SE. Our preoccupation with coronary luminology. The dissociation between clinical and angiographic findings in ischemic heart disease. Circulation 1995; **92**(8): 2333–2342.

23. Nissen SE, Yock P. Intravascular ultrasound: novel pathophysiological insights and current clinical applications. Circulation 2001; **103**(4): 604–616.

24. Mintz GS, Painter JA, Pichard AD, *et al.* Atherosclerosis in angiographically "normal" coronary artery reference segments: an intravascular ultrasound study with clinical correlations. J Am Coll Cardiol 1995; **25**(7): 1479–1485.

25. Glagov S, Weisenberg E, Zarins CK, *et al.* Compensatory enlargement of human atherosclerotic coronary arteries. N Engl J Med 1986; **316**: 1371–1375.

26. Hermiller JB, Tenaglia AN, Kisslo KB, *et al.* In vivo validation of compensatory enlargement of atherosclerotic coronary arteries. Am J Cardiol 1993; **71**(8): 665–668.

27. Losordo DW, Rosenfield K, Kaufman J, *et al.* Focal compensatory enlargement of human arteries in response to progressive atherosclerosis. In vivo documentation using intravascular ultrasound. Circulation 1994; **89**(6): 2570–2577.

28. Nishioka T, Luo H, Eigler NL, *et al.* Contribution of inadequate compensatory enlargement to development of human coronary artery stenosis: an in vivo intravascular ultrasound study. J Am Coll Cardiol 1996; **27**(7): 1571–1576.

29. Mintz GS, Kent KM, Pichard AD, *et al.* Contribution of inadequate arterial remodeling to the development of focal coronary artery stenoses. An intravascular ultrasound study. Circulation 1997; **95**(7): 1791–1798.

30. Schoenhagen P, Ziada KM, Kapadia SR, *et al.* Extent and direction of arterial remodeling in stable versus unstable coronary syndromes : an intravascular ultrasound study. Circulation 2000; **101**(6): 598–603.

31. Pasterkamp G, Schoneveld AH, van der Wal AC, *et al.* Relation of arterial geometry to luminal narrowing and histologic markers for plaque vulnerability: the remodeling paradox. J Am Coll Cardiol 1998; **32**(3): 655–662.

32. Pasterkamp G, Wensing PJ, Post MJ, *et al.* Paradoxical arterial wall shrinkage may contribute to luminal narrowing of human atherosclerotic femoral arteries. Circulation 1995; **91**(5): 1444–1449.

33. Mintz GS, Pichard AD, Popma JJ, *et al.* Determinants and correlates of target lesion calcium in coronary artery disease: a clinical, angiographic and intravascular ultrasound study. J Am Coll Cardiol 1997; **29**(2): 268–274.

34. Ge J, Chirillo F, Schwedtmann J, Gorge G, *et al.* Screening of ruptured plaques in patients with coronary artery disease by intravascular ultrasound. Heart 1999; **81**(6): 621–627.

35. Rioufol G, Finet G, Ginon I, *et al.* Multiple atherosclerotic plaque rupture in acute coronary syndrome: a three-vessel intravascular ultrasound study. Circulation 2002; **106**(7): 804–808.

36. Hong MK, Mintz GS, Lee CW, *et al.* Comparison of coronary plaque rupture between stable angina and acute myocardial infarction: a three-vessel intravascular ultrasound study in 235 patients. Circulation 2004; **110**(8): 928–933.

37. Arnett EN, Isner JM, Redwood DR, *et al.* Coronary artery narrowing in coronary heart disease: comparison of cineangiographic and necropsy findings. Ann Intern Med 1979; **91**(3): 350–356.

38. Waller BF. Anatomy, histology, and pathology of the major epicardial coronary arteries relevant to echocar-

diographic imaging techniques. J Am Soc Echocardiogr 1989; **2**(4): 232–252.

39. Fernandes MR, Silva GV, Caixeta A, *et al.* Assessing intermediate coronary lesions: angiographic prediction of lesion severity on intravascular ultrasound. J Invasive Cardiol 2007; **19**(10): 412–416.

40. Nishioka T, Amanullah AM, Luo H, *et al.* Clinical validation of intravascular ultrasound imaging for assessment of coronary stenosis severity: comparison with stress myocardial perfusion imaging. J Am Coll Cardiol 1999; **33**(7): 1870–1878.

41. Abizaid A, Mintz GS, Pichard AD, *et al.* Clinical, intravascular ultrasound, and quantitative angiographic determinants of the coronary flow reserve before and after percutaneous transluminal coronary angioplasty. Am J Cardiol 1998; **82**(4): 423–428.

42. Takagi A, Tsurumi Y, Ishii Y, *et al.* Clinical potential of intravascular ultrasound for physiological assessment of coronary stenosis: relationship between quantitative ultrasound tomography and pressure-derived fractional flow reserve. Circulation 1999; **100**(3): 250–255.

43. Abizaid AS, Mintz GS, Mehran R, *et al.* Long-term follow-up after percutaneous transluminal coronary angioplasty was not performed based on intravascular ultrasound findings: importance of lumen dimensions. Circulation 1999; **100**(3): 256–261.

44. Hermiller JB, Buller CE, Tenaglia AN, *et al.* Unrecognized left main coronary artery disease in patients undergoing interventional procedures. Am J Cardiol 1993; **71**(2): 173–176.

45. Yamagishi M, Hongo Y, Goto Y, *et al.* Intravascular ultrasound evidence of angiographically undetected left main coronary artery disease and associated trauma during interventional procedures. Heart Vessels 1996; **11**(5): 262–268.

46. Gerber TC, Erbel R, Gorge G, *et al.* Extent of atherosclerosis and remodeling of the left main coronary artery determined by intravascular ultrasound. Am J Cardiol 1994; **73**(9): 666–671.

47. Ge J, Liu F, Gorge G, Haude M, *et al.* Angiographically "silent" plaque in the left main coronary artery detected by intravascular ultrasound. Coron Artery Dis 1995; **6**(10): 805–810.

48. Abizaid AS, Mintz GS, Abizaid A, *et al.* One-year follow-up after intravascular ultrasound assessment of moderate left main coronary artery disease in patients with ambiguous angiograms. J Am Coll Cardiol 1999; **34**(3): 707–715.

49. Fassa AA, Wagatsuma K, Higano ST, *et al.* Intravascular ultrasound-guided treatment for angiographically indeterminate left main coronary artery disease: a long-term follow-up study. J Am Coll Cardiol 2005; **45**(2): 204–211.

50. Jasti V, Ivan E, Yalamanchili V, *et al.* Correlations between fractional flow reserve and intravascular ultrasound in patients with an ambiguous left main coronary artery stenosis. Circulation 2004; **110**(18): 2831–2836.

51. Alfonso F, Macaya C, Goicolea J, *et al.* Intravascular ultrasound imaging of angiographically normal coronary segments in patients with coronary artery disease. Am Heart J 1994; **127**(3): 536–544.

52. Porter TR, Sears T, Xie F, *et al.* Intravascular ultrasound study of angiographically mildly diseased coronary arteries. J Am Coll Cardiol 1993; **22**(7): 1858–1865.

53. Isner JM, Kishel J, Kent KM, *et al.* Accuracy of angiographic determination of left main coronary arterial narrowing. Angiographic—histologic correlative analysis in 28 patients. Circulation 1981; **63**(5): 1056–1064.

54. Detre KM, Wright E, Murphy ML, *et al.* Observer agreement in evaluating coronary angiograms. Circulation 1975; **52**(6): 979–986.

55. DeRouen TA, Murray JA, Owen W. Variability in the analysis of coronary arteriograms. Circulation 1977; **55**(2): 324–328.

56. Cameron A, Kemp HG, Jr., Fisher LD, *et al.* Left main coronary artery stenosis: angiographic determination. Circulation 1983; **68**(3): 484–489.

57. Bech GJ, Droste H, Pijls NH, *et al.* Value of fractional flow reserve in making decisions about bypass surgery for equivocal left main coronary artery disease. Heart 2001; **86**(5): 547–552.

58. Zhou Y, Kassab GS, Molloi S. On the design of the coronary arterial tree: a generalization of Murray's law. Phys Med Biol 1999; **44**(12): 2929–2945.

59. Maehara A, Mintz GS, Ahmed JM, *et al.* An intravascular ultrasound classification of angiographic coronary artery aneurysms. Am J Cardiol 2001; **88**(4): 365–370.

60. Ahmed JM, Mintz GS, Weissman NJ, *et al.* Mechanism of lumen enlargement during intracoronary stent implantation: an intravascular ultrasound study. Circulation 2000; **102**(1): 7–10.

61. Maehara A, Takagi A, Okura H, *et al.* Longitudinal plaque redistribution during stent expansion. Am J Cardiol 2000; **86**(10): 1069–1072.

62. Prati F, Pawlowski T, Gil R, *et al.* Stenting of culprit lesions in unstable angina leads to a marked reduction in plaque burden: a major role of plaque embolization? A serial intravascular ultrasound study. Circulation 2003; **107**(18): 2320–2325.

63. de Feyter PJ, Kay P, Disco C, *et al.* Reference chart derived from post-stent-implantation intravascular ultrasound predictors of 6-month expected restenosis on quantitative coronary angiography. Circulation 1999; **100**(17): 1777–1783.

64. Choi JW, Goodreau LM, Davidson CJ. Resource utilization and clinical outcomes of coronary stenting: a comparison of intravascular ultrasound and angiographical guided stent implantation. Am Heart J 2001; **142**(1): 112–118.

65. Sousa A, Abizaid A, Mintz G, *et al.* The influence of intravascular ultrasound guidance on the in-hospital outcomes after stent implantation: Results from the Brazilian Society of Interventional Cardiology Registry—CENIC. J Am Coll Cardiol 2002; **39**: 54A.

66. Frey AW, Hodgson JM, Muller C, *et al.* Ultrasound-guided strategy for provisional stenting with focal balloon combination catheter: results from the randomized Strategy for Intracoronary Ultrasound-guided PTCA and Stenting (SIPS) trial. Circulation 2000; **102**(20): 2497–2502.

67. Mueller C, Hodgson JM, Schindler C, *et al.* Cost-effectiveness of intracoronary ultrasound for percutaneous coronary interventions. Am J Cardiol 2003; **91**(2): 143–147.

68. Gaster AL, Slothuus U, Larsen J, *et al.* Cost-effectiveness analysis of intravascular ultrasound guided percutaneous coronary intervention versus conventional percutaneous coronary intervention. Scand Cardiovasc J 2001; **35**(2): 80–85.

69. Gaster AL, Slothuus Skjoldborg U, Larsen J, *et al.* Continued improvement of clinical outcome and cost effectiveness following intravascular ultrasound guided PCI: insights from a prospective, randomised study. Heart 2003; **89**(9): 1043–1049.

70. Schiele F, Meneveau N, Vuillemenot A, *et al.* Impact of intravascular ultrasound guidance in stent deployment on 6-month restenosis rate: a multicenter, randomized study comparing two strategies—with and without intravascular ultrasound guidance. RESIST Study Group. REStenosis after Ivus guided STenting. J Am Coll Cardiol 1998; **32**(2): 320–328.

71. Schiele F, Meneveau N, Seronde MF, *et al.* Medical costs of intravascular ultrasound optimization of stent deployment. Results of the multicenter randomized "REStenosis after Intravascular ultrasound STenting" (RESIST) study. Int J Cardiovasc Intervent 2000; **3**(4): 207–213.

72. Oemrawsingh PV, Mintz GS, Schalij MJ, *et al.* Intravascular ultrasound guidance improves angiographic and clinical outcome of stent implantation for long coronary artery stenoses: final results of a randomized comparison with angiographic guidance

73. Mudra H, di Mario C, de Jaegere P, *et al.* Randomized comparison of coronary stent implantation under ultrasound or angiographic guidance to reduce stent restenosis (OPTICUS Study). Circulation 2001; **104**(12): 1343–1349.

74. Orford JL, Denktas AE, Williams BA, *et al.* Routine intravascular ultrasound scanning guidance of coronary stenting is not associated with improved clinical outcomes. Am Heart J 2004; **148**(3): 501–506.

75. de Jaegere P, Mudra H, Figulla H, *et al.* Intravascular ultrasound-guided optimized stent deployment. Immediate and 6 months clinical and angiographic results from the Multicenter Ultrasound Stenting in Coronaries Study (MUSIC Study). Eur Heart J 1998; **19**(8): 1214–1223.

76. Albiero R, Rau T, Schluter M, *et al.* Comparison of immediate and intermediate-term results of intravascular ultrasound versus angiography-guided Palmaz-Schatz stent implantation in matched lesions. Circulation 1997; **96**(9): 2997–3005.

77. Gil RJ, Pawlowski T, Dudek D, *et al.* Comparison of angiographically guided direct stenting technique with direct stenting and optimal balloon angioplasty guided with intravascular ultrasound. The multicenter, randomized trial results. Am Heart J 2007; **154**(4): 669–675.

78. Cheneau E, Leborgne L, Mintz GS, *et al.* Predictors of subacute stent thrombosis: results of a systematic intravascular ultrasound study. Circulation 2003; **108**(1): 43–47.

79. Fujii K, Carlier SG, Mintz GS, *et al.* Stent underexpansion and residual reference segment stenosis are related to stent thrombosis after sirolimus-eluting stent implantation: an intravascular ultrasound study. J Am Coll Cardiol 2005; **45**(7): 995–998.

80. Okabe T, Mintz GS, Buch AN, *et al.* Intravascular ultrasound parameters associated with stent thrombosis after drug-eluting stent deployment. Am J Cardiol 2007; **100**(4): 615–620.

81. Roy P, Steinberg DH, Sushinsky SJ, *et al.* The potential clinical utility of intravascular ultrasound guidance in patients undergoing percutaneous coronary intervention with drug-eluting stents. Eur Heart J 2008; **29**(15): 1851–1857.

82. Maehara A, Mintz GS, Bui AB, *et al.* Incidence, morphology, angiographic findings, and outcomes of intramural hematomas after percutaneous coronary interventions: an intravascular ultrasound study. Circulation 2002; **105**(17): 2037–2042.

83. Abizaid A, Mintz GS, Pichard AD, *et al.* Is intravascular ultrasound clinically useful or is it just a research tool? Heart 1997; **78** Suppl 2: 27–30.

(TULIP Study). Circulation 2003; **107**(1): 62–67.

84. Hoffmann R, Mintz GS, Pichard AD, *et al.* Intimal hyperplasia thickness at follow-up is independent of stent size: a serial intravascular ultrasound study. Am J Cardiol 1998; **82**(10): 1168–1172.

85. Moses JW, Leon MB, Popma JJ, *et al.* Sirolimus-eluting stents versus standard stents in patients with stenosis in a native coronary artery. N Engl J Med 2003; **349**(14): 1315–1323.

86. Sousa JE, Costa MA, Sousa AG, *et al.* Two-year angiographic and intravascular ultrasound follow-up after implantation of sirolimus-eluting stents in human coronary arteries. Circulation 2003; **107**(3): 381–383.

87. Stone GW, Midei M, Newman W, *et al.* Comparison of an everolimus-eluting stent and a paclitaxel-eluting stent in patients with coronary artery disease: a randomized trial. JAMA 2008, **299**(16): 1903–1913.

88. Weissman NJ, Koglin J, Cox DA, *et al.* Polymer-based paclitaxel-eluting stents reduce in-stent neointimal tissue proliferation: a serial volumetric intravascular ultrasound analysis from the TAXUS-IV trial. J Am Coll Cardiol 2005; **45**(8): 1201–1205.

89. Miyazawa A, Ako J, Hongo Y, *et al.* Comparison of vascular response to zotarolimus-eluting stent versus sirolimus-eluting stent: intravascular ultrasound results from ENDEAVOR III. Am Heart J 2008; **155**(1): 108–113.

90. Ormiston JA, Serruys PW, Regar E, *et al.* A bioabsorbable everolimus-eluting coronary stent system for patients with single de-novo coronary artery lesions (ABSORB): a prospective open-label trial. Lancet 2008; **371**(9616): 899–907.

91. Castagna MT, Mintz GS, Leiboff BO, *et al.* The contribution of "mechanical" problems to in-stent restenosis: An intravascular ultrasonographic analysis of 1090 consecutive in-stent restenosis lesions. Am Heart J 2001; **142**(6): 970–974.

92. Shah VM, Mintz GS, Apple S, *et al.* Background incidence of late malapposition after bare-metal stent implantation. Circulation 2002; **106**(14): 1753–1755.

93. Hong MK, Mintz GS, Lee CW, *et al.* Incidence, mechanism, predictors, and long-term prognosis of late stent malapposition after bare-metal stent implantation. Circulation 2004; **109**(7): 881–886.

94. Nakamura M, Kataoka T, Honda Y, *et al.* Late incomplete stent apposition and focal vessel expansion after bare metal stenting. Am J Cardiol 2003; **92**(10): 1217–1219.

95. Serruys PW, Degertekin M, Tanabe K, *et al.* Intravascular ultrasound findings in the multicenter, randomized, double-blind RAVEL (RAndomized study with the sirolimus-eluting VElocity balloon-expandable stent in the treatment of patients with de novo native coronary artery Lesions) trial. Circulation 2002; **106**(7): 798–803.

96. Tanabe K, Serruys PW, Degertekin M, *et al.* Incomplete stent apposition after implantation of paclitaxel-eluting stents or bare metal stents: insights from the randomized TAXUS II trial. Circulation 2005; **111**(7): 900–905.

97. Siqueira DA, Abizaid AA, Costa J de R, *et al.* Late incomplete apposition after drug-eluting stent implantation: incidence and potential for adverse clinical outcomes. Eur Heart J 2007; **28**(11): 1304–1309.

98. Hoffmann R, Morice MC, Moses JW, *et al.* Impact of late incomplete stent apposition after sirolimus-eluting stent implantation on 4-year clinical events: intravascular ultrasound analysis from the multicentre, randomised, RAVEL, E-SIRIUS and SIRIUS trials. Heart 2008; **94**(3): 322–328.

99. Joner M, Finn AV, Farb A, *et al.* Pathology of drug-eluting stents in humans: delayed healing and late thrombotic risk. J Am Coll Cardiol 2006; **48**(1): 193–202.

100. Feres F, Costa JR, Jr., Abizaid A. Very late thrombosis after drug-eluting stents. Catheter Cardiovasc Interv 2006; **68**(1): 83–88.

101. Cook S, Wenaweser P, Togni M, *et al.* Incomplete stent apposition and very late stent thrombosis after drug-eluting stent implantation. Circulation 2007; **115**(18): 2426–2434.

102. Mintz GS, Weissman NJ. Intravascular ultrasound in the drug-eluting stent era. J Am Coll Cardiol 2006; **48**(3): 421–429.

Answers

1. D
2. E
3. A
4. A
5. C

11

CHAPTER 11

Principles of Intra-coronary Optical Coherence Tomography

Peter Barlis[1], Jun Tanigawa[2], Patrick W. Serruys[3], & Evelyn Regar[3]

[1] The University of Melbourne and The Northern Hospital, Melbourne, VIC, Australia
[2] Osaka Medical College, Takatsuki, Osaka, Japan
[3] Thoraxcenter, Erasmus Medical Center, Rotterdam, The Netherlands

Intravascular imaging techniques remain complimentary to assessing vascular structures or results following stent implantation. The recent introduction of optical coherence tomography (OCT) to the coronary circulation has given unique insights into vessel microstructures and responses following stenting. Compared to intravascular ultrasound (IVUS), OCT has a ten-fold higher resolution with fewer artefacts, primarily as a result of the near infrared light used as opposed to sound to generate the image. This advantage has seen OCT successfully applied to the assessment of atherosclerotic plaque (including thin cap fibroatheroma and macrophage distribution within a culprit lesion), stent apposition and tissue coverage, introducing a new era in intravascular coronary imaging [1–11]. This chapter will introduce the principles of OCT and how this novel technology has been implemented into both the clinical and research arenas.

Technical Considerations

Whereas ultrasound produces images from backscattered sound "echoes," OCT uses infrared light waves that reflect off the internal microstructure within the biological tissues. Table 11.1 illustrates

Interventional Cardiology, First Edition. Edited by Carlo Di Mario, George D. Dangas, Peter Barlis.
© 2010 Blackwell Publishing Ltd. Published 2010 by Blackwell Publishing Ltd.

the characteristics of OCT compared to other imaging modalities.

Since the speed of light is much faster than that of sound, an interferometer is required to measure the backscattered light. The interferometer splits the light source into two "arms"—a reference arm and a sample arm, which is directed into the tissue. The frequencies and bandwidths of infrared light (1310 nm broadband super luminescent) are orders of magnitude higher than medical ultrasound. The imaging depth of current OCT systems is approximately 1.5–2.0 mm with an axial and lateral resolution of 15 μm and 25 μm, respectively. The mobile OCT System cart (LightLab Imaging Inc., Westford, MA, USA) contains the optical imaging engine and the computer. The mouse, keyboard, two monitors, two storage drawers, and the patient interface unit (PIU) are all mounted on top of the cart (Figure 11.1).

The ImageWire

The imaging probe (ImageWire™ LightLab Imaging Inc., Westford, MA, USA) has a maximum outer diameter of 0.019″ (with a standard 0.014″ radiolucent coiled tip) and contains a single-mode fiber optic core within a translucent sheath (Figure 11.2). More recently, an OCT system using Fourier-domain technology (C7, LightLab Imaging Inc, Westford, MA, USA) has become licensed in Europe (CE approved). This permits a pullback of up to 20 mm/sec with the imaging wire (DragonFly,

Table 11.1. Overview of image resolution of different coronary imaging modalities.

	OCT	IVUS	Fluoroscopy	Angioscopy	MRI
Resolution (μm)	10–15	80–120	100–200	<200	80–300
Probe size (μm)	140	700	NA	800	NA
Ionizing radiation	No (near infrared light)	No (ultrasound)	Yes	No	No

OCT – optical coherence tomography; INUS – intravascular ultrasound; MRI – magnetic resonance imaging.

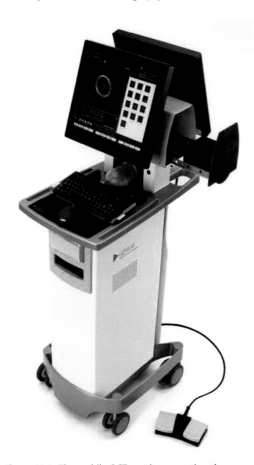

Figure 11.1. The mobile OCT cart incorporating the system console, monitor, and patient interface unit.

LightLab Imaging Inc, Westford, MA, USA) wire passed distal to the region of interest using a simple rapid exchange process.

The image wire is connected at its proximal end to the imaging console that permitted real-time data processing and two-dimensional representation of the backscattered light in a cross-sectional plane. Since the imaging wire is not torquable, it can be advanced distal to the region of interest using the over-the-wire occlusion balloon (for the occlusive

technique, see below) or a simple micro-catheter for the non-occlusive technique (see below, e.g. Transit, Cordis Johnson & Johnson, USA or ProGreat, Terumo Japan, with inner lumens >0.020″). Unlike an IVUS transducer, the optical sensor of the image wire is invisible under fluoroscopy and therefore one must estimate the correct position, using the distal 15 mm radiopaque tip of the ImageWire. As there are no direct radiopaque markers for the infrared sensor, it is possible to inadvertently miss imaging an area of interest resulting in incomplete distal lesion edge assessment. Imaging after stent implantation facilitates positioning because it is sufficient to advance the proximal end of the radiopaque wire tip at least 1 cm distal to the stent struts to image the entire stented segment. In the recently released console (C7), the image wire is advanced using a rapid exchange system over a conventional guidewire. This results in an image wire artefact during acquisition but has significantly simplified the whole process of OCT imaging with even greater pullback speeds (e.g. 20 mm/sec).

Techniques for Blood Removal

As the light used is unable to penetrate red blood cells, OCT requires temporary blood evacuation prior to image acquisition. This remains one of the major limitations precluding the routine use of OCT and warrants further consideration.

Proximal Balloon Occlusion and Flush

The proximal occlusion balloon catheter (Helios, Goodman Co, Japan) is an over-the-wire 4.4Fr catheter (inner diameter 0.025″), compatible with 6Fr guiding catheters (inner lumen diameter ≥0.071″), which is advanced distal to region of interest using a conventional angioplasty guide wire (0.014″). The guidewire is then replaced by the OCT ImageWire™ (0.019″ maximum diameter), and the occlusion balloon catheter is with-

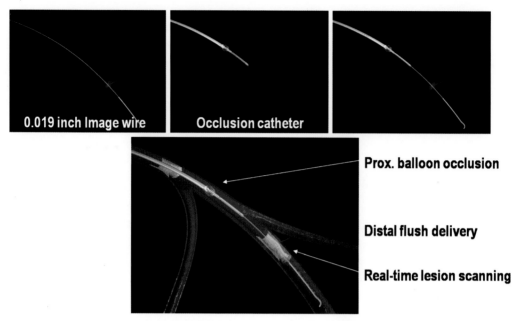

Figure 11.2. The OCT catheter and dedicated optical imaging wire (LightLab Imaging Inc., Westford, MA, USA) of the first generation system (M3). The occlusion balloon is positioned proximal to the region of interest and the imaging wire is then inserted with real-time image acquisition performed at a rate up to 3 mm/sec.

drawn proximal to the segment to be assessed leaving the imaging wire in distal position.

During imaging acquisition, coronary blood flow is removed by continuous flush of Ringer's lactate solution via the end-hole of the occlusion balloon catheter at a flow rate of 0.5–0.7 ml/sec during simultaneous balloon inflation (0.5–0.7 atm). The vessel occlusion time is limited to a maximum of 30 sec to avoid hemodynamic instability or arrhythmias. A 1.0 mm/sec pullback permits the assessment of an up to 30 mm long coronary segment with a frame rate of 15.6 frames/sec.

This technique permits OCT image acquisition without the use of additional contrast for flushing however, as the balloon needs to be positioned in the proximal segment of the vessel, visualization of such regions of the artery is limited. Further, occlusion balloon use is frequently associated with chest discomfort for the patient with associated electrocardiographic ischemia changes.

Non-occlusive Technique

With improvements in the acquisition speeds of OCT data (3.0 mm/sec for the first generation time-domain systems and 20 mm/sec for Fourier-domain OCT), blood can be evacuated by continuous flush through the guiding catheter, thus doing away with the cumbersome proximal balloon occlusion and thereby simplifying the acquisition process. Here, the OCT imaging wire is advanced carefully distal to the region of interest. In the time-domain systems (e.g. M2, M3, LightLab Imaging Inc, Westford, MA, USA) as the fragile wire does not have the properties of a guidewire, it needs to be directed distally using an over the wire catheter (e.g. Transit, Cordis, Johnson & Johnson or ProGreat, Terumo, Japan). With the wire in position, viscous iso-osmolar contrast (Iodixanol, Visipaque™, GE Health Care, Cork, Ireland) at 37° Celsius is used to clear the artery from blood and connected to the standard Y-piece of the guiding catheter. The contrast is either injected manually through the Y-piece or automatically using a pump injector. The pullback is stopped after visualization of the region of interest or in case of significant signs of ischemia, arrhythmia or patient intolerance. Cross sectional images are acquired at 20 frames/sec.

After completion of the OCT study, the image wire is removed, and intra-coronary nitrates are usually administered according to local standards and an angiogram should be taken. The procedure should be terminated if there is any hemodynamic compromise during the infusion and OCT acquisition.

OCT Applications

Although OCT has a number of varied clinical and research uses, the main applications at this present time are the assessment of:

1. Stent apposition.
2. Stent strut tissue coverage at follow-up.
3. Atherosclerotic plaques (including the characterization of vulnerable plaques).

Stent Apposition

OCT is more accurate in assessing strut apposition compared with IVUS because of higher resolution but its poor penetration (approximately 1.5 mm) makes it inferior to IVUS in assessing stent expansion. Stent struts appear as highly reflective surfaces and cast shadows on the vessel wall behind. Even if the stent struts are well apposed to the vessel wall with OCT, the stent may not be optimally expanded given that it is more difficult to identify the external elastic membrane compared with IVUS. Since OCT can show only the endoluminal surface of the strut due to limited penetration through the metal with resulting shadowing (Figure 11.3, arrows), strut and polymer thickness should be considered in assessing apposition for each type of DES design. Table 11.2 lists the thickness of commercially available.

In an evaluation of OCT findings following stent implantation to complex coronary lesions, Tanigawa *et al.* [12] examined a total of 6,402 struts from 23 patients (25 lesions) and found $9.1 \pm 7.4\%$ of all struts in each lesion treated were malapposed. Univariate predictors of malapposition on multilevel logistic regression analysis where: implantation of a sirolimus-eluting stent (SES), presence of overlapping stents, longer stent length and type C lesions. Likely mechanical explanations for malapposition of stent struts include increased strut thickness, closed cell design or acute stent recoil. The latter has been demonstrated in SES to be in the range of 15%, despite the use of high pressure balloon dilatation [13].

Stent Strut Tissue Coverage

One of the "hotly" debated topics currently in the interventional cardiology literature remains stent thrombosis. It appears that this condition is mul-

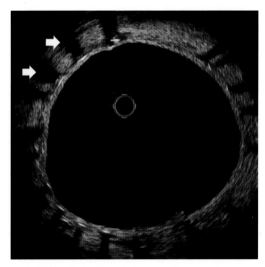

Figure 11.3. This OCT cross-section shows a thin layer of tissue covering the stent struts. As infrared light is unable to penetrate the metal struts, shadowing results (arrows).

tifactorial with premature discontinuation of dual anti-platelet therapy, stent under-expansion, hypersensitivity and lack of endothelial tissue coverage all being implicated [14–18]. Unlike conventional stents which developed circumferential coverage with an average thickness of 500 µm or more, well visualized with IVUS and angiography (corresponding to 1 mm late loss) [6], DES delay and prevent the hyperplastic response so that the average late lumen loss for sirolimus- or paclitaxel-eluting stents can be as low as 0.1 or 0.2 mm [19,20], which means the amount of intimal thickening will not be detectable with IVUS. OCT offers a potential alternative to detect and measure these tiny layers of intimal coverage and to assess late strut malapposition that can be distinguished, if images immediately after implantation are also available, into persistent (present already at the time of stent implantation) and acquired (negative remodeling or disappearance of superficial components behind struts such as thrombus) [6].

Small-scale studies have successfully used OCT to evaluate tissue stent strut coverage at follow-up. Matsumoto *et al.* studied 34 patients following sirolimus-eluting stent (SES) implantation. The mean tissue thickness was 52.5 microns, and the prevalence of struts covered by thin neointima undetectable by IVUS was 64%. The average rate of tissue-covered struts in an individual SES was

Table 11.2. Thickness of stent struts.

Manufacturer	Name	Drug	Metal Strut	Polymer	Total Thickness
Cordis, J&J	Cypher Select	Sirolimus	0.0055″ (140 μm)	0.0003″ (7 μm)	0.0061″ (154 μm)
Boston Scientific	Taxus Liberte	Paclitaxel	0.0038″ (97 μm)	0.0006″ (15 μm)	0.0050″ (127 μm)
Medtronic	Endeavor	Zotarolimus	0.0036″ (91 μm)	0.0003″ (8 μm)	0.0042″ (107 μm)
Abbott	Xience V	Everolimus	0.0032″ (81 μm)	0.0003″ (8 μm)	0.0035″ (89 μm)
Translumina	Yukon	Rapamycin	0.0034″ (87 μm)	NA	0.0034″ (87 μm)
Orbus Neich	Genous	EPC capture	0.0040″ (100 μm)	NA	0.0040″ (100 μm)
Medtronic	Driver	NA	0.0036″ (91 μm)	NA	0.0036″ (91 μm)

NA—not applicable.

89%. Nine SES (16%) showed full coverage by neointima, whereas the remaining stents had no visible strut coverage [5]. Similarly, Takano *et al.* [10] studied 21 patients (4,516 struts) three months following SES implantation. Rates of exposed struts and exposed struts with malapposition were 15% and 6%, respectively. These were more frequent in patients with acute coronary syndrome (ACS) than in those with non-ACS (18% vs. 13%, p < 0.0001; 8% vs. 5%, p < 0.005, respectively). The same group have recently reported 2 year follow-up OCT findings with the thickness of neointimal tissue at two years being greater than that at three months (71 ± 93 μm vs. 29 ± 41 μm, respectively; p < 0.001). Frequency of uncovered struts was found to be lower in the two-year group compared to the three-month group (5% vs. 15%, respectively; p < 0.001) and, in contrast, prevalence of patients with uncovered struts did not differ between the three-month and the two-year group (95% vs. 81%, respectively) highlighting that exposed struts continued to persist at long-term follow-up [21].

Atherosclerotic Plaque Assessment

Several imaging modalities have been used to assess and identify VP including coronary angioscopy, intravascular ultrasound (IVUS) and magnetic resonance imaging. Recently, there has been significant interest in the field of VP detection using OCT [1–4,11,22–25], with the technique able to detect and quantify thin cap fibroatheroma (TCFA) and macrophage distribution [2–4,25]. Several morphologic features described in autopsy series are of particular interest in such

vulnerable plaques. These include the presence of a thin fibrous cap, a necrotic lipid core and the accumulation of macrophages [2,3,25]. Nevertheless, the assessment of plaque by OCT remains largely qualitative with the notable exception of the measurement of the thickness of the fibrous cap covering necrotic areas. The other limitation of OCT for plaque quantification is the inability to provide a full thickness analysis of large plaques because of its limited penetration. OCT however, offers obvious advantages when dealing with superficial structures such as the fibrous cap [6].

Optical coherence tomography is highly sensitive and specific for the characterization of plaques when compared to histological examination. Yabushita *et al.* [26] performed an in-vitro study of more than 300 human atherosclerotic artery segments. When compared to histological examination, OCT had a sensitivity and specificity of 71–79% and 97–98% for fibrous plaques, 95–96% and 97% for fibrocalcific plaques, and 90–94.5% and 90–92% for lipid-rich plaques, respectively. Further, the inter-observer and intra-observer variability of OCT measurements were high (κ values of 0.88 and 0.91 respectively). Table 11.3 highlights the OCT features of fibrous, lipid and calcific plaques. Figure 11.4 demonstrates the OCT appearance of lipid-rich plaque with TCFA.

Recently, Kubo *et al.* [22] used OCT, together with IVUS and angioscopy, to assess plaque characteristics in 30 patients presenting with AMI. The imaging devices were consecutively used following initial mechanical thrombectomy and found the incidence of plaque rupture by OCT to be 73%,

Table 11.3. OCT appearance of different atherosclerotic plaques.

Fibrous	Lipid-rich	Calcified
High reflectivity	Low reflectivity	Low reflectivity
Homogenous	Homogenous	Inhomogeneous
Finely textured	Diffuse margins	Sharp margins
		or
		Isolated, strong reflections in dark background

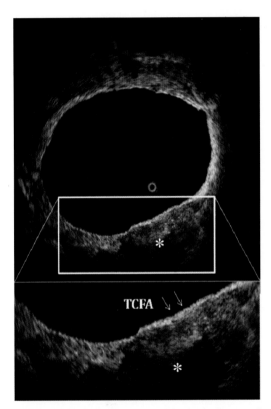

Figure 11.4. The OCT appearance of lipid-rich plaque and thin-capped fibroatheroma (TCFA). This plaque has the typical characteristics of being poorly reflective with diffuse borders (*). The overlying thin fibrous cap is bright and highly reflective. The mean cap thickness was 44 microns. OCT – optical coherence tomography.

significantly higher than that detected by both angioscopy (47%, p = 0.035) and IVUS (40%, p = 0.009). The incidence of TCFA was 83% in this patient population and only OCT was able to estimate the fibrous cap thickness (mean $49 \pm 21\,\mu$m). Further, intracoronary thrombus was observed in all cases by OCT and angioscopy but was identified only in 33% of patients by IVUS (p < 0.001). The potential for OCT in such circumstances is clearly evident with intense research currently ongoing to detect vulnerable lesions early on in their natural history, thereby limiting morbidity and mortality.

OCT Precautions and Limitations

OCT remains a specialized technique that should not be performed unless a thorough proctorship has been undertaken. As the procedure demands temporary blood removal and flush (either lactated ringers or contrast), it should not be performed in patients with poor left ventricular function or those presenting with hemodynamic compromise. Further, it is contra-indicated in patients with single remaining vessel or those with impaired renal function. Lesions that are ostial or proximally located cannot be adequately imaged using proximal balloon occlusion and thus a non-occlusive technique is preferred in these circumstances. Large caliber vessels often preclude complete circumferential imaging and this remains a technological limitation that is currently being refined.

The next generation image wires (e.g. Dragonfly, Lightlab Imaging, Westford, U.S.) offer improved durability and trackability. Frequency-domain OCT now permits extremely fast pullback speeds meaning that long segments of artery can be imaged in only a matter of 5 seconds. Eventually, automated plaque morphology detection will also be included [6]. All these advances will build on an already unique imaging technology that will play a pivotal role in better understanding coronary artery disease well into the future.

References

1. Regar E, Schaar JA, Mont E, *et al.* Optical coherence tomography. Cardiovasc Radiat Med 2003; **4**(4): 198–204.

2. Tearney GJ, Yabushita H, Houser SL, *et al.* Quantification of macrophage content in atherosclerotic plaques by optical coherence tomography. Circulation 2003; **107**(1): 113–119.

3. Jang IK, Tearney GJ, MacNeill B, *et al.* In vivo characterization of coronary atherosclerotic plaque by use of optical coherence tomography. Circulation 2005; **111**(12): 1551–1555.

4. Tearney GJ, Jang IK, Bouma BE. Optical coherence tomography for imaging the vulnerable plaque. J Biomed Opt 2006; **11**(2): 021002.

5. Shite J, Matsumoto D, Yokoyama M. Sirolimus-eluting stent fracture with thrombus, visualization by optical coherence tomography. Eur Heart J 2006; **27**(12): 1389.

6. Tanigawa J, Barlis P, Di Mario C. Intravascular Optical Coherence Tomography: Optimisation of image acquisition and quantitative assessment of stent strut apposition. EuroIntervention 2007; **3**: 128–136.

7. Tanigawa J, Barlis P, Di Mario C. Do unapposed stent struts endothelialise? In vivo demonstration with optical coherence tomography. Heart 2007; **93**(3): 378.

8. Prati F, Zimarino M, Stabile E, *et al.* Does optical coherence tomography identify arterial healing after stenting? An in vivo comparison with histology, on a rabbit carotid model. Heart 2008; **94**(2): 217–221.

9. Tanigawa J, Barlis P, Dimopoulos K, *et al.* Optical coherence tomography to assess malapposition in overlapping drug-eluting stents. EuroIntervention 2008; **3**(13): 580–583.

10. Takano M, Inami S, Jang IK, *et al.* Evaluation by optical coherence tomography of neointimal coverage of sirolimus-eluting stent three months after implantation. Am J Cardiol 2007; **99**(8): 1033–1038.

11. Barlis P, Serruys PW, DeVries A, *et al.* Optical coherence tomography assessment of vulnerable plaque rupture: predilection for the plaque "shoulder". Eur Heart J 2008; **29**(16): 2023.

12. Tanigawa J, Barlis P, Kaplan S, *et al.* Stent strut apposition in complex lesions using optical coherence tomography. Am J Cardiol 2006; **98**(8): Suppl 1: 97M.

13. Regar E, Schaar J, Serruys PW. Images in cardiology. Acute recoil in sirolimus eluting stent: real time, in vivo assessment with optical coherence tomography. Heart 2006; **92**(1): 123.

14. Barlis P, Virmani R, Sheppard MN, *et al.* Angiographic and histological assessment of successfully treated late acute stent thrombosis secondary to a sirolimus-eluting stent. Eur Heart J 2007; **28**(14): 1675.

15. Joner M, Finn AV, Farb A, *et al.* Pathology of drug-eluting stents in humans: delayed healing and late thrombotic risk. J Am Coll Cardiol 2006; **48**(1): 193–202.

16. Virmani R, Guagliumi G, Farb A, *et al.* Localized hypersensitivity and late coronary thrombosis secondary to a sirolimus-eluting stent: should we be cautious? Circulation 2004; **109**(6): 701–705.

17. Park DW, Park SW, Park KH, *et al.* Frequency of and risk factors for stent thrombosis after drug-eluting stent implantation during long-term follow-up. Am J Cardiol 2006; **98**(3): 352–356.

18. Fujii K, Carlier SG, Mintz GS, *et al.* Stent underexpansion and residual reference segment stenosis are related to stent thrombosis after sirolimus-eluting stent implantation: an intravascular ultrasound study. J Am Coll Cardiol 2005; **45**(7): 995–998.

19. Morice MC, Serruys PW, Sousa JE, *et al.* A randomized comparison of a sirolimus-eluting stent with a standard stent for coronary revascularization. N Engl J Med 2002; **346**(23): 1773–1780.

20. Fujii K, Mintz GS, Kobayashi Y, *et al.* Contribution of stent underexpansion to recurrence after sirolimus-eluting stent implantation for in-stent restenosis. Circulation 2004; **109**(9): 1085–1088.

21. Takano M, Yamamoto M, Inami S, *et al.* Long-term follow-up evaluation after sirolimus-eluting stent implantation by optical coherence tomography; do uncovered struts persist? J Am Coll Cardiol 2008; **51**(9): 968–969.

22. Kubo T, Imanishi T, Takarada S, *et al.* Assessment of culprit lesion morphology in acute myocardial infarction: ability of optical coherence tomography compared with intravascular ultrasound and coronary angioscopy. J Am Coll Cardiol 2007; **50**(10): 933–939.

23. Chia S, Christopher Raffel O, Takano M, *et al.* In-vivo comparison of coronary plaque characteristics using optical coherence tomography in women vs. men with acute coronary syndrome. Coron Artery Dis 2007; **18**(6): 423–427.

24. Giattina SD, Courtney BK, Herz PR, *et al.* Assessment of coronary plaque collagen with polarization sensitive optical coherence tomography (PS-OCT). Int J Cardiol 2006; **107**(3): 400–409.

25. Jang IK, Bouma BE, Kang DH, *et al.* Visualization of coronary atherosclerotic plaques in patients using optical coherence tomography: comparison with intravascular ultrasound. J Am Coll Cardiol 2002; **39**(4): 604–609.

26. Yabushita H, Bouma BE, Houser SL, *et al.* Characterization of human atherosclerosis by optical coherence tomography. Circulation 2002; **106**(13): 1640–1645.

CHAPTER 12

Multislice Computed Tomography of Coronary Arteries

Francesca Pugliese, & Pim J. de Feyter

Erasmus MC University Medical Center, Rotterdam, The Netherlands

Introduction

The introduction of 4-slice computed tomography (CT) in 2000 was followed by rapid and revolutionary advances in multislice computed tomography (MSCT) technology. Currently, 64-MSCT and dual source computed tomography (DSCT) are considered state-of-the-art for cardiac MSCT imaging with 320-slice systems also emerging in clinical practice.

Non contrast-enhanced MSCT scans allow visualization of cardiac and coronary artery calcification. After intravenous injection of iodinated contrast agent, MSCT can delineate cardiac chambers, great cardiac vessels and coronary arteries (Figure 12.1).

The evaluation of general cardiac morphology is usually performed by echocardiography and/or magnetic resonance imaging (MRI) without the need for contrast injection or radiation exposure. Nevertheless, MSCT can be clinically helpful in a variety of situations, including the need for cross-sectional imaging in the event of inconclusive findings at echocardiography or in patients with pacemakers or other devices precluding MRI.

Interventional Cardiology, First Edition. Edited by Carlo Di Mario, George D. Dangas, Peter Barlis.
© 2010 Blackwell Publishing Ltd. Published 2010 by Blackwell Publishing Ltd.

Importantly, the main clinical focus of MSCT in cardiac imaging is the evaluation of the coronary arteries.

Coronary MSCT Angiography—Technique

Basic Principles

In MSCT scanners, the X-rays are generated by an X-ray tube mounted on a rotating gantry. The patient is centered within the bore of the gantry such that the array of detectors is positioned to record incident photons after they have traversed the patient. MSCT differs from single detector CT principally by the design of the detector array, which allows the acquisition of multiple adjacent sections simultaneously.

MSCT systems have two principal modes of scanning (Figure 12.2). The first mode is *sequential* scanning, also known as "step-and-shoot," in which the table is advanced in a step-wise fashion. In this mode, the X-rays are generated during an imaging window positioned at a predetermined offset from the R wave (prospective ECG triggering; Figure 12.2, A) whilst the table is stationary. The diastolic phase of the cardiac cycle is usually chosen because cardiac motion is reduced in diastole. Sequential scanning is the current mode for measuring coronary calcium at most centers using MSCT.

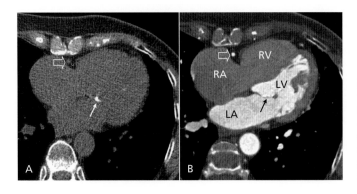

Figure 12.1. Axial images provide four-chamber views of the heart without (A) and with (B) injection of contrast agent. LA: left atrium; LV: left ventricle; RA: right atrium; RV: right ventricle; void arrow: right coronary artery; arrow: mild calcification of the mitral valve.

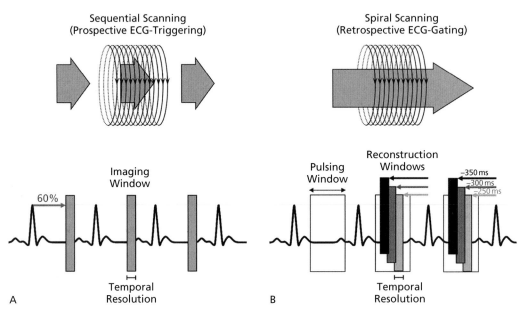

A

B

Figure 12.2. In sequential scanning, data for one axial slice are acquired, after which the table is advanced to the next position (A). Sequential scan protocols use prospective ECG-triggering to synchronize the data acquisition to cardiac motion. Based on the measured duration of previous heart cycles, the scan of one slice is initiated at a pre-specified moment after the R-wave. Diastole is commonly chosen to ensure the least motion artifacts, e.g., 60% of the previous R-R interval. Spiral scanners acquire data continuously and record the patient's ECG while the table moves at a constant speed (B). Images are reconstructed using retrospective ECG-gating. This mode is more flexible to minimize motion artifacts because reconstruction window can be positioned arbitrarily within the R-R interval. If X-ray tube modulation is used, the full output occurs only during an interval of the cardiac cycle (pulsing window) which can eventually be used for image reconstruction.

The second mode is *spiral* or helical scanning, in which the table moves continuously at a fixed speed relative to the gantry rotation. The ECG trace of the patient is recorded during the scan. After data acquisition, the optimal reconstruction window is chosen among all available time positions to minimize motion artifacts (retrospective ECG gating; Figure 12.2, B). Spiral scanning is the current mode for performing coronary MSCT angiography because it allows flexibility in the position of reconstruction windows, which is helpful to ensure the least motion artifacts. However, spiral scanning is associated with a higher X-ray radiation exposure than sequential scanning.

In order to reduce radiation exposure in spiral scanning, the X-ray tube current can be modulated prospectively: guided by the ECG, the full output occurs only during an interval of the cardiac cycle which will be used for image reconstruction (e.g. diastole), whereas the X-ray output will be reduced during the remaining cardiac cycle (Figure 12.2, B).

Temporal resolution is the time for acquiring the data needed for the reconstruction of one image. Temporal resolution depends primarily on gantry rotation time. In particular, because reconstruction of MSCT images requires data acquired over half gantry rotation (180°), temporal resolution equals half of the gantry rotation time (Figure 12.3,

A). The latest development to improve temporal resolution and omit the need to lower patients' heart rates by pre-medication has been the introduction of MSCT scanners with two X-ray sources acquiring different projections simultaneously [1]. In dual-source computed tomography (DSCT), the two X-ray sources are mounted at an angle of 90°, therefore temporal resolution is equal to a quarter of the gantry rotation time, i.e. 330/4 = 83 ms (Figure 12.3, B and Figure 12.4).

Coronary arteries have a diameter of 2–4 mm in their proximal tract and taper distally, therefore high *spatial resolution* is another prerequisite for MSCT coronary imaging. Spatial resolution of MSCT on the transverse plane (x, y) is $0.4 \times 0.4 \, mm^2$.

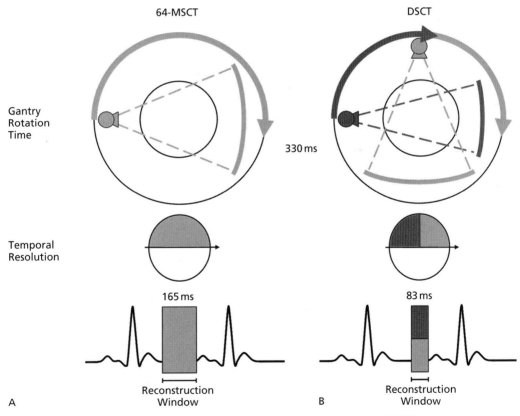

Figure 12.3. Reconstruction of MSCT images (A) uses data acquired over 180°, thus temporal resolution equals half of the gantry rotation time. Because the shortest gantry rotation time currently achievable by a 64-MSCT scanner is 330 ms, the corresponding temporal resolution is 165 ms. Temporal resolution corresponds to the width of reconstruction window. In DSCT (B), two X-ray sources and two corresponding detector arrays are mounted at an angle of 90°, therefore only 90° rotation is needed to provide data from 180°. In DSCT, temporal resolution is equal to a quarter of the gantry rotation time, i.e. 330/4 = 83 ms.

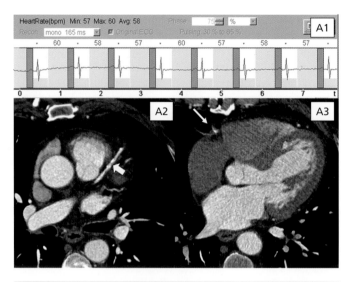

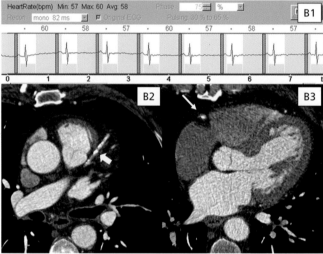

Figure 12.4. MSCT images display the average cardiac motion over the reconstruction window. A 165 mm-wide reconstruction window (A1–A3) averages MSCT views obtained during 180° gantry rotation. This is the reconstruction algorithm employed in 64-MSCT. An 83 mm-wide reconstruction window (B1–B3) averages MSCT views obtained (by 2 detector arrays) during 90° gantry rotation. This is the reconstruction algorithm employed in DSCT. Reconstruction using 180° data (A2) might improve image contrast when compared to reconstruction using 90° data (B2) because more MSCT views are averaged for the reconstruction of the same image (gross arrow = LAD). However, a wider reconstruction window worsens temporal resolution and may cause more blurring (A3) than the use of the narrowest reconstruction window (B3) (thin arrow = RCA).

Spatial resolution along patient's longitudinal axis (z-axis) is determined mainly by the individual detector width, which varies between 0.5–0.625 mm depending on the manufacturer. These features permit reconstruction of high quality images with similar sub-millimeter resolution along the x, y, and z axis. Although catheter angiography has a bi-dimensional spatial resolution of $0.2 \times 0.2\,mm^2$, a major advantage of MSCT over catheter angiography is the ability to perform multi-planar reconstructed images (see below). An overview of major image parameters, patient preparation and contrast administration in catheter angiography, 64-MSCT and DSCT is given in Table 12.1.

Contrast Enhancement

Good contrast enhancement in coronary arteries is essential for the detection of atherosclerotic changes and luminal stenosis. An iodine flow in the range from 1.2–2 g/s is recommended [2]. This can be achieved by either injecting low-concentration contrast material at high flow rates or by injection of high concentration contrast material at lower flow rates. However, it is standard practice to inject contrast agent at rates of at least 5 ml/s. Total contrast volume is determined by contrast injection rate multiplied by the scan time required to cover the heart. Typical injection volumes are in the range 60–100 ml. Dual injection, i.e. iodinated

Table 12.1. Overview of image parameters, patient preparation and contrast administration.

	Catheter Angiography	64-MSCT	DSCT
Spatial resolution	$0.2 \times 0.2\,mm^2$	$0.4 \times 0.4 \times 0.4\,mm^3$	$0.4 \times 0.4 \times 0.4\,mm^3$
Temporal resolution	8 ms	165 ms	83 ms
Preparation			
Beta-blockers	no	if heart rate ≥65 beats/min, metoprolol 100 mg orally 1 hr before scan or/and 5–15 mg i.v. in patients with aortic valve stenosis, severe hypotension, Mobitz heart block consider calcium channel blockers	(optional)
Nitroglycerine	intracoronary	(optional—sublingual)	(optional—sublingual)
Contrast	80–100 ml intracoronary	100 ml intravenous	60–100 ml intravenous

contrast followed by saline (30–50 ml) is recommended for MSCT of the heart. Saline is helpful to avoid dense opacification of the right cardiac chambers and consequent artifacts which might limit the interpretation of the right coronary artery.

Image Post-Processing

With image post-processing, the source axial images are modified and made useful for the observer [3] (Figure 12.5). With isotropic resolution, multiplanar reformats (MPR) and maximum intensity projections (MIP) along the course of the coronary arteries are the routinely methods for assessment of coronaries from MSCT datasets. Three-dimensional volume rendering technique (VRT) provides a helpful overview, e.g. in cases of complex anatomy such as coronary artery bypass grafts (CABG) or anomalous coronary arteries [4]. However, axial images may be best for the detection of coronary stenoses.

Typical Artifacts

It is important to recognize a few typical MSCT artifacts which may lead to image misinterpretation. Motion artifacts (Figure 12.6) typically blur the contours of the heart and coronary arteries. Inconsistent triggering or arrhythmias will lead to misalignment of adjacent image stacks. Partial voluming occurs when a pixel (i.e. smallest portion of an image) contains more than one type of tissue. In this setting, the attenuation value assigned to the pixel is the weighted average of the different atten-uation values. Thus, when a pixel is only partially filled by a structure of very high attenuation (e.g. metal or bone), a high CT number is assigned to the complete pixel, which will thus appear bright on the image. This may lead to overestimation of the size of high-attenuation objects (e.g. coronary calcifications and stents) (Figure 12.7).

Coronary MSCT Angiography—Clinical Applications

Stenosis Detection

Although conventional coronary angiography is still regarded as the reference standard for the detection and quantification of coronary artery stenosis, there are situations where sufficient information may be acquired by a non-invasive technique with benefits in terms of cost, patient risk and discomfort.

Since 1999, when the first studies on MSCT coronary angiography were published, the development of MSCT technology has been tremendous. Numerous studies [5–21] have compared the accuracy of MSCT in the detection of coronary artery stenosis vs. invasive coronary angiography (Table 12.2). Whilst sensitivity and specificity remained similar comparing 16-MSCT and 64-MSCT, 64-MSCT and DSCT became more robust for imaging the coronaries: in the segmental analysis, a decrease was shown for the number of coronary segments that had to be excluded due to insufficient image quality [22] (Figure 12.8, Table 12.2). Importantly, in the per-patient analysis,

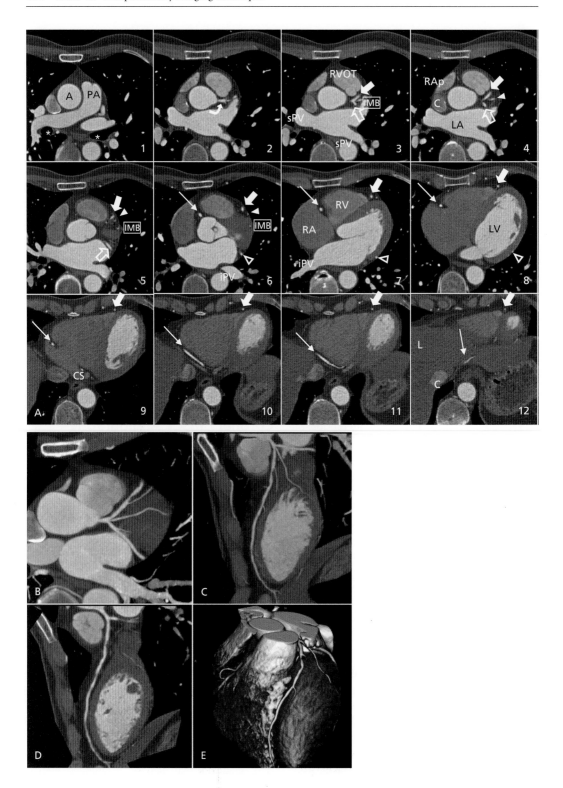

Figure 12.5. A (1–12): The basic information of MSCT is the axial images (A1–A12). Scrolling through them in the cranial to caudal direction shows any structure in the axial plane. The scan starts at the level of the tracheal bifurcation (A1) therefore the main bronchi (asterisks), the ascending aorta (A) and pulmonary artery (PA) are shown. As we scroll caudally, the origin of the left main coronary artery (A2, curved arrow) and its trifurcation (A3) into left anterior descending artery (gross arrow), circumflex artery (void arrow) and intermediate branch (IMB) are seen. The left anterior descending artery (A3–A12, gross arrow) courses along the superior inter-ventricular groove and can be followed down to the apex of the heart. A diagonal branch is also seen (A4-A6, gross arrowhead). The left circumflex artery (A3–A5, void arrow) courses in the left atrio-ventricular groove and gives an obtuse marginal branch (A6–A8, void arrowhead). The proximal right coronary artery (A6, thin arrow) has a short horizontal course. Then the vessel courses caudally (A7–A9, thin arrow) in the right atrio-ventricular groove. The inferior inter-ventricular groove contains the posterior descending artery (A12,

thin arrow). (Abbreviations: A = aorta; PA = pulmonary artery; asterisks = main bronchi; RVOT = right ventricular outflow tract; sPV = superior pulmonary veins; RAp = right appendage; C = cava; LA = left atrium; IMB = intermediate branch; iPV = inferior pulmonary veins; RA = right atrium; RV = right ventricle; LV = left ventricle; CS = coronary sinus; L = liver.)
B–E: Axial images are reconstructed to form a volume. Post-processing is performed on this volume data set. Multiplanar reconstructions (B) cut this volume according to planes arbitrarily tilted in any orientation. When the cut plane is not flat but curved, the result is a curved multiplanar reconstruction (C, D). This image is a flattened representation of the curved plane (D). Maximum intensity projection is an algorithm that visualizes only the structures with the highest attenuation along the observation line (C).
Volume rendering (E) displays the volume based on the density of the structures. Color attribution is arbitrary; therefore the appearance will change when the operator changes the colors of the algorithm.

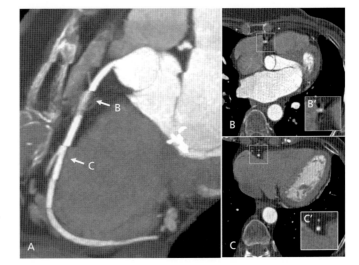

Figure 12.6. Typical artifacts in cardiac MSCT (A) include motion artifacts (B) and stack misalignment due to heart rate variations or slight arrhythmia (C). Whereas motion artifacts cause blurring (B), images within a misaligned stack are not blurred (C).

which is clinically relevant because it explores the ability of MSCT to identify patients with or without significant CAD, the negative predictive value was consistently found to be high, in the range 92–100% (Table 12.2). These findings led to the hypothesis that a normal MSCT may obviate the need for invasive angiography in properly selected clinical circumstances. The reported positive predictive values were lower, indicating the tendency

of MSCT to overestimate the severity of disease in comparison to invasive coronary angiography. Especially in the presence of coronary calcifications and residual motion in the dataset, MSCT is presently limited to accurately grade lesion severity (percentage of stenosis). However, MSCT has a notably high sensitivity and negative predictive value for the detection of significant CAD, thus it may be well suited to clinical situations in which

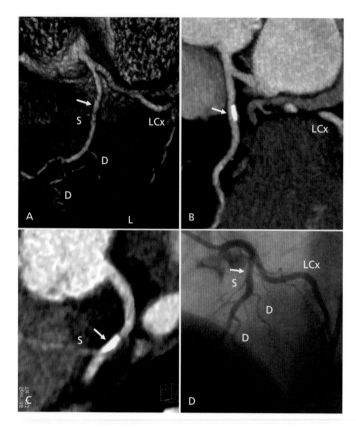

Figure 12.7. Volume rendered image (A), curved maximum intensity projection (B) and multiplanar reconstruction (C) show a calcified plaque (arrow) located in the LAD just proximal to the origin of a septal branch (S). The size of structures with high X-ray attenuation such as calcifications is overestimated in MSCT due to partial voluming. This calcification superimposes most of the coronary artery lumen. The conventional angiogram (D) shows a normal LAD.

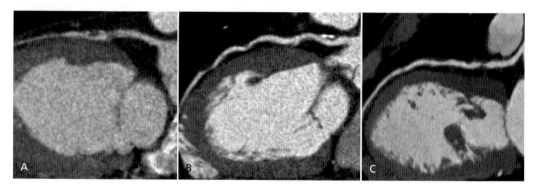

Figure 12.8. Curved multiplanar reconstructions of the LM and LAD arteries obtained in three different patients with 16-MSCT (A), 64-MSCT (B) and DSCT (C) show progressive improvement in image quality. All the patients had heart rates during the scan comprised between 62 and 65 beats/minute.

exclusion of CAD is of paramount concern, e.g. in patients with low to intermediate pretest likelihood of disease [23]. The evolving indications of MSCT of the heart, with emphasis on the evaluation of coronary arteries, are shown in Table 12.3.

Bifurcations and Ostial Lesions

The angiographic evaluation of bifurcation lesions may be hindered by projectional foreshortening, vessels overlap and insufficient vessel opacification; for these reasons, the assessment of the side

Table 12.2. Detection of coronary stenosis—diagnostic performance of MSCT vs. conventional angiography.

	No. patients	Per segment					Per patient			
		Unevaluable segments (%)	Sensitivity (%)	Specificity (%)	PPV (%)	NPV (%)	Sensitivity (%)	Specificity (%)	PPV (%)	NPV (%)
16-MSCT										
Mollet [13]	128	7	92	95	79	98	100	86	97	100
Hoffman [9]	103	6	95	98	87	99	97	87	90	95
Achenbach [5]	50	4	94	96	69	99	100	83	100	86
Mollet [12]	51	0	95	98	87	99	97	84	89	95
Garcia [7]	187	29	85	91	36	99	98	55	50	99
Dewey [6]	129	9	83	86	90	95	93	74	93	92
Hausleiter [8]	129	11	93	87	46	99	—	—	—	—
64-MSCT										
Leschka [11]	53	0	94	97	87	99	100	100	100	100
Raff [18]	70	12	86	95	66	98	95	90	93	93
Leber [10]	59	0	88	97	—	99	94	—	—	—
Pugliese [17]	35	0	99	96	78	99	100	90	96	100
Mollet [14]	52	2	99	95	76	99	100	92	97	100
Ropers [19]	82	4	95	93	56	99	96	91	83	98
Nikolaou [15]	72	10	86	95	72	97	97	72	83	95
Hausleiter [8]	114	8	92	92	54	99	99	75	74	99
320-MSCT										
Dewey [46]	30	0	78	98	75	99	100	94	92	100
DSCT										
Nikolaou [16]	20	4	95	93	79	98	—	—	—	—
Scheffel [20]	30	1	96	98	86	99	—	—	—	—
Weustink [21]	100	0	95	95	75	99	99	87	96	95

Table 12.3. Evolving indications of MSCT of the heart [23] with emphasis on the evaluation of coronary arteries.

Detection of CAD in symptomatic patients
1. Intermediate pre-test probability of CAD + equivocal ECG/unable to exercise
2. Equivocal exercise tests, perfusion imaging, stress echo
3. Evaluation of coronary arteries in patients with heart failure of new onset to assess etiology
Coronary anomalies
Exclusion of CAD prior to cardiac valve surgery/major non-cardiac surgery
Patients with recurrent chest pain after PCI with low probability of in-stent restenosis and large stents (≥3 mm)
Coronary bypass grafts
Acute chest pain
1. Non-ST segment elevation and initial troponin negative
2. Intermediate probability of aortic dissection/aneurysm, pulmonary emboli, obstructive CAD (triple rule out)

branch ostium can be particularly challenging. Errors in diagnosis may lead to consequences for patient management: when CABG surgery is the treatment of choice, underestimation of a side branch lesion may result in the side branch not being grafted; when PCI is preferred, detailed anatomic information will permit to better define intervention strategy. Moreover, conventional angiography does not provide sufficient information on the plaque burden at the level of the bifurcation. In the presence of a high plaque burden, initial treatment of both the main and side branches (e.g. crush or culottes techniques) should be preferred over main branch stenting first followed by provisional balloon angioplasty (with or without stenting) of the side branch.

Van Mieghem et al. [24] compared MSCT to conventional angiography for the detection and classification of coronary bifurcation lesions. In keeping with the available literature on non-bifurcation lesions, they reported 96% sensitivity, 97% specificity, 63% positive predictive value and 99% negative predictive value for the detection of bifurcation lesions (Figure 12.9). MSCT was found to be accurate also in classifying bifurcation lesions according to the Medina classification system [25]. Furthermore, thanks to the three-dimensional

nature of MSCT data, the bifurcation angle between the main vessel and the side branch could be measured accurately. In situations where both branches needed to be stented, information regarding the bifurcation angle was used to support the choice of the stenting technique.

The visualization of ostial lesions (Figure 12.10) may equally be affected by projectional limitations in conventional angiography. Occasionally, ostial lesions can be masked by the engagement of the catheter tip beyond the lesion. At a pre-interventional stage, MSCT can provide information on three-dimensional anatomy of ostial lesions and vessel take-off angle [26].

Chronic Total Occlusion

In the diagnostic work-up of patients with chronically occluded coronary arteries, MSCT can add important information to conventional angiography. Measurement of the length of the occluded segment, which has long been identified as a predictor of failed PCI, can be limited in conventional angiography by foreshortening, calibration limitations and lack of collateral filling (Figure 12.11). Conversely, MSCT is a three-dimensional technique which allows reliable length measurement of coronary segments. Likewise, MSCT permits to evaluate the proximal entry port, the severity of calcification (Figure 12.12) and to delineate occlusion trajectory. Therefore, MSCT may improve the ability to predict the success rate of PCI. Mollet et al. [27] found that a blunt entry point, an occlusion length >15 mm and severe calcification, all determined by MSCT, were independent predictors of procedural failure.

Stents

Coronary stents are notoriously difficult to assess by MSCT. Partial voluming artifacts (see above) enlarge the apparent size of the stent; this is particularly disturbing in smaller stents, where the in-stent lumen might be completely obscured, and in overlapping and bifurcation stents due to an excess of metal. As demonstrated in vitro, types of metal and strut thickness also play an important role for in-stent lumen assessability [28]; generally, stents with thinner struts (e.g. 0.14 mm) are less problematic than stents with thicker struts (e.g. 0.15 mm and above).

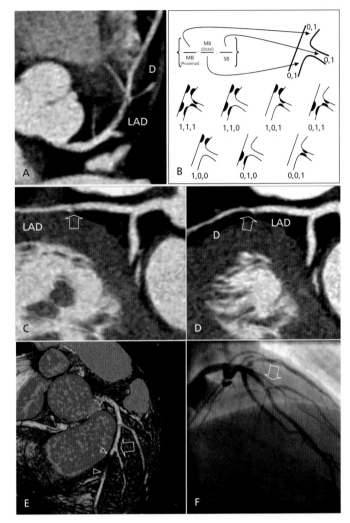

Figure 12.9. The DSCT multiplanar reconstruction (A) shows a proximal bifurcation lesion (arrows) in the LAD artery, also seen on the curved multiplanar reconstructions of the LAD (C) and diagonal branch (E). The lesion is confirmed by the conventional angiogram (F). According the Medina classification system (B), the lesion involves proximal main branch and side branch whereas the distal main branch is unremarkable (1,0,1). The lesion is not clearly detectable in the volume rendered image (E); distally to the bifurcation, the LAD has intramyocardial course (D) (arrowheads).

In the evaluation of coronary stents, the finding of contrast-enhancement distal to the stent is not fool-proof for stent patency, because collateral pathways may fill the vessel retrogradely; if the stent is being evaluated for the presence of non-occlusive in-stent restenosis, direct visualization of the in-stent lumen becomes the mandatory criterion.

Technical requirements for coronary stent imaging are 64-slice MSCT scanners with thin detectors in order to optimize spatial resolution and decrease partial voluming. High temporal resolution is also important because high density

artifacts are exacerbated by the presence of residual motion in the MSCT dataset [29].

Clinical studies compared different generations of MSCT scanners to conventional angiography for the detection of in-stent restenosis, defined as ≥50% luminal narrowing (Table 12.4). Studies performed using 16-MSCT [30], 40-MSCT [31] and 64-MSCT [32–34] reported promising results with variable percentages of unassessable stents. Using DSCT [35], the percentage of unassessable stents was found to be low; whereas the diagnostic performance did not vary significantly between different stent configurations (i.e. single stents vs.

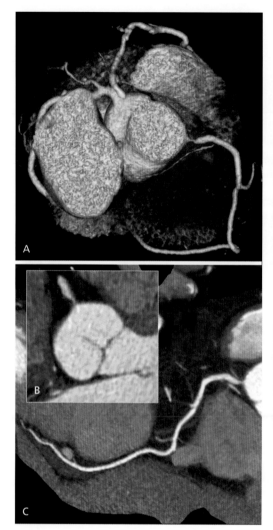

Figure 12.10. The volume rendered view after removal of the right atrium (A), axial image (B) and curved multiplanar reconstruction (C) demonstrate an ostial lesion of the RCA.

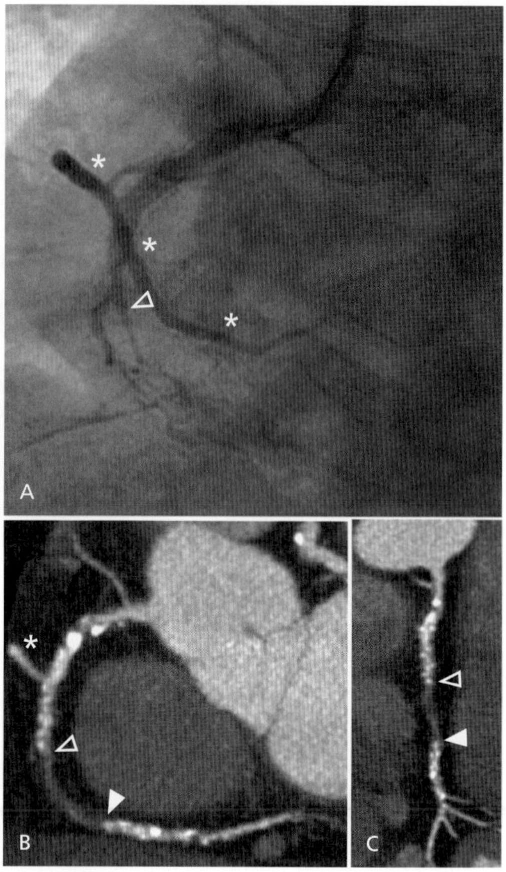

Figure 12.11. Occlusion of the RCA (void arrowheads) is demonstrated by the conventional angiogram (A), DSCT multiplanar reconstruction (B) and curved multiplanar reconstruction (C) of the vessel. The distal patent RCA is not sharply visualized on the angiogram (A). The multiplanar reconstruction (B) and curved multiplanar reconstruction (C) of the RCA permit better visualization of the distal patent vessel (solid arrowheads) and thus of the actual occlusion length. Asterisks: right ventricular branch.

overlapping/bifurcation stenting), the results were influenced importantly by the stent diameter. In particular, the ability of DSCT to exclude with certainty in-stent restenosis in stents with diameters ≤2.75 mm was significantly lower than that observed in larger stents.

Ideally, the stent type and diameter are known prior to the scan, therefore in-stent lumen accessibility in a particular patient could be predicted from the available in-vitro and in-vivo data. However, MSCT was shown to have a constantly high negative predictive value, therefore it may be useful in patients with clinical symptoms but low pre-test probability for in-stent restenosis.

Stent implantation in the left main (LM) and proximal LAD/CX provides a suitable scenario for the use of MSCT in the detection of in-stent restenosis. This is mainly due to the relatively large size of stents implanted in the LM and proximal LAD/CX; moreover, this part of the coronary tree is relatively protected from motion artifacts. Although CABG surgery is still recommended in patients

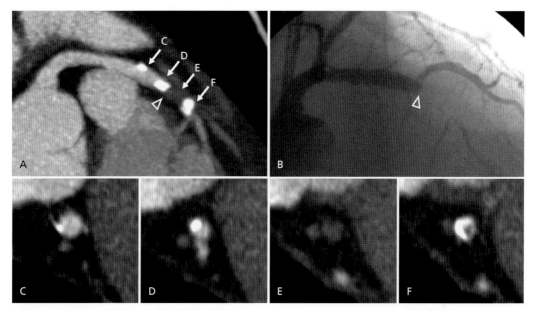

Figure 12.12. Occlusion of the proximal LAD (arrowheads) is demonstrated by the DSCT maximum intensity projection image (A) and conventional angiogram (B). The DSCT cross sections (C–F), obtained as indicated in A, provide information on the severity of lesion calcification. Bulky calcifications are present proximally to the occlusion (C), at the level of the stump (D) and more distally (F).

Table 12.4. Detection of in-stent restenosis—diagnostic performance of MSCT vs. conventional angiography.

	Unevaluable stents (%)	Sensitivity (%)	Specificity (%)	PPV (%)	NPV (%)
16-MSCT					
Gilard [30]					
All diameters	36	—	—	—	—
>3 mm	19	86	100	100	99
≤3 mm	49	54	100	100	94
40-MSCT					
Gaspar [31]					
All diameters	5	89	81	47	97
64-MSCT					
Rixe [34]					
All diameters	42	86	98	86	98
>3 mm	22	100	100	100	100
3 mm	42	83	96	83	96
<3 mm*	92	—	100	—	100
Ehara [33]					
All diameters	12	92	81	54	98
Cademartiri [32]					
All diameters	7	90	86	44	98
DSCT					
Pugliese [35]					
All diameters	5	94	92	77	98
≥3.5 mm	0	100	100	100	100
3 mm	0	100	97	91	100
≤2.75 mm	22	84	64	52	90

*Only 1 stent available, without in-stent restenosis.

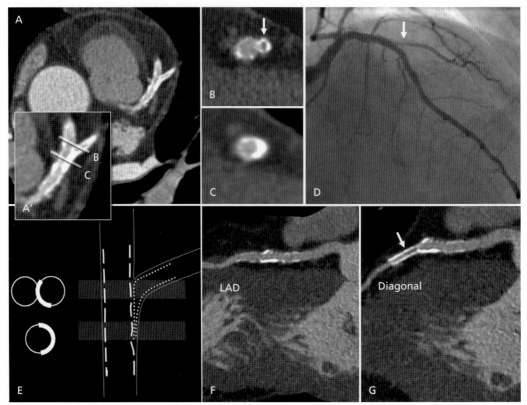

Figure 12.13. The DSCT axial image (A), its magnification (A'), the cross-sectional views (B, C) and the diagram (E) show the typical appearance of the crush stenting technique, characterized by three layers of metal crushed against the ostium of the side branch. The DSCT cross-section obtained at the level of the carina (B) and the curved multiplanar reconstruction of the diagonal branch (G) demonstrate in-stent restenosis in the diagonal branch stent (arrow). The LAD (main branch) is patent (F). The conventional angiogram (D) confirms the findings.

with LM disease, PCI is increasingly performed on the unprotected LM coronary artery in the drug-eluting stent (DES) era. However, in-stent restenosis still occurs with DES and may cause fatal myocardial infarction or sudden death [36], therefore surveillance with routinely angiography six months after PCI for left main stem is highly recommended [37]. A study by Van Mieghem *et al.* [38] showed that MSCT was safe and reliable in excluding in-stent restenosis in patients with LM and proximal LAD/CX stents; this study suggested that MSCT might be an acceptable first-line alternative to conventional angiography for the follow-up of patients after unprotected LM stenting.

MSCT also visualizes the configuration of bifurcation/overlapping stents (Figure 12.13) and the position of stents implanted in ostial lesions. Tissue prolapses, stent malapposition and underexpansion are generally not clearly visualized by MSCT. It is conceivable that stents with thinner struts, absorbable and non-metallic stents (Figure 12.14) will be less affected by high-density artifacts; the introduction of these new devices might increase the utility of MSCT in patients after PCI.

Coronary Artery Bypass Grafts
General Issues

Patients with prior coronary artery bypass graft (CABG) surgery usually present with co-morbidity and have a higher prevalence of valve disease and ventricular dysfunction compared with non-CABG patients. They have a higher incidence of complications during invasive procedures, including cardiac catheterization, and may therefore benefit from non-invasive coronary angiography performed by MSCT.

Generally, bypass grafts are well visualized by MSCT due to their large diameter, limited calcifi-

cation and relative immobility. Surgical opaque material, such as vascular clips, sternal wires and graft orifice indicators may however hinder the evaluability of coronary grafts (Figure 12.15).

Clinical Performance and Limitations (Table 12.5)

64-MSCT permits to evaluate graft patency with a sensitivity approaching 100% in both arterial and venous grafts and without exclusion of grafts due to insufficient image quality [39–42]. However, ischemic symptoms in patients after CABG surgery can be caused by obstruction of bypass grafts or by disease progression in native coronary arteries. Comprehensive evaluation post-CABG surgery should also include the native coronary tree; assessment of the native coronary arteries can be difficult in these patients owing to the diffuse nature of the disease and the presence of severe calcifications [39].

Valve Disease

Whereas the visualization of the tricuspid and pulmonary valves is generally inconsistent, the mitral and aortic valves can reliably be depicted in contrast-enhanced MSCT scans. Whilst MSCT cannot provide measurements of transvalvular flow and pressure gradients, dynamic imaging of the open and closed valve is possible (Figure 12.16). For the

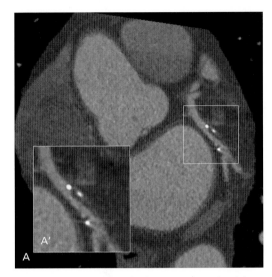

Figure 12.14. The DSCT multiplanar reconstruction (A) and its magnification (A′) show a bioabsorbable stent placed in the LCx artery. The stent is radiolucent with radiopaque markers at the stent edges.

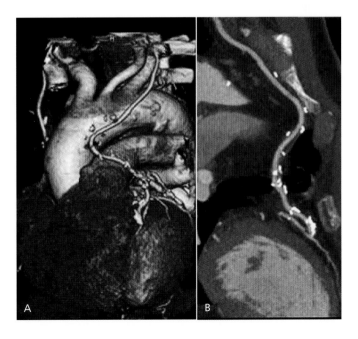

Figure 12.15. In a patient after coronary artery bypass graft surgery, the DSCT volume rendered image (A) and the curved multiplanar reconstruction (B) show patency of the left internal mammary artery graft and of the anastomosis of the graft onto the LAD. Notice the hyper-dense appearance of the surgical clips.

Table 12.5. Detection of coronary graft and native vessel stenosis—diagnostic performance of 64-MSCT vs. conventional angiography.

	Unevaluable (%)	Sensitivity (%)	Specificity (%)	PPV (%)	NPV (%)
Malagutti [39]					
All grafts	0	100	98	98	100
arterial	—	100	100	100	100
venous	—	100	96	98	100
Distal run-offs	0	89	93	50	99
Non-grafted natives	0	97	86	66	99
Ropers [42]					
All grafts	0	100	94	92	100
Distal run-offs	7	86	90	50	98
Non-grafted natives	9	86	76	44	96
Meyer [40]					
All grafts	2	97	97	93	99
arterial	—	93	97	86	98
venous	—	99	98	96	99
Pache [41]					
All grafts	3	98	89	90	98
arterial	—	—	—	—	92
venous	—	—	—	—	100

normal and stenotic aortic valve, recent studies have demonstrated the ability of MSCT to measure the orifice area with close correlation to transesophageal echocardiography and invasive assessment of the aortic orifice area [43,44]. However, in the setting of severely calcified stenosis, measurements of the opening area by CT may become unreliable. Non-enhanced CT scans can be used to quantify aortic valve calcium [45].

Coronary Anomalies

It may sometimes be difficult during invasive coronary angiography to define the origin and course of anomalous coronary arteries. MSCT is extremely reliable to visualize the origin and course of anomalous coronary vessels and is well suited for investigating patients with known or suspected congenital coronary artery anomalies. MSCT permits morphological analysis with very high resolution; moreover, this technique is not restricted by "echo windows" or by implanted devices such as pacemakers or implantable cardioverter defibrillators, which are frequently encountered in patients with congenital heart disease.

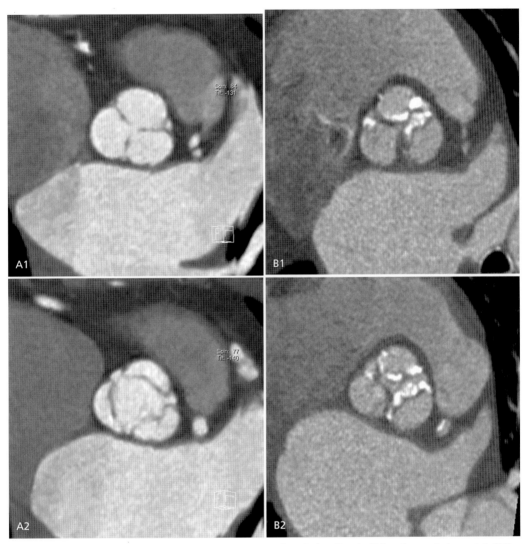

Figure 12.16. The MSCT multiplanar images were obtained in two different patients (A and B) parallel to the aortic valve. Images in the upper row (A1, B1) were obtained during diastole. Images in the lower row (A2, B2) were obtained in systole. In patient A, the cusps adapt during diastole (A1) and open during systole (A2); the aortic valve is normal. In patient B, aortic cusps are thickened and calcified (B1, B2). Opening is incomplete during systole (B2); the patient has aortic valve stenosis.

References

1. Flohr TG, McCollough CH, Bruder H, *et al.* First performance evaluation of a dual-source CT (DSCT) system. Eur Radiol 2006; **16**: 256–268.

2. Cademartiri F, Mollet NR, van der Lugt A, *et al.* Intravenous contrast material administration at helical 16-detector row CT coronary angiography: effect of iodine concentration on vascular attenuation. Radiology 2005; **236**: 661–665.

3. Fishman EK, Magid D, Ney DR, *et al.* Three-dimensional imaging. Radiology 1991; **181**: 321–337.

4. Vogl TJ, Abolmaali ND, Diebold T, *et al.* Techniques for the detection of coronary atherosclerosis: multidetector row CT coronary angiography. Radiology 2002; **223**: 212–220.

5. Achenbach S, Ropers D, Pohle FK, *et al.* Detection of coronary artery stenoses using multi-detector CT with 16 × 0.75 collimation and 375 ms rotation. Eur Heart J 2005; **26**: 1978–1986.

6. Dewey M, Teige F, Schnapauff D, *et al.* Noninvasive detection of coronary artery stenoses with multislice computed tomography or magnetic resonance imaging. Ann Intern Med 2006; **145**: 407–415.

7. Garcia MJ, Lessick J, Hoffmann MH. Accuracy of 16-row multidetector computed tomography for the assessment of coronary artery stenosis. JAMA 2006; **296**: 403–411.

8. Hausleiter J, Meyer T, Hadamitzky M, *et al.* Noninvasive coronary computed tomographic angiography for patients with suspected coronary artery disease: the Coronary Angiography by Computed Tomography with the Use of a Submillimeter resolution (CACTUS) trial. Eur Heart J 2007; doi:10.1093/eurheartj/ehm150. Available online http://eurheartj.oxfordjournals.org/cgi/content/full/ehm150v1. (Accessed 25 September 2007.)

9. Hoffmann MH, Shi H, Schmitz BL, *et al.* Noninvasive coronary angiography with multislice computed tomography. JAMA 2005; **293**: 2471–2478.

10. Leber AW, Knez A, von Ziegler F, *et al.* Quantification of obstructive and nonobstructive coronary lesions by 64-slice computed tomography: a comparative study with quantitative coronary angiography and intravascular ultrasound. J Am Coll Cardiol 2005; **46**: 147–154.

11. Leschka S, Alkadhi H, Plass A, *et al.* Accuracy of MSCT coronary angiography with 64-slice technology: first experience. Eur Heart J 2005; **26**: 1482–1487.

12. Mollet NR, Cademartiri F, Krestin GP, *et al.* Improved diagnostic accuracy with 16-row multi-slice computed tomography coronary angiography. J Am Coll Cardiol 2005; **45**: 128–132.

13. Mollet NR, Cademartiri F, Nieman K, *et al.* Multislice spiral computed tomography coronary angiography in patients with stable angina pectoris. J Am Coll Cardiol 2004; **43**: 2265–2270.

14. Mollet NR, Cademartiri F, van Mieghem CA, *et al.* High-resolution spiral computed tomography coronary angiography in patients referred for diagnostic conventional coronary angiography. Circulation 2005; **112**: 2318–2323.

15. Nikolaou K, Knez A, Rist C, *et al.* Accuracy of 64-MDCT in the diagnosis of ischemic heart disease. AJR Am J Roentgenol 2006; **187**: 111–117.

16. Nikolaou K, Saam T, Rist C, *et al.* Pre- and postsurgical diagnostics with dual-source computed tomography in cardiac surgery. Radiologe 2007; **47**: 310–318.

17. Pugliese F, Mollet NR, Runza G, *et al.* Diagnostic accuracy of non-invasive 64-slice CT coronary angiography in patients with stable angina pectoris. Eur Radiol 2006; **16**: 575–582.

18. Raff GL, Gallagher MJ, O'Neill WW, *et al.* Diagnostic accuracy of noninvasive coronary angiography using 64-slice spiral computed tomography. J Am Coll Cardiol 2005; **46**: 552–557.

19. Ropers D, Rixe J, Anders K, *et al.* Usefulness of multidetector row spiral computed tomography with 64- x 0.6-mm collimation and 330-ms rotation for the non-invasive detection of significant coronary artery stenoses. Am J Cardiol 2006; **97**: 343–348.

20. Scheffel H, Alkadhi H, Plass A, *et al.* Accuracy of dual-source CT coronary angiography: First experience in a high pre-test probability population without heart rate control. Eur Radiol 2006; **16**: 2739–2747.

21. Weustink AC, Meijboom WB, Mollet NR, *et al.* Reliable high-speed coronary computed tomography in symptomatic patients. J Am Coll Cardiol 2007; **50**: 786–794.

22. Pugliese F, Mollet NR, Hunink MG, *et al.* Diagnostic performance of computed tomography coronary angiography using different generation multislice scanners. Single-centre experience. Radiology. In press.

23. Hendel RC, Patel MR, Kramer CM, *et al.* ACCF/ACR/SCCT/SCMR/ASNC/NASCI/SCAI/SIR 2006 appropriateness criteria for cardiac computed tomography and cardiac magnetic resonance imaging: a report of the American College of Cardiology Foundation Quality Strategic Directions Committee Appropriateness Criteria Working Group, American College of Radiology, Society of Cardiovascular Computed Tomography, Society for Cardiovascular Magnetic Resonance, American Society of Nuclear Cardiology, North American Society for Cardiac Imaging, Society for Cardiovascular Angiography and Interventions, and Society of Interventional Radiology. J Am Coll Cardiol 2006; **48**: 1475–1497.

24. Van Mieghem CA, Thury A, Meijboom WB, *et al.* Detection and characterization of coronary bifurcation lesions with 64-slice computed tomography coronary angiography. Eur Heart J 2007; **28**: 1968–1976.

25. Medina A, Suarez de Lezo J, Pan M. A new classification of coronary bifurcation lesions. Rev Esp Cardiol 2006; **59**: 183.

26. Aviram G, Shmilovich H, Finkelstein A, *et al.* Coronary ostium-straight tube or funnel-shaped? A computerized tomographic coronary angiography study. Acute Card Care 2006; **8**: 224–248.

27. Mollet NR, Hoye A, Lemos PA, *et al.* Value of preprocedure multislice computed tomographic coronary angiography to predict the outcome of percutaneous recanalization of chronic total occlusions. Am J Cardiol 2005; **95**: 240–243.

28. Maintz D, Seifarth H, Raupach R, *et al.* 64-slice multidetector coronary CT angiography: in vitro evaluation of 68 different stents. Eur Radiol 2006; **16**: 818–826.

29. Pugliese F, Cademartiri F, van Mieghem C, *et al.* Multidetector CT for visualization of coronary stents. Radiographics 2006; **26**: 887–904.

30. Gilard M, Cornily JC, Pennec PY, *et al.* Assessment of coronary artery stents by 16 slice computed tomography. Heart 2006; **92**: 58–61.

31. Gaspar T, Halon DA, Lewis BS, *et al.* Diagnosis of coronary in-stent restenosis with multidetector row spiral computed tomography. J Am Coll Cardiol 2005; **46**: 1573–1579.

32. Cademartiri F, Schuijf JD, Pugliese F, *et al.* Usefulness of 64-slice multislice computed tomography coronary angiography to assess in-stent restenosis. J Am Coll Cardiol 2007; **49**: 2204–2210.

33. Ehara M, Kawai M, Surmely JF, *et al.* Diagnostic accuracy of coronary in-stent restenosis using 64-slice computed tomography: comparison with invasive coronary angiography. J Am Coll Cardiol 2007; **49**: 951–959.

34. Rixe J, Achenbach S, Ropers D, *et al.* Assessment of coronary artery stent restenosis by 64-slice multidetector computed tomography. Eur Heart J 2006; **27**: 2567–2572.

35. Pugliese F, Weustink AC, Van Mieghem C, *et al.* Dual-source coronary computed tomography angiography for detecting in-stent restenosis. Heart 2007; doi:10.1136/hrt.2007.126474. Available online http://heart.bmj.com/cgi/content/abstract/hrt.2007.126474v1?papetoc. (Accessed 25 September 2007).

36. Takagi T, Stankovic G, Finci L, *et al.* Results and long-term predictors of adverse clinical events after elective percutaneous interventions on unprotected left main coronary artery. Circulation 2002; **106**: 698–702.

37. Smith SC, Jr., Feldman TE, Hirshfeld JW, Jr., *et al.* ACC/AHA/SCAI 2005 Guideline Update for Percutaneous Coronary Intervention—summary article: a report of the American College of Cardiology/American Heart Association Task Force on Practice Guidelines (ACC/AHA/SCAI Writing Committee to Update the 2001 Guidelines for Percutaneous Coronary Intervention). Circulation 2006; **113**: 156–175.

38. Van Mieghem CA, Cademartiri F, Mollet NR, *et al.* Multislice spiral computed tomography for the evaluation of stent patency after left main coronary artery stenting: a comparison with conventional coronary angiography and intravascular ultrasound. Circulation 2006; **114**: 645–653.

39. Malagutti P, Nieman K, Meijboom WB, *et al.* Use of 64-slice CT in symptomatic patients after coronary bypass surgery: evaluation of grafts and coronary arteries. Eur Heart J 2007; **28**: 1879–1885.

40. Meyer TS, Martinoff S, Hadamitzky M, *et al.* Improved noninvasive assessment of coronary artery bypass grafts with 64-slice computed tomographic angiography in an unselected patient population. J Am Coll Cardiol 2007; **49**: 946–950.

41. Pache G, Saueressig U, Frydrychowicz A, *et al.* Initial experience with 64-slice cardiac CT: non-invasive visualization of coronary artery bypass grafts. Eur Heart J 2006; **27**: 976–980.

42. Ropers D, Pohle FK, Kuettner A, Pflederer T, *et al.* Diagnostic accuracy of noninvasive coronary angiography in patients after bypass surgery using 64-slice spiral computed tomography with 330-ms gantry rotation. Circulation 2006; **114**: 2334–2341; quiz 2334.

43. Alkadhi H, Wildermuth S, Plass A, *et al.* Aortic stenosis: comparative evaluation of 16-detector row CT and echocardiography. Radiology 2006; **240**: 47–55.

44. Feuchtner GM, Dichtl W, Friedrich GJ, *et al.* Multislice computed tomography for detection of patients with aortic valve stenosis and quantification of severity. J Am Coll Cardiol 2006; **47**: 1410–1417.

45. Willmann JK, Weishaupt D, Lachat M, *et al.* Electrocardiographically gated multi-detector row CT for assessment of valvular morphology and calcification in aortic stenosis. Radiology 2002; **225**: 120–128.

46. Dewey M, Zimmermann E, Deissenrieder F, *et al.* Noninvasive coronary angiography by 320-row computed tomography with lower radiation exposure and maintained diagnostic accuracy: comparison of results with cardiac catheterization in a head-to-head pilot investigation. Circulation 2009; **120**: 867–875.

CHAPTER 13

Cardiac Magnetic Resonance Imaging

Amgad N. Makaryus[1], & Steven D. Wolff[2]

[1] North Shore University Hospital, NYU School of Medicine, Manhasset, New York, NY, USA
[2] Columbia University, College of Physicians and Surgeons, New York, NY, USA

Introduction

Cardiovascular magnetic resonance (CMR) provides diagnostic morphologic and functional information for the evaluation and management of patients with cardiovascular disease. CMR has improved substantially over the past decade, and it has now entered the mainstream of diagnostic imaging. CMR has long been considered the procedure of choice in the evaluation of pericardial disease and intracardiac and pericardiac masses, for imaging the right ventricle and pulmonary vessels, and for assessing many forms of congenital heart disease. More recently, CMR has become increasingly recognized as a valuable tool for assessing patients with ischemic heart disease. CMR is gaining widespread use due to its superior diagnostic accuracy and ability to perform a complete anatomical and functional assessment in a single study without ionizing radiation [1–4].

This chapter details the complementary nature of the various CMR sequences for the planning of interventions and assessment of patients undergoing cardiac interventional procedures. We focus our comments on the pertinent information that CMR can provide the interventional cardiologist in the management of their patients. A discussion of the CMR assessment of cardiac function, cardiac perfusion, cardiac viability, atherosclerotic plaque, and CMR in interventional procedures is undertaken.

MRI Techniques

Technical Concepts

CMR is based on the detection of the magnetic spin direction of protons from water and fat in the body. Each proton contains molecular magnets that align with the magnetic field of the MRI scanner. The intrinsic angular momentum of each prtoton results in rotation (or precession) around the axis of the scanner's magnetic field. This is referred to as "spin." When a perpendicular field is applied transiently then the proton spins rotate together, emitting a coherent oscillating signal that decays in amplitude and coherence with time. The decay of amplitude (T1 relaxation) and coherence (T2 relaxation) is unique to each specific tissue and generates an energy which is measured by the receiver coils positioned near the region of interest (in our case a cardiac coil is positioned near the heart on the anterior chest wall) [5].

There are a variety of MRI techniques that can be used to image the heart. Spin-echo (SE) MRI provides black blood images of the heart which are useful for its anatomic assessment. Gradient-echo (GE) and steady-state free precession (SSFP) techniques can be applied to create bright blood cine

Interventional Cardiology, First Edition. Edited by Carlo Di Mario, George D. Dangas, Peter Barlis.
© 2010 Blackwell Publishing Ltd. Published 2010 by Blackwell Publishing Ltd.

images to assess cardiac function and blood flow. GE and SSFP allow quantitative evaluation of ventricular function, valvular regurgitation or stenosis, and abnormal hemodynamics. The images may be reconstructed in different phases of the cardiac cycle and can be displayed in cine format. Another MRI imaging technique is Phase Contrast (Blood Velocity) Mapping. When a pulse sequence is applied to a patient in an MRI scanner, two sets of data are obtained. The magnitude data provides the map of protons within the slice, giving the conventional cross-sectional image. The other set of data obtained is the phase data. This data set provides a map of the velocity of the protons within the slice. The intensity of a pixel in a phase image reflects the velocity of the protons within that pixel. Evaluation of the intensity of a region of pixels provides quantitative data reflecting the flow of blood through a portion of the heart or artery [6–9].

Practical Concepts

To prepare a patient for a CMR exam, absence of major contraindications such as cerebrovascular clips, cochlear implants, ocular metallic fragments and pacemakers and defibrillators must be assured. Most coronary and peripheral stents are safe for CMR, even immediately after implantation, as are many nitinol-based devices, such as septal occluders. Serum creatinine must be assessed since patients with severe renal insufficiency (i.e. a eGFR <30) are at increased risk for Nephrogenic Systemic Fibrosis or Nephrogenic Fibrosing Dermopathy (NSF/NFD) (see http://www.fda.gov/cder/drug/advisory/gadolinium_agents.htm). Patients undergoing CMR stress imaging should withhold heart rate-reducing medications or caffeine-containing substances if dobutamine or adenosisne/persantine agents will be employed. Placement of a 20 gauge intravenous catheter in an arm vein is undertaken for the administration of the contrast agent. A second intravenous line is placed in the contralateral arm if a pharmacologic stress agent will be employed. Vectorcardiographic chest leads are placed for ECG gating. The phased array cardiac receiver coil is then placed on the precordium. Brachial cuff pressure and digital pulse oximetry may be periodically measured throughout the study. During the 20–45 minute examination (depending on the indication), most of the

sequences are performed during repeated 5–10 second breath-holds on expiration [10–13].

Cardiac Function and Volume Assessment

Volumetric Assessment

CMR provides accurate volumetric quantification of global and regional systolic ventricular function. CMR is well validated for quantifying the volumes of the ventricles, and it has become the clinical standard of reference against which other techniques are measured because of its 3D nature and no need for geometrical assumptions. The accuracy and reproducibility of the measurements make CMR useful for the longitudinal follow-up of patients [6].

An important feature of CMR is the excellent interstudy reproducibility of volume and mass measurements. The interstudy reproducibility for volumes and mass by CMR is excellent for both the left [14] and right ventricle [15], and is considerably superior to that of two-dimensional echocardiography. This reproducibility has allowed several drug trials to use CMR as a primary endpoint measure.

Volumetric Flow Quatitation

In the assessment of the MR signal, phase can be used to encode flow information [16]. Since its was first used [17], gated flow quantification has been studied extensively in the heart and great vessels and has been applied successfully to valvular heart disease, congenital heart disease, and disease secondary to pulmonary hypertension. Flow quantification with MR imaging has features in common with pulsed Doppler ultrasonography in that it samples discretely and is therefore vulnerable to aliasing if the flow velocities are too high. However, unlike Doppler ultrasonography, MR flow quantification is not limited by acoustic windows. The velocity-encoding value (VENC) is defined as the velocity that produces a phase shift of 180°. If the highest velocity in the vessel of interest is less than the VENC, it can be measured without aliasing. If, however, flow velocity slightly exceeds the VENC, high-velocity flow in one direction may be erroneously encoded as fast flow in the opposite direction (aliasing). Using phase contrast imaging, stroke volumes of both the RV and LV may be assessed. Further, regurgitant volumes may be calculated in patients with valvular regurgitation [18–22].

Regional Myocardial Function Assessment

CMR is valuable for assessment of regional contractile function by visual inspection of cines in standard imaging planes. Standardized measurement of global and regional left (LV) and right ventricular (RV) function is performed in sequential short axis slices of 5–10 mm thickness with 0–10 mm gaps. In end-systole and end-diastole, endocardial and epicardial borders are traced in each of the short axis slices, and the LV is segmented following the 17 segment model of the AHA/ASE. The modified Simpson's rule is then applied and LV and RV end-systolic and end-diastolic volumes, ejection fraction, and cardiac output are calculated. LV mass is derived from the volume difference between the epicardium and the endocardium. CMR can also provide 3D images of the ventricular cavity that can be rotated into all planes to assist interventionalists in the planning of percutaneous valvular procedures [23].

Functional Imaging in Ischemic Heart Disease

Stress CMR using dobutamine is now clinically established for diagnosing obstructive coronary artery disease through induction of new wall motion abnormalities. Stress CMR is effective in the diagnosis of CAD in patients who are unsuitable for dobutamine echocardiography. Fast gradient-echo techniques provide high contrast images with high temporal and spatial resolution which can be obtained within the time of a single breath-hold. This allows evaluation of regional myocardial contraction, ventricular filling and ejection, valve motion and vascular flow patterns. Excellent visualization of the endo- and epicardial surfaces of ventricular myocardium on cine MRI displays changes in regional wall thickening and wall motion throughout the cardiac cycle [24].

Myocardial Tagging

A newer CMR technique is tagging, which directly assesses myocardial strain and other deformations

as a measure of contractility [25]. LV regional wall thickening is determined per segment. Quantification of wall motion and thickening using conventional techniques is possible for both the LV and the RV. A newer CMR technique to assess regional myocardial function is myocardial tagging using spatial modulation magnetization (SPAMM), which directly assesses myocardial strain and other deformations as a measure of contractility. This technique non-invasively creates a grid of tag lines on the myocardium. These tag lines track deformation of underlying myocardium through the cardiac cycle. Myocardial tagging can be used to non-invasively perform a myocardial strain analysis and decompose gross wall deformation into more fundamental units of deformation such as principal strains or fiber strains. This technique has been used to depict functional recovery after thrombolytic therapy in infarcted myocardium, to elucidate the mechanism of remote myocardial dysfunction, to discriminate between viable and non-viable myocardium using stress myocardial tagging, and to measure the efficacy of medication on LV dysfunction [26–29].

Tagging CMR has been validated using sonomicrometer studies and can be applied for full three-dimensional myocardial analysis by collective modeling of the numerous small individual myocardial elements. Recently, advanced tagging CMR acquisitions have greatly increased the spatial and temporal resolution and considerably simplified postprocessing. Myocardial tagging also offers insights into wall strain patterns revealing intrinsic mechanisms of ventricular function. Velocity encoding techniques accurately assess blood flow to measure valvular function, shunts, and to validate volumetric assessments [30].

Cardiac Perfusion Assessment

Stress Perfusion Technique in Patients with Ischemic Heart Disease

Myocardial perfusion MRI uses a first-pass technique to assess areas of decreased perfusion (Figure 13.1). A fast intravenous bolus of gadolinium contrast agent is given using a power injector, and the myocardial signal changes during the first pass are measured. Each slice is usually imaged with each cardiac cycle to maximize the quality of the

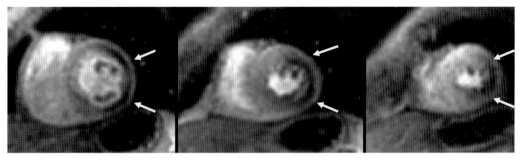

Figure 13.1. First-pass adenosine stress myocardial perfusion MRI imaging (going from basal to apical slices from left to right) showing inducible ischemia (arrows) in a 68 year old man who was later found to have a severe mid left circumflex coronary stenosis on invasive coronary angiography.

analysis. Low signal areas representing reduced perfusion can be visualized directly or computer quantification of parameters can be used to generate perfusion maps or measures of perfusion difference at rest and stress [31].

Perfusion CMR protocols employ commonly used pharmacological stress agents such as adenosine and dipyridamole. There are two principle approaches for assessing myocardial perfusion with MRI. The first method acquires perfusion images only during stress and uses late gadolinium contrast enhancement to define areas of non-viability (discussed below) [32]. The other approach is to perform both stress and resting myocardial perfusion CMR to produce perfusion reserve measurements [33]. Another technique that does not require ultrafast imaging or gadolinium contrast has been described and called T2*blood oxygen level dependent (BOLD) [34], but the sensitivity of T2*BOLD to perfusion change may be quite low and its clinical role is not yet defined.

Comparison with other Modalities

Several clinical reports have endorsed the accuracy of first-pass myocardial perfusion CMR, mostly in combination with adenosine or dipyridamole stress. Wolff *et al.* [35] showed a sensitivity, specificity, and accuracy of 93%, 75%, and 85, respectively. A study by Chiu *et al.* [36] from 2003 reports an accuracy of 90% for detection of angiographically significant coronary artery disease by using first-pass CMR. Other reports show very good results for the detection of CAD in comparison with coronary angiography, PET, and SPECT [37]. Several groups have used myocardial perfusion reserve or myocardial perfusion reserve index to assess patients with coronary artery disease. The reserve index may be more reliable than determination of coronary flow reserve since the effect of (protective) myocardial collateral flow supply is taken into account. Al-Saadi *et al.* [38] found the diagnostic sensitivity, specificity, and diagnostic accuracy for the detection of coronary artery stenosis (≥50%) were 90%, 83%, and 87%, respectively. Nandalur *et al.* performed a meta-analysis of 37 studies (2191 patients) using stress-induced wall motion abnormalities and perfusion imaging to assess the diagnostic performance of stress cardiac magnetic resonance imaging in the detection of coronary artery disease. Stress-induced wall motion abnormalities imaging demonstrated a sensitivity of 83% and specificity of 86% on a patient level (disease prevalence = 70.5%). Perfusion imaging demonstrated a sensitivity of 91% and specificity of 81% on a patient level (disease prevalence = 57.4%) [39].

Cardiac Infarction, Viability, and Scar Assessment

Delayed Contrast Enhancement

Earliest clinical observations that myocardial infarcts enhance with extracellular contrast agents were made in the late 1980s [40–42]. Gadolinium is administered intravenously and CMR is performed (typically after a 5–20 minute delay) using an inversion recovery sequence. In normal myocardium, gadolinium is excluded from the intracellular space by cell membranes. In regions of acute necrosis or infarction, the extracellular compartment is expanded due to cell membrane rupture, and therefore the concentration of gadolinium contrast is greater in these areas, making them brighter on the MR image. In the chronic case, areas of necrosis are replaced with scar tissue, which also has more extracellular space than normal myocardium. The transmural distribution of scar can be visualized using this technique [43].

Assessment of Myocardial Infarction and Viability in Patients with Coronary Artery Disease

Delayed gadolinium CMR images are useful in the assessment of myocardial viability to determine the likely benefit from revascularization (Figure 13.2). Late gadolinium enhancement is useful for predic-

tion of functional recovery in cases of acute MI. There is high concordance of late gadolinium enhancement CMR with PET, and superior results have been shown in comparison with thallium-201 SPECT [44–50].

Over the past few years, delayed contrast enhancement CMR viability imaging has become widely accepted for the detection and characterization of acute and chronic myocardial infarction. Validation of this technique has been performed in pathological models in animals and gadolinium enhancement CMR has been found in humans to be able to detect Q wave and non-Q wave MI accurately [51]. In the acute setting, the extent of late gadolinium enhancement is related to the magnitude of cardiac enzyme release and the functional

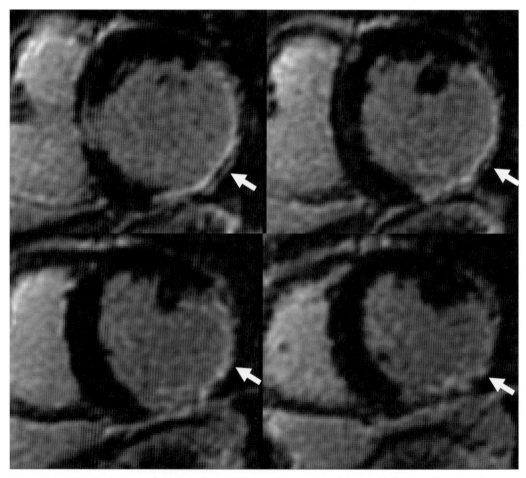

Figure 13.2. Delayed enhancement MRI imaging in a 75 year old man with a history of inferior and lateral wall infarction shown as enhanced and thinned myocardial segments in the figure (arrows).

outcome after recovery. This technique has been found to be very sensitive that small infarcts can be demonstrated that are not apparent using gated perfusion SPECT [52], and microinfarcts can be shown after percutaneous coronary intervention [53–55]. Compared with radionuclide imaging, delayed enhancement CMR provides clear advantages, particularly for non-transmural infarction, such that CMR is now considered by some to outperform nuclear tomography [56,57].

Vascular Imaging

Magnetic Resonance Angiography

Vascular imaging with MRI has been decribed as Magentic Resonance Angiography (MRA). MRA has the abilty to define arterial anatomy throughout the body. In patients with congenital heart disease, MRA is often used to define great vessel anatomy (Figure 13.3). Studies are often performed with contrast. Time resolved angiography can show the dynamic passage of contrast with time which can be helpful in assessing patients with shunts [58].

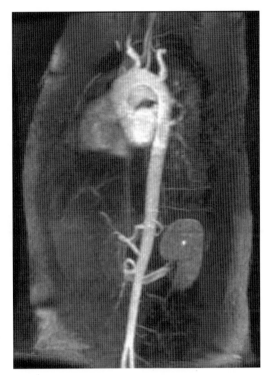

Figure 13.3. CMR angiography (MRA) evaluates the aorta and large vessels of the chest and abdomen.

Atherosclerotic Plaque Assessment

Research studies have shown that MRI can be used to identify total plaque burden within the arterial wall. Quantification of the vessel wall volume over the imaging stack can be achieved by summation planimetry of the difference in each image between the outer and inner vessel boundary [59]. CMR may be used as is intravascular ultrasound to measure the effectiveness of antiatheroma therapy such as statin treatment [60]. Plaque composition can be assessed using a combination of proton density-weighted imaging sequences, which allows assessment of plaque vulnerability. "Soft" plaque deposits have been described as having low signal on the images, with a fibrous cap identified overlying this. Thin or disrupted caps on CMR which may portend more "vulnerability" to the plaque have been identified. The high resolution of MR imaging and the development of sophisticated contrast agents offer the promise of molecular imaging techniques of the plaque. Coronary artery plaque imaging with MRI remains a highly promising, but not yet clinically adequate diagnostic tool. Large-scale prospective studies addressing

its use for risk stratification are currently being planned and performed [61–63].

Coronary Artery Imaging

Coronary CMR angiography is still technically challenging for the assessment of the presence and severity of coronary stenosis owing to small arterial size, tortuosity, complex anatomy, and cardiac and respiratory motion. By using optimized 3-D acquisitions, there has been gradual improvement in resolution and clinical robustness using both breathhold and respiratory navigator techniques. A recent multicenter study showed good results for the exclusion of multivessel proximal CAD requiring operative intervention [64].

Although there are limitations in the assessment of luminal stenosis, CMR is highly efficacious for the evaluation of the course of anomalous coronary arteries. The relationship between the great vessels and the course of coronary arteries is better depicted by CMR than by conventional coronary

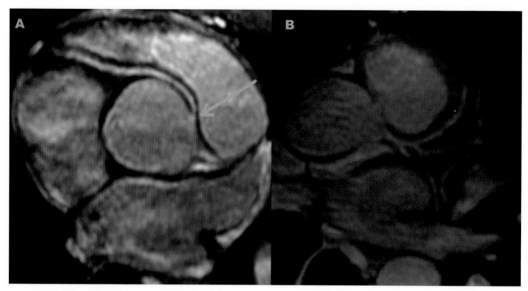

Figure 13.4. Oblique tomographic CMR images from a 36 year old woman who presented originally for the evaluation of syncope on strenuous exertion. Panel A shows the origin of the right coronary artery (arrow) and the left coronary artery is shown in panel B. In (A), the right coronary artery is noted to course between the aorta and the main pulmonary artery (unfavorable geometry).

angiography because of the three-dimensional CMR tomograms in comparison with two-dimensional X-ray projections with overlapping structures (Figure 13.4). CMR has the benefit of clarifying the spatial relationship of these arteries, most importantly whether the proximal portion runs between the aorta and the pulmonary artery, which is associated with sudden death [65].

Utility of CMR in Other Cardiac Conditions

Pericardial Disease

CMR can be very useful for assessing patients with pericardial disease. Pericardial effusions are well defined with CMR. On spin-echo examination, a hemorrhagic pericardial effusion presents as areas of mixed low, intermediate, and high signal, depending upon the age of the blood. Non-hemorrhagic effusions on spin-echo MR have predominantly low signal intensity. Inflammatory effusion, as seen in uremia, tuberculosis, or trauma, may have medium signal intensity components on spin-echo MR, especially in dependent areas. Pericardial constriction is usually associated with pericardial thickening, which is well depicted with

both spin-echo and gradient-echo imaging. Further, real-time CMR imaging can very nicely depict the presence of ventricular interdependence [66].

Dilated Cardiomyopathy

The direct demonstration of the ventricular myocardium by CMR provides a reproducible means of identifying the distribution of abnormal muscle, and characterizing the nature of the cardiomyopathy. Cine acquisition displays the epicardial and endocardial borders of the ventricular myocardium, providing temporally resolved images from which myocardial mass and ventricular chamber volumes and stroke volume can be computed [67].

Hypertrophic Cardiomyopathy (HCM)

Use of MRI in HCM allows accurate characterization of the distribution of apical hypertrophy; distribution can be described as symmetric, asymmetric, or only involving the cardiac apex [68,69]. In patients with HCM, cine MRI has been used to quantitate LV mass, volumes, and ejection fraction as well as right ventricular function. Suzuki *et al.* [70] found increased RV mass, reduced peak filling rate, and decreased RV filling fractions in these patients. Velocity-encoded cine MRI has been used to study coronary sinus blood flow in patients with HCM [71]. Resting coronary blood flow was not significantly different from that found in normal individuals. However, after dipyridamole administration, coronary sinus blood flow in patients with HCM increased to a much lower level than that seen in the healthy volunteers, indicating decreased coronary flow reserve. Impaired diastolic function due to non-uniform hypertrophy with subsequent loss of myocardial contractile elements, myocardial perfusion abnormalities, and change in LV geometry has been demonstrated [72].

With contrast CMR imaging, most patients have no gadolinium enhancement, and a common benign pattern is an area of focal enhancement in the junction of the right ventricular insertion into the left ventricle. More extensive gadolinium enhancement can be dense and plaque-like or diffuse. The greater the gadolinium enhancement, the higher the risk of heart failure or sudden death, presumably because of reentrant tachycardias and systolic failure from myocyte replacement [73].

Restrictive Cardiomyopathy

Amyloidosis frequently causes restrictive cardiomyopathy. It may be recognized by widespread thickening of all chamber walls and atrioventricular valve leaflets in face of decreased ejection fraction and abnormal segmental wall motion. Amyloid infiltration of the myocardium generally shows increased signal with late gadolinium enhancement due to expansion of the extracellular compartment. In addition, mitral and tricuspid regurgitation frequently associated with restrictive cardiomyopathy, can be demonstrated and quantified on MRI [74]. In patients with cardiomyopathy due to cardiac sarcoidosis, loci of high myocardial signal intensity can be found after administration of intravenous gadolinium [75,76].

Arrhythmogenic Right Ventricular Dysplasia (ARVD)

CMR is widely used for the investigation of ARVD. The diagnostic criteria of ARVD are well defined, and MRI provides an excellent assessment of right ventricular morphology and function. Fatty infiltration which has long been described as being associated with ARVD is not considered a definitive sign of disease, because it can occur in other circumstances [77–79].

Myocarditis

By CMR assessment early in the course of the disease, myocardial enhancement using gadolinium-enhanced spin-echo CMR images with early imaging at one to two minutes tends to be localized, reflecting the focal nature of the myocardial inflammation. However, as the disease progresses, the enhancement can be seen throughout the muscle, depicting evolution of myocarditis into a diffuse process. Signal intensity normalization occurs with healing. Contrast enhancement four weeks after the onset of symptoms is due to scarring and is predictive for functional and clinical long-term outcomes [80].

Valvular Heart Disease

Echocardiography is usually the initial imaging technique in the work-up of cardiac murmurs. Because echocardiography is the first-line clinical test to investigate valve disease, CMR is used when acoustic windows are poor or when discordant imaging and invasive results occur. CMR can be useful for direct demonstration of the jets of valvular dysfunction, as well as the quantitation of the dysfunction. CMR is useful for the assessment of valve morphology, quantification of turbulence and jets, valvular regurgitation and stenosis, as well as the assessment of prosthetic valves. Although metallic valve components produce artifacts and signal loss, CMR of all prosthetic heart valves at 1.5 T is safe, because there is no substantial magnetic interaction and heating is negligible [81].

Accurate estimation of the severity of a valvular lesion is crucial for timing surgical intervention. With CMR, quantitative assessment of regurgitation can be obtained in a number of ways. If a single valve is affected on either side of the heart, the regurgitant volume can be calculated from the difference of right ventricular and left ventricular stroke volumes using the volumetric technique of contiguous short-axis cine slices of the ventricles. This method compares favorably with catheterization and Doppler echocardiography [82,83]. CMR quantification of stenosis can be assessed by measuring the velocity of a jet through a valve

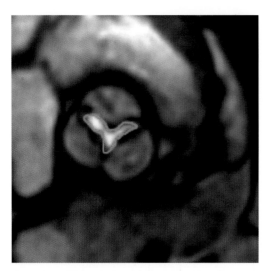

Figure 13.5. Short axis view of the aortic valve of a 72 year old man with poor acoustic windows on transthoracic echocardiography. Planimetric assessment (green tracing) was made possible by CMR.

provide whole-body imaging capability in any plane without exposure to radiation. Interventional CMR requires the combination of real-time image acquisition and reconstruction, angiography, and image guidance. For the cardiovascular system, a key component is the tracking of the intravascular and intracardiac catheter and guidewire. This has been attempted by incorporating a small receive-only coil in the tip of the device. The coil generates a signal that can be rapidly localized in three dimensions and shown on a previously acquired MR image, and different coils and receivers can be used for multiple devices. This technique has been applied in renal angiography [87], femoral angioplasty, wall imaging, placement of stents, coronary angiography [88], and assessment of radiofrequency ablation procedures [89]. Advances in this area are currently being studied and the future of this technology seems promising.

stenosis by employing phase contrast techniques. Turbulence around the jet core is usual, appears dark on the cine image, and does not interfere with measurements within the jet. There is good agreement between CMR and other techniques in evaluating mitral and aortic valve stenosis. The valve area can also be directly planimetered (Figure 13.5) or calculated using the continuity equation in patients with aortic stenosis. The pressure gradient across a valve can be indirectly quantitated using the modified Bernoulli equation [84–86].

Intravascular and Interventional CMR

New techniques are currently being investigated which incorporate CMR for intravascular and interventional applications. The push for this type of technique is due to the fact that CMR can

Conclusion

Cardiac MR imaging, although still evolving rapidly, has matured to the point where it is now a powerful tool with a range of clinical and research applications in the field of interventional cardiology. For evaluation of complex anatomy, cardiac function, myocardial viability, valvular disease, myocardial perfusion, and congenital heart disease, MR imaging is especially effective. Although there has been recently increasing advances in multislice computed tomography with regard to the assessment of coronary artery anatomy, CMR will meet the challenge through continued developments in machine hardware, pulse sequences, motion compensation, and the use of novel contrast agents, and will continue to provide pertinent information to the interventional cardiologist with respect to perfusion, viability, and flow quantification.

Questions

1. **Advantages of cardiovascular magnetic resonance over other invasive imaging techniques include all the following, except:**
   A Utilizes no ionizing radiation
   B MR contrast agents are more nephrotoxic than iodinated preparations
   C Fewer geometric assumptions regarding mass/volume determinations
   D Facilitates acquisition of true tomographic images

2. **MRI has NOT been shown to have a valuable clinical role in the assessment of:**
   A Quantification of epicardial calcium
   B Left ventricular mass
   C Left ventricular regional and global systolic function
   D Calculation of intracardiac shunts

3. **Among patients with simple and complex congenital heart disease, CMR has a clinical role for all except:**
   A Determination of Qp/Qs ratios and flow through various conduits
   B Assessment of anomalous coronary artery disease
   C Assessment of pulmonary artery pressures
   D Identification of anomalous pulmonary venous drainage

4. **For quantification of regurgitant fraction and Qp/Qs ratio in an adult with multivalvular regurgitation, the most accurate noninvasive modality is:**
   A MRI with assessment of left and right ventricular stroke volume from cine data
   B MRI with phase velocity mapping
   C First-pass radionuclide angiography
   D Transthoracic Doppler echocardiography

References

1. Lieberman JM, Alfidi RJ, Nelson AD, *et al.* Gated magnetic resonance imaging of the normal and diseased heart. Radiology 1984; **152**: 465–470.

2. Ray T, Biederman RW, Doyle M, *et al.* Magnetic resonance imaging in the assessment of coronary artery disease. Curr Atheroscler Rep 2005; **7**(2): 108–114.

3. Lanzer P, Botvinick EH, Schiller NB, *et al.* Cardiac imaging using gated magnetic resonance. Radiology 1984; **150**: 121–127.

4. Lanzer P, Barta C, Botvinick EH, *et al.* ECG-synchronized cardiac MR imaging: Method and evaluation. Radiology 1985; **155**: 681–686.

5. Firmin DN, Nayler GL, Klipstein RH, *et al.*: In vivo validation of magnetic resonance velocity imaging. J Comput Assist Tomogr 1987; **11**: 751.

6. Walsh TF, Hundley WG. Assessment of ventricular function with cardiovascular magnetic resonance. Cardiol Clin 2007; **25**(1): 15–33.

7. Kim HW, Klem I, Kim RJ. Detection of myocardial ischemia by stress perfusion cardiovascular magnetic resonance. Cardiol Clin. 2007 February; **25**(1): 57–70.

8. Weinsaft JW, Klem I, Judd RM. MRI for the assessment of myocardial viability. Cardiol Clin 2007; **25**(1): 35–56.

9. Haacke EM, Li D, Kaushikkar S. Cardiac MR imaging: Principles and techniques: Top Magn Reson Imaging. 1995; **7**(4): 200–217.

10. Scott NA, Pettigrew RI. Absence of movement of coronary stents after placement in a magnetic resonance imaging field. Am J Cardiol 1994; **73**: 900.

11. Strohm O, Kivelitz D, Gross W, *et al.* Safety of implantable coronary stents during H-1 magnetic resonance imaging at 1.0 and 1.5 T. J Cardiovasc Magn Reson 1999; **1**: 239.

12. 1Schroeder AP, Houlind K, Pedersen EM, *et al.* Magnetic resonance imaging seems safe in patients with intracoronary stents. J Cardiovasc Magn Reson 2000; **2**: 43.

13. Finn JP, Nael K, Deshpande V, *et al.* Cardiac MR imaging: State of the technology. Radiology 2006; **241**(2): 338–354.

14. Grothues F, Smith GC, Moon JCC, *et al.* Comparison of interstudy reproducibility of cardiovascular magnetic resonance with two-dimensional echocardiography in normal subjects and in patients with heart failure or left ventricular hypertrophy. Am J Cardiol 2002; **90**: 29.

15. Grothues F, Moon JCC, Bellenger NG, *et al.* Interstudy reproducibility of right ventricular volumes, function and mass with cardiovascular magnetic resonance. Am Heart J 2004; **147**: 218.

16. Stahlberg F, Nordell B, Ericsson A, *et al.* Method for quantification of low flow velocities by magnetic resonance phase imaging. Acta Radiol Suppl 1986; **369**: 486–489.

17. Matthaei D, Haase A, Merboldt KD, *et al.* ECG-triggered arterial FLASH-MR flow measurement using an external standard. Magn Reson Imaging 1987; **5**: 325–330.

18. Mitchell L, Jenkins JP, Watson Y, Rowlands DJ, Isherwood I. Diagnosis and assessment of mitral and aortic valve disease by cine-flow magnetic resonance imaging. Magn Reson Med 1989; **12**: 181–197.

19. Hundley WG, Li HF, Willard JE, *et al.* Magnetic resonance imaging assessment of the severity of mitral

regurgitation: comparison with invasive techniques. Circulation 1995; **92**: 1151–1158.

20. Hartiala JJ, Foster E, Fujita N, *et al.* Evaluation of left atrial contribution to left ventricular filling in aortic stenosis by velocity-encoded cine MRI. Am Heart J 1994; **127**: 593–600.

21. Boxt LM. Magnetic resonance and computed tomographic evaluation of congenital heart disease. J Magn Reson Imaging 2004; **19**: 827–847.

22. Kruger S, Haage P, Hoffmann R, *et al.* Diagnosis of pulmonary arterial hypertension and pulmonary embolism with magnetic resonance angiography. Chest 2001; **120**: 1556–1561.

23. Bloomgarden DC, Fayad ZA, Ferrari VA, *et al.* Global cardiac function using breath-hold MRI: Validation of new acquisition and analysis techniques. Magn Reson Med 1997; **37**: 683.

24. Kuijpers D, Ho KY, van Dijkman PR, *et al.* Dobutamine cardiovascular magnetic resonance for the detection of myocardial ischemia with the use of myocardial tagging. Circulation 2003; **107**: 1592.

25. Scott CH, St. John Sutton MG, Gusani N, *et al.* Effect of dobutamine on regional left ventricular function measured by tagged magnetic resonance imaging in normal subjects. Am J Cardiol 1999; **83**: 412.

26. Bogaert J, Maes A, Van de Werf F, *et al.* Functional Recovery of subepicardial myocardial tissue in transmural myocardial infarction after successful reperfusion. Circulation 1999; **99**: 36–43.

27. Kramer CM, Lima JA, Reichek N, *et al.* Regional differences in function within noninfarcted myocardium during left ventricular remodeling. Circulation 1993; **88**: 1279–1288.

28. Kramer CM, Rogers WJ, Theobald TM, *et al.* Remote noninfarcted region dysfunction soon after first anterior myocardial infarction: A magnetic resonance tagging study. Circulation 1996; **94**: 660–666.

29. Bogaert J, Bosmans H, Maes A, Suetens P, *et al.* Remote myocardial dysfunction after acute anterior myocardial infarction: Impact of left ventricular shape on regional function. A magnetic resonance myocardial tagging study. J Am Coll Cardiol 2000; **35**: 1525–1534.

30. Young AA, Axel L. Three dimensional motion and deformation of the heart wall: Estimation with spatial modulation of magnetisation—A model based approach. Radiology 1992; **185**: 241.

31. Panting JR, Gatehouse PD, Yang GZ, *et al.* Abnormal subendocardial perfusion in cardiac syndrome-X detected by cardiovascular magnetic resonance imaging. N Engl J Med 2002; **346**: 1948.

32. Schwitter J, Nanz D, Kneifel S, *et al.* Assessment of myocardial perfusion in coronary artery disease by magnetic resonance: A comparison with positron emission tomography and coronary angiography. Circulation 2001; **103**: 2230.

33. Al-Saadi N, Nagel E, Gross M, *et al.* Noninvasive detection of myocardial ischemia from perfusion reserve based on cardiovascular magnetic resonance. Circulation 2000; **101**: 1379.

34. Wacker CM, Hartlep AW, Pfleger S, *et al.* Susceptibility-sensitive magnetic resonance imaging detects human myocardium supplied by a stenotic coronary artery without a contrast agent. J Am Coll Cardiol **41**:834, 2003.

35. Wolff SD, Schwitter J, Coulden R, *et al.* Myocardial first-pass perfusion magnetic resonance imaging: a multicenter dose-ranging study. Circulation. 2004; **110**(6): 732–737.

36. Chiu CW, So NM, Lam WW, *et al.* Combined first-pass perfusion and viability study at MR imaging in patients with non-ST segment-elevation acute coronary syndromes: feasibility study. Radiology 2003; **226**: 717–722.

37. Schwitter J, Nanz D, Kneifel S, *et al.* Assessment of myocardial perfusion in coronary artery disease by magnetic resonance: A comparison with positron emission tomography and coronary angiography. Circulation 2001; **103**: 2230.

38. Al Saadi N, Nagel E, Gross M, *et al.* Improvement of myocardial perfusion reserve early after coronary intervention: Assessment with cardiac magnetic resonance imaging. J Am Coll Cardiol 2000; **36**: 1557.

39. Nandalur KR, Dwamena BA, Choudhri AF, *et al.* Diagnostic performance of stress cardiac magnetic resonance imaging in the detection of coronary artery disease: a meta-analysis. J Am Coll Cardiol. 2007; **50**(14): 1343–1353.

40. Cullen JH, Horsfield MA, Reek CR, *et al.* A myocardial perfusion reserve index in humans using first-pass contrast-enhanced magnetic resonance imaging. J Am Coll Cardiol. 1999; **33**: 1386–1394.

41. van der Wall EE, van Dijkman PR, de Roos A, *et al.* Diagnostic significance of gadolinium-DTPA (diethylenetriamine penta-acetic acid) enhanced magnetic resonance imaging in thrombolytic treatment for acute myocardial infarction: its potential in assessing reperfusion. Br Heart J 1990; **63**: 12–17.

42. van Dijkman PR, van der Wall EE, de Roos A, *et al.* Gadolinium-enhanced magnetic resonance imaging in acute myocardial infarction. Eur J Radiol 1990; **11**: 1–9.

43. Judd RM, Kim RJ. Imaging time after Gd-DTPA injection is critical in using delayed enhancement to determine infarct size accurately with magnetic resonance imaging. Circulation 2002; **106**: e6.

44. Baer FM, Voth E, Schneider CA, *et al.* Comparison of low-dose dobutamine-gradient-echo magnetic resonance imaging and positron emission tomography with [18F]fluorodeoxyglucose in patients with chronic coronary artery disease: A functional and morphological approach to the detection of residual myocardial viability. Circulation 1995; **91**: 1006.

45. Ramani K, Judd RM, Holly TA, *et al.* Contrast magnetic resonance imaging in the assessment of myocardial viability in patients with stable coronary artery disease and left ventricular dysfunction. Circulation 1998; **98**: 2687.

46. Kim RJ, Wu E, Rafael A, *et al.* The use of contrast enhanced magnetic resonance imaging to identify reversible myocardial dysfunction. N Engl J Med 2000; **16**: 1445.

47. Kitagawa K, Sakuma H, Hirano T, *et al.* Acute myocardial infarction: Myocardial viability assessment in patients early thereafter—Comparison of contrast enhanced MR imaging with resting 201-Tl SPECT. Radiology 2003; **226**: 138.

48. Eichenberger AC, Schuiki E, Kochli VD, *et al.* Ischemic heart disease: Assessment with gadolinium-enhanced ultrafast MR imaging and dipyridamole stress. J Magn Reson Imaging 1994; **4**: 425–431.

49. Hartnell G, Cerel A, Kamalesh M, *et al.* Detection of myocardial ischemia: value of combined myocardial perfusion and cineangiographic MR imaging. Am J Roentgenol 1994; **163**: 1061–1067.

50. Wintersperger BJ, Penzkofer HV, Knez A, et al. Perfusion imaging and regional myocardial function analysis: Complimentary findings in chronic myocardial ischemia. Int J Card Imaging 1999; **15**: 425–434.

51. Wu E, Judd RM, Vargas JD, *et al.* Visualisation of presence, location and transmural extent of healed Q-wave and non-Q-wave myocardial infarction. Lancet 2001; **357**: 21.

52. Wagner A, Mahrholdt H, Holly TA, *et al.* Contrast-enhanced MRI and routine single photon emission computed tomography (SPECT) perfusion imaging for detection of subendocardial myocardial infarcts: An imaging study. Lancet 2003; **361**: 374.

53. Ricciardi MJ, Wu E, Davidson CJ, *et al.* Visualization of discrete microinfarction after percutaneous coronary intervention associated with mild creatine kinase-MB elevation. Circulation 2001; **103**: 2780.

54. Moon JC, De Arenaza DP, Elkington AG, *et al.* The pathologic basis of Q-wave and non-Q-wave myocardial infarction: A cardiovascular magnetic resonance study. J Am Coll Cardiol. 2004; **44**(3):554–60.

55. Mahrholdt H, Wagner A, Holly TA, *et al.* Reproducibility of chronic infarct size measurement by contrast enhanced magnetic resonance imaging. Circulation 2002; **106**: 2322.

56. Lee VS, Resnick D, Tiu SS, *et al.* MR imaging evaluation of myocardial viability in the setting of equivocal SPECT results with 99mTc sestamibi. Radiology 2004; **230**(1): 191–197.

57. Klein C, Nekolla SG, Bengel FM, *et al.* Assessment of myocardial viability with contrast-enhanced magnetic resonance imaging: Comparison with positron emission tomography. Circulation 2002; **105**: 162–167.

58. Silber HA, Bluemke DA, Ouyang P, *et al.* The relationship between vascular wall shear stress and flow-mediated dilation: Endothelial function assessed by phase-contrast magnetic resonance angiography. J Am Coll Cardiol 2001; **38**: 1859.

59. Yuan C, Beach KW, Smith LH, *et al.* Measurement of atherosclerotic carotid plaque size in-vivo using high resolution magnetic resonance imaging. Circulation 1998; **98**: 2666.

60. Corti R, Fuster V, Fayad ZA, *et al.* Lipid lowering by simvastatin induces regression of human atherosclerotic lesions: Two years' follow-up by high-resolution non-invasive magnetic resonance imaging. Circulation 2002; **106**: 2884.

61. Fayad ZA. MR imaging for the non-invasive assessment of atherothrombotic plaques. Magn Reson Imaging Clin N Am 2003; **11**(1): 101–113.

62. Yuan C, Mitsumori LM, Ferguson MS, *et al.* In vivo accuracy of multispectral magnetic resonance imaging for identifying lipid-rich necrotic cores and intraplaque hemorrhage in advanced human carotid plaques. Circulation 2001; **104**: 2051.

63. Yuan C, Zhang SX, Polissar NL, *et al.* Identification of fibrous cap rupture with magnetic resonance imaging is highly associated with recent transient ischemic attack or stroke. Circulation 2002; **105**: 181.

64. Kim WY, Danias PG, Stuber M, *et al.* Coronary magnetic resonance angiography for the detection of coronary stenosis. N Engl J Med 2001; **345**: 1863.

65. Taylor AM, Thorne SA, Rubens MB, *et al.* Coronary artery imaging in grown-up congenital heart disease: Complementary role of MR and x-ray coronary angiography. Circulation 2000; **101**: 1670.

66. Sechtem U, Tscholakoff D, Higgins CB. MRI of the abnormal pericardium. Am J Roentgenol 1986; **147**: 245–252.

67. Wagner S, Aufferman W, Buser P, *et al.* Functional description of the left ventricle in patients with volume overload, pressure overload, and myocardial disease using cine nuclear magnetic resonance imaging (NMR). Am J Cardiol Imaging 1991; **5**: 87–97.

68. McCrohon JA, Moon JC, Prasad SK, *et al* Differentiation of heart failure related to dilated cardiomyopathy and coronary artery disease using gadolinium-enhanced cardiovascular magnetic resonance. Circulation 2003; **108**: 54.

69. Soler R, Rodriguez E, Rodriguez JA, *et al.* Magnetic resonance imaging of apical hypertrophic cardiomyopathy. Thorac Imaging 1997; **12**: 221–222.

70. Suzuki J, Chang JM, Caputo GR, *et al.* Evaluation of right ventricular early diastolic filling by cine nuclear magnetic resonance imaging in patients with hypertrophic cardiomyopathy. J Am Coll Cardiol 1991; **18**: 120–126.

71. Kawada N, Sakuma H, Yamakado T, *et al.* Hypertrophic cardiomyopathy: MR measurement of coronary blood flow and vasodilator flow reserve in patients and healthy subjects. Radiology 1999; **211**: 129–135.

72. Yamanari H, Kakishita M, Fujimoto Y, *et al.* Regional myocardial perfusion abnormalities and regional myocardial early diastolic function in patients with hypertrophic cardiomyopathy. Heart Vessels 1997; **12**: 192–198.

73. Moon JCC, McKenna WJ, McCrohon JA, *et al.* Toward clinical risk assessment in hypertrophic cardiomyopathy with gadolinium cardiovascular magnetic resonance. J Am Coll Cardiol 2003; **41**: 1561.

74. Didier D, Ratib O, Lerch R, Friedli B. Detection and quantification of valvular heart disease with dynamic cardiac MR imaging. Radiographics 2000; **20**(5): 1279–1299.

75. Vignaux O, Dhote R, Duboc D, *et al.* Clinical significance of myocardial magnetic resonance abnormalities in patients with sarcoidosis: A 1-year follow-up study. Chest 2002; **122**: 1895.

76. Chandra M, Silverman ME, Oshinski J, *et al.* Diagnosis of cardiac sarcoid aided by MRI. Chest 1996; **110**: 524–526.

77. Blake LM, Scheinman MM, Higgins CB. MR features of arrhythmogenic right ventricular dysplasia. Am J Roentgenol 1994; **162**: 809.

78. Burke AP, Farb A, Tashko G, *et al.* Arrhythmogenic right ventricular cardiomyopathy and fatty replacement of the right ventricular myocardium: Are they different diseases? Circulation 1998; **97**: 1571.

79. Tandri H, Saranathan M, Rodriguez ER, *et al.* Invasive detection of myocardial fibrosis in arrhythmogenic right ventricular cardiomyopathy using delayed-enhancement magnetic resonance imaging. J Am Coll Cardiol 2005; **45**(1): 98–103.

80. Wagner A, Schulz-Menger J, Dietz R, Friedrich MG. Long-term follow-up of patients with acute myocarditis by magnetic resonance imaging. MAGMA 2003; **16**: 17.

81. Edwards MB, Taylor KM, Shellock FG. Prosthetic heart valves: Evaluation of magnetic field interactions, heating, and artifacts at 1.5 T. J Magn Reson Imaging 2000; **12**: 363.

82. Globits S, Frank H, Mayr H, *et al.* Quantitative assessment of aortic regurgitation by magnetic resonance imaging. Eur Heart J 1992; **13**: 78.

83. Kizilbash AM, Hundley WG, Willett DL, *et al.* Comparison of quantitative Doppler with magnetic resonance imaging for assessment of the severity of mitral regurgitation. Am J Cardiol 1998; **81**: 792.

84. Kilner PJ, Manzara CC, Mohiaddin RH, *et al.* Magnetic resonance jet velocity mapping in mitral and aortic valve stenosis. Circulation 1993; **87**: 1239.

85. Friedrich MG, Schulz-Menger J, Poetsch T, *et al.* Quantification of valvular aortic stenosis by magnetic resonance imaging. Am Heart J 2002; **144**: 329.

86. Tanaka K, Makaryus AN, Wolff SD. Correlation of Aortic Valve Area Obtained by the Velocity-Encoded Phase Contrast Continuity Method to Direct Planimetry using Cardiovascular Magnetic Resonance. J Cardiovasc Magn Res 2007; **9**(5): 799–805.

87. Serfaty JM, Yang X, Foo TK, *et al.* MRI-guided coronary catheterization and PTCA: A feasibility study on a dog model. Magn Reson Med 2003; **49**: 258.

88. Wildermuth S, Debatin JF, Leung DA, *et al.* MR imaging-guided intravascular procedures: Initial demonstration in a pig model. Radiology 1997; **202**: 578.

89. Lardo AC, McVeigh ER, Jumrussirikul P, *et al.* Visualization and temporal/spatial characterization of cardiac radiofrequency ablation lesions using magnetic resonance imaging. Circulation 2000; **102**: 698.

Answers

1. B
2. A
3. C
4. B

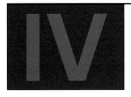

PART IV

Indications in Acute and Chronic Syndromes

CHAPTER 14

Stable Angina

Abhiram Prasad, & Bernard J. Gersh

Mayo Clinic and Mayo Foundation, Rochester, MN, USA

The main objectives of treatment for stable angina are the relief of symptoms related to myocardial ischemia and improvement in prognosis. Significant progress has been made over the past three decades in drug therapy, percutaneous coronary intervention (PCI) and coronary artery bypasses grafting (CABG). Whilst this chapter will focus on percutaneous revascularization, it is important to remember that medical therapy and secondary prevention play a central role in the management of coronary atherosclerosis. Secondary prevention via lifestyle modification, treatment of conventional risk factors (Table 14.1), and drug therapy (Figure 14.1) [1–3] reduces cardiovascular mortality, myocardial infarction, unstable angina, onset of heart failure, and the need for revascularization, likely by plaque stabilization and limiting the progression of atherosclerosis.

Guidelines on the Management of Stable Angina

The most recent guidelines on the management of stable angina have been published by the European Society of Cardiology in 2006 (Tables 14.2–14.4) [4] as well as by the American College of Cardiology (ACC) and the American Heart Association (AHA)

Interventional Cardiology, First Edition. Edited by Carlo Di Mario, George D. Dangas, Peter Barlis.
© 2010 Blackwell Publishing Ltd. Published 2010 by Blackwell Publishing Ltd.

in 2002 [5]. Additional relevant guidelines include the ACC/AHA 2004 Guideline Update for Coronary Artery Bypass Graft Surgery [6], and the ACC/AHA/SCAI 2005 Guideline Update for Percutaneous Coronary Intervention (Tables 14.5, 14.6) [7]. These guidelines are evidence based and should be the basis for clinical practice. However, there are several fundamental limitations of the trial data available on the management of stable angina. First, as with many clinical trials, the rigorous inclusion and exclusion criteria have resulted in a small number of the screened patients being enrolled into the studies. This significantly limits the ability to generalize the findings to the larger population in daily practice. Moreover, clinical trials have generally excluded high risk patients with severe angina, severe atherosclerosis, severely reduced left ventricular systolic function or multiple comorbid conditions. Second, the findings of clinical trials comparing treatment strategies often become outdated quickly due to the rapid evolution in clinical practice.

Indications for Coronary Angiography

The decision regarding whether to treat a patient with medical therapy or revascularization is based on the fundamental principal of risk stratification. The spectrum of risk for myocardial infarction and cardiovascular death is wide even in "stable" coronary artery disease (CAD). Initial risk stratification and thereby the decision to perform coronary angiography can be determined by a combination of

Table 14.1. Optimal secondary prevention in stable angina.

Risk factor	Goal/Recommended intervention
Lipid management	LDL cholesterol <70 mg/dL (<2 mmol/L) Low fat-low cholesterol diet and a statin Secondary goal is non-HDL cholesterol <130 mg/dL (<3.2 mmol/L) in pts with triglycerides >200 mg/dL (>2.2 mmol/L).
Blood pressure control	<130/80 mmHg Lifestyle modification and drug therapy (beta-blockers and ACE-inhibitors preferred)
Diabetes management	Hemoglobin A_{1c} < 6.5% Lifestyle modification ± drug therapy
Smoking	Complete cessation. No environmental exposure
Weight management	Body mass index 18.5 to 24.9 Kg/m², waist circumference: men <40 inches (<100 cm), and women <35 inches (88 cm) Regular physical exercise and restrict caloric intake
Physical activity	30 minutes, minimum 5 days per week

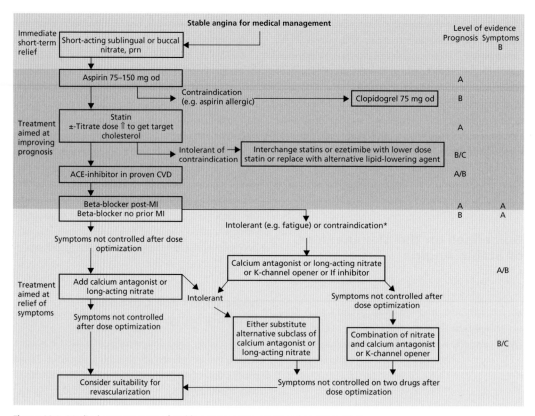

Figure 14.1. Medical management of stable angina ESC guidelines (see Table 14.2).

Table 14.2. ESC guidelines for percutaneous coronary intervention in stable angina.

Class I: Evidence and/or general agreement that PCI is beneficial, useful and effective
Assuming suitable coronary anatomy and procedural risks do not outweigh the potential benefits
1. Moderate to severe symptoms despite medical therapy in patients with single vessel disease
2. Moderate to severe symptoms despite medical therapy in patients with multi-vessel disease who do not have high risk coronary anatomy

Class IIa: Evidence/opinion is in favour of usefulness/efficacy-PCI reasonable
Assuming suitable coronary anatomy and procedural risks do not outweigh the potential benefits
1. Mild to moderate symptoms in patients with single vessel disease which are unacceptable to the patient
2. Mild to moderate symptoms in patients with multi-vessel disease which are unacceptable to the patient

ESC = European Society of Cardiology.

Table 14.3. ESC guidelines for coronary artery bypass graft surgery (CABG) to improve prognosis in patients with stable angina.

Class I: Evidence and/or general agreement that CABG is useful and effective
1. Significant left main coronary artery stenosis or its equivalent
2. Left main equivalent disease (severe ostial stenoses of the LAD and circumflex arteries)
3. Proximal stenosis of 3 major vessels. Particularly in the presence of left ventricular dysfunction, or early/extensive reversible ischemia
4. One- or two-vessel disease high-grade stenosis of the proximal LAD with reversible ischemia on non-invasive testing
5. Significant disease with impaired left ventricular function and viability demonstrated on non-invasive testing

Class IIa: Evidence/opinion is in favor of usefulness/efficacy of CABG
1. One- or two-vessel disease without significant proximal LAD stenosis in patients who have survived sudden cardiac death or sustained ventricular tachycardia
2. Significant three-vessel disease in diabetics with reversible ischemia on functional testing
3. CABG or PCI for patients with reversible ischemia on functional testing and evidence of frequent episodes of ischemia during daily activities

ESC = European Society of Cardiology; LAD = Left Anterior Descending Artery.

Table 14.4. ESC guidelines for coronary artery bypass graft surgery (CABG) to relieve symptoms in patients with stable angina.

Class I: Evidence and/or general agreement that CABG is useful and effective
Assuming suitable coronary anatomy and surgical risks do not outweigh the potential benefits
1. Multi-vessel disease in patients with moderate to severe symptoms despite medical therapy

Class IIa: Evidence/opinion is in favor of usefulness/efficacy of CABG
1. One-vessel disease in patients with moderate to severe symptoms despite medical therapy
2. Multi-vessel disease in patients with mild to moderate symptoms that are unacceptable to the patient

Class IIb: Usefulness/efficacy of CABG is less well established by evidence/opinion
1. One-vessel disease in patients with mild to moderate symptoms that are unacceptable to the patient in whom the operative risk is not greater than the estimated annual mortality

Table 14.5. ACC/AHA/SCAI guideline for percutaneous coronary intervention (PCI) in asymptomatic patients or Canadian Classification System Class I or II angina.

Class I: there is evidence and/or general agreement that PCI is useful and effective
None

Class IIa: weight of evidence/opinion is in favor of usefulness/efficacy-PCI reasonable
1. 1 or 2 coronary arteries suitable for PCI with a high likelihood of success and a low risk of morbidity and mortality. The vessels to be dilated must subtend a moderate to large area of viable myocardium or be associated with a moderate to severe degree of ischemia on noninvasive testing.
2. Recurrent stenosis after PCI with a large area of viable myocardium or high risk criteria on noninvasive testing.
3. Significant left main disease (>50% diameter stenosis) who are candidates for revascularization but are not eligible for CABG.

Class IIb: Usefulness/efficacy is less well established by evidence/opinion- PCI may be considered
1. 2- or 3-vessel disease with significant proximal LAD disease CAD who are otherwise eligible for CABG with 1 arterial conduit and who have treated diabetes or abnormal LV function is not well established.
2. Non-proximal LAD disease that subtends a moderate area of viable myocardium and demonstrates ischemia on noninvasive testing.

Class III: there is evidence and/or general agreement that the procedure/treatment is not useful/effective and in some cases may be harmful- PCI not recommended
1. A small area of viable myocardium at risk.
2. No objective evidence of ischemia.
3. Lesions that have a low likelihood of successful
4. Mild symptoms that are unlikely to be due to myocardial ischemia.
5. Factors associated with increased risk of morbidity or mortality.
6. Left main disease and eligibility for CABG.
7. Insignificant disease (less than 50% coronary stenosis).

Table 14.6. ACC/AHA/SCAI guideline for percutaneous coronary intervention (PCI) in Canadian Classification System Class III angina.

Class I: there is evidence and/or general agreement that PCI is useful and effective
None

Class IIa: weight of evidence/opinion is in favor of usefulness/efficacy-PCI reasonable
1. Single-vessel or multivessel disease who are undergoing medical therapy and who have 1 or more significant lesions in 1 or more coronary arteries suitable for PCI with a high likelihood of success and low risk of morbidity or mortality.
2. Single-vessel or multivessel disease who are undergoing medical therapy with focal saphenous vein graft lesions or multiple stenoses who are poor candidates for reoperative surgery.
3. Significant left main CAD (>50% diameter stenosis) who are candidates for revascularization but are not eligible for CABG.

Class IIb: Usefulness/efficacy is less well established by evidence/opinion- PCI may be considered
1. Single-vessel or multivessel CAD who are undergoing medical therapy and who have 1 or more lesions to be dilated with a reduced likelihood of success.
2. No evidence of ischemia on noninvasive testing or who are undergoing medical therapy and have 2- or 3-vessel CAD with significant proximal LAD CAD and treated diabetes or abnormal LV function.

Class III: there is evidence and/or general agreement that the procedure/treatment is not useful/effective and in some cases may be harmful- PCI not recommended
No evidence of myocardial injury or ischemia on objective testing, and no trial of medical therapy, or who have 1 of the following:
1. A small area of myocardium at risk.
2. Lesion morphology that conveys a low likelihood of success.
3. A high risk of procedure-related morbidity or mortality.
4. Insignificant disease (less than 50% coronary stenosis).
5. Significant left main disease and CABG candidate

clinical evaluation, and in most cases stress testing and an assessment of left ventricular function (Figure 14.2). Those with high risk features on clinical evaluation such as severe angina, unstable angina, and severe heart failure should proceed directly to coronary angiography without being subjected to a stress test. Coronary angiography is not indicated in low risk patients. The decision in intermediate risk patients should be based on severity of symptoms, response to initial medical therapy, functional status, lifestyle, and occupation. Moreover, a detailed discussion with the

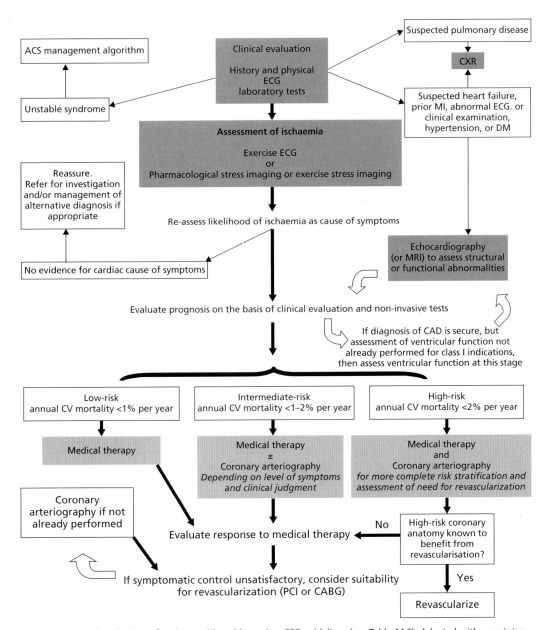

Figure 14.2. Initial evaluation of patients with stable angina. ESC guidelines (see Table 14.2). Adapted with permission from N Engl J Med 2007; **356**: 1503–1516. Copyright © 2007, Massachusetts Medical Society.

patient regarding the risks, benefits, alternatives and goals of invasive assessment is required prior to proceeding with coronary angiography. Coronary angiography is indicated in patients with high risk features on non-invasive assessment irrespective of symptoms, severe angina (Class 3 of

Canadian Cardiovascular Society Classification (CCS)), diagnostic uncertainty after non-invasive evaluation, and patients with the possibility of restenosis following PCI in a coronary distribution supplying a moderate to large amount of myocardium.

Percutaneous Coronary Intervention for Stable Angina

Several randomized trials have compared the outcomes following PCI vs. medical management for stable angina [8–11]. These include the studies from the balloon angioplasty era such as the second Randomized Intervention Treatment of Angina (RITA-2) [9] and the Angioplasty Compared to Medicine (ACME) trials [10]. The studies and meta-analyses of the randomized trials [12,13] have consistently demonstrates that PCI does not reduce the likelihood of death or myocardial infarction, but is more effective in relieving angina in patients with single and multivessel disease. Notably, there was an early hazard associated with PCI in the RITA-2 trial in which there was a greater likelihood of myocardial infarction related to the procedure, but the rate of death and myocardial infarction at seven years was similar in both arms of the trial. In addition, studies conducted in the balloon angioplasty era had shown that there was an increased risk for emergency CABG in the PCI treated group, but this was not reported in the recent Clinical Outcomes Utilizing Revascularization and Aggressive Drug Evaluation (COURAGE) trial, presumably due to the routine use of stent [14].

The COURAGE trial is the largest study to compare medical therapy to PCI and its findings are consistent with previous studies. The trial enrolled 2287 patients (approximately two-thirds with two or three vessel disease) with stable CAD. The inclusion criteria were either a coronary stenosis ≥80% and classic angina without provocative stress testing, or a stenosis ≥70% in at least one proximal epicardial coronary artery and objective evidence of myocardial ischemia. A large number of patients were excluded from the trial because of high risk features such as a strongly positive stress test, persistent CCS class IV angina, an ejection fraction of <30%, refractory heart failure or cardiogenic shock, revascularization within the previous six months, and those with coronary anatomy unsuitable for PCI. The randomization was to either optimal medical therapy alone or PCI with optimal medical therapy. During a median follow-up duration of 4.6 years, there was no difference in the primary composite endpoint of death and nonfatal myocardial infarction (19.0% vs. 18.5%, p = 0.62) (Figure 14.3). These findings must be to be interpreted in light of the facts that less than 10% of the patients screened met eligibility criteria for enrollment (as is the case in virtually all revascularization trials), 85% of patients were male, and that randomization was performed in the cardiac catheterization laboratory following angiography, which may have contributed to selection bias. The percentage of those requiring revasularization during follow-up were 21.1% of patients in the PCI arm, compared with 32.6% in the medical arm. The repeat revascularization rates in the PCI group would likely have been lower had drug eluting stents (DES) been used. PCI was associated with a small reduction in the requirement for anti-anginal therapy and greater likelihood of freedom from angina, however, this benefit diminished over time. Of note, approximately one-third of the patients in the medical arm had to cross over to PCI due to inadequate control of symptoms with optimal medical therapy. Finally, it is important to recognize that the findings of the COURAGE trial are also in keeping with earlier studies comparing CABG with medical therapy in which surgical revascularization did not improve survival or prevent myocardial infarction in patients with stable disease who had mild to moderate symptoms and good LV function.

Despite the overall conclusion of the COURAGE trial, the importance of risk stratification based on the magnitude of ischemic burden was highlighted by the results of the nuclear perfusion stress test substudy. The findings indicated that medical therapy alone was associated with a higher risk of mortality and infraction in patients who had a reversible perfusion defect involving more than 10% of the myocardium. These data suggest that a more sophisticated approach than subjective visual estimation of coronary stenoses and their ischemic potential is required in the management of stable CAD [15]. Measurement of fractional flow reserve (FFR) appears to be beneficial in the triage of patients with an intermediate stenosis who have not had a stress test prior to the angiogram. In the DEFER trial, patients with single vessel disease and an intermediate stenosis, an FFR

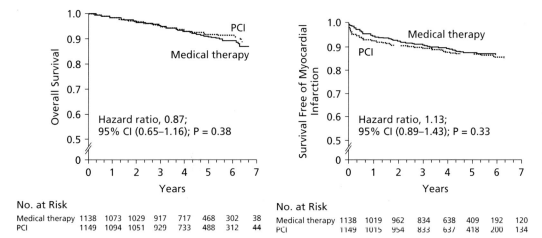

Figure 14.3. Kaplan Meier estimate for survival (left) and survival free of myocardial infarction (right) in the COURAGE trial. Adapted with permission from N Engl J Med 2007; 356: 1503-1516. Copyright © 2007 Massachusetts Medical Society.

≥0.75 identified a low risk group of patients who did not benefit from angioplasty at a follow-up of five years.

The Medicine, Angioplasty, or Surgery Study (MASS) and MASS II trials have compared medical therapy with PCI and CABG in stable angina. The MASS trial enrolled patients with single vessel disease (>80% proximal left anterior descending artery stenosis) [16] axp03. Whilst balloon angioplasty and medical therapy were associated with greater need for revascularization, there was no difference in rate of death or myocardial infarction in the three groups during follow-up. The trial was conducted in the pre-stent era without modern medical therapy which limits the applicability of the findings to contemporary practice. The MASS II trial, however, was conducted in patients with multivessel disease, and had a similar design except that PCI was performed with bare metal stents in most patients, and more contemporary medical therapy was implemented. At five years, the results were similar to the MASS trial in that there was no difference in death or myocardial infarction between the three treatment strategies, but the need for revascularization for refractory angina during follow-up was much higher with medical therapy and PCI [17].

A unique study in elderly patients with stable angina was the Trial of Invasive vs. Medical therapy in Elderly patients (TIME). At one year, the primary endpoint of quality of life was equally improved with both strategies. The invasive approach was associated with an early hazard, but there was no difference with regards to reduction in symptoms, death or nonfatal infarction at-one-year. PCI did reduce the likelihood of subsequent hospitalization for uncontrolled symptoms [18].

A significant number of patients with CAD have asymptomatic or "silent" ischemia which is associated with an increased risk of cardiovascular events. The Asymptomatic Cardiac Ischemia Pilot (ACIP) study investigated the efficacy of three treatment strategies among patients with stable disease who had angina or silent ischemia due to single or multivessel disease. Patients were randomized to angina-guided medical therapy, angina plus ischemia-guided medical therapy, or revascularization by either balloon angioplasty or CABG. At two years following randomization, revascularization was associated with a lower mortality and a reduction in the composite endpoint of death, myocardial infarction, recurrent hospitalization [19]. Another important study that evaluated treatment of silent ischemia is the Swiss Interventional Study on Silent Ischemia Type II (SWISS II) trial which compared medical therapy with balloon angioplasty among patients who had suffered a myocardial infarction, and had one or two vessel disease [20]. A surprising finding was that cardiac death and myocardial infarction were significantly lower in the group randomized to balloon angioplasty. Whilst the findings of the

ACIP and SWISS II trials are significant, they need to be interpreted with the knowledge that both enrolled relatively small number of patients and that optimal medical therapy, as defined in the COURAGE trial, was not implemented.

The studies to date have had significant cross over to revascularization in those originally randomized to medical therapy and hence have been trials of "initial treatment strategies" rather than specific treatments. Thus, based on the evidence from the COURAGE trial and the preceding randomized clinical trials, it is reasonable to conclude that medical therapy is an appropriate *initial strategy* for a substantial proportion of patients with mild to moderately severe stable angina. PCI is suitable for those patients who are significantly symptomatic despite optimal medical therapy, have a positive stress test at low workload, or have a moderate to large ischemic territory. Aggressive secondary prevention is essential regardless of the treatment strategy utilized. The findings of the Atorvastatin versus Revascularization Treatment (AVERT) trial showed that PCI in combination with inadequate lipid lowering therapy is associated with worse outcomes in patients with angina when compared to a strategy of optimal lipid management and medical therapy alone [11].

Despite the individual clinical trials not showing a mortality reduction with PCI, a large meta-analysis of 7513 patients with stable angina or silent ischemia enrolled in 17 prospective randomized trials of medical therapy vs. PCI recently reported that revascularization was associated with a 20% reduction in the relative risk of all-cause death (odds ratio: 0.80; 95% confidence interval [CI]: 0.64 to 0.99 [21]. The report contradicts the general dogma that PCI has no impact on mortality. The findings are especially notable because the randomized trials have generally limited the enrolment to patients with single vessel disease and have excluded high risk patients with left main disease or chronic total occlusion for whom revascularization may offer greater benefit.

Comparison of Percutaneous and Surgical Revascularization

The available evidence suggests that PCI and CABG are equivalent for the treatment of single vessel disease. This was specifically investigated in the MASS trial at a single center in which patients with significant (>80%) proximal LAD stenosis were randomized to balloon angioplasty, CABG or medical therapy. The data demonstrated that there was similar relief of symptoms with both forms of revascularization. However, revascularization resulted in a lower incidence of inducible ischemia compared to medical therapy alone, and all three strategies resulted in the effective treatment of limiting angina [16]. Similar findings have been reported from another small study of 134 patients with isolated proximal LAD stenosis in which angioplasty and CABG produced comparable results [22] also when the follow-up is prolonged to 10 years [23]. Importantly, the need for repeat revascularization during follow-up was greater with percutaneous revascularization using balloon angioplasty in both trials.

In the assessment of trials comparing surgery and PCI, an important premise is that none of these studies have specifically addressed the functional significance of the lesions treated. With respect to PCI in multivessel disease, the Fractional Flow Reserve vs. Angiography for Multivessel Evaluation (FAME) trial has recently demonstrated that a targeted strategy guided by measurement of FFR provides superior outcomes at one year compared to treatment of all vessels with visually estimated significant stenoses [24]. Several randomized clinical trials [25–29] and meta-analyses of the data [30] have compared PCI directly with CABG for the treatment of single and multivessel disease. The studies are predominantly from the pre-stent era among relatively low risk patients with multivessel disease and preserved left ventricular function. By design, the inclusion criteria for these trials had mandated that the coronary anatomy was suitable for both forms of revascularization, thereby excluding most patients with very complex coronary anatomy or chronic total occlusions.

The largest of these studies is the Bypass Angioplasty Revascularization Investigation (BARI) trial in which 1829 patients were enrolled. PCI was performed with balloon angioplasty which was associated with similar frequency of death, myocardial infarction, and recurrent angina when compared to CABG during 10 years of follow-up in the overall study population [31]. Not surprisingly, repeat revascularization was significantly less in patients randomized to surgery. One notable finding that has influenced current practice is that cardiac mortality was significantly lower (19.4% vs. 34.5%, p = 0.003) amongst diabetics requiring glucose lowering therapy who were randomized to CABG and received at least one mammary graft. A potential explanation for this observation is that CABG may offer complete revascularization and hence mitigate some of the adverse impact of the greater atherosclerotic burden, and the greater likelihood of restenosis and disease progression in diabetics. This finding has been confirmed in a more contemporary study [32] but the clinical relevance and applicability of the BARI study results have been somewhat contradicted by the findings from the BARI registry, which highlights the importance of clinical judgment. The patients in the registry had clinical characteristics that were similar to those in the randomized trial, but the survival among diabetics was similar regardless of whether angioplasty or CABG was performed. It has been speculated that the conflicting results between the registry and the trial may have been due to the fact that the treatment assignment in the registry was at the discretion of the physicians who might have selected the most appropriate form of revascularization for each patient [33].

The Arterial Revascularization Therapy Study Part I (ARTS I) and the Stent or Surgery (SoS) trials have compared bare metal stent based PCI with CABG [34,35]. In the ARTS I trial, death and myocardial infarction were similar with both treatment strategies, but as one might expect, complete revascularization was less often achieved and repeat revascularization was more frequent with percutaneous revascularization. The results of the SoS trial were similar, but for reasons that are unclear, there was an unexpected higher mortality associated with PCI (5% vs. 2% p = 0.01), likely unrelated to the treatment selection as the difference was entirely due to non cardiac deaths. The long-term results (5 to 6 years) of the ARTS, ERACI II and SoS trials and a large (7812 patients) meta-analysis including 10 randomized trials of balloon angioplasty or stenting vs. surgery with a median follow-up of 5.9 years have recently been published [36–39]. In the meta-analysis, long-term mortality was similar after CABG and PCI in patients with multivessel coronary artery disease (hazard ratio 0.91, 95% CI 0.82–1.02; p = 0.12). CABG was associated with a significantly lower mortality in patients with diabetes (HR 0.98, 0.86–1.12; p = 0.014 for interaction) and patients aged 65 years or older (0.82 (0.70–0.97, p = 0.002 for interaction).

DES account for approximately 50–70% of stents used for contemporary PCI around the world but there are limited data comparing the outcomes between PCI using DES and CABG. There are only two large randomized clinical trials but their follow-up is limited to one year (SYNTAX and CARDia) and the data from CARDIA has not been published [40]. Multicenter registry data from ARTS II (Arterial Revascularization Therapies Study Part II) has compared PCI using the sirolimus DES to historical controls from the ARTS I trial [41]. The incidence of the composite primary endpoint of all-cause death, any cerebrovascular event, nonfatal myocardial infarction, or any repeat revascularization at one year in the DES group was similar to the CABG treatment arm of ARTS 1. The rate of repeat revascularization was 8.5% in DES group compared to 4.1% and 21.3 % in CABG and PCI arms, respectively, of ARTS I. The three year results were consistent and confirmed, in patients with and without diabetes, the absence of significant differences in the combined endpoint when compared with the historical control of ARTS I surgical arm [42]. Whilst the data has inherent limitations of using historical controls, it suggests that PCI using DES might result in comparable outcomes to CABG, predominantly by decreasing repeat revascularization.

The Synergy Between PCI with TAXUS and Cardiac Surgery (SYNTAX) trial randomized 1800 patients with three vessel and/or left main disease to either CABG or PCI after a local interventional cardiologist and cardiac surgeon at each site prospectively evaluated eligible patients and determined that equivalent anatomical revascularization could be achieved with either strategy [40]. A score of anatomical complexity (SYNTAX score) was prospectively calculated. Unlike most previous trials where a small minority of patients who were screened were ultimately enrolled, almost half of the 4337 screened were randomized, with the majority of those excluded were unsuitable for PCI. The rates of death and myocardial infarction at 12 months were similar in the two groups. Stroke was significantly more frequent in the CABG group (2.2% vs. 0.6%, p = 0.003) whilst the incidence of stent thrombosis and symptomatic graft occlusion at 12 months were similar in the two groups (3.3 and 3.4%, respectively). An increased rate of repeat revascularization in the PCI group (13.5% vs. 5.9%, p < 0.001) led to an excess of major cardiac and cardiovascular events in the PCI group, with the endpoint of the trial (non-inferiority of PCI using DES) not being met. Subgroup analysis based on the predetermined SYNTAX score showed that the negative outcome was confined to patients with high scores (>33, 10.9% in the surgical arm vs. 23.4% in the PCI arm). The patients with left main disease had similar incidence of 12 month MACCE in the surgical and PCI groups (13.7 vs. 15.8%, p = 0.44). Whilst the overall superiority of CABG is undeniable if the goal is to reduce repeat revascularization, interventionalists may argue that patients are more interested in hard endpoints which were similar with both forms of revascularization, and that the excess of strokes in the surgical group offsets the advantage of CABG over PCI with respect to revascularization. A major limitation of the SYNTAX trial to date is the short duration of follow-up. Based on the data available, it is reasonable to conclude that the traditional practice of all left main and three vessel disease being treated surgically is not supported by the results of SYNTAX trial, and attention should be paid to the individual characterization of the patient's coronary anatomy and surgical risk. Those with low to intermediate SYNTAX scores should be offered both revascularization options, but PCI would be the preferred strategy in patients with high surgical risk. In patients with a high SYNTAX score, the potential advantages of surgery should be stressed, but PCI should not be denied to patients who have a strong preference or a very high surgical risk. The results of CARDia and the subgroup analysis of SYNTAX, reported but not yet published, have confirmed that diabetic patients achieve similar outcomes, at least at one year.

Coronary Artery Bypass Surgery for Stable Angina

The European Coronary Surgery Study (ECSS), Coronary Artery Surgery Study (CASS), and Veterans Administration Cooperative Study (VA Study) are large randomized trials that have compared CABG with medical therapy among patients with mild to moderate angina [43–45]. The consistent finding from these studies was that surgical revascularization provides better symptomatic relief from angina but the benefit is lost over time, most likely because of vein graft failure and subsequent cross-over to CABG in the medical treatment arm. The randomized trials and a meta-analysis [46] indicate that an initial strategy of surgical revascularization does not improve survival in the general population of CAD, but that there are specific subsets that either have a large amount of ischemic myocardium or significant left ventricular dysfunction. Thus, patients with significant left main disease, three vessel disease (especially in those with abnormal left ventricular function), two or three vessels disease with >75% stenosis of the left anterior descending artery (LAD) or a markedly positive stress test derive prognostic benefit from CABG. In general, patients with severe symptoms have been excluded from the trials, but an analysis from registry data of the CASS study indicates that surgical revascularization probably improves prognosis in patients with severe angina who have multivessel disease, even in the absence of left ventricular function or proximal LAD stenosis [47]. It is important to be aware that this evidence which has been used to craft current guidelines is limited by the fact that the randomized trials were all conducted in the early years of bypass surgery, and are not representative of the contemporary surgical techniques such as the routine use of internal mammary grafts or minimally invasive and off-pump surgery [48]. Conversely, the medical group did not benefit of the aggressive preventive measures which are now is routine nor did they consistently receive beta-blockers or ACE-inhibitors. Furthermore, the general applicability of these trials is limited by the fact that they did not enroll many women or patients over 65 years old.

Recommendations for Revascularization in Stable Angina

Broadly speaking revascularization is appropriate for patients with limiting symptoms despite optimal medical therapy, strongly positive stress tests, proximal multivessel disease, and those who prefer an interventional approach over medical therapy. The choice between PCI and CABG in any one patient is determined by the risks of the procedure, likelihood of success, and ability to achieve complete revascularization with the two strategies as well diabetic status and patient preference. Contraindications to PCI are as listed as class III recommendations of the ACC/AHA/SCAI guidelines (Tables 14.4,14.5). Whilst medical therapy is the cornerstone of treatment of stable angina, it is important to remember that there is no evidence that medical therapy alone improves prognosis in high risk patients, as defined in the clinical trials of medical treatment vs. CABG.

Patients with significant *proximal left anterior descending artery disease* have a survival advantage with CABG compared to medical therapy, even in the absence of severe symptoms, LV dysfunction or other lesions. PCI provides similar results among patients who have suitable anatomy for PCI of the proximal LAD and normal LV function CABG offers a survival advantage over medical therapy in patients with severe symptoms and *three vessel disease*, even in the absence of LAD involvement or LV dysfunction. Patients with three vessel disease and LV dysfunction should have CABG. PCI is an alternative to CABG in those with angiographically suitable targets and normal LV function.

In patients with *diabetes mellitus*, particularly in the setting of multivessel or diffuse disease, there is a survival advantage with CABG compared to PCI with balloon angioplasty or bare metal stents. PCI is reasonable for diabetics with discrete *two vessel disease* and preserved LV function.

For the majority of patients with stable CAD who do not fall into the subgroups described above, there is no survival advantage with revascularization. PCI and CABG should be offered for the treatment of symptoms refractory to medical therapy. The guidelines state that both forms of revascularization are suitable for two vessel disease, but in current practice the majority of these patients and those with single vessel disease are treated with PCI unless the lesions are angiographically unsuitable, or involve the proximal LAD [49]. Revascularization in asymptomatic patients should only be considered with the goal of improving prognosis. The guidelines for the treatment of asymptomatic patients are similar to those for symptomatic patients. However, the level of evidence for asymptomatic patients is weaker as the clinical trials have mainly included symptomatic patients. But ischemia is an important therapeutic target in contemporary practice over and above the treatment of symptoms.

Conclusions

Unlike PCI for acute coronary syndromes, percutaneous revascularization does not prevent death or myocardial infarction in patients with stable angina. There remains the possibility that PCI may reduce hard endpoints in high risk patients, but clinical trials in these patient subsets have not been conducted. For patients in low risk subgroups, the main advantage of PCI is the ability to effectively and more rapidly relieve symptoms In general, therefore, PCI is indicated for the treatment of symptomatic coronary atherosclerosis, particularly in patients who remain symptomatic limited despite optimal medical therapy. PCI is preferred revascularization strategy for single vessel disease, younger patients (age <50 years), elderly patients with significant comorbid conditions, and those who are not surgical candidates. There is no clear indication for PCI in the treatment of asymptomatic disease.

CABG is also highly effective in relieving symptoms, but importantly it reduces mortality in high risk patients. This benefit is proportional to baseline risk profile of the patient. Complete revascularization is more likely to be achieved with CABG. Thus, CABG is preferred for high risk patients such as those with multivessel disease where complete revascularization is an important goal, particularly in three vessel disease, and in the presence of significant left ventricular systolic dysfunction. Subgroups that should be considered for surgery include significant unprotected left main disease, three vessel disease, especially if there is impaired left ventricular function, diffuse atherosclerosis, or one or more chronic total occlusion. Another important group of patients who may benefit with CABG are diabetics with severe or diffuse three vessel disease. However, as with PCI, CABG does not reduce the incidence of non-fatal myocardial infarction. Balloon angioplasty and the use bare metal stents for multivessel disease is associated with higher rates of repeat revascularization compared to CABG, but this may no longer be the case with DES because the need for repeat target vessel revascularization for restenosis has decreased markedly with the use of DES.

Rapid developments in medical therapy, PCI and CABG result in limited data being available from clinical trials that reflect contemporary practice, especially in high risk patients. With regards to PCI, the initial optimism for the current generation of DES has been tempered by the concerns of late stent thrombosis and the potential need for long-term dual antiplatelet therapy. There are several clinical trials in progress that will provide important insight into the efficacy of DES in multivessel disease and diabetes. The SYNTAX trial has completed the primary endpoint of one year follow-up but only the analyses at three and five years will offer sufficient support for a modification of the current preferential indication to surgery in left main and multivessel disease [40]. The Bypass Angioplasty Revascularization Investigation 2 Diabetes (BARI 2D) sponsored by the National Institutes of Health and the Future Revascularization Evaluation in Patients With Diabetes Mellitus: Optimal Management of Multivessel Disease (FREEDOM) trials are comparing treatment strategies involving PCI, CABG and optimal medical management in patients with diabetes mellitus. The data from these trials will provide much needed information regarding optimal revascularization strategies in high risk patients with multivessel disease and diabetics and the role of DES.

Questions

1. **An 80 year-old man presents with precordial ST depression and ongoing ischemic pain He had undergone prior CABG surgery with a LIMA to the LAD and a SVG to the left circumflex OM1 branch. Two years ago a bare metal stent (4.0 × 16 mm) was placed in the body of the left circumflex graft with an excellent result. The most likely cause of his current symptoms is:**

    A The development of a new lesion in the native LAD beyond the LIMA touchdown

    B Stent thrombosis in the SVG graft

    C Disease progression with a new ruptured plaque outside the previously placed stent

    D Development of a distal anastamotic lesion at the LIMA/LAD insertion

2. **All of the following statements about diabetic patients are true, except:**

    A Compared to non-diabetics, patients with diabetes have 2- to 3-fold higher rate of coronary disease and are at increased risk of myocardial infarction, congestive heart failure, and death

    B Compared with non-diabetics undergoing bypass surgery, diabetics have more in-hospital stroke, late myocardial infarction, and repeat revascularization

    C Acute procedural successful rates for PTCA are similar between diabetics and non-diabetics

    D In the BARI trial, 5-year mortality rates for diabetics with multivessel disease were independent of the mode of initial revascularization

3. **Which of the following statements regarding the randomized control trials of coronary bypass surgery (CABG) versus medical therapy are correct?**

    A Survival differences in favor of CABG are noted in all subgroups.

    B The incidence of myocardial infarction is reduced by CABG.

    C Relief of angina is better with CABG.

    D Patients with left ventricular dysfunction do better with medical therapy.

    E The use of "statins" improved outcomes in both groups.

References

1. Graham I, Atar D, Borch-Johnsen K, *et al.* European guidelines on cardiovascular disease prevention in clinical practice: executive summary: Fourth Joint Task Force of the European Society of Cardiology and Other Societies on Cardiovascular Disease Prevention in Clinical Practice. Eur Heart J 2007; **28**: 2375–2414.

2. Rosendorff C, Black HR, Cannon CP, *et al.* Treatment of hypertension in the prevention and management of ischemic heart disease: a scientific statement from the American Heart Association Council for High Blood Pressure Research and the Councils on Clinical Cardiology and Epidemiology and Prevention. Circulation 2007; **115**: 2761–2788.

3. Smith SC Jr, Allen J, Blair SN, *et al.* AHA/ACC guidelines for secondary prevention for patients with coronary and other atherosclerotic vascular disease: 2006 update: endorsed by the National Heart, Lung, and Blood Institute. Circulation 2006; **113**: 2363–2372.

4. Fox K, Garcia MA, Ardissino D, *et al.* Guidelines on the management of stable angina pectoris: executive summary: the Task Force on the Management of Stable Angina Pectoris of the European Society of Cardiology. Eur Heart J 2006; **27**: 1341–1381.

5. Gibbons RJ, Abrams J, Chatterjee K, *et al.* ACC/AHA 2002 guideline update for the management of patients with chronic stable angina: a report of the American College of Cardiology/ American Heart Association Task Force on Practice Guidelines (Committee to Update the 1999 Guidelines for the Management of Patients with Chronic Stable Angina). 2002. Available at www.acc.org/clinical/guidelines/stable/stable.pdf.

6. Eagle KA, Guyton RA, Davidoff R, *et al.* ACC/AHA 2004 guideline update for coronary artery bypass graft surgery: a report of the American College of Cardiology/ American Heart Association Task Force on Practice Guidelines (Committee to Update the 1999 Guidelines for Coronary Artery Bypass Graft Surgery). Circulation 2004; **110**: e340.

7. Smith SC Jr, Feldman TE, Hirshfeld JW Jr, *et al.* ACC/AHA/SCAI 2005 guideline update for percutaneous coronary intervention: a report of the American College of Cardiology/American Heart Association Task Force on Practice Guidelines (ACC/AHA/SCAI Writing Committee to Update 2001 Guidelines for Percutaneous Coronary Intervention). Circulation 2006; **113**: e166–286.

8. Parisi AF, Folland ED, Hartigan P. A comparison of angioplasty with medical therapy in the treatment of single-vessel coronary artery disease. N Engl J Med 1992; **326**: 10–16.

9. Anonymous. Coronary angioplasty versus medical therapy for angina: the second Randomised Intervention Treatment of Angina (RITA-2) trial. RITA-2 trial participants. Lancet 1997; **350**: 461–468.

10. Folland ED, Hartigan PM, Parisi AF. Percutaneous transluminal coronary angioplasty versus medical therapy for stable angina pectoris: outcomes for patients with double-vessel versus single-vessel coronary artery disease in a Veterans Affairs Cooperative randomized trial. Veterans Affairs ACME InvestigatorS. J Am Coll Cardiol 1997; **29**: 1505–1511.

11. Pitt B, Waters D, Brown WV, *et al*. Aggressive lipid-lowering therapy compared with angioplasty in stable coronary artery disease. Atorvastatin versus Revascularization Treatment Investigators. N Engl J Med 1999; **341**: 70–76.

12. Bucher HC, Hengstler P, Schindler C, *et al*. Percutaneous transluminal coronary angioplasty versus medical treatment for non-acute coronary heart disease: meta-analysis of randomised controlled trials. BMJ 2000; **321**: 73–77.

13. Katritsis DG, Ioannidis JP. Percutaneous coronary intervention versus conservative therapy in nonacute coronary artery disease: a meta-analysis. Circulation 2005; **111**: 2906–2912.

14. Boden WE, O'Rourke RA, Teo KK, *et al*. Optimal medical therapy with or without PCI for stable coronary disease. N Engl J Med 2007; **356**: 1503–1516.

15. Shaw LJ, Berman DS, Maron DJ, *et al*. COURAGE Investigators. Optimal medical therapy with or without percutaneous coronary intervention to reduce ischemic burden: results from the Clinical Outcomes Utilizing Revascularization and Aggressive Drug Evaluation (COURAGE) trial nuclear substudy. Circulation 2008; **117**(10): 1283–1291.

16. Hueb WA, Soares PR, Almeida De Oliveira S, *et al*. Five-year follow-op of the medicine, angioplasty, or surgery study (MASS): A prospective, randomized trial of medical therapy, balloon angioplasty, or bypass surgery for single proximal left anterior descending coronary artery stenosis. Circulation 1999; **100** (Suppl): II 107–113.

17. Hueb W, Lopes NH, Gersh BJ, Soares P, *et al*. Five-year follow-up of the Medicine, Angioplasty, or Surgery Study (MASS II): A randomized controlled clinical trial of 3 therapeutic strategies for multivessel coronary artery disease. Circulation 2007; **115**: 1082–1089.

18. Pfisterer M, Buser P, Osswald S, *et al*. Outcome of elderly patients with chronic symptomatic coronary artery disease with an invasive versus optimized medical treatment strategy: one-year results of the randomized TIME trial. JAMA 2003; **289**: 1117–1123.

19. Davies RF, Goldberg AD, Forman S, Pepine CJ, Knatterud GL, Geller N, *et al*. Asymptomatic Cardiac Ischemia Pilot (ACIP) study two-year follow-up: outcomes of patients randomized to initial strategies of medical therapy versus revascularization. Circulation 1997; **95**: 2037–2043.

20. Erne P, Schoenenberger AW, Burckhardt D, *et al*. Effects of percutaneous coronary interventions in silent ischemia after myocardial infarction: the SWISSI II randomized controlled trial. JAMA 2007; **297**: 1985–1991.

21. Schömig A, MD, Mehilli J, MD, de Waha A, MD, Seyfarth M, Pache J, Kastrati AA. Meta-Analysis of 17 Randomized Trials of a Percutaneous Coronary Intervention-Based Strategy in Patients With Stable Coronary Artery Disease. J Am Coll Cardiol 2008; **52**: 894–904.

22. Goy JJ, Eeckhout E, Burnand B, *et al*. Coronary angioplasty versus left internal mammary artery grafting for isolated proximal left anterior descending artery stenosis. Lancet 1994; **343**: 1449–1453.

23. Goy JJ, Kaufmann U, Hurni M, *et al*. SIMA Investigators 10-year follow-up of a prospective randomized trial comparing bare-metal stenting with internal mammary artery grafting for proximal, isolated de novo left anterior coronary artery stenosis the SIMA (Stenting versus Internal Mammary Artery grafting) trial. J Am Coll Cardiol. 2008; **52**(10): 815–817.

24. Tonino PA, De Bruyne B, Pijls NH, *et al*. FAME Study Investigators. Fractional flow reserve versus angiography for guiding percutaneous coronary intervention. N Engl J Med. 2009; **360**(3): 213–224.

25. Comparison of coronary bypass surgery with angioplasty in patients with multivessel disease. The Bypass Angioplasty Revascularization Investigation (BARI) Investigators. N Engl J Med 1996; **335**: 217–225. Anonymous. Coronary angioplasty versus coronary artery bypass surgery: the Randomized Intervention Treatment of Angina (RITA) trial. Lancet 1993; **341**: 573–580.

26. Hamm CW, Reimers J, Ischinger T, *et al*. A randomized study of coronary angioplasty versus bypass-surgery in patients with symptomatic multivessel coronary disease. N Engl J Med 1994; **331**: 1037–1043.

27. King, SB III, Lembo, NJ, Weintraub WS, *et al*. A randomized trial comparing coronary angioplasty with coronary bypass surgery. N Engl J Med 1994; **331**: 1044–1050.

28. Anonymous. First-year results of CABRI (Coronary Angioplasty versus Bypass Revascularisation Investigation). CABRI Trial Participants. Lancet 1995; **346**: 1179–1184.

29. Rodriguez A, Boullon F, Perez-Balino N, *et al*. Argentine randomized trial of percutaneous transluminal coro-

nary angioplasty versus coronary artery bypass surgery in multivessel disease (ERACI): in-hospital results and 1-year follow-up. ERACI Group. J Am Coll Cardiol 1993; **22**: 1060–1067.

30. Hoffman SN, TenBrook JA, Wolf MP, *et al*. A meta-analysis of randomized controlled trials comparing coronary artery bypass graft with percutaneous trans-luminal coronary angioplasty: one- to eight-year out-comes. J Am Coll Cardiol 2003; **41**: 1293–1304.

31. BARI Investigators. The final 10-year follow-up results from the BARI randomized trial. J Am Coll Cardiol 2007; **49**: 1600–1606.

32. Niles NW, McGrath PD, Malenka D, Quinton H, Wennberg D, Shubrooks SJ, *et al*. Survival of patients with diabetes and multivessel coronary artery disease after surgical or percutaneous coronary revasculariza-tion: results of a large regional prospective study. Northern New England Cardiovascular Disease Study Group. J Am Coll Cardiol 2001; **37**: 1008–1015.

33. Gersh BJ, Frye RL. Methods of coronary revasculariza-tion–things may not be as they seem. N Engl J Med 2005; **352**: 2235–2237.

34. Serruys PW, Unger F, Sousa JE, *et al*. Comparison of coronary-artery bypass surgery and stenting for the treatment of multivessel disease. N Engl J Med 2001; **344**: 1117–1124.

35. Legrand VM, Serruys PW, Unger F, *et al*. Three-year outcome after coronary stenting versus bypass surgery for the treatment of multivessel disease. Circulation 2004; **109**: 1114–1120.

36. Serruys PW, Ong ATL, van Herwerden LA, *et al*. Five-year outcomes after coronary stenting versus bypass surgery for the treatment of multivessel disease. The final analysis of the Arterial Revascularization Therapies (ARTS) randomized trial. J Am Coll Cardiol 2005; **46**: 575–581.

37. Rodriguez AE, Baldi J, Pereira CF, *et al*. Five-year fol-low-up of the Argentine randomized trial of coronary angioplasty with stenting versus coronary bypass surgery in patients with multiple vessel disease (ERACI II). J Am Coll Cardiol 2005; **46**: 582–588.

38. Booth J, Clayton T, Pepper J, *et al*. Randomized, con-trolled trial of coronary artery bypass surgery versus percutaneous coronary intervention in patients with multivessel coronary artery disease. Six-year follow-up from the Stent or Surgery trial (SoS). Circulation 2008; **118**: 381–388.

39. Hlatky MA, Boothroyd DB, Bravata DM, *et al*. Percutaneous coronary interventions for multivessel disease: a collaborative analysis of individual patient data from ten randomised trials. Lancet 2009; **373**: 1190–1197.

40. Serruys PW, Morice MC, Kappetein AP, *et al*. Percutaneous coronary intervention versus coronary-artery bypass grafting for severe coronary artery disease. N Engl J Med 2009; **360**: 961–972.

41. Valgimigli M, Dawkins K, Macaya C, *et al*. Impact of stable versus unstable coronary artery disease on 1-year outcome in elective patients undergoing multivessel revascularization with sirolimus-eluting stents: a suba-nalysis of the ARTS II trial. J Am Coll Cardiol 2007; **49**: 431–441.

42. The VA Coronary Artery Bypass Surgery Cooperative Study Group. Eighteen-year follow-up in the Veterans Affairs Cooperative Study of Coronary Artery Bypass Surgery for stable angina. Circulation 1992; **86**: 121–130.

43. Varnauskas E. Twelve-year follow-up of survival in the randomized European Coronary Surgery Study. N Engl J Med 1988; **319**: 332–337.

44. Passamani E, Davis KB, Gillespie MJ, Killip T. A rand-omized trial of coronary artery bypass surgery. Survival of patients with a low ejection fraction. N Engl J Med 1985; **312**: 1665–1671.

45. Yusuf S, Zucker D, Peduzzi P, *et al*. Effect of coronary artery bypass graft surgery on survival: overview of 10-year results from randomised trials by the Coronary Artery Bypass Graft Surgery Trialists Collaboration. Lancet 1994; **344**: 563–570.

46. Myers WO, Schaff HV, Gersh BJ, *et al*. Improved sur-vival of surgically treated patients with triple vessel coronary artery disease and severe angina pectoris. A report from the Coronary Artery Surgery Study (CASS) registry. J Thorac Cardiovasc Surg 1989; **97**: 487–495.

47. Rihal CS, Raco DL, Gersh BJ, Yusuf S. Indications for coronary artery bypass surgery and percutaneous coronary intervention in chronic stable angina: review of the evidence and methodological considerations. Circulation 2003; **108**: 2439–2445.

48. Hannan EL, Racz MJ, Walford G, *et al*. Long-term out-comes of coronary-artery bypass grafting versus stent implantation. N Engl J Med 2005; **352**: 2174–2183.

49. Ong AT, Serruys PW, Mohr FW, *et al*. The SYNergy between percutaneous coronary intervention with TAXus and cardiac surgery (SYNTAX) study: Design, rationale, and run-in phase. Am Heart J 2006; **151**: 1194–1204.

Answers

1. C
2. D
3. C

CHAPTER 15

Indications in Acute Coronary Syndromes Without ST Elevation (NSTE-ACS)

Christian W. Hamm[1], & Albrecht Elsaesser[2]
[1] Heart and Thoraxcenter, Kerckhoff Klinik, Bad Nauheim, Germany
[2] Heart Center, Oldenburg Medical Centre, Oldenburg, Germany

The optimal treatment for patients with acute coronary syndromes without ST-elevation has been under discussion for almost two decades. The therapeutic aim is to relieve angina and ongoing myocardial ischemia, as well as to prevent progression to myocardial infarction or death. The basic questions in this context are when to choose an invasive or conservative strategy and what is the preferred timing.

Invasive vs. Conservative Strategy

The question of an invasive vs. conservative approach on short term outcome has been investigated in numerous small or mid-size controlled trials. The effects on hard endpoints like death and myocardial infarction have been elucidated in several meta-analyses [1,2,3]. Long term follow-up data are available from RITA-3 at five years [4] and FRISC-2 at two and five years [5,6].

The meta-analysis of Mehta *et al.* [1] of 7 randomized trials includes early studies prior to the routine use of stents and multidrug adjunctive therapy and compares routine angiography (n = 4608) followed by revascularization with a more conservative strategy (invasive care only in

patients with recurrent or inducible ischemia, n = 4604). A reduced rate of death and myocardial infarction was shown at the end of follow-up (12.2% vs. 14.4%, OR 0.82, 95% CI 0.72–0.93, P = 0.001). There was a non-significant trend towards fewer deaths (5.5% vs. 6.0%, OR 0.92, 95% CI 0.77–1.09), while a significant reduction in infarction rate alone was observed (7.3% vs. 9.4%, OR 0.72, 95% CI 0.65–0.88, p < 0.001). These results were obtained despite an early hazard observed during initial hospitalization in the routine invasive group. There was a significantly higher risk of death, and death/ myocardial infarction (1.8% vs. 1.1%, OR 1.6, 95% CI 1.14–2.25, p = 0.007 for death; 5.2% vs. 3.8%, OR 1.36, 95% CI 1.12–1.66, p = 0.002 for death and myocardial infarction). The beneficial effect was actually achieved from hospital discharge to end of follow-up, when a significant risk reduction in death and death/ myocardial infarction was observed (3.8% vs. 4.9%, OR 0.76, 95% CI 0.62–0.94, p = 0.01 for death; 7.4% vs. 11.0%, OR 0.64, 95% CI 0.55–0.75, p < 0.001 for death and myocardial infarction). Over a mean follow-up of 17 months, recurrent angina was reduced by 33% and re-hospitalization by 34% in the routine invasive group.

Many of the trials analyzed in the meta-analysis by Mehta *et al.* were not contemporary in terms of adjunctive therapy and use of stents. In four of the trials, namely TIMI-3B, VANQWISH, MATE and FRISC-2, the use of stents and GP IIb/IIIa

Interventional Cardiology, First Edition. Edited by Carlo Di Mario, George D. Dangas, Peter Barlis.
© 2010 Blackwell Publishing Ltd. Published 2010 by Blackwell Publishing Ltd.

inhibitors was low or non existent [6,7,8,9]. However, a review of the more contemporary trials by the Cochrane collaboration confirmed the initial observations reported by Mehta and co-workers. This meta-analysis confirmed the existence of a trend towards an early excess of mortality with invasive strategy (RR 1.59, 95% CI 0.96–2.54), but with a significant long-term benefit in terms of death (RR 0.75, 95% CI 0.62–0.92) or myocardial infarction (RR 0.75, 95% CI 0.62–0.91) with invasive vs. conservative at 2–5 year follow-up [3].

A more recent meta-analysis (Figure 15.1) by Bavry et al. [2] including seven trials with 8375 patients available for analysis showed after a mean follow-up of two years a significant risk reduction for all-cause mortality (4.9% vs. 6.5%, RR 0.75, 95% CI 0.63–0.90, p = 0.001) of early invasive vs. conservative management, without excess of death at one month (RR = 0.82, 95% CI 0.50–1.34, p = 0.43). At two years of follow-up, the incidence of nonfatal myocardial infarction was 7.6% vs. 9.1% (RR = 0.83, 95% CI 0.72–0.96, p = 0.012), without excess at 1 month (RR = 0.93, 95% CI 0.73–1.19, p = 0.57).

In a meta-analysis reported in the recent ESC guidelines [10] including six contemporary trials, the risk reduction for death and myocardial infarction was 16% (OR 0.84 95%, CI 0.73–0.97 early invasive vs. conservative strategy) (Figure 15.2). The benefit of the routine invasive strategy was present in patients with elevated troponins at baseline, but not in troponin-negative patients (from the analysis of the three most recently performed trials with available troponin data) [5,11,6].

In contrast to the results of the meta-analyses, the ICTUS trial challenges the paradigm of superior outcome with routine invasive strategy [12]. In this trial, 1200 patients were randomized to an early invasive strategy vs. a selective invasive approach. There was no difference in the incidence of the primary composite endpoint of death, myocardial infarction or re-hospitalization for angina within 1 year (22.7% vs. 21.2%, RR 1.07, 95% CI 0.87–1.33, p = 0.33) with early vs. selective invasive strategy. These results were maintained at three-year follow-up [13]. Routine intervention was associated with a significant early hazard, because myocardial infarction was significantly more frequent in the early invasive group (15.0% vs. 10.0%,

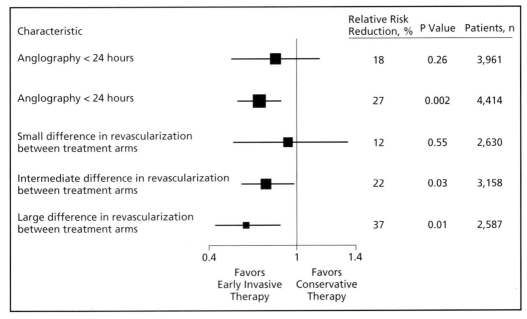

Figure 15.1. Meta-analysis of contemporary randomized trial comparing invasive vs. conservative management in ACS [2]. Reprinted with permission from J Am Coll Cardiol 2006; 48: 1319–1325.

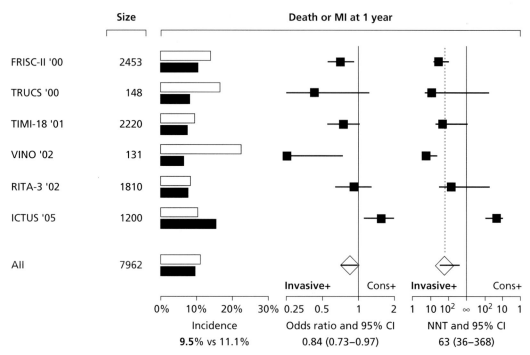

Figure 15.2. Death or myocardial infarction in six contemporary randomized trials comparing early invasive (dark bars) vs. conservative strategy (open bars). NNT = number of patients who needed to be treated to avoid one event [2]. Reprinted with permission from J Am Coll Cardiol 1998; 32: 596–605.

RR 1.5, 95% CI 1.10–2.04, p = 0.005). The majority (67%) of myocardial infarction (defined as ≥1–3 times ULN CPK-MB) were directly associated with revascularization procedures. The discrepancy between this and prior trials could be attributed in part to the small difference in revascularization rates between the two study groups and the high overall rate of revascularization before discharge (76% in the routine invasive and 40% in the selective group). In addition, the criterion for diagnosis of myocardial infarction (any CK-MB elevation above ULN as opposed to >3 times ULN) differs between studies. Furthermore, the selection of patients may have been biased, as some studies included all consecutive patients admitted while others did not enter severely unstable patients.

In all trials, a large proportion of patients initially assigned to conservative management eventually underwent revascularization ("cross-over") such that the true benefit of revascularization is skewed [14]. When comparing the relative mortality benefit between routine and selective revascularization strategies with the actual difference in the revascularization rates between arms, a linear relationship emerges. The greater the difference in the rate of revascularisation, the greater is the benefit on mortality (Figure 15.3).

Timing of an Invasive Strategy

There is in general, no debate for emergency angiography and revascularization in patients with ongoing chest pain and severe, particularly dynamic ST-T changes. Controversy exists, however, as to the optimal timing between hospital admission, initiation of medical therapy, and invasive evaluation for the majority of chest pain patients. The question is to whether "cooling-down" the patient may result in a better procedural outcome.

No early hazard was observed in TACTICS-TIMI-18 (mean delay for PCI was 22 hours) with upstream treatment with the GP IIb/IIIa inhibitor tirofiban [15]. The question of these two strategies was systematically investigated in the ISAR-COOL study [16] in 410 consecutive, high-risk patients with either ST-segment depression (65%) or elevated cTnT (67%). Deferral of the interven-

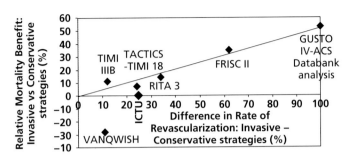

Figure 15.3. The ability to demonstrate relative mortality benefit with the revascularization strategy depends on the gradient in rates of revasularization between both randomization arms [2]. Reprinted with permission from J Am Coll Cardiol 1998; 32: 596–605.

tion did not improve outcome. Patients assigned to immediate PCI (on average 2.4 hours after admission) had a lower incidence of death or myocardial infarction at 30 days than patients randomized to deferred PCI (86 hours after admission and medical therapy including triple antiplatelet treatment) (5.9% vs. 11.6%, RR 1.96, 95% CI 1.01–3.82, p = 0.04). In contrast to these findings, early routine invasive care in the ICTUS trial within 48 hours of randomization in 56% and during initial hospitalization in 76% of cases was associated with an excess of myocardial infarction (15.0% vs. 10.0%, RR 1.5, 95% CI 1.10–2.04, p = 0.005). Expedite catheterization was also associated with worse outcome in FRISC-2 as well as in the GRACE and CRUSADE registry [6,17–19]. Two trials have further modified our approach towards early interventions in non-ST elevation myocardial infarction. The Canadian TIMACS study performed angiography in 1593 patients randomized to an early strategy of revascularization at a median of 14 hrs (IQR 3-21) after admission and compared them with a group of 1438 patients treated with a delayed strategy at 50 (IQR 41-81) hours. The primary endpoint of the trial was negative. Death, myocardial infarction and stroke at 180 days were lowered by the early strategy but the hazard ratio was 0.85 (CI 0.68–1.06, p = 0.15). Still the reduction became highly significant when refractory ischemia was added to the combined endpoint and bleeding was not higher in the early revascularization group. The significant cost reduction with an early approach was another element which turned this trial potentially negative for an early revascularization strategy into a powerful driver to rapid treatment [20]. A recently published trial followed an even more radical approach randomizing patients with a TIMI score greater or equal to 3 to immediate

angiography (1.10 hours (IQR 0.51–2.03) vs. next day angiography (20.5 hours, 17.3–24.3). This small study did not reach the endpoint (peak troponin I) but drastically reduced hospital stay (almost 1 day) with no indicators of safety concerns [21].

Accordingly, current evidence does not mandate a systematic approach of immediate angiography in NSTE-ACS patients stabilized with a contemporary pharmacological approach. Likewise, a routine practice of immediate transfer of stabilized patients admitted in hospitals without on site catheterization facilities is not mandatory, but should be organized within 72 hours.

Choice of Best Revascularization Modality

Invasive coronary angiography is prerequisite for determining suitability for percutaneous and/or surgical revascularization. The intracoronary administration of vasodilators (nitrates) in order to attenuate vasoconstriction and offset the dynamic component that is frequently present is advised. In hemodynamically compromised patients (pulmonary oedema, cardiogenic shock, severe arrhythmias), it may be advantageous to perform the examination after placement of an intra-aortic balloon pump. The angiographic findings in conjunction with ECG finding and wall motion abnormalities frequently allows the identification the culprit lesion that often shows eccentricity, irregular borders, ulceration, haziness and filling defects suggestive of intracoronary thrombus [22]. Diffuse atherosclerotic infiltration without significant narrowing is found in 14% to 19% of cases [23].

About one third of patients with unstable coronary syndromes have single vessel and approximately 50% have multivessel disease (>50% diameter stenosis). [7,24] The incidence of critical left main lesions varies from 4% to 8%. With the exception of an urgent procedure, the choice of revascularization technique in NSTE-ACS is the same as for elective revascularization procedures. The proportion of patients with NSTE-ACS requiring bypass surgery during the initial hospitalization is about 10% [12].

PCI is the best treatment option for the majority of patients. In patients with single vessel disease, PCI with stenting of the culprit lesion is the first choice. In patients with multivessel disease the decision for PCI or CABG must be made individually. A sequential approach with treating the culprit lesion by PCI followed by elective CABG may in some patients be advantageous. In other patients a staged PCI procedure may be considered.

Outcome after PCI in NSTE-ACS has been markedly improved with the use of intracoronary stenting and contemporary antithrombotic and antiplatelet therapy. Closure devices and the radial approach may be considered to reduce the risk of bleeding complications. However, a femoral approach is preferred in hemodynamically compromised patients to permit the use of intra-aortic balloon counterpulsation. As for all patients undergoing PCI, stent implantation in this setting helps to reduce the threat of abrupt closure and restenosis. The safety and efficacy of drug-eluting stents has not been prospectively tested in the ACS population, although patients with NSTE-ACS represent up to 50% of patients included in most PCI trials.

Currently there is no outcome data supporting PCI in non-significant culprit or non-culprit coronary obstructions on angiography ("plaque sealing") [25]. Non-significant culprit lesions presenting features of plaque rupture (e.g. haziness, irregular borders, dissections) may justify a mechanical intervention only exceptionally.

Adjunctive Pharmacological Treatment

The appropriate adjunctive treatment in patients undergoing PCI is covered in separate chapters. The anticoagulant and antiplatelet treatment for NSTEMI-ACS patients is therefore here only summarized. PCI in patients with NSTEMI-ACS

must be performed under effective anticoagulant and antithrombotic treatment to avoid thrombotic complications in this active state of disease [10].

In ACS unfractionated heparin, enoxaparin, fondaparinux, bivalirudin are available as anticoagulants. The anticoagulant should be selected according to the risk of both ischemic and bleeding risks as well as the initial strategy. Bivalirudin and fondaparinux have been shown to reduce the risk of bleeding [26,27]. In an urgent invasive strategy (<120 min) unfractionated heparin, enoxaparin or bivalirudin should be immediately started. At PCI procedures the initial anticoagulant should be maintained also during the procedure regardless whether this treatment is unfractionated heparin, enoxaparin or bivalirudin, while addititional unfractionated heparin in standard dose (50–100 IU/kg bolus) is necessary in case of fondaparinux to avoid catheter thombus formation. Anticoagulation may be stopped within 24 hours after the invasive procedure.

Dual antiplatelet treatment with aspirin and clopidogrel is recommended for all patients presenting with ACS. In patients considered for an invasive procedure/PCI, a loading dose of 600 mg of clopidogrel may be used to achieve more rapid (~2 hours) and more potent inhibition of platelet function. In patients at intermediate to high risk, particularly patients with elevated troponins, ST-depression, or diabetes, either eptifibatide or tirofiban for initial upstream treatment is recommended in addition to oral antiplatelet agents ("triple antiplatelet therapy"). Patients who received initial treatment with eptifibatide or tirofiban prior to angiography, should be maintained on the same drug during and after PCI. In high risk patients not pretreated with GP IIb/IIIa inhibitors and proceeding to PCI, abciximab is recommended immediately following angiography. The use of eptifibatide or tirofiban in this setting is less well established. Bivalirudin may be used as an alternative to GP IIb/IIIa inhibitors plus heparins.

Strategy Recommended by Guidelines (Figure 15.4)

According to the recent ESC Guidelines on NSTE-ACS [10], the need for and timing of angiography

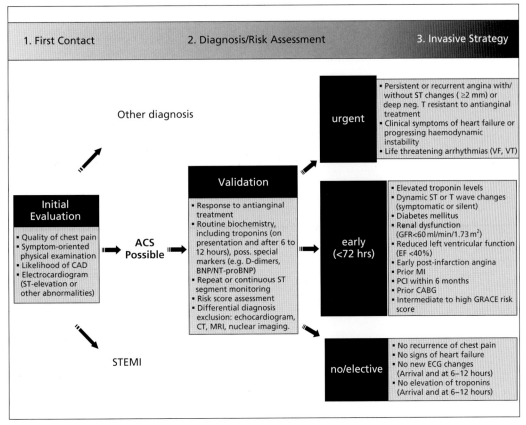

Figure 15.4. Decision making algorithm for the management of patients with NSTE-ACS [2]. Reprinted with permission from J Am Coll Cardiol 1998; 32: 596–605.

has to be tailored into three categories: urgent invasive, early invasive, or conservative.

Urgent Invasive Strategy

This is advised for patients who are early in the process of developing major myocardial necrosis escaping the ECG (e.g. occlusion of the circumflex artery) or are estimated to be at high risk of rapid progression to vessel occlusion. These patients are characterized by:

- Refractory angina (e.g. evolving infarction without ST abnormalties)
- Recurrent angina despite intense antianginal treatment associated with ST depression (≥2 mm) or deep negative T waves
- Clinical symptoms of heart failure or haemodynamic instability ("shock")

- Life threatening arrhythmias (ventricular fibrillation or ventricular tachycardia).

Coronary angiography should be planned as soon as possible in such patients who represent 2% to 15% of the patients admitted with NSTE-ACS [28–30].

Early Invasive Strategy

Some patients initially respond to the anti-anginal treatment, but are at increased risk and need early angiography. The timing depends on the local circumstances, but it should be performed within 72 hours. The decision about the timing of catheterization must continuously be re-evaluated and modified according to clinical evolution and occurrence of new clinical findings.

The following features indicate patients that should undergo routine early angiography:

- Elevated troponin levels
- Dynamic ST or T wave changes (symptomatic or silent) (≥0.5 mm)
- Diabetes mellitus
- Reduced renal function (GFR < 60 ml/min/ 1.73 m^2)
- Depressed LVEF < 40%
- Early post infarction angina
- PCI within six months
- Prior CABG
- Intermediate to high risk according to a GRACE risk score.

A GP IIb/IIIa inhibitor (tirofiban, eptifibatide) should be added to the standard treatment prior to catheterization in case of elevated troponins, dynamic ST/T changes, or diabetes provided there is no overt excessive bleeding risk.

Conservative Strategy

Patients that fulfill all the following criteria may be regarded as low risk and should not be submitted to early invasive evaluation:

- No recurrence of chest pain
- No signs of heart failure
- No abnormalities in the initial ECG or a second ECG (6–12 hours)
- No elevation of troponins (arrival and at 6–12 hours).

Low risk as assessed by a risk score can support the decision making process for a conservative strategy. The further management in these patients is according to the evaluation of stable CAD [31]. Before discharge a stress test for inducible ischemia is useful for further decision making.

Questions

1. A 58 year old woman is seen by you in the ER with 5 days of intermittent fatigue, nausea and dyspnea. Risk factors include hypertension, hyperlipidemia and a positive family history (mother died suddenly at age 55). Initial EKG and troponin are negative. In the ER she develops another episode of severe SOB and her EKG show new non-specific T wave abnormalities. Physical exam is normal. Her BP increased to 150/85 with the episode of SOB. How would you manage her?

   A D/C home with follow-up in pulmonary clinic

   B Admit to the CP unit with repeat ECG and troponin in 6 hours

   C Admit to the hospital for observation

   D Admit for urgent cardiac catheterization

2. A 66 year old man is admitted with typical angina and anterior ST depression. He was on no medication prior to admission. Initial troponin is elevated. He is given NTG, ASA, clopidogrel, heparin, abciximab and metoprolol with a fall in his BP from 165/100 to 130/80, relief of symptoms and normalization of his ECG. He is taken the cath lab and he is found to have an EF of 40%, a 75% hazy stenosis of the LAD, and total occlusions of the mid RCA and distal circumflex. How would you manage this patient?

   A Immediate PCI of the LAD only

   B Immediate PCI of the LAD and attempted PCI of RCA and Circ

   C Urgent CABG

   D Emergency CABG

3. Which of the following is true about troponin elevation in unstable angina?

   A Elevations occur in about 30% to 50% of patients with rest pain

   B Troponin release suggests embolization of thrombus distally

   C Troponin release worsens prognosis

   D All of the above

   E None of the above

4. What is the most appropriate therapy for a 68-year-old diabetic male who presents with 40 minutes of persistent severe chest pain, ST depression and a positive troponin?

   A Cool off with a GPIIb/IIIa inhibitor and stress after stabilization

   B Coronary angiography urgently and use abciximab if PCI is performed

   C Half dose thrombolytics and IIb/IIIa inhibitors

   D All are appropriate

   E None are appropriate

References

1. Mehta SR, Cannon CP, Fox KA, *et al.* Routine vs. selective invasive strategies in patients with acute coronary syndromes: a collaborative meta-analysis of randomized trials. JAMA 2005; **293**: 2908–2917.

2. Bavry AA, Kumbhani DJ, Rassi AN, *et al.* Benefit of early invasive therapy in acute coronary syndromes: a meta-analysis of contemporary randomized clinical trials. J Am Coll Cardiol 2006; **48**: 117–1325.

3. Hoenig MR, Doust JA, Aroney CN, *et al.* Early invasive versus conservative strategies for unstable angina & non-ST-elevation myocardial infarction in the stent era. Cochrane Database Syst Rev 2006; **3**: CD004815.

4. Fox KA, Poole-Wilson P, Clayton TC, *et al.* Five-year outcome of an interventional strategy in non-ST-elevation acute coronary syndrome: the British Heart Foundation RITA 3 randomized trial. Lancet 2005; **366**: 914–920.

5. Lagerqvist B, Husted S, Kontny F, *et al.* Five-year outcomes in the FRISC-II randomized trial of an invasive versus a non-invasive strategy in non-ST-elevation acute coronary syndrome: a follow-up study. Lancet 2006; **368**: 998–1004.

6. Lagerqvist B, Husted S, Kontny F, *et al.* A long-term perspective on the protective effects of an early invasive strategy in unstable coronary artery disease: two-year follow-up of the FRISC-II invasive study. J Am Coll Cardiol 2002; **40**: 1902–1914.

7. TIMI IIIB Investigators. Effects of tissue plasminogen activator and a comparison of early invasive and conservative strategies in unstable angina and non-Q-wave myocardial infarction. Results of the TIMI IIIB Trial. Thrombolysis in Myocardial Ischemia. Circulation 1994; **89**: 1545–1556.

8. Boden WE, O'Rourke RA, Crawford MH, *et al.* Outcomes in patients with acute non-Q-wave myocardial infarction randomly assigned to an invasive as compared with a conservative management strategy. Veterans Affairs Non-Q-Wave Infarction Strategies in Hospital (VANQWISH) Trial Investigators. N Engl J Med 1998; **338**: 1785–1792.

9. McCullough PA, O'Neill WW, Graham M, *et al.* A prospective randomized trial of triage angiography in acute

coronary syndromes ineligible for thrombolytic therapy. Results of the medicine versus angiography in thrombolytic exclusion (MATE) trial. J Am Coll Cardiol 1998; **32**: 596–605.

10. Bassand JP, Hamm CW, Ardissino D, et al.., for the Task Force for the Diagnosis and Treatment of Non-ST-Segment Elevation Acute Coronary Syndromes of the European Society of Cardiology: Guidelines for the diagnosis and treatment of non-ST-segment elevation acucte coronary syndromes. Eur Heart J 2007; **28**: 1598–1660.

11. Diderholm E, Andren B, Frostfeldt G, et al. The prognostic and therapeutic implications of increased troponin T levels and ST depression in unstable coronary artery disease: the FRISC II invasive troponin T electrocardiogram substudy. Am Heart J 2002; **143**: 760–767.

12. de Winter RJ, Windhausen F, Cornel JH, et al. Early invasive versus selectively invasive management for acute coronary syndromes. N Engl J Med 2005; **353**: 1095–1104.

13. Hirsch A, Windhausen F, Tijssen JG, et al. Long-term outcome after an early invasive versus selective invasive treatment strategy in patients with non-ST-elevation acute coronary syndrome and elevated cardiac troponin T (the ICTUS trial): A follow-up study. Lancet 2007; **369**: 827–835.

14. Cannon CP. Revascularisation for everyone? Eur Heart J 2004; **25**: 1471–1472.

15. Cannon CP, Weintraub WS, Demopoulos LA, et al. Comparison of early invasive and conservative strategies in patients with unstable coronary syndromes treated with the glycoprotein IIb/IIIa inhibitor tirofiban. N Engl J Med 2001; **344**: 1879–257.

16. Neumann FJ, Kastrati A, Pogatsa-Murray G, et al. Evaluation of prolonged antithrombotic pretreatment ("cooling-off" strategy) before intervention in patients with unstable coronary syndromes: a randomized controlled trial. JAMA 2003; **290**: 1593–1599.

17. Fox KA, Anderson FA, Dabbous OH, et al. Intervention in acute coronary syndromes: Do patients undergo intervention on the basis of their risk characteristics? The global registry of acute coronary events (GRACE). Heart 2007; **93**: 177–182.

18. Mehta RH, Roe MT, Chen AY, et al. Recent trends in the care of patients with non-ST-segment elevation acute coronary syndromes: insights from the CRUSADE initiative. Arch Intern Med 2006; **166**: 2027–2034.

19. Van de Werf F, Gore JM, Avezum A, et al. Access to catheterisation facilities in patients admitted with acute coronary syndrome: multinational registry study. BMJ 2005; **330**: 441.

20. Mehta SR, Granger CB, Boden WE, et al. TIMACS Investigators. Early versus delayed invasive intervention in acute coronary syndromes. N Engl J Med. 2009; **360**: 2165–75.

21. Montalescot G, Cayla G, Collet JP, et al. ABOARD Investigators. Immediate vs delayed intervention for acute coronary syndromes: a randomized clinical trial. JAMA. 2009; **302**: 947–54.

22. Avanzas P, Arroyo-Espliguero R, Cosin-Sales J, et al. Markers of inflammation and multiple complex stenoses (pancoronary plaque vulnerability) in patients with non-ST segment elevation acute coronary syndromes. Heart 2004; **90**: 847–852.

23. Lenzen MJ, Boersma E, Bertrand ME, et al. Management and outcome of patients with established coronary artery disease: the Euro Heart Survey on coronary revascularization. Eur Heart J 2005; **26**: 1169–1179.

24. FRISC II Investigators. Invasive compared with non-invasive treatment in unstable coronary-artery disease: FRISC II prospective randomised multicentre study. FRagmin and Fast Revascularisation during InStability in Coronary artery disease Investigators. Lancet 1999; **354**: 708–715.

25. Mercado N, Maier W, Boersma E, et al. Clinical and angiographic outcome of patients with mild coronary lesions treated with balloon angioplasty or coronary stenting. Implications for mechanical plaque sealing. Eur Heart J 2003; **24**: 541–551.

26. Yusuf S, Mehta SR, Chrolavicius S, et al. Efficacy and Safety of Fondaparinux compared to Enoxaparin in 20,078 patients with acute coronary syndromes without ST segment elevation. The OASIS (Organization to Assess Strategies in Acute Ischemic Syndromes)-5 Investigators. N Engl J Med 2006; **354**: 1464–1476.

27. Stone GW, McLaurin BT, Cox DA, et al. Bivalirudin for patients with acute coronary syndromes. N Engl J Med 2006; **355**: 2203–2216.

28. Al-Khatib SM, Granger CB, Huang Y, et al. Sustained ventricular arrhythmias among patients with acute coronary syndromes with no ST-segment elevation: incidence, predictors, and outcomes. Circulation 2002; **106**: 309–312.

29. Srichai MB, Jaber WA, Prior DL, et al. Evaluating the benefits of glycoprotein IIb/IIIa inhibitors in heart failure at baseline in acute coronary syndromes. Am Heart J 2004; **147**: 84–90.

30. Yan AT, Yan RT, Tan M, et al. ST-segment depression in non-ST elevation acute coronary syndromes: quantitative analysis may not provide incremental prognostic value beyond comprehensive risk stratification. Am Heart J 2006; **152**: 270–276.

31. Fox K, Garcia MA, Ardissino D, et al. Guidelines on the management of stable angina pectoris: executive summary: The Task Force on the Management of Stable Angina Pectoris of the European Society of Cardiology. Eur Heart J 2006; **27**: 1341–1381.

Answer

1. B
2. C
3. D
4. Answer B. Thrombolytics are contraindicated in USA. This patient has several high risk features: DM, male >65 yrs old, +troponin, rest pain, and ST depression. Early invasive strategy with abciximab if PCI performed is the correct management.

CHAPTER 16

Primary and Rescue PCI in Acute Myocardial Infarction

Neil Swanson[1], & Anthony Gershlick[2]

[1] James Cook University Hospital, Middlesbrough, UK

[2] Glenfield Hospital, Leicester, UK

Introduction

Acute myocardial infarction (AMI) remains a common and life-threatening event. Case fatality rates in patients after AMI are poor (up to 45% in some series), mainly due to death before reaching hospital [1,2,3]. Real-world registries of those reaching hospital show one-year survival rates of around 20%, considerably worse than the cohorts recruited to randomized control trials [4,5].

The underlying pathology is the abrupt occlusion of a coronary artery caused by plaque rupture and consequent thrombus formation. Treatment for this catastrophic event is primarily aimed at the restoration of flow to the infarct-related artery. It is assumed that restoration of flow reduces adverse outcomes—the so-called open artery hypothesis [6]. Long-term survival does correlate with the presence of an open artery. Post-infarct patients with TIMI grade 0/1 early had a 12-year survival of 54%; those with TIMI 3 flow, 72% [7].

Prompt thrombolysis achieves reperfusion in 50–60% of patients (compared to 15% spontaneously reperfusing) [8]. Since PCI achieves patency rates of around 95% [9], there is an obvious hypothetical benefit to PCI over thrombolysis.

Interventional Cardiology, First Edition. Edited by Carlo Di Mario, George D. Dangas, Peter Barlis.
© 2010 Blackwell Publishing Ltd. Published 2010 by Blackwell Publishing Ltd.

Primary Angioplasty in Acute Myocardial Infarction (PAMI)

Primary angioplasty in acute myocardial infarction (PAMI) or primary PCI (PPCI) are terms for the use of balloon angioplasty (usually with stent) to open a blocked coronary artery in acute myocardial infarction, *instead* of thrombolysis.

A series of trials comparing prompt thrombolysis with coronary angioplasty and/or stenting have shown PPCI to be superior to thrombolysis [10,11,12,13,14]. Meta-analysis of 23 such trials (n = 7739 patients) [15] has confirmed the benefits of PPCI over thrombolysis, if performed quickly, reducing the combined end point at 30 days (8% vs. 14%), 30 day mortality (7% vs. 9%), re-infarction (3% vs. 7%) and stroke (1% vs. 2%). Hospital stay is also reduced [16].

These benefits appear durable, with data out to five years showing sustained benefit and five year survival rates around 80% [17,18,19]. Over longer term, mortality rates (at least for anterior MIs) continue to diverge, perhaps due to better preservation of LV function [18]. Costs of PPCI appear similar to thrombolysis [20].

Time Considerations in PPCI

The main apparent weakness of a PCI approach in comparison to thrombolysis is the relative complexity of the process, requiring a multiskilled team at all hours and a well-equipped catheterization lab, which may be remote from the patient.

Bringing a patient to cath lab, often out of normal working hours, leads to inevitable delay compared to thrombolysis. These delays are usually defined as the door-to-balloon time (D2B) time—the time from hospital arrival to establishment of reperfusion by angioplasty balloon inflation and the door to needle time. Time of *administration* of thrombolysis does not of course equate to time of *reperfusion* with thrombolysis, which may take much longer to occur.

It would seem intuitive that excessive delay in D2B time may reduce the efficacy of PCI, even to the point where it becomes less effective than speedy thrombolysis.

This appears borne out in most (but not all [21]) of the trial literature—the longer the door to balloon time (although interestingly, not the *symptom onset* to balloon time [22]), the higher the mortality rate becomes [23,24,25] (see Figure 16.1). In an analysis of published trials between 1993 and 2003, delays are evident in the delivery of reperfusion, with little sign of improvement over 10 years (see Figure 16.2). Median door to needle times were 65 min, door-to-balloon times 81 min [26]. In the USA, delay, especially for patients requiring inter-hospital transfer for PCI [27], has been far longer than recommended in guidelines. Such transfer-related delay can be overcome with effective development of a network of services. Randomized trials of transfer where effective transfer networks exist still show a superiority of PPCI over thrombolysis in the initial hospital [13,28].

Current guidelines [29] recommend that the delay to performing PPCI is no longer than 90 minutes, although this may be a fairly crude cutoff time. Analysis of the 192,500 patient NRMI registry of acute MI showed that the maximum delay before the benefit of PPCI over thrombolysis might be lost varied greatly according to clinical factors. These factors included age, the time taken to presentation and the infarct territory [30].

How the admission process for PPCI can be accelerated has been studied [31] by the D2B Alliance. This is an association of professionals interested in improving D2B times in the USA, including the American Heart Association, health insurers, emergency physicians and cardiologists. They studied 28 strategies used by various large hospitals using primary angioplasty to treat STEMI. Six were associated with significantly reduced D2B times (see Table 16.1).

Whilst it seems logical to accelerate D2B times, data exist to suggest that PPCI is superior to thrombolysis *despite* delays. Analysis of 25 randomized control trials comparing lytic therapy with PPCI [23] has suggested that even with PPCI-related delay relative to thrombolysis of up to two hours, there was a consistent mortality benefit to an invasive strategy. Data beyond this delay point are lacking in the randomized trials. The RIKS-HIA Swedish database [16] has shown benefit to PPCI even if the procedure-related delay is many hours.

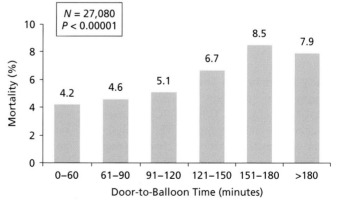

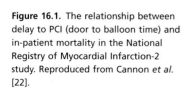

Figure 16.1. The relationship between delay to PCI (door to balloon time) and in-patient mortality in the National Registry of Myocardial Infarction-2 study. Reproduced from Cannon *et al.* [22].

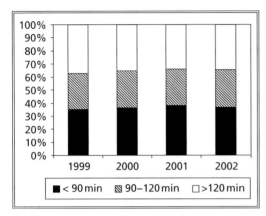

Figure 16.2. Real-world (US NRMI registry) reperfusion times: Proportion patients (%) receiving PPCI within ACC/AHA recommended times. Only 35% Achieve Door To Balloon <90 minutes. Reproduced from McNamara RL, Herrin J, Bradley EH, *et al.* Hospital Improvement in Time to Reperfusion in Patients With Acute Myocardial Infarction, 1999 to 2002. J Am Coll Cardiol 2006; **47**(1): 45–51.

Table 16.1. Strategies found to be associated with shorter door-to-balloon (D2B) times.

Strategy	Mean reduction in D2B (min)
ED activates the cath lab while patient still *en route*	19.3
ED physicians activates the cath lab	8.2
Single call to a central page operator activate cath lab	13.8
Expecting cath lab staff to arrive <20 minutes after page	19.3
Attending cardiologist always on site	14.6
Having staff use and receive real-time feedback	8.6

ED = Emergency Department. Adapted from Bradley *et al.* [31].

Early Reperfusion Therapy

Retrospective subgroup analyses from the PRAGUE-2 [13] and CAPTIM (Comparison of Angioplasty and Prehospital Thrombolysis In acute Myocardial infarction) [32] studies suggest no improvement in outcome with PPCI over lysis within the first 2–3 hours of symptom onset. CAPTIM found that patients thrombolysed within

two hours were less likely to develop cardiogenic shock (1.3% vs. 5.3%, p = 0.032) and had a trend toward improved mortality at 30 days compared to PPCI (2.2% vs. 5.7%, p = 0.058).

If there are benefits to very early thrombolysis, it may be logical to provide that thrombolysis at the earliest opportunity, pre-hospital. CAPTIM is the largest study (884 patients) to compare this strategy to PPCI. The rate of the primary endpoint was not significantly different (8.2% with lysis and 6.2% with PPCI, risk difference 1.96, 95% CI -1.53 to 5.46). Rescue angioplasty was done in 26% of the fibrinolysis patients [33]. The smaller (304 patient) WEST study (Which Early ST-elevation myocardial infarction Therapy) [34] recruited high-risk patients within 6h of symptom onset, emphasizing pre-hospital treatment and randomized to one of three groups: tenecteplase, tenecteplase and mandatory invasive study 24h, including rescue PCI for reperfusion failure, and PPCI. The primary composite outcome at 30 days were equal (around 25%). Lysis alone fared worse in terms of death and recurrent MI compared to PPCI (13.0 vs. 4.0%, respectively, P-logrank = 0.021), but not when supported by liberal, early use of angiography and/or rescue PCI (difference 6.7% vs.4.0%, P-logrank = 0.378).

Late Perfusion Therapies

Patients presenting 12 hours or more after symptom onset have generally a poor response to lysis (presumably because of organization of clot). Several trials have examined the effect of PCI at various late time points after the initial MI.

The Bavarian Reperfusion Alternatives Evaluation (BRAVE)-2 investigators randomized 365 patients with STEMI (12–48 hours from symptom onset) to PCI with abciximab vs. conservative care [8]. Infarct size measured by sestamibi was smaller in the invasive group (8% vs. 13%, p < 0.001). Differences in clinical endpoints did not however reach statistical significance.

The SWISS-II trial suggested that, in the presence of significant silent ischemia, revascularization by PCI of the IRA, distant from the initial event, reduced adverse event rates ten years on [35]. This was a small (201 patient) trial with much less aggressive medical therapy than in contemporary trials such as COURAGE [36].

Re-opening of occluded infarct-related arteries distant from the initial MI in the *absence* of ongoing ischemia has not been shown to have any meaningful clinical benefit [37,38,39,40], despite the appeal of the open artery hypothesis.

Selecting Patients for Primary PCI

Although there appears to be a consistent overall benefit of PPCI over thrombolysis, the benefit is heterogeneous amongst subgroups. The benefit of PPCI is not absolute, but relates to the relative speed with which the two different strategies can be performed.

Patient characteristics are important in determining the relative benefit (or harm) of PPCI compared to lysis. Certain patient groups appear to benefit strongly from PPCI over thrombolysis—those in cardiogenic shock [41], anterior MIs [18], diabetics [42] or those presenting later [16].

Conversely, mortality benefits have been lacking in clinical trials in other groups. The Senior Primary Angioplasty in Myocardial Infarction trial [43] randomized 483 elderly (>70 years old) patients to PPCI or thrombolytic. The primary end point (death or disabling stroke at 30 days) was 11.3% and 13.0% (p = NS) in the PCI and thrombolytic arms, respectively, and the secondary endpoint (death, re-infarction or disabling stroke) was 11.6% and 18% (p < 0.05). Benefit was seen with PPCI in patients aged 70–80 (37% reduction in death, 55% reduction in death, myocardial infarction, or stroke [p < 0.001]). However, among patients >80, no benefit was seen with PPCI and both arms had very high adverse event rates.

Attempts have been made to score patients on admission to determine the likely mortality benefit from PPCI relative to lysis [44]. Simple risk assessment, based on the TIMI criteria, can be done quickly on admission to identify the patients likely to benefit from PPCI—mainly those with hemodynamic upset or pulmonary congestion. Patients without such findings (74% of the study population in the DANAMI-2 trial) constitute a lower-risk group in whom no benefit in mortality or composite endpoints was demonstrated with PPCI over thrombolysis.

Since there appear to be subgroups who benefit less (or not at all) from PPCI vs. thrombolysis, it may seem reasonable to adopt a selective policy for PPCI. This might target the higher-risk patients with most to gain from PPCI (approximately 25% of admissions in the DANAMI-2 cohort) and give thrombolysis (with possible rescue PCI as required) to the remainder.

Techniques to Improve Outcome in PPCI

The main drawbacks of PPCI are poor perfusion following vessel reopening (the no-reflow phenomenon), bleeding complications consequent to adjunctive therapy and stent (or balloon) restenosis and thrombosis, as in other areas of PCI practice. Other complications include vascular access site complications (reduced by radial PCI) and contrast nephropathy or reaction [20].

Stents

Initial experience with PPCI was in the pre-stent era. Early experience with stents was not promising [45]. Despite decreased restenosis and re-infarction, a trend was seen to *increased* mortality, associated with worse TIMI3 flow rates (i.e. more no-reflow) than with PTCA alone [12]. Subsequent trials (see Figure 16.3) have confirmed benefit in favor of routine stenting, in terms of reduced restenosis and re-infarction [9,46].

The routine use of stenting in PPCI has been analysed in a meta-analysis of nine trials by the Cochrane group [47]. They found no mortality benefit (indeed a non-significant increase in mortality was observed) with stent use, but confirmed a benefit in terms of reduced risk of re-infarction (OR 0.67, 95% CI 0.45 to 0.98) or target vessel revascularization (OR 0.47, 95% CI 0.38 to 0.57) at one year. Similar results have been found in a more recent meta-analysis [48].

Routine stenting is recommended in European guidelines, with a class 1A evidence [49].

Drug Eluting Stents

The TYPHOON (Trial to Assess the Use of the Cypher Stent in Acute Myocardial Infarction Treated with Balloon Angioplasty) (50) reported reduced (7.3% vs. 14.3%, p < 0.01) target vessel failure in the sirolimus eluting stent (SES) group at one year. By comparison, the PASSION

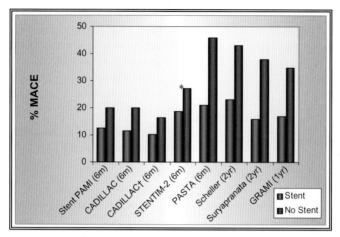

Figure 16.3. MACE rates with the routine use of stents vs. balloon angioplasty in primary PCI trials. All differences statistically significant except * p = NS. Reduced MACE rates were due to reduced revascularization and re-infarction. No improvements in mortality have been demonstrated. Note differing lengths of follow-up in the quoted trials. Trial references (numbers of stented patients enrolled): STENT-PAMI [12] (452); CADILLAC [9] (512); CADILLACt(with abciximab) (524); STENTIM-2, Maillard et al., J Am Coll Cardiol 2000; **35**(7): 1729–1736 (124); PASTA, Saito et al., Catheter Cardiovasc Interv **48**(3): 262–268 (67); Scheller et al., Am J Med 2001; **101**(1): 1–6 (127); Suryapranata et al., Heart 2001; **85**(6): 667–671 (112); GRAMI, Rodriguez et al., Am J Cardiol 1998; **81**(11): 1286–1291 (130).

(Paclitaxel-Eluting Stent versus Conventional Stent for STEMI) study [51] of the paclitaxel eluting stent (PES) failed to demonstrate superiority over bare metal stents (BMS).

The STRATEGY (High-dose Bolus Tirofiban and Sirolimus-Eluting Stent vs. Abciximab and Bare Metal Stent in AMI) study randomized 175 AMI patients to receive SES plus tirofiban or BMS plus abciximab [52]. MACE rates with SES plus tirofiban at eight months showed a significant reduction (19% vs. 50%), entirely due to a reduced need for revascularization. In the SESAMI trial (Sirolimus Eluting Stenting in Acute Myocardial Infarction) [53] of 320 patients the SES group had lower MACE (6.8% vs. 16.8%; p = 0.005), driven by revascularization rates than BMS. In the e-CYPHER registry, SES use in MI had MACE rate of 5.3% at 180 days [54]. In the RESEARCH registry PPCI with SES in 186 consecutive patients and compared to historical controls. At 300 days, MACE rates were 9.4% (SES) vs. 17% (controls) [55].

The longer-term risks of DES in PPCI are unclear, although use in PPCI is a risk factor for DES stent thrombosis [56]. This may relate to the presence of acute thrombus, delayed healing of the vessel or polymer-related inflammation, which may all predispose to later stent thrombosis [57].

In summary, DES may lead to lower MACE rates after PPCI compared to BMS, mainly due to a lower need for further revascularization, rather than death. Late stent thrombosis may be more likely in this setting than in stable angina.

Adjunctive devices

The large thrombus load often seen in STEMI patients is partly responsible for the no-reflow phenomenon and consequent impairment of myocardial function. Removal of this thrombus might therefore be beneficial. Trials of devices to achieve this have had mixed, often disappointing results. Distal protection (filter) devices appear ineffective [58,59], thrombectomy devices have had mixed results—negative or harmful in some cases [60,61], of benefit (in surrogate endpoints) in others [62,63,64]. Meta-analysis of 18 such trials found wide variations in efficacy, with an overall trend in favour of their use. No benefits in hard endpoints were demonstrated [65].

Adjunctive Pharmacotherapy

Glycoprotein GIIb/IIIa inhibitors (GPI), most commonly abciximab, are often given during or prior to PCI in acute MI. This is discussed in detail later in this chapter in the context of "facilitated" PCI.

Pre-hospital i.v. enoxaparin in a small registry gave a 40% TIMI 2/3 flow seen in the infarct-related vessel at subsequent PCI [66]. Nicorandil i.v. bolus pre-PCI lowers readmission rates with heart failure after MI (3.2% vs.10.9% compared to placebo, p < 0.01) in a 368 patient trial. Cardiovascular death rates were non-significantly reduced. [67]. The proposed mechanism of action is a combination of ischemic pre-conditioning and reduction in no-reflow due to improved microvascular flow.

Other factors to improve reperfusion or reduce reperfusion injury have generally been disappointing. Adenosine [68] and GIK (Glucose-insulin-potassium) [69,70] failed to show significant differences in the primary outcome measures. Stem cell therapy or the use of G-CSF (granulocyte-colony stimulating factor) has generally been disappointing in the context of AMI [71], although multiple studies are ongoing.

PCI for Non-culprit Vessels

In general, the trials of PCI in acute MI have treated only the infarct-related artery. Randomized data are scarce [72] and underpowered to advise on the wisdom or otherwise of tackling other significant lesions. One retrospective analysis of a US registry has suggested that better outcomes may be achieved with multivessel PCI than with treating the infarct vessel alone [73], another has strongly suggested not [74]. In the setting of cardiogenic shock, there is expert consensus that non-culprit vessels should be revascularized where possible [49]. Outside of this area, guidelines recommend *not* to intervene acutely on other lesions [75], preferring a more objective, ischemia-driven approach in the recovery period after the initial event.

Guidelines for the Use of PPCI

ESC and ACC/AHA guidelines for the management of STEMI have been updated in the most recent PCI guidelines [49,75]. European guidelines recommend PPCI over thrombolysis in patients presenting 3–12 hours after symptom onset (Class I C evidence). The main benefit justifying this advice was felt to be the reduction in stroke, as well as myocardial salvage. US Guidelines are less emphatic, saying only that PPCI is an "alternative" to lysis. Both guidelines emphasize the importance of speedy performance of PCI, by skilled teams in high volume centers.

Conclusions for PPCI

Primary PCI has been tested against thrombolysis in a wide range of clinical situations and been found to be superior in clinical trials and registries. The use of PPCI improves mortality, reduces re-infarction, stroke and hospital stay with sustained long-term benefits. These benefits vary according to numerous patient characteristics and are attenuated when delay to PCI is longer.

PPCI (when available) is appropriate for a wider range of patients than thrombolysis (i.e. those with late presentation or high bleeding risks).

A strategy of PPCI for all infarcts increases the proportion of infarct patients offered reperfusion, with superior long-term results compared to a selective strategy, pre-hospital or in-hospital thrombolysis, even when that PCI is delayed by many hours.

Evidence therefore supports the use of timely and expert PCI as the preferred revascularization option in acute STEMI.

Facilitated PCI (FPCI)

Facilitated PCI is the use of treatment—either thrombolytic, GPI or both—given at earliest possible moment after diagnosis of STEMI as a first step to be followed by urgent PCI. This concept overcomes, in principal, the unavoidable delay to PCI over lytic therapy. Such a strategy would enhance early patency in keeping with the open artery hypothesis (see Figure 16.4).

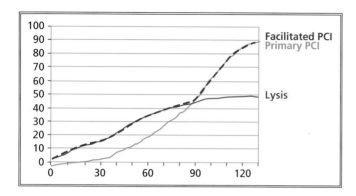

Figure 16.4. Principles of facilitated-PCI: Percentage likelihood of TIMI 3 flow is shown against time according to reperfusion strategy: Early reperfusion with lytic can be complemented with optimal patency and prevention of re-infarction with PCI. Reproduced from Gersh *et al.*, JAMA 2005; **293**(8): 979–986.

FPCI with Lytic Alone

Early studies of FPCI used lytics and suggested that infarct artery patency rates were higher in patients given thrombolysis in advance of cath lab arrival.

More recently, the ASSENT-4 study [76] randomized STEMI patients presenting <6 hours after symptoms to either PPCI (n = 838) or FPCI with full dose tenecteplase given 1–3 hours prior to PCI. The trial was stopped early because of higher in-hospital mortality in the facilitated arm compared to the PPCI group (6% vs. 3%, p = 0.0105). The primary composite end point at 90 days was 19% in the FPCI group vs. 13% in the PPCI group (p = 0.0045). There was also higher incidence of in-hospital stroke (1.8% vs. 0, p < 0.0001), re-infarction (6% vs. 4%, p = 0.0279) and revascularization (7% vs. 3%, p = 0.0041) in the FPCI arm.

FPCI with Lytic and GPI

Since the thrombus that forms after plaque rupture is platelet rich, the efficacy of thrombolysis might be improved with concurrent antiplatelet medication (on top of aspirin).

The SPEED pilot trial (n = 323) [77] examined outcomes when PCI was undertaken quickly after administration of lytic and GPI. An 86% incidence of TIMI grade 3 flow was seen at 90 min with a trend toward improved clinical outcomes (30-day MACE rate of 5.6%).

The FINESSE (Facilitated Intervention with Enhanced Reperfusion Speed to Stop Events) trial [78] was a 2452 patient multicenter, randomized trial, comparing three PCI reperfusion strategies: FPCI with combination half-dose lytic and abciximab vs. FPCI with upstream abciximab only vs. PPCI with adjunctive abciximab given at the time of PCI. Final results of FINESSE are awaited. Where half-dose lytic was given with abciximab, a poorer outcome was seen compared to primary PCI alone in terms of bleeding, without any clinical benefit.

GPI Alone

Routine, up-stream use of GPI (predominantly abciximab) has been studied in a number of key trials. Although aggressive clot dissolution may assist in PCI, the results have been mixed. Despite promising 30-day reductions in overall MACE rates [79] and improved left ventricular function [80] in patients treated with abciximab, sustained (one year) benefit to PCI with abciximab was non-significantly different, with excess bleeding risk [81].

The CADILLAC trial [9] reported an overall benefit to abciximab use, but this was only significant in the patients undergoing PTCA alone. In the stent group, ReoPro use gave no additional benefit (six-month MACE 11.5% with stent alone vs. 10.2% stent plus abciximab, p = ns).

Three metanalyses of PPCI trials using abciximab have been reported. de Luca *et al.* found that abciximab led to a significant reduction in short-term (30-day) (2.4% vs. 3.4%, p = 0.047) and long-term (6–12 months) mortality (4.4% vs. 6.2%, p = 0.01) compared to controls [82]. A second meta-analysis of up-stream GPI [83] showed improved outcomes if abciximab was given early, rather than at the time of PCI. Mortality was not significantly different, although re-infarction was reduced (5.5% vs. 2.3%, p = 0.013). Benefit was more striking in the diabetic subgroup. The most recent meta-analysis of outcomes to three years has shown that when abciximab is given in acute MI in *stented* patients [84], a borderline significant reduction in mortality is seen (14.3% vs. 10.9%, p = 0.052), with a significant reduction in re-infarction (5.5% vs. 2.3%, p = 0.013). Again, benefits were more marked in diabetics.

The most recent large trial using upstream abciximab routinely was FINESSE (as described above) [78]. As with the combined facilitation arm, abciximab alone led to no noticeable improvement in outcomes, with higher bleeding risks than with primary PCI alone.

Guidelines on the Use of FPCI

US guidelines [75] give FPCI a IIbB level of evidence, saying that it "might be performed as a reperfusion strategy in higher-risk patients when PCI is not immediately available." ESC guidelines [49] are more dismissive, saying, "there is no evidence to recommend facilitated PCI."

Conclusions of FPCI

A meta-analysis of 17 FPCI trials (lytic, GPI, or both) showed that although pre-PCI TIMI flows were improved with FPCI, post-PCI flow was the same. Adverse outcomes were higher in the FPCI arms (death 5% vs. 3%, p = 0.04, re-infarction 3% vs. 2%, p = 0.006, revascularization 4% vs. 1%, p = 0.01, stroke 1.1% vs. 0.3%, p = 0.0008, major bleeding 7% vs. 5%, p = 0.01). These increased event rates were seen in FPCI trials using lytics. Trials using GPI showed equivalent adverse rates to PPCI.

Overall, on the currently available evidence, there are clear indications of harm if PCI is facilitated with thrombolytic agents routinely pre-PCI. GPI use routinely has not been shown to have marked overall benefit, although in stented patients or diabetics, especially when used early (i.e. pre-hospital), they do appear beneficial.

Rescue PCI (RPCI)

Rescue PCI (RPCI) is the use of PCI in patients with AMI in whom primary treatment has been thrombolysis, which has been unsuccessful in achieving reperfusion.

The weight of evidence currently available supports the use of PPCI as the reperfusion therapy of choice in acute MI. In the developed world, registries have shown that PPCI rates have begun to overtake thrombolysis in cases where a reperfusion therapy was used [71,85,86]. However, thrombolysis remains an extremely common reperfusion technique worldwide. This seems likely to be the case for some time, because of resource limitations and difficulties reorganizing services to provide universal PPCI. Geographical constraints will continue to create situations where transfer is likely to be greatly delayed.

If thrombolysis is going to be widely used as first treatment for acute MI, but is only successful in restoring artery patency in 60% or so of patients, effective strategies are required for the remainder who "fail" lysis. Failed fibrinolysis approximately doubles the risk of in-hospital mortality [87].

Repeat fibrinolysis in such patients has not improved outcomes compared to conservative treatment in three randomized trials [24–26]. A meta-analysis of these studies [88] showed that further thrombolytic therapy failed to reduce the rates of all-cause mortality (Relative risk [RR] 0.68; 95% CI, 0.41 to 1.14; p = 0.14) or re-infarction (RR 1.79; 95% CI, 0.92–3.48; p = 0.09). RPCI has been found to maintain this mortality benefit through longer-term (median 4.4 years) follow up [89].

By contrast, successful RPCI restores outcomes to the level seen after successful thrombolysis [90].

Pathophysiology of Failed Fibrinolysis

High thrombin levels in certain individuals may promote a resistant fibrin architecture. Access of fibrinolytic to all parts of the formed clot may be impaired if there is total coronary occlusion or if there is coronary hypoperfusion due to cardiogenic shock. After four hours, fibrin cross-links mature and thrombus becomes organized, reducing the likelihood of effective thrombolysis [91]. Fibrinolytic agents have even been shown to induce a transient pro-coagulant effect by increasing thrombin activity [92].

Diagnosing Failed Fibrinolysis

Clinical markers of failed reperfusion are largely unhelpful [93]. *Complete* relief of chest pain is a guide to successful reperfusion [93–95] but may be affected by opiates, anxiety or subjective differences in pain appreciation. It occurs in a minority of patients [93], limiting its usefulness. Biochemical indices can predict poor vessel patency [96,97], but are not widely or rapidly available.

ST-resolution to detect reperfusion has the advantage of objectivity and ease of use. Differing degrees of ST-resolution (complete, >70%, partial, 30% to 70% or absent) have been correlated with reperfusion and outcome [98]. The optimal timing of when to assess the degree of ST resolution is unclear and varies in trials of RPCI.

Clinical Trials of Rescue PCI

Trials of RPCI have generally struggled to recruit patients, limiting the data in this field. However, multiple trials have now reported, sufficient to give some indication of likely benefits of RPCI.

Early RPCI trials used balloon angioplasty only. The Thrombolysis and Angioplasty in Myocardial Infarction [99] trial (575 patients) compared immediate coronary angiography, with RPCI in the event of lytic failure to delayed angiography +/− PCI after 5–10 days. Patients treated immediately showed a modest reduction in in-hospital adverse outcomes (67% vs. 55%, p = 0.004). RESCUE-1 and RESCUE-2 [100,101] both targeted patients with large (anterior) infarcts, randomizing those with angiographic failure of reperfusion to RPCI or conservative treatment. Both showed improvements in mortality and the development of heart failure.

In the "post-stent" era, the Middlesborough Early Revascularization to Limit Infarction (MERLIN) trial [102] randomized 307 patients (instead of the planned 3000, due to recruitment difficulties) with persistent >50% ST-elevation at 60 minutes post-fibrinolysis (90% with streptokinase) to RPCI or conservative management. There was no difference in all-cause mortality at 30 days [103], although the trial was under-powered to show mortality difference. There was a reduction in the composite secondary end-point at 30 days in the RPCI group (27.3% vs. 50%, p = 0.02), driven almost exclusively by revascularization. This benefit persisted at one year (43.1% vs. 57.8%, p = 0.01) (35). An increase in stroke (4.6% vs. 0.6%, p = 0.03) and transfusion, mainly due to groin complications (11.1% vs. 1.3%, p = 0.01) was seen following RPCI.

In the RPCI arm, only 66% actually had PCI. The remainder (who had a further 18.1% incidence of unplanned revascularization within one year) were included in the RPCI intention-to-treat analysis. Low rates of stent (50.3%) and GPI (3.3%) use may have increased adverse events in the RPCI group, while an early 60 minute time-point at which to declare lytic failure may have lowered mortality in the conservative-treatment arm.

Three meta-analyses of RPCI have been published. Wijeysundra *et al.* [88] analyzed data from six trials (908 patients) randomized to RPCI or conservative care. RPCI reduced re-infarction (RR 0.58; 95% CI 0.35 to 0.97; p = 0.04) and the development of heart failure (RR 0.73; 95% CI, 0.54 to 1.00; p = 0.05). There was a trend to reduced all-cause mortality (RR 0.69; 95% CI, 0.46 to 1.05; p = 0.09), but RPCI increased the risk of stroke (RR 4.98; 95% CI, 1.10 to 22.5; p = 0.04) and minor bleeding (RR 4.58; 95% CI, 2.46 to 8.55; p-0.001). Patel *et al.* [104] demonstrated a reduced risk of death (RR 0.64; 95% CI, 0.41 to 1.00; p = 0.048) with RPCI with a trends towards reduced risk of heart failure (RR 0.72; 95% CI,0.51 to 1.01; p = 0.06) and increased risk of thrombo-embolic stroke in the RPCI groups (RR 3.61; 95% CI, 0.91 to 14.27; p = 0.07). Collet *et al.* [105] found a borderline-significant reduction in mortality following RPCI (RR 0.63; 95% CI, 0.39 to 0.99; p = 0.055), and a reduction in the risk of death or re-infarction at 30 days (RR 0.60; 95% C,I 0.41 to 0.89; p = 0.012), with an increased risk of major (mostly sheath-related) non-fatal bleeding (see Figure 16.5).

Guidelines on Rescue PCI

ESC guidelines [49] support the (routine) use of RPCI, with a 1B level of evidence, US guidelines [75] are less supportive with a class C evidence when evidence of ongoing ischemia is present, and discouraging rescue in the absence of ischemia.

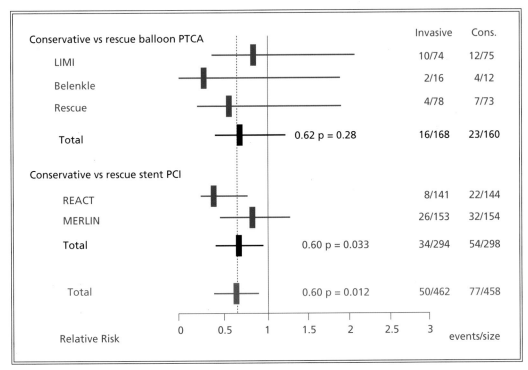

Figure 16.5. Metanalysis of 30-day outcomes following RPCI in 920 patients, Overall OR 0.60; 95% CI, 0.41–0.89. LIMI = Limburg Myocardial Infarction trial, Vermeer *et al.*, Heart 1999; **82**(4): 426–431; Belenkie *et al.*, Can J Cardiol 1992; **8**(4): 357–362; RESCUE [100]; REACT, Gershlick *et al.*, Heart 2002; **93**: Suppl I–A5; MERLIN [102]. Reproduced with permission from Collet *et al.* [105].

Rescue PCI Conclusions

The three meta-analyses, which were not adequately powered to detect significant mortality differences, give an impression of benefit in terms of reduced re-infarction and trends towards improved mortality and lower heart failure. This comes at the cost of an increase in non-fatal bleeding, and a possible increase in the rate of stroke, largely driven by the MERLIN RPCI cohort. Many of the patients in the meta-analysis were selected for their high-risk profile—i.e. anterior infarcts. These nuanced findings have led some to advocate the use of RPCI only in patients with large infarcts where the risks of mortality or heart failure are high [71] and clinical considerations on an individual patient basis are needed to weigh the potential risks and benefits of RPCI [106].

The balance of evidence would seem to favor RPCI in reducing adverse cardiac outcomes in patients with STEMI following failure of fibrino-lytic therapy (while repeat administration of lytic offers little or no clinical benefit).

Routine PCI After Thrombolysis

Going further than the issues surrounding "failed" thrombolysis, is the argument that *all* patients should undergo early angiography, irrespective of the outcome of thrombolysis.

SIAM-III (Southwest German Interventional Study in Acute Myocardial Infarction) [107] was a small (163 patient) study comparing immediate stenting after thrombolysis with delayed PCI at two weeks. Strong reductions in the composite end-points were seen in the immediate stenting group (25.6% vs. 50.6%, p = 0.001). CAPITAL AMI (Combined Angioplasty and Pharmacological Intervention versus thrombolysis Alone in Acute Myocardial Infarction) [108] was a small trial looking at high-risk patients (anterior MI, heart failure or hypotension). Tenecteplase plus immediate angioplasty was superior to tenecteplase alone. MACE rates at six months were lower for PCI (11.6% vs. 24.4%, p = 0.04), largely due to reductions in recurrent unstable ischemia and re-infarction. GRACIA-1 (Grupo de Analisis de la Cardiopatia Isquemica Aguda) [109] was the largest (500 patient) contemporary trial of routine PCI after thrombolysis. A trend towards reduced death/re-infarction (7% vs. 12%, p = 0.07) was seen at one year. When unplanned revasculariza-tion was included, the composite endpoint reached significance (9% vs. 21, p = 0.0008).

Recent meta-analysis [105] of trials comparing routine, early PCI after thrombolysis (irrespective of reperfusion status) showed, in recent "stent-era" trials, a trend towards reduced mortality at 30 days (OR 0.56, CI 0.29–1.05, p = 0.07). This benefit was not seen in earlier "balloon-era" trials, or when both groups of trials were analyzed together. A similar pattern was seen when death and re-infarction were measured together—the recent trials showed clear benefit (OR 0.53, CI 033–083, p = 0.0067), which was diluted when older trials were included.

Three recent randomized trials have convinc-ingly confirmed the advantage of early angioplasty. In The Combined Abciximab Reteplase Stent Study in Acute Myocardial Infarction (CARESS-in-AMI) multicentre trial (109), 600 patients aged <75 years with high risk STEMI admitted to a non PCI-hospital were randomly assigned to immedi-ate transfer for PCI (n = 299) or to standard treat-ment with rescue PCI if needed (n = 301). In all patients the fibrinolytic regimen was represented by half-dose reteplase (5 units bolus followed by another 5 units after 30 min) and abciximab (0.25 mg/kg bolus followed by 0.125 µg/kg/min over 12 h). Patients in the invasive arm underwent angiography after a median time of 135 min (inter-quartile range [IQR] 96-175). A total of 85.6% received PCI.

At 30 days patients in the invasive arm had a significantly lower rate of primary endpoint as compared to the conservative arm (4.4% vs.10.7%, HR 0.40 95%CI 0.21–0.76; log rang 0.004). No differences in terms of stroke or major bleeding were observed whilst patients undergoing immedi-ate PCI had higher rates of minor bleeding (occur-ring especially in the arterial access site) as compared to patients in the conservative group (10.8% vs. 4.0%; p = 0.002).

The Trial of Routine Angioplasty and Stenting After Fibrinolysis to Enhance Reperfusion in Acute Myocardial Infarction (TRANSFER-AMI) (110) is a multicentre trial designed to address the issue whether patients with STEMI treated by fibrinoly-sis should be transferred to undergo routine and early catheterization and PCI. Before randomiza-tion all patients were treated with Tenecteplase plus aspirin plus heparin or enoxaparin plus clopidrogel (bolus of 300 mg). A total of 1,030 patients were randomly assigned to either a phar-macoinvasive strategy of transfer for routine early PCI within 6 h after fibrinolysis (n = 508) or a conservative strategy with transfer for rescue PCI in case of FT or hemodynamic instability or for elective angiography/PCI after 24 h (n = 522). The interval between symptoms onset and fibrinolysis was similar in the two groups.

In the pharmacoinvasive arm 97% of patients underwent coronary angiography with a median time of 3 hours (IQR 2-4). PCI was performed in 84% of cases and glycoprotein IIb/IIIa inhibitor used in 73%. In the conservative arm 82% of patients underwent coronary angiography with a median time of 27 h (IQR 4-69). PCI was per-formed in 62% of cases and glycoprotein IIb/IIIa inhibitor used in 53%.

At 30 days patients in the pharmacoinvasive group had a significantly lower incidence of all the adverse events listed in the combined primary end-point (10.6% vs. 16.6% OR 0.537 95%CI 0.368–0.783, p = 0.0013) and a significantly lower incidence of each individual adverse except death and cardiogenic shock.

No significant differences were observed with reference to the rate of bleeding as evaluated by either TIMI or GUSTO scale.

The NORDISTEMI (NORwegian study on District treatment of ST-Elevation Myocardial Infarction) trial (111) randomized patients with acute (<6 hours) STEMI admitted to district general hospitals in an area of central-eastern Norway remote from primary angioplasty centres. Consequently, tenecteplase was administered to all patients, with half (132 pts) treated conservatively in the centre of initial admission and the remaining 134 immediately transported for an average of 158

Km to the nearest angioplasty centre. The primary endpoint of death, re-MI, recurrent ischemia and stroke at 12 months was not met (20.9% vs. 27.3%, p = 0.18) but the secondary endpoint of death, re-MI and stroke was in favour of an immediate transfer. No increase in bleeding was observed in the group of immediate transfer.

Guidelines for Routine PCI Post-thrombolysis

2005 recommendations from the ESC support a strategy of "lyse now, stent later," whereby all patients should be transferred for early angiography and PCI as appropriate, with an evidence level of 1A [49]. In marked contrast, US guidelines [75] support routine PCI after thrombolysis much less strongly, with a category C evidence level. The US guidelines do however support routine PCI where there is evidence of impaired LV function or symptomatic heart failure, as well as those with ongoing ischemia or hemodynamic instability post-lysis.

Conclusions for Routine PCI Post-thrombolysis

Guidelines differ on the importance of a routine strategy for early PCI after thrombolysis. There is consensus that it is beneficial in patients with ongoing ischemia, hemodynamic instability or extensive infarction. A blanket strategy of such intervention has not been shown to have a mortality benefit, only to reductions in repeat interventions and trends toward reduction in re-infarction.

Conclusions

Primary-PCI (as early as possible, by a skilled team) is the optimal treatment for STEMI, even when delays are long or transfer is required. A non-selective PPCI strategy is associated with the best results, even though subgroups of infarct patients appear to have little absolute benefit of PCI over thrombolysis. Up-stream GPI and stent use improve PPCI outcomes. Multivessel disease should probably best be staged, with objective testing for ischemia. Late (>24 hours) PCI to occluded vessels in the absence of objective ischemia is not beneficial.

If PPCI cannot be provided, early (ideally pre-hospital) lysis with rescue PCI for high-risk failed thrombolysis may approach the same outcomes.

Routine early PCI after *successful* thrombolysis is of marginal benefit.

Facilitated-PCI (with lytic) brings worse outcomes than PPCI, although combinations of GPI and lower dose lytics may prove beneficial in patients with potentially long delays to reperfusion.

Questions

1. **A 48 year old man presents with 6 hours of chest pain and anterior ST segment elevation. You perform an emergent coronary angiogram and find a 50% ostial LAD lesion and an occluded mid LAD. You successfully open and stent the mid LAD. Your colleague asks what the best strategy is regarding the ostial LAD? You tell him:**
   A You will measure FFR down the LAD and if <0.75–0.80, you will stent the ostial LAD lesion.
   B You will allow the patient to recover from his MI for at least a week and then either perform a stress imaging study or perform FFR.
   C You will IVUS the ostial LAD lesion and if the MLA is <6.0 mm2 you will stent the lesion.
   D You will stent the lesion because you are there and the risks for stenting intermediate lesions are low.

2. **Drug eluting stents vs. bare metal stents in STEMI have been shown to be associated with of the following?**
   A Improved short-term mortality
   B Increased sub-acute thrombosis rate
   C Increased distal embolization rates
   D Reduced TLR

3. **A 70 year old female with hypertension and DM presents to a local ER complaining of diaphoresis and dyspnea of 3 hour duration. Her exam is remarkable for BP 140/77, HR 86, clear lung fields, regular heart exam and appropriate pulses in her lower extremities. Admission EKG shows 2 mm ST segment elevation in the anterolateral leads. The hospital does not have PCI capabilities and the nearest catheterization laboratory is approximately 20 minutes away. She is given an aspirin, IV metoprolol, and morphine for analgesia. What is the best next step in her care?**
   A Administer full dose TNK, IV heparin, and transfer for immediate PCI
   B Administer ½ dose TNK, IV heparin, and eptifibatide and transfer for immediate PCI
   C Give IV heparin and transfer for immediate PCI

   D Give full dose abciximab and enoxaparin then reassess symptoms ST segments
   E Give IV heparin and eptifibitide alone as risk of transfer or thrombolytic therapy is high

References

1. Abildstrom SZ, Rasmussen S, Rosen M, *et al.* Trends in incidence and case fatality rates of acute myocardial infarction in Denmark and Sweden. Heart 2003; **89**(5): 507–511.
2. Gillum RF. Sudden coronary death in the United States: 1980–1985. Circulation 1989; **79**(4): 756–765.
3. Norris RM. Fatality outside hospital from acute coronary events in three British health districts, 1994–5. UK Heart Attack Study Collaborative Group. BMJ 1998; **316**(7137): 1065–1070.
4. Bjorklund E, Lindahl B, Stenestrand U, *et al.* Outcome of ST-elevation myocardial infarction treated with thrombolysis in the unselected population is vastly different from samples of eligible patients in a large-scale clinical trial. Am Heart J 2004; **148**(4): 566–573.
5. Mandelzweig L, Battler A, Boyko V, *et al.* The second Euro Heart Survey on acute coronary syndromes: Characteristics, treatment, and outcome of patients with ACS in Europe and the Mediterranean Basin in 2004. Eur Heart J 2006; **27**(19): 2285–2293.
6. Yousef ZR, Marber MS. The open artery hypothesis: Potential mechanisms of action. Prog Cardiovasc Dis 2000; **42**(6): 419–438.
7. French JK, Hyde TA, Patel H, *et al.* Survival 12 years after randomization to streptokinase: The influence of thrombolysis in myocardial infarction flow at three to four weeks. J Am Coll Cardiol 1999; **34**(1): 62–69.
8. Stone GW, Cox D, Garcia E, *et al.* Normal flow (TIMI-3) before mechanical reperfusion therapy is an independent determinant of survival in acute myocardial infarction: Analysis from the primary angioplasty in myocardial infarction trials. Circulation 2001; **104**(6): 636–641.
9. Stone GW, Grines CL, Cox DA, *et al.* Comparison of Angioplasty with Stenting, with or without Abciximab, in Acute Myocardial Infarction. N Engl J Med 2002; **346**(13): 957–966.
10. A clinical trial comparing primary coronary angioplasty with tissue plasminogen activator for acute myocardial infarction. The Global Use of Strategies to Open Occluded Coronary Arteries in Acute Coronary Syndromes (GUSTO IIb) Angioplasty Substudy Investigators. N Engl J Med 1997; **336**(23): 1621–1628.
11. Grines CL, Browne KF, Marco J, *et al.* A Comparison of Immediate Angioplasty with Thrombolytic Therapy

for Acute Myocardial Infarction. N Engl J Med 1993; **328**(10): 673–679.

12. Grines CL, Cox DA, Stone GW, *et al.* Coronary Angioplasty with or without Stent Implantation for Acute Myocardial Infarction. N Engl J Med 1999; **341**(26): 1949–1956.

13. Widimsky PF, Budesinsky TF, Vorac DF, *et al.* Long distance transport for primary angioplasty vs. immediate thrombolysis in acute myocardial infarction. Final results of the randomized national multicentre trial—PRAGUE-2 (0195-668X (Print)).

14. Zijlstra F, Hoorntje JCA, de Boer MJ, *et al.* Long-Term Benefit of Primary Angioplasty as Compared with Thrombolytic Therapy for Acute Myocardial Infarction. N Engl J Med 1999; **341**(19): 1413–1419.

15. Keeley EC, Boura JA, Grines CL. Primary angioplasty versus intravenous thrombolytic therapy for acute myocardial infarction: A quantitative review of 23 randomised trials. Lancet 2003; **361**(9351): 13–20.

16. Stenestrand U, Lindback J, Wallentin L. Long-term outcome of primary percutaneous coronary intervention vs prehospital and in-hospital thrombolysis for patients with ST-elevation myocardial infarction. JAMA 2006; **296**(14): 1749–1756.

17. Parodi G, Memisha G, Valenti R, *et al.* Five year outcome after primary coronary intervention for acute ST elevation myocardial infarction: results from a single centre experience. Heart 2005; **91**(12): 1541–1544.

18. Henriques JPS, Zijlstra F, van't Hof AWJ, *et al.* Primary percutaneous coronary intervention versus thrombolytic treatment: long term follow up according to infarct location. Heart 2006; **92**(1): 75–79.

19. Widimsky P, Bilkova D, Penicka M, *et al.* Long-term outcomes of patients with acute myocardial infarction presenting to hospitals without catheterization laboratory and randomized to immediate thrombolysis or interhospital transport for primary percutaneous coronary intervention. Five years' follow-up of the PRAGUE-2 Trial. Eur Heart J 2007; **28**(6): 679–684.

20. Keeley EC, Hillis LD. Primary PCI for myocardial infarction with ST-segment elevation. N Engl J Med 2007; **356**(1): 47–54.

21. De Luca G, Suryapranata H, Zijlstra F, *et al.* Symptom-onset-to-balloon time and mortality in patients with acute myocardial infarction treated by primary angioplasty. J Am Coll Cardiol 2003; **42**(6): 991–997.

22. Cannon CP, Gibson CM, Lambrew CT, *et al.* Relationship of Symptom-Onset-to-Balloon Time and Door-to-Balloon Time With Mortality in Patients Undergoing Angioplasty for Acute Myocardial Infarction. JAMA 2000; **283**(22): 2941–2947.

23. Boersma E. The Primary Coronary Angioplasty vs. Thrombolysis (PCAT). Does time matter? A pooled analysis of randomized clinical trials comparing primary percutaneous coronary intervention and in-hospital fibrinolysis in acute myocardial infarction patients. Eur Heart J 2006; **27**(7): 779–788.

24. Brodie BR, Stuckey TD, Wall TC, *et al.* Importance of time to reperfusion for 30-day and late survival and recovery of left ventricular function after primary angioplasty for acute myocardial infarction. J Am Coll Cardiol 1998; **32**(5): 1312–1319.

25. McNamara RL, Wang Y, Herrin J, *et al.* Effect of Door-to-Balloon Time on Mortality in Patients With ST-Segment Elevation Myocardial Infarction. J Am Coll Cardiol 6 A.D.; **47**(11): 2180–2186.

26. Barbagelata A, Perna ER, Clemmensen P, *et al.* Time to reperfusion in acute myocardial infarction. It is time to reduce it! J Electrocardiol 2007; **40**(3): 257–264.

27. Nallamothu BK, Bates ER, Herrin J, *et al.* Times to Treatment in Transfer Patients Undergoing Primary Percutaneous Coronary Intervention in the United States: National Registry of Myocardial Infarction (NRMI)-3/4 Analysis. Circulation 2005; **111**(6): 761–767.

28. Andersen HR, Nielsen TT, Rasmussen K, *et al.* A comparison of coronary angioplasty with fibrinolytic therapy in acute myocardial infarction. N Engl J Med 2003; **349**(8): 733–742.

29. Antman EM, Anbe DT, Armstrong PW, *et al.* ACC/AHA Guidelines for the Management of Patients With ST-Elevation Myocardial Infarction. Circulation 2004; **110**(9): e82–292.

30. Pinto DS, Kirtane AJ, Nallamothu BK, *et al.* Hospital Delays in Reperfusion for ST-Elevation Myocardial Infarction: Implications When Selecting a Reperfusion Strategy. Circulation 2006; **114**(19): 2019–2025.

31. Bradley EH, Herrin J, Wang Y, *et al.* Strategies for Reducing the Door-to-Balloon Time in Acute Myocardial Infarction. N Engl J Med 2006; NEJMsa063117.

32. Steg PG, Bonnefoy E, Chabaud S, *et al.* Impact of time to treatment on mortality after prehospital fibrinolysis or primary angioplasty: Data from the CAPTIM randomized clinical trial. Circulation 2003; **108**(23): 2851–2856.

33. Bonnefoy E, Lapostolle F, Leizorovicz A, *et al.* Primary angioplasty versus prehospital fibrinolysis in acute myocardial infarction: A randomised study. Lancet 2002; **360**(9336): 825–829.

34. Armstrong PW, WEST Steering Committee. A comparison of pharmacologic therapy with/without timely

coronary intervention vs. primary percutaneous intervention early after ST-elevation myocardial infarction: the WEST (Which Early ST-elevation myocardial infarction Therapy) study. Eur Heart J 2006; **27**(13): 1530–1538.

35. Erne P, Schoenenberger AW, Burckhardt D, *et al.* Effects of percutaneous coronary interventions in silent ischemia after myocardial infarction: the SWISSI II randomized controlled trial. JAMA 2007; **297**(18): 1985–1991.

36. Boden WE, O'Rourke RA, Teo KK, *et al.* Optimal medical therapy with or without PCI for stable coronary disease. N Engl J Med 2007; **356**(15): 1503–1516.

37. Steg PG, Thuaire C, Himbert D, *et al.* DECOPI (DEsobstruction COronaire en Post-Infarctus): A randomized multi-centre trial of occluded artery angioplasty after acute myocardial infarction. Eur Heart J 2004; **25**(24): 2187–2194.

38. Yousef ZR, Redwood SR, Bucknall CA, *et al.* Late intervention after anterior myocardial infarction: effects on left ventricular size, function, quality of life, and exercise tolerance: Results of the Open Artery Trial (TOAT Study). J Am Coll Cardiol 2002; **40**(5): 869–876.

39. Dzavik V, Buller CE, Lamas GA, *et al.* Randomized Trial of Percutaneous Coronary Intervention for Subacute Infarct-Related Coronary Artery Occlusion to Achieve Long-Term Patency and Improve Ventricular Function: The Total Occlusion Study of Canada (TOSCA)-2 Trial. Circulation 2006; **114**(23): 2449–2457.

40. Hochman JS, Lamas GA, Buller CE, *et al.* Coronary intervention for persistent occlusion after myocardial infarction. N Engl J Med 2006; **355**(23): 2395–2407.

41. Hochman JS, Sleeper LA, Webb JG, *et al.* Early Revascularization in Acute Myocardial Infarction Complicated by Cardiogenic Shock. N Engl J Med 1999; **341**(9): 625–634.

42. Timmer JR, Ottervanger JP, de Boer MJ, *et al.* Primary Percutaneous Coronary Intervention Compared With Fibrinolysis for Myocardial Infarction in Diabetes Mellitus: Results From the Primary Coronary Angioplasty vs. Thrombolysis-2 Trial. Arch Intern Med 2007; **167**(13): 1353–1359.

43. A prospective randomized trial of primary angioplasty and thrombolytic therapy in elderly patients with acute myocardial infarction (SENIOR-PAMI): 5 A.D.

44. Thune JJ, Hoefsten DE, Lindholm MG, *et al.* Simple Risk Stratification at Admission to Identify Patients With Reduced Mortality From Primary Angioplasty. Circulation 2005; **112**(13): 2017–2021.

45. Hannan EL, Racz MJ, Arani DT, *et al.* Short- and long-term mortality for patients undergoing primary angioplasty for acute myocardial infarction. J Am Coll Cardiol 2000; **36**(4): 1194–1201.

46. Stone GW, Brodie BR, Griffin JJ, *et al.* Clinical and Angiographic Follow-Up After Primary Stenting in Acute Myocardial Infarction: The Primary Angioplasty in Myocardial Infarction (PAMI) Stent Pilot Trial. Circulation 1999; **99**(12): 1548–1554.

47. Nordmann AJ, Bucher H, Hengstler P, *et al.* Primary stenting versus primary balloon angioplasty for treating acute myocardial infarction. Cochrane Database Syst Rev 2005; (2). DOI: 10.1002/14651858.CD005313.

48. De Luca G, Suryapranata H, Stone GW, *et al.* Coronary stenting versus balloon angioplasty for acute myocardial infarction: A meta-regression analysis of randomized trials. Int J Cardiol 2008; **126**(1): 37–44.

49. Silber S, FAU-Albertsson P, Albertsson PF, *et al.* Guidelines for percutaneous coronary interventions. The Task Force for Percutaneous Coronary Interventions of the European Society of Cardiology. (0195-668X (Print)).

50. Spaulding C, Henry P, Teiger E, *et al.* Sirolimus-Eluting versus Uncoated Stents in Acute Myocardial Infarction. N Engl J Med 2006; **355**(11): 1093–1104.

51. Laarman GJ, Suttorp MJ, Dirksen MT, *et al.* Paclitaxel-eluting versus uncoated stents in primary percutaneous coronary intervention. N Engl J Med 2006; **355**(11): 1105–1113.

52. Valgimigli M, Percoco G, Malagutti P, *et al.* Tirofiban and Sirolimus-Eluting Stent vs. Abciximab and Bare-Metal Stent for Acute Myocardial Infarction: A Randomized Trial. JAMA 2005; **293**(17): 2109–2117.

53. Menichelli M, Parma A, Pucci E, *et al.* Randomized Trial of Sirolimus-Eluting Stent Versus Bare-Metal Stent in Acute Myocardial Infarction (SESAMI). J Am Coll Cardiol 2007; **49**(19): 1924–1930.

54. Urban P, Gershlick AH, Guagliumi G, *et al.* Safety of coronary sirolimus-eluting stents in daily clinical practice: one-year follow-up of the e-Cypher registry. Circulation 2006; **113**(11): 1434–1441.

55. Lemos PA, Serruys PW, van Domburg RT, *et al.* Unrestricted Utilization of Sirolimus-Eluting Stents Compared With Conventional Bare Stent Implantation in the "Real World": The Rapamycin-Eluting Stent Evaluated At Rotterdam Cardiology Hospital (RESEARCH) Registry. Circulation 2004; **109**(2): 190–195.

56. Park DW, Park SW, Park KH, *et al.* Frequency of and risk factors for stent thrombosis after drugeluting stent implantation during long-term follow-up. Am J Cardiol 2006; **98**(3): 352–356.

57. Luscher TF, Steffel J, Eberli FR, *et al.* Drug-Eluting Stent and Coronary Thrombosis: Biological Mechanisms and Clinical Implications. Circulation 2007; **115**(8): 1051–1058.

58. Stone GW, Webb J, Cox DA, *et al.* Distal Microcirculatory Protection During Percutaneous Coronary Intervention in Acute ST-Segment Elevation Myocardial Infarction: A Randomized Controlled Trial. JAMA 2005; **293**(9): 1063–1072.

59. Gick M, Jander N, Bestehorn HP, *et al.* Randomized Evaluation of the Effects of Filter-Based Distal Protection on Myocardial Perfusion and Infarct Size After Primary Percutaneous Catheter Intervention in Myocardial Infarction With and Without ST-Segment Elevation. Circulation 2005; **112**(10): 1462–1469.

60. Ali A, Cox D, Dib N, *et al.* Rheolytic thrombectomy with percutaneous coronary intervention for infarct size reduction in acute myocardial infarction: 30-day results from a multicenter randomized study. J Am Coll Cardiol 2006; **48**(2): 244–252.

61. Kaltoft A, Bottcher M, Nielsen SS, *et al.* Routine thrombectomy in percutaneous coronary intervention for acute ST-segment-elevation myocardial infarction: a randomized, controlled trial. Circulation 2006; **114**(1): 40–47.

62. Burzotta F, Trani C, Romagnoli E, *et al.* Manual Thrombus-Aspiration Improves Myocardial Reperfusion: The Randomized Evaluation of the Effect of Mechanical Reduction of Distal Embolization by Thrombus-Aspiration in Primary and Rescue Angioplasty (REMEDIA) Trial. J Am Coll Cardiol 2005; **46**(2): 371–376.

63. Lefevre T, Garcia E, Reimers B, *et al.* X-Sizer for Thrombectomy in Acute Myocardial Infarction Improves ST-Segment Resolution: Results of the X-Sizer in AMI for Negligible Embolization and Optimal ST Resolution (X AMINE ST) Trial. J Am Coll Cardiol 2005; **46**(2): 246–252.

64. Silva-Orrego P, Colombo P, Bigi R, *et al.* Thrombus aspiration before primary angioplasty improves myocardial reperfusion in acute myocardial infarction: The DEAR-MI (Dethrombosis to Enhance Acute Reperfusion in Myocardial Infarction) study. J Am Coll Cardiol 2006; **48**(8): 1552–1559.

65. Burzotta F, Testa L, Giannico F, *et al.* Adjunctive devices in primary or rescue PCI: A meta-analysis of randomized trials. Int J Cardiol 2008; **123**(3): 313–321.

66. Labeque JN, Jais C, Dubos O, *et al.* Prehospital administration of enoxaparin before primary angioplasty for ST-elevation acute myocardial infarction. Catheter Cardiovasc Interv 2006; **67**(2): 207–213.

67. Ishii H, Ichimiya S, Kanashiro M, *et al.* Impact of a single intravenous administration of nicorandil before reperfusion in patients with ST-segment-elevation myocardial infarction. Circulation 2005; **112**(9): 1284–1288.

68. Ross AM, Gibbons RJ, Stone GW, *et al.*, for the AMISTAD-II Investigators. A Randomized, Double-Blinded, Placebo-Controlled Multicenter Trial of Adenosine as an Adjunct to Reperfusion in the Treatment of Acute Myocardial Infarction (AMISTAD-II). J Am Coll Cardiol 2005; **45**(11): 1775–1780.

69. van der Horst, I, Zijlstra F, van't Hof AW, *et al.* Glucose-insulin-potassium infusion inpatients treated with primary angioplasty for acute myocardial infarction: The glucose-insulin-potassium study: a randomized trial. J Am Coll Cardiol 2003; **42**(5): 784–791.

70. The CREATE-ECLA Trial Group. Effect of Glucose-Insulin-Potassium Infusion on Mortality in Patients With Acute ST-Segment Elevation Myocardial Infarction: The CREATE-ECLA Randomized Controlled Trial. JAMA 2005; **293**(4): 437–446.

71. Dixon SR, Grines CL, O'Neill WW. The Year in Interventional Cardiology. J Am Coll Cardiol 2007; **50**(3): 270–285.

72. Di Mario C, Mara S, Flavio A, *et al.* Single vs. multivessel treatment during primary angioplasty: results of the multicentre randomised HEpacoat for cuLPrit or multivessel stenting for Acute Myocardial Infarction (HELP AMI) Study. Int J Cardiovasc Intervent 2004; **6**(3–4): 128–133.

73. Kong JA, Chou ET, Minutello RM, *et al.* Safety of single versus multi-vessel angioplasty for patients with acute myocardial infarction and multi-vessel coronary artery disease: report from the New York State Angioplasty Registry. Coron Artery Dis 2006; **17**(1): 71–75.

74. Corpus RA, House JA, Marso SP, *et al.* Multivessel percutaneous coronary intervention in patients with multivessel disease and acute myocardial infarction. Am Heart J 2004; **148**(3): 493–500.

75. Smith SC, Jr., Feldman TE, Hirshfeld JW, Jr., *et al.* ACC/AHA/SCAI 2005 Guideline Update for Percutaneous Coronary Intervention—Summary Article: A Report of the American College of Cardiology/American Heart Association Task Force on Practice Guidelines (ACC/AHA/SCAI Writing Committee to Update the 2001 Guidelines for Percutaneous Coronary Intervention). Circulation 2006; **113**(1): 156–175.

76. Primary versus tenecteplase-facilitated percutaneous coronary intervention in patients with ST-segment elevation acute myocardial infarction (ASSENT-4 PCI): Randomised trial. Lancet 2006; **367**(9510): 569–578.

77. Herrmann HC, Moliterno DJ, Ohman EM, *et al.* Facilitation of early percutaneous coronary intervention after reteplase with or without abciximab in acute myocardial infarction: Results from the SPEED (GUSTO-4 Pilot) trial. J Am Coll Cardiol 2000; **36**(5): 1489–1496.

78. Ellis SG, Armstrong P, Betriu A, *et al.* Facilitated percutaneous coronary intervention versus primary percutaneous coronary intervention: Design and rationale of the Facilitated Intervention with Enhanced Reperfusion Speed to Stop Events (FINESSE) trial. Am Heart J 2004; **147**(4): E16.

79. Neumann FJ, Kastrati A, Schmitt C, *et al.* Effect of glycoprotein IIb/IIIa receptor blockade with abciximab on clinical and angiographic restenosis rate after the placement of coronary stents following acute myocardial infarction. J Am Coll Cardiol 2000; **35**(4): 915–921.

80. Neumann FJ, Blasini R, Schmitt C, *et al.* Effect of glycoprotein IIb/IIIa receptor blockade on recovery of coronary flow and left ventricular function after the placement of coronary-artery stents in acute myocardial infarction. Circulation 1998; **98**(24): 2695–2701.

81. Brener SJ, Barr LA, Burchenal JEB, *et al.* Randomized, Placebo-Controlled Trial of Platelet Glycoprotein IIb/IIIa Blockade With Primary Angioplasty for Acute Myocardial Infarction. Circulation 1998; **98**(8): 734–741.

82. De Luca G, Suryapranata H, Stone GW, *et al.* Abciximab as adjunctive therapy to reperfusion in acute ST-segment elevation myocardial infarction: a meta-analysis of randomized trials. JAMA 2005; **293**(14): 1759–1765.

83. Montalescot G, Borentain M, Payot L, *et al.* Early vs. late administration of glycoprotein IIb/IIIa inhibitors in primary percutaneous coronary intervention of acute ST-segment elevation myocardial infarction: A meta-analysis. JAMA 2004; **292**(3): 362–366.

84. Montalescot G, Antoniucci D, Kastrati A, *et al.* Abciximab in primary coronary stenting of ST-elevation myocardial infarction: A European meta-analysis on individual patients' data with long-term follow-up. Eur Heart J 2007; **28**(4): 443–449.

85. Nallamothu B, Fox KA, Kennelly BM, *et al.* Relationship of treatment delays and mortality in patients undergoing fibrinolysis and primary percutaneous coronary intervention. The Global Registry of Acute Coronary Events. Heart 2007; **93**(12): 1552–1555.

86. Mandelzweig L, Battler A, Boyko V, *et al.* The second Euro Heart Survey on acute coronary syndromes: Characteristics, treatment, and outcome of patients with ACS in Europe and the Mediterranean Basin in 2004. Eur Heart J 2006; **27**(19): 2285–2293.

87. Anderson JL, Karagounis LA, Califf RM. Meta-analysis of five reported studies on the relation of early coronary patency grades with mortality and outcomes after acute myocardial infarction. Am J Cardiol 1996; **78**(1): 1–8.

88. Wijeysundera HC, Vijayaraghavan R, Nallamothu BK, *et al.* Rescue angioplasty or repeat fibrinolysis after failed fibrinolytic therapy for ST-segment myocardial infarction: a meta-analysis of randomized trials. J Am Coll Cardiol 2007; **49**(4): 422–430.

89. Steg PG, Francois L, Iung B, *et al.* Long-term clinical outcomes after rescue angioplasty are not different from those of successful thrombolysis for acute myocardial infarction. Eur Heart J 2005; **26**(18): 1831–1837.

90. Tomaru T, Uchida Y, Masuo M, *et al.* Experimental canine arterial thrombus formation and thrombolysis: a fiberoptic study. Am Heart J 1987; **114**(1 Pt 1): 63–69.

91. Gulba DC, Barthels M, Westhoff-Bleck M, *et al.* Increased thrombin levels during thrombolytic therapy in acute myocardial infarction. Relevance for the success of therapy. Circulation 1991; **83**(3): 937–944.

92. Califf RM, O'Neil W, Stack RS, *et al.* Failure of simple clinical measurements to predict perfusion status after intravenous thrombolysis. Ann Intern Med 1988; **108**(5): 658–662.

93. Shah PK, Cercek B, Lew AS, *et al.* Angiographic validation of bedside markers of reperfusion. J Am Coll Cardiol 1993; **21**(1): 55–61.

94. Christenson RH, Ohman EM, Topol EJ, *et al.* Assessment of Coronary Reperfusion After Thrombolysis With a Model Combining Myoglobin, Creatine KinaseûMB, and Clinical Variables. Circulation 1997; **96**(6): 1776–1782.

95. Tanasijevic MJ, Cannon CP, Antman EM, *et al.* Myoglobin, creatine-kinase-MB and cardiac troponin-I 60-minute ratios predict infarct-related artery patency after thrombolysis for acute myocardial infarction: Results from the thrombolysis in myocardial infarction study (TIMI) 10B. J Am Coll Cardiol 1999; **34**(3): 739–747.

96. Stewart JT, French JK, Theroux P, *et al.* Early noninvasive identification of failed reperfusion after intravenous thrombolytic therapy in acute myocardial infarction. J Am Coll Cardiol 1998; **31**(7): 1499–1505.

97. Schroder R, Wegscheider K, Schroder K, *et al.* Extent of early ST segment elevation resolution: a strong predictor of outcome in patients with acute myocardial infarction and a sensitive measure to compare thrombolytic regimens. A substudy of the International Joint

Efficacy Comparison of Thrombolytics (INJECT) trial. J Am Coll Cardiol 1995; **26**(7): 1657–1664.

98. Califf RM, Topol EJ, Stack RS, et al. Evaluation of combination thrombolytic therapy and timing of cardiac catheterization in acute myocardial infarction. Results of thrombolysis and angioplasty in myocardial infarction—phase 5 randomized trial. TAMI Study Group. Circulation 1991; **83**(5): 1543–1556.

99. Ellis SG, da Silva ER, Heyndrickx G, et al. Randomized comparison of rescue angioplasty with conservative management of patients with early failure of thrombolysis for acute anterior myocardial infarction. Circulation 1994; **90**(5): 2280–2284.

100. Ellis SG, da Silva ER, Spaulding CM, et al. Review of immediate angioplasty after fibrinolytic therapy for acute myocardial infarction: insights from the RESCUE I, RESCUE II, and other contemporary clinical experiences. Am Heart J 2000; **139**(6): 1046–1053.

101. Kunadian B, Sutton AG, Vijayalakshmi K, et al. Early invasive versus conservative treatment in patients with failed fibrinolysis—no late survival benefit: The final analysis of the Middlesbrough Early Revascularisation to Limit Infarction (MERLIN) randomized trial. Am Heart J 2007; **153**(5): 763–771.

102. Sutton AGC, Campbell PG, Graham R, et al. One year results of the Middlesbrough early revascularisation to limit infarction (MERLIN) trial. Heart 2005; **91**(10): 1330–1337.

103. Patel TN, Bavry AA, Kumbhani DJ, et al. A meta-analysis of randomized trials of rescue percutaneous coronary intervention after failed fibrinolysis. Am J Cardiol 2006; **97**(12): 1685–1690.

104. Collet JP, Montalescot G, Le May M, et al. Percutaneous coronary intervention after fibrinolysis: A multiple meta-analyses approach according to the type of strategy. J Am Coll Cardiol 2006; **48**(7): 1326–1335.

105. Grines CL, O'Neill WW. Rescue angioplasty: Does the concept need to be rescued? J Am Coll Cardiol 2004; **44**(2): 297–299.

106. Scheller B, Hennen B, Hammer B, et al. Beneficial effects of immediate stenting after thrombolysis in acute myocardial infarction. J Am Coll Cardiol 2003; **42**(4): 634–641.

107. Le May MR, Wells GA, Labinaz M, et al. Combined Angioplasty and Pharmacological Intervention Versus Thrombolysis Alone in Acute Myocardial Infarction (CAPITAL AMI Study). J Am Coll Cardiol 2005; **46**(3): 417–424.

108. Fernandez-Aviles F, Alonso JJ, Castro-Beiras A, et al. Routine invasive strategy within 24 hours of thrombolysis versus ischaemia-guided conservative approach for acute myocardial infarction with ST-segment elevation (GRACIA-1): A randomised controlled trial. Lancet 2004; **364**(9439): 1045–1053.

109. Di Mario C, Dudek D, Piscione F, et al. Immediate angioplasty versus standard therapy with rescue angioplasty after thrombolysis in the Combined Abciximab REteplase Stent Study in Acute Myocardial Infarction (CARESS-in-AMI): an open, prospective, randomised, multicentre trial. Lancet 2008 Feb 16; **371**(9612): 559–568.

110. Cantor WJ, Fitchett D, Borgundvaag B, et al. TRANSFER-AMI Trial Investigators. Routine early angioplasty after fibrinolysis for acute myocardial infarction. N Engl J Med. 2009 Jun 25; **360**(26): 2705–2718.

111. Bøhmer E, Hoffmann P, Abdelnoor M, Arnesen H, Halvorsen S HYPERLINK "/pubmed/19747792?itool= EntrezSystem2.PEntrez.Pubmed.Pubmed_ ResultsPanel.Pubmed_RVDocSum&ordinalpos=3" Efficacy and Safety of Immediate Angioplasty Versus Ischemia-Guided Management After Thrombolysis in Acute Myocardial Infarction in Areas With Very Long Transfer Distances Results of the NORDISTEMI (NORwegian study on DIstrict treatment of ST-Elevation Myocardial Infarction). J Am Coll Cardiol. 2009 Sep 4. [Epub ahead of print]

Answers

1. B
2. D
3. C

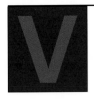

PART V

Approaching Complex Coronary Interventions

CHAPTER 17

Chronic Total Coronary Occlusion

Gerald S. Werner

Cardiology & Intensive Care, Klinikum Darmstadt, Darmstadt, Germany

Introduction

Coronary chronic total occlusions (CTO) are not infrequently discovered during diagnostic angiography with reports that around one third of patients have at least one coronary artery occlusion [1]. The term CTO had not been rigidly defined in recent years [2], with studies and reports on CTO comprising lesions of various duration and degree of occlusion. Some have included lesions as early as three days after a documented acute myocardial infarction [3]. More common is the inclusion of lesions greater than 2–4 weeks after the presumed event of the occlusion [4]. Furthermore, these occlusions also included lesions termed "functional" occlusions when there was still flow (TIMI-grade I) through the actual lesion. This variety of definitions in clinical practice has a strong bearing on the perception of lesion morphology, the discussion of residual luminal channels within occluded lesions and the advice as to which technical approach to take to achieve successful recanalization. Further, this also influences the long-term outcome of successfully treated lesions [5].

In order to find a common ground for future development and discussion of techniques and patient outcomes, a consensus was recently published by a group of experts suggesting a firm defi-

nition of CTO as those with a documented duration of occlusion of at least three months, and with absolutely no flow through the lesion itself (TIMI 0 flow) [2]. Occlusions within 1–3 months' duration can therefore be addressed as recent occlusions, and within a period of four weeks or less following an acute myocardial infarction, as subacute occlusions (e.g. lesions that were treated in the Occluded Artery Trial [6]).

Another important characteristic of a CTO is the length of the actually occluded segment. This can only be assessed through simultaneous visualization of the proximal (ipsilateral) segment and the distal segment through collateral filling. As the majority of collaterals originate from the contralateral artery, this requires double injection (see below).

For the interventional strategy of entering, crossing, and exiting the occluded segment, the basic patho-anatomical features of a CTO have to be kept in mind [7,8,9] (Figure 17.1). We discriminate a proximal cap of the occlusion, which is often fibrotic or calcified and may provide considerable resistance to guidewire advancement. Then, along the occlusion follows a segment of loose fibrous tissue or organized thrombus. Especially in longstanding occlusions, it may include islets of calcification, which provide an obstacle to the advancement of the wire through this part of the occlusion until the distal cap is encountered. The resistance of the distal cap is usually lower than the proximal cap, presumably because of the lower pressure of about 30—40 mmHg existing in this collateralized segment of the occluded artery [10].

Interventional Cardiology, First Edition. Edited by Carlo Di Mario, George D. Dangas, Peter Barlis.
© 2010 Blackwell Publishing Ltd. Published 2010 by Blackwell Publishing Ltd.

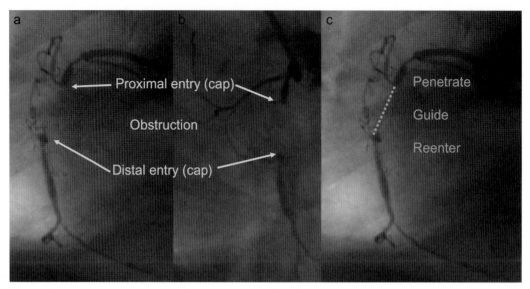

Figure 17.1. The basic features of a chronic total coronary occlusion (a and b) and the technical steps of recanalization (c).

Indication for Treatment

The CTO is a unique set of lesions with regard to the complexity of the required interventional technique, but also with regard to the discordant view on the indication to treat these lesions. The latter is reflected by the low representation of CTOs among lesions treated by PCI, while on the other hand the presence of a CTO appears to bear a specific additional prognostic risk if left untreated [11,12]. In general, patients with a CTO present with stable angina pectoris except if other coronary lesions progress and lead to unstable angina. They are at particularly high risk if the collateral supplying artery is involved in an acute myocardial infarction as the territory at risk is larger than in patients with non-occluded vessels [13].

One hindrance to accept CTOs as a unanimous target for PCI is the lack of a randomized study to answer this issue. However, the wealth of data from prospective registries already provides considerable evidence to treat CTOs. The indication is based on three basic goals:
1. to relieve exercise limiting symptoms of angina or dyspnoea, especially in patients with preserved left ventricular function, or to resolve ischemia caused by the CTO, similar to the indi-

cation in stable angina caused by non-occlusive lesions;
2. to improve regional left ventricular (LV) dysfunction in the territory of the occluded artery, provided there is residual viability; the latter can nowadays readily be assessed by magnetic resonance imaging with late contrast enhancement [14,15];
3. to improve patient prognosis, as there is considerable risk of future progression of coronary artery disease in the remaining patent arteries [16,17].

A specific problem arises with CTOs in the context of multivessel coronary artery disease. These patients may become progressively symptomatic because of progression of non-occlusive lesions, and in the situation of an acute coronary syndrome, a target lesion may be attended to before considering the recanalization of a CTO. In non-acute patients however, complete revascularization should be the ultimate goal, and coronary artery bypass grafting (CABG) is often a viable alternative. Therefore, a staged PCI approach should begin with the CTO as the first target lesion, especially as lesions in the collateral supplying artery would be treated at increased risk if the CTO were not treated [11]. If the CTO procedure fails, the patient may still be referred for CABG for complete revascularization [16].

Basic Rules of Engagement

When a CTO is attempted, the complications inherent in a regular PCI are not smaller because the artery is already occluded from the outset, as considerable damage could be inflicted on the supplying collaterals during the procedure, similar to an acute occlusion during a non-occlusive procedure with ensuing infarction [5].

A CTO is a lesion where the distal segment is not clearly visible, where the actual course of the vessel is completely obstructed and cannot be readily assessed by angiography, especially in long occlusions. To cross a CTO we need to visualize the distal segment in order to direct our guidewire progress, and we often need to resort to more rigid wires than in non-occlusive lesions. The latter go along with a potential to cause damage to the arterial wall, deviation into the subintimal vascular space, or even perforate towards the pericardium, which requires special emphasis on control of the wire progress and position during every step of wire manipulation (Figure 17.2).

The absolute prerequisite for a CTO procedure is to reduce risk and avoid complications. The indication is a mere symptomatic one, as prognostic considerations are not backed by a randomized study. Therefore the CTO procedure should not harm the patient in any way, and the *first rule of engagement* is to always be absolutely sure where the tip of the wire is positioned. A second sheath for injection of contrast to visualize the collateral filling from the contra-lateral artery is therefore always mandatory except in those cases where a left coronary occlusion is approached with filling from one of the other branches. But the most frequent

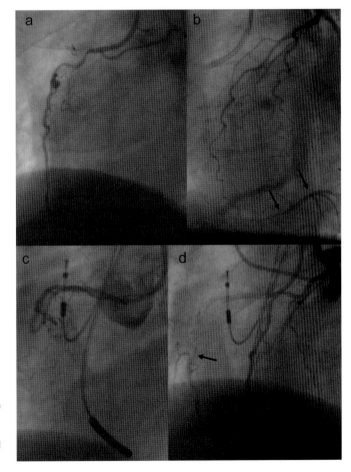

Figure 17.2. Bilateral contrast injection is essential for control of the wire position and advancement and direction. Examples. Proximal RCA occlusion (a) with recanalization wire in a posterolateral sidebranch (b, arrows). Proximal RCA occlusion (c) with recanalization wire outside of the distal vessel lumen (d, arrow).

occlusion, the right coronary and the left anterior descending artery, usually require such a double, simultaneous injection. For a regular antegrade recanalization approach, it is sufficient to use a small diagnostic sheath (4 or 5 Fr) for the contralateral visualization. This also minimizes contrast use compared to use of larger diameter catheters. The *second rule of engagement* is to provide optimum backup for the procedure. Even if a wire may be passed rather effortlessly, the passage of balloons and stents may fail because of poor guide support. Especially for the right coronary artery the regular Judkins guide may not provide adequate support. However, there is a balance to be made between catheter size and shape, and this requires careful planning right at the start of the procedure. A large diameter such as 8Fr (often preferred by Japanese colleagues) will provide enforced support even with less aggressive shapes such as the JR, and it provides ample working space for complex techniques of double wire, double balloon, etc. This approach is especially important for proximal or ostial occlusions, where deep guide engagement is not possible or counterproductive. In non-ostial lesions, a smaller guide size of 6Fr will require deeper engagement for adequate support. This can be ideally achieved by an AL1 shape in most cases. A good rule of thumb is to use catheters with side holes, especially for the right coronary artery, to avoid local dissections during contrast injection into the occluded proximal artery, and to avoid hypoperfusion of proximal sidebranches.

For the left coronary artery the guide catheter has to be selected according to the length of the left main artery, and the angle of takeoff of the occluded artery. Provided that CTOs worthwhile for treatment will generally be located in the main arteries, the LAD occlusion recanalization may be well supported by an extra-backup shape, while occasionally the classic AL2 or 3 may be ideal for proximal circumflex occlusions.

The *third rule of engagement* is to select the guidewire wisely, and not to damage the proximal arterial segments with aggressive rigid wires. Therefore, this author strongly advises the use of a support catheter or microcatheter in an over-the-wire technique as it facilitates the wire manipulation greatly. For example, a sharp angled take-off from the LCA may require soft hydrophilic wires

to negotiate it, whereas the required angle and the wire stiffness will be inadequate for the actual occlusion. The advancement of a microcatheter through the difficult proximal angulation will be always possible, and once positioned at the proximal end of the CTO, the soft wire can be exchanged for a dedicated recanalization wire without damage to the risk of proximal artery.

Guidewire Selection and Handling

Guidewire selection incorporates a great deal of personal preferences and experience. For a detailed description of available wires see [2] or [5]. In general, however, one can discriminate and advice on the use of the two basic guidewire features, that is hydrophilic PTFE wires and metal wires, which may have a hydrophilic coating to a various extent.

There is not a single wire that serves all lesions and all circumstances, and a familiarity with several wires from each family is mandatory.

For CTO procedures, two features of guidewires are of utmost importance, the *tip stiffness*, and the *torque control*. Wires may be used in incremental fashion with increasing tip stiffness when the previous wire encounters resistance. The torque control is a major feature of dedicated CTO wires in order to facilitate maneuvering of the wire in long, resistive lesions.

The wire selection depends on the planned approach to the occlusion, which is determined by the angiographic features of the lesion. Basically, three technical approaches are discriminated, the *drilling* technique, the *penetrating* and the *sliding* technique. Each of them may be selected from the onset but often needs to be changed during the procedure. Flexibility and adaptation is required throughout the whole procedure.

Before the wire is advanced, the tip has to be shaped. This is the first and basic step of wire manipulation, and often requires modification during the progress of the procedure. In non-occlusive lesions a basic rule of thumb is to adapt the radius of the tip angle to the size of the artery in which the wire is to be advanced. A major difference with tip shapes in CTOs is that the vessel diameter at the lesion site is practically zero, because it is occluded. Therefore the length of the

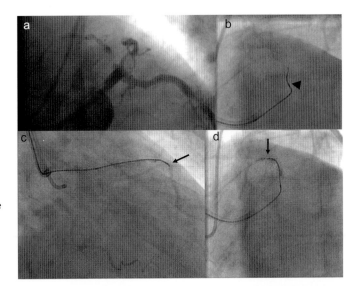

Figure 17.3. Proximal LAD occlusion with tapered entry (a). The tip shape for entering the LAD is different from what is required for navigation within the occlusion. After advancing in to the LAD, a microcatheter (b, arrow tip) is advanced, and the tip reshaped. Further advancement is controlled by bilateral contrast injection in two planes (c and d).

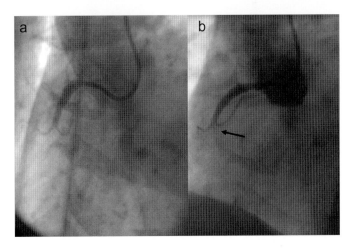

Figure 17.4. Proximal RCA occlusion with two sidebranches (a). Perforation of the proximal cap is required with a Confianza wire (Asahi Intecc, Japan) (b arrow).

proximal tip angle is as short as possible with a moderate 30 to 45° angle. A secondary angle is added about 5 to 10 mm distally to enable wire manipulation in the vessel segment proximal to the occlusion, and to facilitate the tip engagement. These considerations apply in general to all wire types and techniques in CTOs.

The drilling approach is ideal for occlusions with a distinct entry point (Figure 17.3). Typical wires for this approach are moderately stiff wires with high torque-control such as the Miracle Bros (Asahi Intec, Japan) family of wires. The tip diameter of these wires is like normal work horse wires 0.014″, but the enforcement of tip strength is incremental. The 3G wire may be used initially and

increasing strength used in case of problems with progress. The wire strength cannot be increased by the aforementioned microcatheters, but the ease of manipulation will be improved as the friction within the catheter is lower than within a long proximal arterial segment. The wire handling with drilling consists of a very slow advancement of the wire into the occlusion with a turning movement on the torque handle less than 90° degrees in each direction in alternative ways.

The penetrating approach is ideal for occlusions without any discernible entry point, typically at the site of sidebranches (Figure 17.4). The penetration requires smaller tip wires such as the Cross-it family (Abbott Vascular) with 0.010″ tip diameter

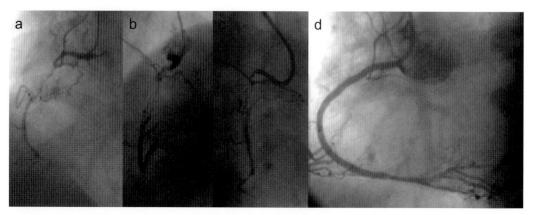

Figure 17.5. Proximal RCA occlusion with a long intracoronary channel (possibly the result of spontaneous secondary recanalization). A Whisper LS wire is gently advanced (a) and (b) and successfully reaches the distal vessel lumen (c) and the procedure is concluded successfully (d).

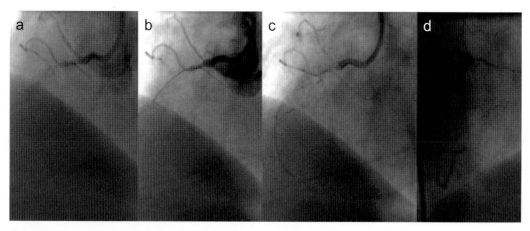

Figure 17.6. A proximal RCA occlusion with sidebranch and no visible entry (a). Still, a Pilot 50 (Abbott Vascular) wire can be successfully advanced gently (b) and reaches the distal vessel (c and d), as confirmed by contrast staining around the wire.

or the Confianza family of wires with 0.009″ tip diameter (Asahi Intec, Japan). Both families provide increasing tip stiffness, and with the latter, additional hydrophilic coating except for the wire tip reduces friction of the wire and enhances the penetration force.

The sliding technique rests on the low friction advancement of PTFE coated wires and is ideal for occlusions with suspected residual lumen (Figure 17.5). These wires include, among others, the Choice PT, Whisper, Pilot, Fielder (regular, FC and the recently introduced Fielder XT with a tapered 0.09″ tip, the last two widely used to navigate through tortuous collateral channels in the retro-grade approach). In general, these wires can often be overused and misused as they promise a fast approach because of the low friction, but they are poorly steerable and will easily leave the vessel lumen. However, occasionally they can be used gently and carefully as an alternative approach and will also be successful in crossing even inadvertently looking occlusions (Figure 17.6). Their better use is as a step down option, once the proximal occlusion cap is passed, e.g. by a Confianza wire, and the softer distal occlusion poses resistance to the advancement of the shafts of the rigid wires, not to their tips. Exchange over a microcatheter is ideal in these cases.

No single technique serves all lesions, and all approaches should be utilized and combined as required.

Advanced Wire Techniques

The basic approach is to advance a single wire gently with just enough force for a slow advancement. The tip of the wire can give information to the experienced operators about the intravascular position; however, this is not reliable, and requires checking by monitoring of the wire advancement in at least two orthogonal projections and occasional contralateral contrast injection. Not infrequently, the first wire enters a subintimal space which is recognized by missing the distal entry of the occlusion outside of the contrast filled lumen.

At that time the first wire can be used as a helpful guide of the general direction of the vessel course and may enable the manipulation of a second *parallel wire* slightly deviating from the initial course to successfully enter the distal lumen.

This is called the parallel wire technique (Figure 17.7). Often, the first wire is a moderately stiff wire, and the second wire is of increased stiffness, or tapered (e.g. Miracle in combination with Confianza). This technique can be accommodated by modern 6Fr guide catheters. However, if both wires are supported by a microcatheter or over-the-wire balloon (then termed the "see-saw technique"), a larger diameter of 7 or 8Fr is required. If necessary even a third wire may be introduced.

The deviation of the primary wire from the true vessel lumen may occur at every point during advancement, particularly when there is a large sidebranch at the level of the occlusion. A refined technique to control this and modify the entry point is the use of *intravascular ultrasound (IVUS)*. An IVUS probe is advanced, after intentional dilatation of the wrong channel, into this false lumen, and under IVUS imaging and orientation of the relative wire positions and the IVUS catheter on fluoroscopy a wire may be redirected into the true lumen [18,19,20].

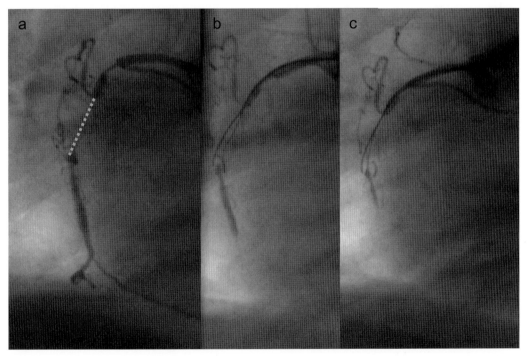

Figure 17.7. Typical example of the advantage of parallel wiring with a Miracle 3G (a, left wire) and a Confianza Pro (b, right wire), where the Confianza Pro can be redirected successfully into the lumen (c) which was confirmed in a second plane.

Retrograde Approach

The success rate of conventional and advanced wire techniques was increased in dedicated centers in unselected CTOs to more than 80%. However, there remain limitations in long and calcified occlusions, and those with inadequate guide catheter support. Often it is difficult to determine the entry into the occlusion, and therefore, alternative approaches would be desirable. The so-called retrograde approach provides such an enhancement of technical means by taking the reverse route of occlusion passage from the distal to the proximal cap. As the distal cap is often softer than the proximal cap, the advancement of the wire may be easier than the antegrade approach. To reach the distal part of an occlusion the initial way was to use a bypass graft and use this access to steer the wire upward to the proximal vessel site. This is, of course a rare coincidence, but it was the first actual application of this approach.

It is to the credit of our Japanese colleagues, and, in particular Dr Osamo Katoh from the Toyohashi Heart Center, Toyohashi, Japan who pioneered the development of this retrograde approach for a wider patient population by using atraumatic PTFE wires to navigate within collaterals from the donor artery to the distal segment of an occluded artery [21,22]. In principal several pathways may be used, but the septal connections are those best

approached with the least danger to the patient in case of collateral damage. Ideally, small trans-septal thread-like collateral connections (CC1 collateral connections [23]) should be used for the approach to either the occluded RCA or LAD. This approach should be used only after extensive experience with the antegrade approach and hence is only briefly covered in this chapter. (Figure 17.8).

In principle, three different methods are used incrementally as required: (1) a wire is placed through a collateral at the distal end of the occlusion to provide a constant aim for the antegrade wire navigation (marker wire). Thus, contrast use can be reduced considerably. (2) The retrograde wire is advanced through the occlusion as far as possible to get contact with the antegrade wire as a kissing wire approach. A more aggressive wire than the soft PTFE types may be required and exchange can be accomplished by use of a support catheter such as a long OTW balloon (shaft length more or equal to 145 cm is required) or microcatheter (for instance the Terumo Finecross or Cordis Prowler and others) or the recently introduced dedicated Asahi Corsair microcatheter, with a tapered flexible tip which can be rotated to facilitate progression. The catheter needs to be advanced into the distal artery beyond the collaterals, as no stiff wire must be manoeuvered within the collateral channel. It may be necessary to facilitate this exchange by dilating the septal collateral channels with a 1 to

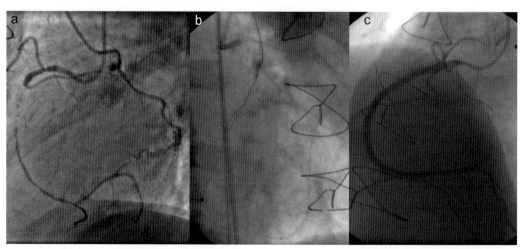

Figure 17.8. A proximal RCA occlusion in a post CABG patient which was tried twice before antegradely (a), but could not be crossed with successful distal reentry. A retrograde approach is chosen (b) and a wire passed through a septal perforator into the posterior descending artery and the advanced towards the distal cap of the occlusion. In a time consuming manouever, the recanalization was completed with the CART technique (c).

1.25 mm balloon at very low pressures of 2–3 atm. (3) If the antegrade passage is still not possible, a balloon may be advanced retrogradely. If a dissection is caused both by the antegrade and retrograde advancement, such balloon inflation will lead to a connection of these dissection planes and facilitate the distal reentry of the wire into the true lumen. This is known as the combined antegrade and retrograde subintimal tracking (CART) technique. However, it is preferable to pass the occlusion without creating a dissection.

Balloon Dilatation

Improving Guide Catheter Support

There are several techniques available to increase support if even a small balloon cannot be advanced [24,25]. They are intended to improve and stabilize the guide catheter position in the ostium. In order of increasing complexity the respective methods are (1) try to deeply engage the guide catheter without damage to the proximal vessel segments; (2) add a second wire introduced into a sidebranch proximal to the occlusion, preferably with a stiff shaft to increase support; (3) advance a second balloon into a sidebranch and inflate this balloon to trap the guide catheter during advancement of the first balloon through the occlusion.

In some instances with heavily calcified lesions, rotational atherectomy is required. However, it may be extremely difficult to exchange the recanalization wire for the delicate 0.010″ rotablator guidewire with the aid of a support catheter, which is advanced as far as possible into the occlusion. If this can be achieved, a small rotablator burr will be advanced. Another specific device useful in this situation would be a laser catheter, but due to high hardware costs and limited applications these devices are rarely found in catheterization laboratories [26,27]. A new device which may help in getting the initial headway through the occlusion is the Tornus support catheter (ASAHI Intec Inc. Japan) which can be screwed across the occlusion once a guidewire is in position [28].

The decision on the correct balloon size for subsequent full lesion pre-dilatation is often difficult and also holds true for the selection of the proper stent size. Therefore, nitroglycerine is given frequently intracoronary to increase the distal vessel size which is always constricted after the recanaliza-tion, as with collateral supply the existing pressure in that system had been in the range of 30–40 mmHg, and the vasodilatory response to the increased antegrade pressure takes time and may lead to underestimation of actual distal vessel diameters. The balloon length is chosen to facilitate the subsequent stent advancement. Stent implantation is mandatory in CTOs [29], and there may be rare exceptions in very small vessels and short occlusions, where a stent is not implanted, but there the question arises on the functional relevance of these CTOs in secondary small coronary arteries.

Stent Placement

The long-term patency after balloon angioplasty, before the advent of stents was below 50% with a high rate of reocclusion. Several randomized studies with bare metal stents had proven a clear advantage over balloon angioplasty, however, the need for more than one stent increases the risk of lesion recurrence considerably, and if more than two stents are required, the target vessel failure rate increases to two out of three [30,31].

The recent amendments of guidelines considered several studies with DES in CTOs and gave a clear indication for their use. The need for long and multiple stents no longer appears to have a considerable impact on vessel patency, although the issue of long-term freedom from very late stent thrombosis is not yet established in this specific lesion subset. When comparing results of previous studies with more recent ones on the use of stents for CTO, it needs to be kept in mind that parallel to the introduction of DES, the complexity of CTO lesions successfully recanalized has also increased in dedicated centers with improved techniques.

When planning stent implantation, a liberal coverage and maximizing stent expansion may be advantageous to avoid focal restenosis at the edges of the stent when they are implanted within severely atherosclerotic segments, and to reduce flow turbulence to avoid stent thrombosis. There is no strong evidence for this advice, and support by prospective studies is needed.

Intravascular Ultrasound in CTOs

Intravascular ultrasound (IVUS) can be of use during several steps of the interventional procedure. As an advanced adjunctive technique requiring considerable expertise, it may be used to locate the entry into an occlusion if a sidebranch is located at the site of the proximal cap [19,20]. If the guidewire is advanced into the subintimal space, an IVUS catheter advanced into this false space may help reentry into the true lumen [18], again a technique only for the experienced.

Where IVUS may be of general advantage, even with less experience, is for the assessment of stent placement and optimized stent expansion [32,33]. As mentioned above, diffuse atherosclerosis makes it difficult to place the proximal and distal stent borders within a less diseased segment to avoid edge stenosis, and to expand the stent fully due to the underestimation of the actual media to media vessel diameter. Full lesion coverage and expansion may be key factors to obtain also persistent long-term success in these lesions.

Basic Rules of Disengagement

The success rate in CTOs will remain lower than in non-occlusive lesions, and the important question arises when to stop the procedure, either to opt for a subsequent second attempt, which is often a feasible choice, or to opt for alternative methods like surgical revascularization. There may be technical reasons to stop the procedure, and safety aspects. From the outset it must be clear that CTO recanalization requires considerable laboratory time, typically 90–120 minutes, but may extend well beyond these limits. Therefore, a sufficient time slot must be reserved, to avoid the abortion of a potentially successful procedure because of logistical reasons.

The typical reason to stop the procedure is a dissection caused by the guidewire which by itself is not reason enough to stop, but to resort to advanced parallel wire techniques. However, when the dissection occurs together with a subintimal hematoma close to the distal reentry it may lead to obstruction of the distal vessel lumen with reduced or complete loss of collateral filling. A retrograde approach may still be possible, but generally a second attempt after 4–6 weeks and resolution of the dissection will be the best approach, also to limit contrast load [34].

The patient's safety is the preeminent consideration regarding the amount of radiation and con-

trast media. Radiation will run typically into 40–60 min fluoroscopic time, sometimes even longer. To avoid radiation damage to the patient's skin, the angulation must be changed and adjusted frequently to avoid a single spot radiation [35,36]. The maximum amount of contrast for each individual patient should be set before the start of the procedure with respect to the patient's age and renal function. The contrast use can be reduced by using smaller guide catheters and diagnostic catheters for contralateral injection and in critical patients, may be an indication to use the retrograde marker wire technique to avoid repetitive contrast injections during the wire manipulation.

Complications

The published data show no difference in complication rates between occlusive and non-occlusive lesions, but these comparisons were not made with advanced techniques and new dedicated guidewires [4,37]. In view of the often disputed indication to recanalize a CTO, and the viable option of surgical revascularization, the interventional procedure must be kept a safe procedure.

Some complications are typical for a CTO procedure, including perforating a vessel during wire advancement, but this is harmless as long as it is correctly recognized. Therefore every care has to be used to recognize and correct false wire positions, and never to follow these wires with balloons without absolute certainty of the correct intraluminal wire position. Dissection and perforation may lead to contrast staining of the myocardium, which is not necessarily a reason to stop the procedure as long as it does not hemodynamically compromise the patient or collateral vessel supply.

The wire may leave the lumen also once it had passed the occlusion and is positioned distally. The stiff wires may easily damage the distal vessel lumen when they are left in place during the balloon and stent procedure. Therefore the distal wire tip should be always kept in view, and very stiff wires should be exchanged for regular guidewires with soft tips as soon as possible, e.g. after the first balloon dilatation.

But as vessel damage and pericardial effusion is an intrinsic risk, a basic rule is to avoid any other anticoagulant than heparin during the procedure, which can be readily reversed by protamine sulfate. There is also no data to support the use of other means like glycoprotein IIb/IIIa antagonists in CTO PCI.

In case of wire perforation, most frequently a distal one, with leakage into the pericardium, the patient runs the danger of pericardial tamponade [38,39]. The operator needs to be experienced in placing a pericardial drainage if needed, but often this can be avoided by rapidly obstructing the leakage with a balloon inflated for several (more than 10) minutes to seal the damage (Figure 17.9). If this does not work, negative pressure suction on a microcatheter advanced far into the distal vessel may help, or thrombus injection through this microcatheter. The problem will be difficult to control if the leakage is fed not only by the antegrade course, but also via collaterals. Then reversal of heparin anticoagulation with protamine sulfate and a pericardial drainage for some time may be the only option, and in case of continuing effusion a surgical repair.

Other complications observed are inflicted on neighboring vessels during the approach towards the occlusion. Here, particular care is required as damage with partial vessel occlusion may put the patient at severe risk as one artery is already chronically occluded. Stiff wires should not be advanced through the left main artery across angles to avoid such damage, and rather be advanced through over-the-wire catheters which are put into position with the help of regular floppy guidewires.

New types of complications may be inflicted through the application of the retrograde wire technique. Particular care and foresight is required not to use the singular principal supplying collateral as any damage would immediately lead to severe ischemia. Furthermore, epicardial and specifically apical collateral connections are prone to be damaged and may even be ruptured, leading to a life-threatening acute tamponade. On the other hand, damage inflicted within the transseptal pathways is rarely severe and resolves without sequelae. These advanced techniques should be reserved to the most experienced operators after extensive experience in safe application of conventional and advanced antegrade wire techniques.

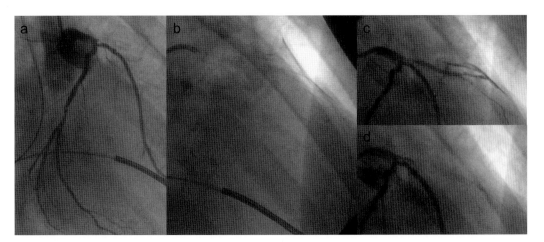

Figure 17.9. Proximal LAD occlusion at the entry of a bare metal stent (a). A Pilot 50 wire was easily advanced through the occluded stent and further distally. No bilateral injection was done as the wire was believed to be in the correct lumen (b). But after balloon inflation immediate staining of the pericardium and chest pain occurred (c). The perforation was sealed after prolonged balloon inflation (d), and the procedure was successfully concluded 4 weeks later with bilateral injections.

Questions

1. **Successful percutaneous recanalization of a chronic total occlusion may have which of the following benefits:**
   i   Improvement in symptoms of ischemia
   ii   Improved long-term survival
   iii Improved left ventricular function
   iv   Reduced predisposition for arrhythmic event
   v   Increased tolerance of progressive CAD
   A All of the above except (iii)
   B All of the above except (iv)
   C All of the above except (v)
   D All of the above except (iv & v)
   E All of the above

2. **The following are predictor of lower success for recanalizing CTOs except:**
   A Occlusion of longer duration
   B Longer length of chronic total occlusion
   C Bridging collaterals
   D Origin at side branch
   E Non-tapered stump

3. **Which of the following statement about chronic total occlusions is not true?**
   A The most common cause of failure to recanalize a CTO is failure to cross with a guidewire
   B PCI is indicated for a CTO if the occluded artery is responsible for the ischemic symptoms, CTO territory is viable, likelihood of success is >60%, death < 1% and MI < 5%
   C Capillary density and angiogenesis decrease with occlusion age
   D In chronic total occlusions <1 year, new capillary formation is greatest in the adventia
   E Aging of fibrotic CTOs generally have negative remodeling; however, plaque hemorrhage and inflammation can result in positive remodeling

References

1. Kahn JK. Angiographic suitability for catheter revascularization of total coronary occlusions in patients from a community hospital setting. Am Heart J 1993; **126**(3 Pt 1): 561–564.

2. Di Mario C, Werner GS, Sianos G, *et al.* European perspective in the recanalisation of Chronic Total Occlusions (CTO): consensus document from the EuroCTO Club. EuroIntervention 2007; **3**: 30–43.

3. Buller CE, Dzavik V, Carere RG, *et al.* Primary stenting versus balloon angioplasty in occluded coronary arteries: the Total Occlusion Study of Canada (TOSCA). Circulation 1999; **100**: 236–242.

4. Sirnes PA, Golf S, Myreng Y, *et al.* Stenting in Chronic Coronary Occlusion (SICCO): a randomized, controlled trial of adding stent implantation after successful angioplasty. J Am Coll Cardiol 1996; **28**: 1444–1451.

5. Stone GW, Colombo A, Teirstein PS, *et al.* Percutaneous recanalization of chronically occluded coronary arteries: procedural techniques, devices, and results. Catheter Cardiovasc Interv 2005; **66**: 217–236.

6. Hochman JS, Lamas GA, Buller CE, *et al.* Coronary intervention for persistent occlusion after myocardial infarction. N Engl J Med 2006; **355**: 2395–2407.

7. Katsuragawa M, Fujiwara H, Miyamae M, *et al.* Histologic studies in percutaneous transluminal coronary angioplasty for chronic total occlusion: comparison of tapering and abrupt types of occlusion and short and long occluded segments. J Am Coll Cardiol 1993; **21**: 604–611.

8. Srivatsa S, Holmes D, Jr. The Histopathology of Angiographic Chronic Total Coronary Artery Occlusions N Changes in Neovascular Pattern and Intimal Plaque Composition Associated with Progressive Occlusion Duration. J Invasive Cardiol 1997; **9**: 294–301.

9. Stone GW, Kandzari DE, Mehran R, *et al.* Percutaneous recanalization of chronically occluded coronary arteries: a consensus document: part I. Circulation 2005; **112**: 2364–2372.

10. Werner GS, Ferrari M, Betge S, *et al.* Collateral function in chronic total coronary occlusions is related to regional myocardial function and duration of occlusion. Circulation 2001; **104**: 2784–2790.

11. Hannan EL, Racz M, Holmes DR, *et al.* Impact of completeness of percutaneous coronary intervention revascularization on long-term outcomes in the stent era. Circulation 2006; **113**: 2406–2412.

12. Abbott JD, Kip KE, Vlachos HA, *et al.* Recent trends in the percutaneous treatment of chronic total coronary occlusions. Am J Cardiol 2006; **97**: 1691–1696.

13. van der Schaaf RJ, Vis MM, Sjauw KD, *et al.* Impact of Multivessel Coronary Disease on Long-Term Mortality in Patients With ST-Elevation Myocardial Infarction Is Due to the Presence of a Chronic Total Occlusion. Am J Cardiol 2006; **98**: 1165–1169.

14. Werner GS, Surber R, Kuethe F, *et al.* Collaterals and the recovery of left ventricular function after recanaliza-

tion of a chronic total coronary occlusion. Am Heart J 2005; **149**: 129–137.

15. Baks T, van Geuns RJ, Duncker DJ, *et al.* Prediction of left ventricular function after drug-eluting stent implantation for chronic total coronary occlusions. J Am Coll Cardiol 2006; **47**: 721–725.

16. Suero JA, Marso SP, Jones PG, *et al.* Procedural outcomes and long-term survival among patients undergoing percutaneous coronary intervention of a chronic total occlusion in native coronary arteries: a 20-year experience. J Am Coll Cardiol 2001; **38**: 409–414.

17. Hoye A, van Domburg RT, Sonnenschein K, *et al.* Percutaneous coronary intervention for chronic total occlusions: the Thoraxcenter experience 1992–2002. Eur Heart J 2005; **26**: 2630–2636.

18. Werner GS, Diedrich J, Scholz KH, *et al.* Vessel reconstruction in total coronary occlusions with a long subintimal wire pathway: use of multiple stents under guidance of intravascular ultrasound. Cathet Cardiovasc Diagn 1997; **40**: 46–51.

19. Ito S, Suzuki T, Ito T, *et al.* Novel technique using intravascular ultrasound-guided guidewire cross in coronary intervention for uncrossable chronic total occlusions. Circ J 2004; **68**: 1088–1092.

20. Surmely JF, Suzuki T. Intravascular ultrasound-guided recanalization of a coronary chronic total occlusion located in a stent implanted subintimally: a case report. J Cardiol 2006; **48**: 95–100.

21. Surmely JF, Katoh O, Tsuchikane E, *et al.* Coronary septal collaterals as an access for the retrograde approach in the percutaneous treatment of coronary chronic total occlusions. *Catheter* Cardiovasc Interv 2007; **69**: 826–832.

22. Surmely JF, Tsuchikane E, Katoh O, *et al.* New concept for CTO recanalization using controlled antegrade and retrograde subintimal tracking: the CART technique. J Invasive Cardiol 2006; **18**: 334–338.

23. Werner GS, Ferrari M, Heinke S, *et al.* Angiographic assessment of collateral connections in comparison with invasively determined collateral function in chronic coronary occlusions. Circulation 2003; **107**: 1972–1977.

24. Takahashi S, Saito S, Tanaka S, *et al.* New method to increase a backup support of a 6 French guiding coronary catheter. Catheter Cardiovasc Interv 2004; **63**: 452–456.

25. Hirokami M, Saito S, Muto H. Anchoring technique to improve guiding catheter support in coronary angioplasty of chronic total occlusions. Catheter Cardiovasc Interv 2006; **67**: 366–371.

26. Werner GS, Buchwald A, Unterberg C, *et al.* Recanalization of chronic total coronary arterial occlusions by percutaneous excimer-laser and laser-assisted angioplasty. Am J Cardiol 1990; **66**: 1445–1450.

27. Taylor K, Reiser C. Next generation catheters for excimer laser coronary angioplasty. Lasers Med Sci 2001; **16**: 133–140.

28. Tsuchikane E, Katoh O, Shimogami M, *et al.* First clinical experience of a novel penetration catheter for patients with severe coronary artery stenosis. Catheter Cardiovasc Interv 2005; **65**: 368–373.

29. Stone GW, Reifart NJ, Moussa I, *et al.* Percutaneous recanalization of chronically occluded coronary arteries: a consensus document: part II. Circulation 2005; **112**: 2530–2537.

30. Agostoni P, Valgimigli M, Biondi-Zoccai GG, *et al.* Clinical effectiveness of bare-metal stenting compared with balloon angioplasty in total coronary occlusions: insights from a systematic overview of randomized trials in light of the drug-eluting stent era. Am Heart J 2006; **151**: 682–689.

31. Werner GS, Bahrmann P, Mutschke O, *et al.* Determinants of target vessel failure in chronic total coronary occlusions after stent implantation. The influence of collateral function and coronary hemodynamics. J Am Coll Cardiol 2003; **42**: 219–225.

32. Werner GS, Gastmann O, Ferrari M, *et al.* Determinants of stent restenosis in chronic coronary occlusions assessed by intracoronary ultrasound. Am J Cardiol 1999; **83**: 1164–1169.

33. Hong MK, Mintz GS, Lee CW, *et al.* Late stent malapposition after drug-eluting stent implantation: an intravascular ultrasound analysis with long-term follow-up. Circulation 2006; **113**: 414–419.

34. Pradhan J, Niraj A, Afonso L. Determinants of amount of contrast utilized in patients undergoing percutaneous coronary procedures. Coron Artery Dis 2007; **18**: 275–282.

35. Bell MR, Berger PB, Menke KK, *et al.* Balloon angioplasty of chronic total coronary artery occlusions: what does it cost in radiation exposure, time, and materials? Cathet Cardiovasc Diagn 1992; **25**: 10–15.

36. Suzuki S, Furui S, Kohtake H, *et al.* Radiation Exposure to Patient's Skin During Percutaneous Coronary Intervention for Various Lesions, Including Chronic Total Occlusion. Circ J 2006; **70**: 44–48.

37. Stone GW, Rutherford BD, McConahay DR, *et al.* Procedural outcome of angioplasty for total coronary artery occlusion: an analysis of 971 lesions in 905 patients. J Am Coll Cardiol 1990; **15**: 849–856.

38. Kinoshita I, Katoh O, Nariyama J, *et al.* Coronary angioplasty of chronic total occlusions with bridging collateral vessels: immediate and follow-up outcome from a large single-center experience. J Am Coll Cardiol 1995; **26**: 409–415.

39. Gunning MG, Williams IL, Jewitt DE, *et al.* Coronary artery perforation during percutaneous intervention: incidence and outcome. Heart 2002; **88**: 495–498.

Answers

1. E
2. C
3. C

CHAPTER 18

Percutaneous Coronary Intervention in Unprotected Left Main

Alaide Chieffo[1], Valeria Magni[1], & Antonio Colombo[2]

[1] San Raffaele Hospital, Milan, Italy

[2] San Raffaele Scientific Institute and EMO Centro Cuore Columbus, Milan, Italy

Left main coronary artery (LMCA) disease is present in 3–5% of the patients undergoing cardiac catheterization for ischemic chest pain, heart failure or cardiogenic shock [1]. Since the first pathological description in 1912, the natural outcome of this subset of patients is considered poor, with <50% survival rate at three years in patients treated with medical therapy [2].

Evaluation of LMCA Stenosis

As discussed in Chapter 4, the assessment of an LMCA stenosis with angiography is sometimes difficult and unreliable. Ostial lesions can be missed because of deep engagement beyond the ostium or overestimated because of catheter-induced spasm or too rapid withdrawal of the catheter because of pressure dumping resulting in an insufficient number of projections examined to evaluate eccentric lesions. Similarly visualization of bifurcation stenoses can be impaired by vessel overlapping while the degree of involvement of the distal LMCA in ostial stenoses of the left anterior descending artery (LAD) or left circumflex (LCX) is nearly impossible to judge angiographically in most cases. Not surprisingly, autopsy studies or repeat angiog-

raphy have demonstrated mild LMCA stenoses in patients unnecessarily treated with bypass surgery [3].

Despite the widespread use of intravascular ultrasound (IVUS) to determine the significance of an LMCA stenosis in patients with an angiographically ambiguous stenosis, physiological correlations of IVUS parameters have only recently been studied and the cut-off values of IVUS parameters that predict the physiological significance of the LMCA stenosis assessed. In a study by Jasti *et al.* [4], 55 patients with an angiographically ambiguous LMCA stenosis, underwent pressure guide wire as well as IVUS examination. A strong correlation was found between fractional flow reserve (FFR) and minimal lumen diameter (MLD, $r = 0.79$, $P < 0.0001$) and FFR and minimal cross-sectional area (CSA, $r = 0.74$, $P < 0.0001$). Compared with FFR as the "gold standard," an MLD of 2.8 mm had the highest sensitivity and specificity (93% and 98%, respectively) for determining the significance of a LMCA stenosis, followed by a CSA of 5.9 mm^2 (93% and 95%, respectively).

Percutaneous Coronary Intervention in Unprotected LMCA

Despite improvements in the safety and long-term efficacy of percutaneous coronary intervention (PCI) for coronary revascularization in recent

Interventional Cardiology, First Edition. Edited by Carlo Di Mario, George D. Dangas, Peter Barlis.

years, the presence of a significant narrowing in the LMCA has remained one of the last bastions of surgical dominance over PCI. The poor immediate and short-term outcome of the first attempts of percutaneous transluminal coronary angioplasty (PTCA) with balloon angioplasty led Gruentzig to list LMCA as exclusion criterion for elective percutaneous balloon angioplasty. The introduction of stents led to demonstrable short-term efficacy and safety of PCI for LMCA revascularization, there have been residual concerns regarding the use of PCI for LMCA revascularization due to restenosis following bare metal stent (BMS) implantation and possibly manifesting itself as sudden cardiac death. Although studies performed with BMS demonstrated a low rate of in-hospital mortality, the incidence of in-stent restenosis remained high (Figure 18.1), forcing the patients to repeat routine angiographic controls.

In these series, the overall in-hospital mortality and immediate revascularization averaged respectively 6% and 4%. Mortality at one to two years varied between 3.1% and 20.1% and repeated revascularization between 15% and 34% [5–9]. However, several authors have also reported more favorable results in "low-risk" patients (younger patients, normal left ventricular function, and predominantly ostial or midshaft lesions) with one-year mortality rate of 3.4% to 7% [6], and a three-year mortality rate of 7.4% [10]. Even in these patients, however, repeat revascularization rates were 28% to 32%.

Accordingly, current guidelines afford PCI of unprotected LMCA stenosis a class IIa or IIb recommendation if coronary artery bypass grafting (CABG) is not a viable option and a class III recommendation (contra-indication) if the patient is eligible for CABG [11,12].

Drug Eluting Stent Implantation in Unprotected LMCA

With the availability of drug eluting stents (DES) and the dramatic reduction in restenosis rates they have provided, the results of LMCA stenting have certainly improved. Encouraging results have been reported at mid-term clinical follow-up in some observational registries with elective DES implantation in LMCA and a one-year mortality of 0 to 5% [13–17] (Table 18.1 and Figure 18.2). In these registries, the need for target lesion revascularization (TLR) varied from 0% to 14% and target vessel revascularization (TVR) from 0% to 19%.

From these preliminary results it is clear that patient selection as well as lesion location could be responsible for the differences in outcome reported in the different experiences [15]. Another important finding from these registries is the fact that in all of them, the major contributor to major adverse cardiac events (MACE) is the need for a repeat procedure with no apparent increase in the incidence of myocardial infarction (MI) or death, albeit with the limitations of one-year follow-up and a total of only 489 patients. There is no doubt that further progress has been made: 6- to 12-month mortality rates of 2% to 4% following PCI are now similar to the ones reported for surgery for LMCA disease in-hospital (1.7 to 7.0%) and at one year (6–14%) [18–21].

Sabik *et al.* reported the 20-year outcomes for surgical treatment of LMCA disease in 3803

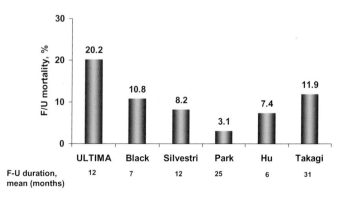

Figure 18.1. Mortality in observational registries evaluating bare metal stent implantation in unprotected left main coronary artery lesions.

| F-U duration, mean (months) | ULTIMA 12 | Black 7 | Silvestri 12 | Park 25 | Hu 6 | Takagi 31 |

Table 18.1. Observational registries evaluating drug eluting stent implantation in non-bifurcation left main coronary artery lesions.

Study	Number of patients	Type of DES	Distal location of LMCA stenosis, %	Restenosis or TLR or TVR, %	Cardiac death, %
De Lezo et al. [13]	52	SES	42	6/2	0
Park et al. [14]	102	SES	71	7/2	0
Valgimigli et al. [25]	95	SES and PES	65	6 (TVR)	14
Chieffo et al. [15]	85	SES and PES	81.2	19/14.1	3.5
Lefevre et al. [24]	291	PES	78.4	7.9 (TVR)	5.2
Mehran et al. [30]	63	SES and PES	73	16 (TLR)	5

DES = drug eluting stent; LMCA = left main coronary artery; TLR = target lesion revascularization; TVR = target vessel revascularization; SES = sirolimus eluting stent; PES = paclitaxel eluting stent.

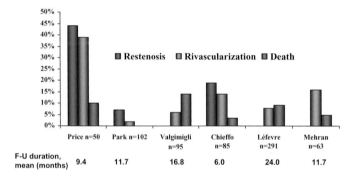

Figure 18.2. Angiographic and clinical outcome in observational registries evaluating drug eluting stent implantation in unprotected left main coronary artery lesions.

patients with LMCA stenosis ≥5.0% (out of a total of 26,927 patients treated with CABG) [22]. In this study, survival at 30 days, 1, 5, 10, 15, and 20 years was 97.6%, 93.6%, 83%, 64%, 44%, and 28% respectively, and freedom from coronary re-intervention was 99.7%, 98.9%, 96.6%, 89%, 76%, and 61% respectively. Buszman et al. [23] recently published their multicenter prospective registry (LE MANS) including 252 patients after unprotected LMCA stenting. Drug-eluting stents were implanted in 36.2% of patients. Major adverse cardiovascular and cerebral events (MACCE) occurred in 12 (4.8%) patients during the 30-day period, which included 4 (1.5%) deaths. After 12 months there were 17 (12.1%) angiographically confirmed cases of restenosis. During long-term follow-up (1 to 11 years, mean 3.8 years) there were 64 (25.4%) MACCE and 35 (13.9%) deaths. The 5- and 10-year survival rates were 78.1% and 68.9%, respectively. Despite differences in demographical and clinical data in favor of BMS patients, unmatched analysis showed a significantly lower MACCE rate in DES patients (25.9% vs. 14.9%, p = 0.039). This difference was strengthened after propensity score

matching with DES lowering both mortality and MACCE for distal ULMCA lesions when compared with BMS.

An important limitation to PCI is that the majority of LMCA lesions treated are located in the distal LMCA bifurcation, shown to be associated with worse clinical outcome [24] and for which we still do not have an ideal stenting approach. The ostium of the LCX appears particularly vulnerable to restenosis, accounting for about one-half of the restenosis cases in these series.

Restenosis has been rare for ostial and mid-shaft LMCA lesions, but it has been significantly higher (8% to 17%) for distal LMCA lesions, especially with the two-stent techniques which are needed for about 50% of the distal lesions in one series [25]. Indeed, results from DES registries demonstrated that restenosis after LMCA drug eluting stenting was essentially confined to distal bifurcation lesions [14,15,26].

Korean Experience

Park et al. have compared the clinical and angiographic outcome of selected patients (preserved left ventricular ejection fraction [LVEF]) electively treated for *de novo* unprotected LMCA stenosis with PCI and sirolimus eluting stent (SES) implantation (n = 102) vs. BMS (n = 121), during the preceding two years [14]. Compared to the BMS group, the SES group received more direct stenting, fewer debulking procedures with rotational or directional atherectomy, a greater number of stents implanted, more segments stented, and more bifurcation stenting. The procedural success rate was 100% for both groups. There were no deaths, stent thrombosis, Q-wave MI, or emergent CABG during hospitalization in either group. The net balance of a lower acute gain (2.06 ± 0.56 mm vs. 2.7 ± 0.73 mm, P < 0.001) and a lower late lumen loss (0.05 ± 0.57 mm vs. 1.27 ± 0.90 mm, P < 0.001) in the SES group, was in favor of the SES patients who showed and a lower six-month angiographic restenosis rate (7.0% vs. 30.3%, P < 0.001) vs. the BMS group. At 12 months, the rate of freedom from death, MI, and TLR was 98.0 ± 1.4% in the SES group and 81.4 ± 3.7% in the BMS group (P = 0.0003). Recently, Kim *et al.* [27] published the results of a multicenter registry evaluating outcomes among patients with unprotected LMCA stenosis undergoing stenting with either BMS or DES. A total of 1217 consecutive patients were divided into 2 groups: 353 who received only BMS and 864 who received at least 1 DES. The 3-year outcomes were compared by use of the adjustment of inverse-probability-of-treatment-weighted method. Patients receiving DES were older and had a higher prevalence of diabetes mellitus, hypertension, hyperlipidemia, and multi-vessel disease. In the overall population, with the use of DES, the 3-year adjusted risk of death (8.0% versus 9.5%; hazard ratio, 0.71; 95% confidence interval, 0.36 to 1.40; P = 0.976) or death or myocardial infarction (14.3% versus 14.9%; hazard ratio, 0.83; 95% confidence interval, 0.49 to 1.40; P = 0.479) was similar compared with BMS. However, the risk of TLR was significantly lower with the use of DES than BMS (5.4% versus 12.1%; hazard ratio, 0.40; 95% confidence interval, 0.22 to 0.73; P = 0.003). When patients were classified according to lesion location, DES was still associated with lower risk of TLR in patients with bifurcation (6.9% versus 16.3%; hazard ratio, 0.38; 95% confidence interval, 0.18 to 0.78; P = 0.009) or non-bifurcation (3.4% versus 10.3%; hazard ratio, 0.39; 95% confidence interval, 0.17 to 0.88; P = 0.024) lesions with a comparable risk of death or MI.

Rotterdam Experience

Valgimigli *et al.*, in 2005, reported the results of the "Rapamycin-Eluting and Taxus Stent Evaluated At Rotterdam Cardiology Hospital Registries (RESEARCH and T-SEARCH)" [28]: from April 2001 to December 2003, 181 patients underwent PCI for LMCA stenosis. Patients with acute MI and cardiogenic shock were included. The first cohort consisted of 86 patients (19 protected LMCA) treated with BMS (pre-DES group); the second cohort of 95 patients (15 protected LMCA) treated exclusively with DES. The two cohorts were well balanced for all baseline characteristics. At a median follow-up of 503 days (range, 331 to 873 days), the cumulative incidence of MACE was lower in the DES cohort than in patients in the pre-DES group (24% vs. 45%, respectively; hazard ratio (HR), 0.52 [95% CI, 0.31–0.88]; P = 0.01). Total mortality did not differ between cohorts; however, there were significantly lower rates of both MI (4% vs. 12%, respectively; HR, 0.22 [95% CI, 0.07–0.65]; P = 0.006) and TVR (6% vs. 23%, respectively; HR, 0.26 [95% CI, 0.10–0.65]; P = 0.004) in the DES group. On multivariate analysis, use of DES, Parsonnet classification, Troponin elevation at entry, distal LMCA location, and reference vessel diameter were independent predictors of MACE.

In further analyses from this registry with a slightly greater number of patients, while lesion location in the distal bifurcation was clearly an independent predictor of outcome (driven primarily by repeat revascularization of the target lesion) [24], the use of either a single stent technique or a two-stent technique were associated with similar clinical and angiographic outcomes [28]. Additionally, both SES as well paclitaxel eluting stent (PES) were associated with similar outcomes when assessed separately.

Milan Experience

In this series, 85 consecutive patients electively treated with DES (both SES and PES) for *de novo* lesions on unprotected LMCA were compared with the historical group of consecutive patients treated with BMS (n = 64) [15]. Patients treated with DES had lower LVEF (51.1 ± 11% vs.

57.4 ± 13%, P = 0.002) and more often were diabetics (21.2% vs. 10.9%, P = 0.12) and more frequently had distal LMCA involvement (81.2% vs. 57.8%, P = 0.003). Furthermore, in the DES group, smaller vessels (3.33 ± 0.6 vs. 3.7 ± 0.7 mm, respectively; P = 0.0001) with more severe lesions (2.94 ± 1.6 vs. 2.25 ± 1.3, P = 0.004) and more frequent multivessel involvement (number of vessels with >50% DS 2.03 ± 0.69 vs. 1.8 ± 0.72, P = 0.05) were treated with longer stents (24.3 ± 12 vs. 15.8 ± 8.6 mm, P = 0.0001). Despite the higher-risk patient and lesion profiles in the DES group, the incidence of MACE at a six-month clinical follow-up was lower in the DES than in the BMS group (20.0% vs. 35.9%, respectively; P = 0.039). Moreover, cardiac deaths occurred in three DES patients (3.5%), as compared to six (9.3%) in the BMS group (P = 0.17).

More recently four-year results from a cohort of 107 patients with unprotected LMCA disease treated with DES were presented at Transcatheter Cardiovascular Therapeutics (TCT) 2008, Washington DC [29]. At four years 13 (12%) patients died, among them 8 (7.4%) were adjudicated as cardiac deaths according to Academic Research Consortium (ARC) definition. Five of the cardiac deaths could be considered as possible late stent thrombosis (ST). Only one patient had a definite late ST at 3.9 months whilst on double antiplatelet therapy (DAT). TVR (defined as any revascularization in left coronary system) occurred in 30 (28.0%) patients and TLR (defined as any revascularization in the stented segment) in 21 (19.6%): of them 25 had a re-PCI whilst five patients underwent CABG.

Scripps Clinic Experience

Price *et al.*, enrolled all consecutive patients (n = 50) who underwent elective, urgent, or emergent implantation of SES for unprotected LMCA lesions between February 2003 and July 2004 [17].

Patients were predominantly at high risk for cardiac surgery, with 58% having an estimated Euroscore operative mortality of ≥5%. The procedure was elective for stable angina or ischemia in 33 patients (66%), and was urgent or emergent in 17 patients (34%). Cardiogenic shock was present in four patients (8%). This series has the highest

percentage (94%) of distal LMCA. In-lesion restenosis occurred in 21 patients (42%); in 85% of cases was focal, and in 82% involved the ostium of the branch. TLR occurred in 19 patients (38%) over a mean follow-up of 276 ± 57 days; but interestingly, TLR was ischemia-driven only in seven patients (14%). Late loss was significantly greater within the LCX ostium compared to the parent vessel (PV) of the LMCA bifurcation (0.83 ± 0.89 mm vs. 0.49 ± 0.72 mm, P = 0.04). Late loss continued to increase between three- and nine-month follow-up.

Turin Experience

Sheiban *et al.* prospectively evaluated the long-term results of consecutive patients with LMCA disease treated with SES implantation from November 2002 to December 2004 [30]. The primary end point of the study was the occurrence of MACE. In total, 85 patients were treated and followed for 595 ± 230 days. Event-free survival rates at one year and two years were 85.5% and 78.6%, respectively. Only two deaths occurred overall (2.4%), the first in-hospital in a very high-risk patient according to the Euroscore [31] and the second in a patient with severe systolic dysfunction already at the index procedure. MI was adjudicated in three patients (3.6%), two occurring peri-procedural and one during follow-up for a *de novo* non-target lesion. There were seven (10.8%) TLR at 24 months. At nine-month angiography, late loss was 0.15 ± 0.81 mm and restenosis rate was 8.2%. No case of ST was reported.

French Experience

The "Mid Term Results of the French Multicenter Taxus Left Main Registry," a feasibility and safety study from four experienced centers, evaluated 291 consecutive patients treated between May 2003 to June 2005 for *novo* LMCA lesions [25] Patients presenting with acute MI and cardiogenic shock were excluded. The median age of this cohort was 68.8 ± 11.4 years; diabetes was present in 28.9%, renal failure in 27.6% and presentation with unstable angina (UA) in 35.4% of patients. LVEF was 60 ± 13% and lesion location was distal LMCA in 78.4% of cases. Additive Euroscore was 4.8 ± 3.4. In-hospital death occurred in 0.7%, MI in 2.7%,

TVR in 0.3% of patients. Two years follow-up was completed in 289 patients (99.3%), with angiographic follow-up in 64% of patients. All cause mortality was 9.3% (5.2% were cardiac deaths), MI 3.5%, TVR 7.9% (CABG 1.4%) and stroke 0.3%. Definite ST occurred in one patient (0.34%): it was an early ST accounting for one death during PCI. Probable ST occurred in one patient (0.34%): the event occurred early and was adjudicated because of the occurrence of sudden death within eight days from the procedure. Possible ST was adjudicated in nine patients (3.1%, all late and very late ST): four sudden deaths (one after stopping antiplatelets treatment) and five in whom the cause of death was unexplained (one after stopping antiplatelets treatment).

Columbia University Experience

Kim *et al.* studied 63 patients [32] with unprotected LMCA stenosis treated at Columbia University Medical Center, mean age was 67 years, with a 30% prevalence of diabetes mellitus. Mean LVEF was 50%, with a mean Parsonnet score of 21. Distal LMCA lesion location was observed in 73% of patients, with true bifurcation lesions treated in the majority (54%) of cases. The majority of bifurcation lesions were treated with crossover stenting (78%), with IVUS guidance in the majority of cases. Long-term outcomes were favorable, with three deaths overall (5%), 10 TLR events (16%), and seven non-Q-wave MI (11%). In this series, the involvement of the LMCA bifurcation was highly associated with adverse events (37% rate of MACE vs. 6% for non-bifurcation lesions, P = 0.03). This appeared to be driven by numerically higher rates of all components of the composite end point, including death (three events with bifurcation involvement vs. 0 events without bifurcation involvement), MI (six events vs. one event, respectively), and TVR (11 events vs. one event, respectively).

ISAR Left Main

Results from "A Randomized Clinical Trial on Drug-Eluting Stents for Unprotected Left Main Lesions study" (the ISAR-LEFT MAIN) were reported in the Late Breaking Clinical Trial Session at TCT 2008 [33]. In the ISAR left main, 607 patients with ischemic symptoms or evidence of myocardial ischemia in the presence of >50% stenosis located in unprotected LMCA were randomized to receive a PES or SES. The primary end-point of the study was the incidence of MACE defined as the composite of death, MI, TLR at one-year follow-up (the study hypothesis was that PES is not inferior to SES in terms of MACE). No differences were reported in clinical and lesion characteristics between SES and PES: distal LMCA was present in 63% of the patients and Euroscore was respectively 4.7 ± 3.5 in PES and 4.4 ± 3.2 in SES. Two-stent technique was used in 51% in PES vs. 49% in SES (predominantly "Culotte" technique was used). The primary end-point of non inferiority was met at one year (MACE was 13.6% in PES vs. 15.8% in SES; RR = 0.85; 95% CI 0.56–1.29). Moreover, two years results were also presented in the same session confirming that MACE were comparable between PES and SES (RR = 0.99; 95% CI, 0.69-1.42). No differences were observed also in two-year mortality (RR 1.14, 95% CI, 1.94-0.66, P = 0.64), ST rates (in PES definite ST 0.3%, probable ST 0.0%, in SES definite ST 0.7%, probable ST 0.3%) and TLR (in PES 9.2% vs. 10.7% in the SES; P = 0.47).

Multicenter Registries and Studies: DES in Non Bifurcation LMCA

A multicenter registry conducted in five international centers has addressed the issue of unprotected LMCA non-bifurcation lesions [34]. In the registry were included 147 consecutive patients who had a stenosis in the ostium and/or the midshaft of an unprotected LMCA (not requiring the treatment of the bifurcation) electively treated with PCI and SES (n = 107) or PES (n = 40). Patients with ST or non-ST elevation MI (STEMI and NSTEMI) were excluded from the analysis.

In 72 (almost 50%) patients IVUS guidance was performed. Procedural success was achieved in 99% of the patients; in one patient with stenosis in the LMCA ostium, more than 30% residual stenosis persisted at the end of the procedure and the patient was referred for CABG. During hospitalization no patients experienced a Q wave MI or died. At long-term clinical follow-up (886 ± 308 days), five (2.7%) patients died. Seven patients required

Table 18.2. In-hospital and long-term outcome in the multicenter registry evaluating drug eluting stent implantation in non-bifurcation left main coronary artery lesions (n = 147).

	In-Hospital	886 ± 308 days
Death, n (%)	1 (0.7)	5 (3.4)
Cardiac Death, n (%)	0	4 (2.7)
TLR, n (%)	1 (0.7)	1 (0.7)
MI, n (%)	5 (3.4)	0
MACE, n (%)	6 (4.0)	11 (7.4)

TLR = target lesion revascularization; MI = myocardial infarction; MACE = major adverse cardiac event.

TVR (five were treated with PCI and two with CABG) of these only one patient required TLR because of in Taxus-restenosis in the shaft of LMCA (Table 18.2). Angiographic follow-up was performed in 106 patients (73%): restenosis rate was only 0.9% with a late loss of −0.01 mm.

In our multicenter series, no cases of angiographically proven ST were observed but it could not be excluded in the four (2.7%) patients who died of unknown cause (all of them had a LVEF <40% and with a Euroscore [31] ≥6 and/or Parsonnet ≥13 [35]). Therefore, in the worst possible scenario, we could assume a cumulative thrombosis rate at a mean of 886 days of 2.7% (95% CI: 1%–7%).

This finding is mostly explained by the favourable anatomical location. Nevertheless, an important factor could have been that in almost 50% of our patients IVUS guidance was used. IVUS guidance in DES era is still debated and controversial especially in this particular subset of lesions. Agostoni *et al.* reported in a small series that IVUS guidance, used in 41% (of the total 58 patients) of the procedures, was not associated with additional clinical benefit with respect to angiographic-assisted stent deployment in patients with LMCA stenosis [36]. Conversely, the Korean group reported that in the BMS era, IVUS guidance could optimize the immediate procedural results and in patients treated with DES and concomitant IVUS guidance a restenosis rate of 7% (the lowest reported) was observed [7,14]. These data were replicated and reinforced in the "Revascularization for Unprotected Left Main Coronary Artery Stenosis: Comparison of Percutaneous Coronary

Angioplasty versus Surgical Revascularization" (the MAIN COMPARE Registry) [37]. In the MAIN-COMPARE registry, 756 patients with unprotected LMCA stenosis underwent elective stenting under the guidance of IVUS vs. 219 under conventional angiography. In 201 matched pairs of overall population, there was a tendency of lower risk of three-year morality with IVUS-guidance compared with angiography-guidance (6.0% vs. 13.6%, log-rank P = 0.063; hazard ratio (HR), 0.54; 95% confidence interval (CI), 0.28–1.03). In particular, in 145 matched pairs of patients receiving drug-eluting stent, the three-year incidence of mortality was lower with IVUS-guidance as compared with angiography-guidance (4.7% vs. 16.0%, log-rank P = 0.048; HR, 0.39; 95% CI, 0.15–1.02). In contrast, the use of IVUS-guidance did not reduce the risk of mortality in 47 matched pairs of patients receiving bare-metal stent (8.6% vs. 10.8%, log-rank P = 0.346; HR, 0.59; 95% CI, 0.18–1.91).

Long-term Results with DES

In the "Drug Eluting stent for LeFT main" (DELFT Registry) [38], 358 consecutive patients who underwent PCI with DES implantation for *de novo* lesions on unprotected LMCA have been retrospectively selected and analyzed in seven European and US tertiary care centers. No patients were excluded from the analysis and all patients had a minimum follow-up of three years. After three years, MACE free survival in the whole population was 73.5%. According to the ARC definitions, cardiac death occurred in 9.2% of patients and re-infarction, TLR and TVR occurred in 8.6%, 5.8% and 14.2% of patients, respectively. Definite ST occurred in two patients (specifically at 0 and 439 days). In elective patients, the three-year MACE-free survival was 74.2%, with a mortality, re-infarction, TLR and TVR rate of 6.2%, 8.3%, 6.6 and 16%, respectively. In the emergent group the three-year MACE-free survival was 68.2%, with a mortality, re-infarction, TLR and TVR rate of 21.4%, 10%, 2.8 and 7.1%, respectively (Figure 18.3).

These results were confirmed in a two-center registry from San Raffaele Hospital, Milan, Italy and Columbia University Medical Center, New

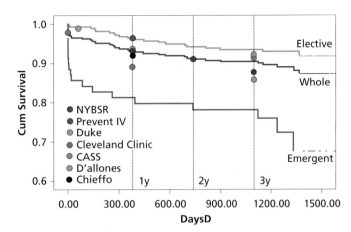

Figure 18.3. Cumulative freedom from death in elective (green line), emergent (red line) and overall (blue line) patients treated with PCI in "Drug Eluting Stent for LeFT main" Registry as compared with the major surgical vs. drug eluting stent studies. Courtesy of Dr E. Meliga.

York, NY which analyzed 267 consecutive patients who had SES or PES electively implanted in de novo lesions on unprotected LMCA between March 2002 and July 2006 [39]. Among them 223 (83.5%) had a distal LMCA lesion location and, in this subset of lesions, a double stent technique was used in 108 (48.8%) of the patients. At two years' clinical follow-up 21 (7.8%) patients died; among them 13 (4.8%) were adjudicated as cardiac death; there were six MI (2.2%), 40 (14.9%) TLR and 54 (20.2%) TVR. As far as ST is concerned, three (1.1%) were adjudicated as definite ST (one sub-acute and two late ST whilst on DAT, none of them died from the thrombotic event), two (0.7%) as probable ST and six (2.2%) as p ST.

Recently, results from the j-Cypher registry were published [40]. In this multi-center Japanese registry, consecutive patients receiving stenting to unprotected left main were included. At 3 years follow-up, among 476 patients whose LMCA lesions were treated exclusively with a sirolimus-eluting stent, patients with ostial/shaft lesions (n = 96) compared to those with bifurcation lesions (n = 380) had a significantly lower rate of TLR (3.6% versus 17.1%, P = 0.005), with similar cardiac death rates at 3 years (9.8% versus 7.6%, P = 0.41). Among patients with bifurcation lesions, patients with stenting of both the main and side branches (n = 119) had significantly higher rates of cardiac death (12.2% versus 5.5%; P = 0.02) and TLR (30.9% versus 11.1%; P < 0.0001) than those with main-branch stenting alone (n = 261). The authors concluded that the higher unadjusted mortality rate of patients undergoing LMCA stent-

ing with a sirolimus-eluting stent did not appear to be related to the LMCA treatment itself but rather to the patients' high-risk profile.

Observational Non randomized Registries Evaluating DES vs. CABG

There have been a number of observational studies evaluating DES vs. CABG reported [16,41–43]. They all found no difference in the occurrence of MACE between patients treated with DES compared to the ones treated with CABG. The most important limitations of these registries were the different baseline clinical characteristics of the two populations (PCI and CABG) and the duration of follow-up (limited to one year).

Lee *et al.* evaluated the clinical outcomes of consecutive, selected patients treated with CABG or PCI with DES for LMCA disease [16].In this study 173 patients were included: 50 were treated with DES and 123 with CABG. Those treated with SES numbered 42, and those treated with PES, 8. High-risk patients (Parsonnet score >15) were present in 46% of the CABG and 64% of the PCI group (P = 0.04).

The 30-day major adverse cardiac and cerebrovascular event (MACCE) rate for CABG and PCI was 17% and 2% (P < 0.01), respectively. The estimated MACCE-free survival at six months and one year was 83% and 75% in the CABG group vs. 89% and 83% in the PCI group (P = 0.20). By multivariable Cox regression, Parsonnet score, diabetes, and CABG were independent predictors of MACCE.

However, the small number of patients included, the absence of a systematic post-procedure surveillance for MI, the low rate of angiographic follow-up (only 42% after PCI), the one-month shorter clinical follow-up in PCI compared to the CABG cohort and the overall clinical follow-up (less than one year) raise several concerns about the possibility to extend these results.

A single center retrospective study in the treatment of unprotected LMCA lesions has compared 249 patients with LMCA stenosis treated with PCI and DES implantation (n = 107) or CABG (n = 142) between March 2002 and July 2004 [41]. In the PCI group, 87 (81.3%) patients treated had distal LMCA stenosis: 77 were bifurcations and 10 were trifurcations. A propensity analysis was performed to adjust for baseline differences between the two cohorts.

During hospitalization, MI occurred in 10 (9.3%) patients after PCI vs. 37 (26.0%) in the CABG group; of these, Q-wave MI occurred in five patients after CABG vs. none after PCI. Three (2.1%) patients died after CABG, whereas there were no deaths in the PCI group. Two patients had cerebrovascular events after CABG and none after PCI.

At one year, nine (6.4%) in the CABG group vs. 3 (2.8%) in the PCI group died, and one (0.9%) patient had MI vs. two (1.4%) in the CABG group. The rate of angiographic follow-up was higher in the PCI group (85% vs. 6% in CABG). There was a lower rate of TLR (3.6% in CABG vs. 15.8% in PCI) as well as TVR (3.6% in the CABG group vs. 19.6% in the PCI group) in the CABG group.

At one year, there was no statistical difference in the occurrence of death in PCI vs. CABG both for the unadjusted (OR = 0.291; 95% CI = 0.054–1.085; P = 0.0710) and adjusted analyses (OR = 0.331; 95% CI = 0.055–1.404; P = 0.1673). PCI was correlated to a lower occurrence of the composite end points of death and MI (unadjusted OR = 0.235; 95% CI = 0.048–0.580; P = 0.0002; adjusted OR = 0.260; 95% CI = 0.078–0.597; P = 0.0005) and death, MI, and cerebrovascular events (unadjusted OR = 0.300; 95% CI = 0.102–0.617; P = 0.0004; adjusted OR = 0.385; 95% CI = 0.180–0.819; P = 0.01). No difference was found in the occurrence of MACCE in the unadjusted (OR = 0.675; 95% CI = 0.371–1.189; P = 0.1891) and adjusted analyses (OR = 0.568; 95% CI = 0.229–1.344; P = 0.2266, Figure 18.4 A–B).

No differences in the rate of mortality and myocardial infarction between PCI and CABG for the treatment of unprotected LMCA were reported by Palmerini et al. [42].

Ellis et al. reported a matched comparison of PCI vs. CABG in unprotected LMCA lesions: 97 patients who underwent PCI were matched in a 1:2 ratio with a cohort that underwent CABG (n = 190) [43]. The groups were similar for age, gender, European System for Cardiac Operative Risk Evaluation (EUROSCORE), LVEF, history of MI, and presence of renal disease. Kaplan-Meier estimates of three-year mortality were similar for the PCI and CABG groups at 80% (95% confidence interval (CI) 68–88) vs. 85% (95% CI 79–89, P = 0.14), respectively. Propensity score-adjusted three-year mortality did not differ between groups (P = 0.22). Multivariable modelling identified only higher European System for Cardiac Operative Risk Evaluation (hazard rate 1.33, 95% CI 1.16–1.54, P < 0.001) and the presence of diabetes mellitus (hazard rate 1.96, 95% CI 1.24–3.09, P = 0.004) as independent predictors of mortality at three years.

Recently, in the "Revascularization for Unprotected Left Main Coronary Artery Stenosis: Comparison of Percutaneous Coronary Angioplasty versus Surgical Revascularization" (the MAIN COMPARE Registry) [44], 1102 patients with unprotected LMCA who underwent stent implantation and 1138 patients who underwent CABG in Korea between January 2000 and June 200 were analyzed. Adverse outcomes (death; a composite outcome of death, Q-wave MI or stroke; TVR) were evaluated with the use of propensity-score matching in the overall cohort and in separate subgroups according to type of stent.

In the overall matched cohort, there was no significant difference between the stenting and CABG groups in the risk of death (hazard ratio for the stenting group, 1.18; 95% CI, 0.77–1.80) or the risk of the composite outcome (hazard ratio for the stenting group, 1.10; 95% CI, 0.75–1.62). The rates of TVR were significantly higher in the group that received stents than in the group that underwent CABG (hazard ratio, 4.76; 95% CI, 2.80–8.11).

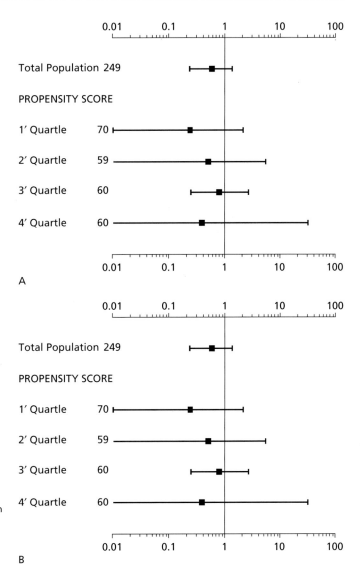

Figure 18.4. Cumulative major adverse cardiac and cerebrovascular events with (Panel A) and without (Panel B) revascularization at one year in Milan registry evaluating drug eluting stent vs. CABG.

Comparisons of the group that received BMS with the group that underwent CABG and of the group that received DES with the group that underwent CABG produced similar results, although there was a trend toward higher rates of death and the composite end point in the group that received DES mostly due to higher risk patient and lesion characteristics.

A small randomized study comparing stenting vs. CABG in unprotected LMCA was conducted in Poland: 52 patients were randomized to PCI and 53 to CABG [45]. Because of the small number of patients it was chosen a surrogate primary end point such as the change in LVEF at 12 months after the intervention. Secondary end points included 30-day major adverse events (MAE), MACCE, length of hospitalization, target vessel failure (TVF), angina severity and exercise tolerance after one year, and total and MACCE-free survival. A significant increase in LVEF at the 12-month follow-up was noted only in the PCI group (3.3 +/− 6.7% after PCI vs. 0.5 +/− 0.8% after CABG; P = 0.047). Patients performed equally well on stress tests, and angina status improved similarly in the two groups. PCI was associated with a lower 30-day risk of MAE (P < 0.006) and MACCE

(P = 0.03) and shorter hospitalizations (P = 0.0007). Total and MACCE-free one-year survival was comparable. Left main TVF was similar in the two groups. During the 28.0 +/– 9.9-month follow-up, there were three deaths in the PCI group and seven deaths in the CABG group (P = 0.08).

Syntax Left Main

In the "Synergy between Percutaneous Coronary Intervention with TAXUS and Cardiac Surgery (SYNTAX) Study", first presented at the European Society of Cardiology (ESC) Congress 2008, Berlin, patients with three-vessel disease and/or unprotected LMCA lesions were randomized to CABG vs. PCI with TAXUS® (Boston Scientific Corporate, Natick, MA) stent implantation [46]; the patients were stratified according to the presence of an unprotected LMCA and diabetes mellitus. The subgroup analysis of the LMCA lesions enrolled in SYNTAX trial were presented at TCT Congress 2008, Washington DC, by Patrick W. Serruys [47]. Seven hundred and five (39.2%) patients were included in LMCA subgroup. The primary end point of this study was the 12-month major cardiovascular or cerebrovascular event rate (MACCE, composite of death, stroke [CVA], MI, and repeat revascularization) which was not different between PCI and CABG in this subgroup of patients (15.8% and 13.7%, P = 0.44). Equivalent MACCE rates also were shown with CABG and PCI in patients with isolated LMCA disease (8.5% vs. 7.1%; P = 1.0) as well as patients with LMCA disease plus single-vessel disease (13.2% vs. 7.5%; P = 0.27), double-vessel disease (14.4% vs. 19.8%; P = 0.29), and triple-vessel disease (15.4% vs. 19.3%; P = 0.42). No differences were found between PCI and CABG in this subgroup of patients in terms of all-cause death (4.2% vs. 4.4%, P = 0.88), MI (4.3% vs. 4.1, P = 0.97), the composite end point of Death/CVA/MI (7.0% vs. 9.1%, P = 0.29) and symptomatic graft occlusion and ST (2.7% vs. 3.7%, P = 0.49); a significant difference was found in terms of revascularization up to 12 months in favor of CABG (12.0% vs. 6.7%, P = 0.02) and in terms of CVA in favor of PCI (0.3% vs. 2.7%, P = 0.009).

Despite these very encouraging results, we should take into account that the subgroup analysis of left main patients had no power to detect a non inferiority of PCI vs. CABG. Therefore these results should be interpreted with some caution and mostly should be considered as hypothesis generating rather than conclusive.

Issues Relating to PCI Technique

Several aspects of the LMCA anatomy should be taken into account when performing PCI. One is lesion location. Disease isolated to the ostium or body of the LMCA (non-bifurcation LMCA stenosis) tends to be the most straightforward to treat: it generally allows the operator to avoid treatment of the distal bifurcation, and as reported above LMCA ostial/body stenoses are associated with excellent short and mid-term results when treated with DES. Nonetheless, there are several noteworthy technical issues to treatment of stenoses located at the LMCA ostium/body. Balloon predilation is used only for severely stenotic and/or calcified lesions, in order to ensure adequate stent expansion. We also in almost all cases try to place the stent back to the ostium of the vessel when treating LMCA body stenoses to prevent proximal edge restenosis occurring within the LMCA itself.

The treatment of bifurcation (or trifurcation) LMCA disease with PCI adds to the higher risk of LMCA lesion location in general, the further complexity of a bifurcation lesion, and thus should only be attempted by experienced operators with a sound knowledge of the treatment of coronary bifurcation disease. Park and colleagues have suggested a LMCA-specific algorithm to determine the stenting strategy for LMCA bifurcation lesions which is based upon both the size of the LMCA as well the presence/absence of LCX disease: in this algorithm, if there is minimal LCX disease, a crossover strategy with a single stent (from LMCA to LAD) is the favored strategy; if there is significant LCX disease, a two-stent strategy is favored (with kissing stents if the LMCA is large or crush/minicrush if the LMCA is small) [48]. The outcomes with such a strategy compared to others have not been rigorously compared, and whilst there are no head-to-head studies demonstrating superiority of one technique of bifurcation stenting over another for LMCA disease, simpler strategies such as crossover (provisional stenting) do appear to produce reliable results in non-LMCA bifurcation lesions if there is minimal disease in the sidebranch and an adequate lumen and flow within the sidebranch can be achieved [49]. Nonetheless, on a case-by-case basis, consideration can be given to any of a variety of bifurcation stenting techniques (crossover, V-stenting, Culotte stenting, crush stenting, mini-crush/T-stenting). In our practice, irrespective of which strategy is used, we typically re-cross the sidebranch and perform a high-pressure inflation (18–20 atmospheres) followed by a final kissing balloon inflation in both branches.

One unresolved question with regards to LMCA bifurcation stenting that remains is why a relatively high rate of restenosis is still observed when bifurcation LMCA are treated, despite the use of DES. Whether this is specific to stenting technique (related to final stent geometry differences occurring with specific stenting strategies such as two stents compared to one), or related to other factors such as underutilization of adjunctive IVUS or inadequate high-pressure sidebranch postdilation is unknown. Whilst the high rate of routine angiographic follow-up in registry series might have contributed to the increased use of repeat revascularization in these studies, some have argued that few patients overall in these studies underwent routine non-invasive testing for ischemia, and focal restenotic lesions that were subsequently treated may not have been clinically significant. In comparison, in most surgical series of LMCA revascularization, angiographic follow-up is not routinely performed and as such, progressive lesions/graft failures do not tend to be identified in the absence of a change in clinical symptoms. A further issue specifically related to the identification of restenotic disease following LMCA PCI is the difficulty in angiographic characterization of bifurcations; due to vessel overlap and angulation, angiography can often over-estimate the severity of disease (relative to its functional significance) at sidebranches [50]. A final as yet unanswered fundamental question is why the majority of LMCA restenoses tend to occur focally at the ostium of the sidebranch in distal bifurcation lesions. Our preliminary observations indicate that focal stent recoil at the ostium of the sidebranch might be one cause.

Stent Thrombosis

In a recent multicenter registry [51] with clinical follow-up of 29.5 ± 13.7 months obtained in 731 consecutive patients electively treated for unprotected LMCA stenosis with DES, the rate of definite and probable ST was 0.9% with a MACE rate of 19%. It is important to point that 3/4 definite ST occurred within 30 days from stenting and that all the patients were on DAT at the time of thrombotic event highlighting the importance of procedural factors and responsiveness to DAT.

Conclusions

Encouraging results have been reported at midterm clinical follow-up in some observational registries with elective DES implantation in LMCA. However, longer term clinical follow-up are warranted in order to assess the efficacy and safety of DES implantation in LMCA lesions and to confirm the encouraging results observed in the subgroup of patients with ostium and shaft lesions. Moreover, for distal LMCA lesions, the evidence is uncertain pending results from large randomized trials evaluating DES implantation vs. CABG. However, the recently presented results of the subgroup analyses from the SYNTAX trial showed that for patients with LMCA disease, revascularization with PCI has comparable safety and efficacy to CABG and eventually that PCI is a reasonable treatment alternative in this patient population, in particular when the SYNTAX score is low or intermediate. Such a view has also been put forth by the American College of Cardiology Interventional Scientific Council in their recently published white paper [52]. Additionally, the PRECOMBAT (PREmier of randomized COMparison of Bypass surgery and AngioplasTy using sirolimus eluting stent in patients with unprotected left main coronary artery disease) trial of 600 patients with LMCA disease randomized to PCI with Cypher DES or CABG is approximately two-thirds complete with recruitment ongoing in Korea.

The complex issue of left main revascularization has been recently addressed by the Interventional Scientific Council of the American College of Cardiology and the respective expert committee published a document (ref) indicating the need to move the guidelines for performing percutaneous stent implantation away from the current class III. The appropriate committees of the European and American societies are expected to formally address this subject this year. In addition, a large multi-center study is being initiated in order to prospectively test the non-inferiority of stent implantation to coronary bypass surgery for left main coronary artery disease [52].

Questions

1. **Stenting of the *distal* left main compared with the ostium or body is associated with:**
   A Similar rates of clinical restenosis
   B Lower rates of death or MI
   C A greater need for repeat revascularization
   D Less fluoroscopic and procedural time
2. **Which is true regarding drug-eluting vs. bare metal stents when used in the left main coronary artery?**
   A Death rates are significantly lower for DES
   B MACE rates (death, MI, TVR) are all not significantly different
   C Stent thrombosis rates are significantly higher for DES
   D TVR is significantly lower for DES
3. **When left main PCI is considered, which is an important correlate of mortality?**
   A Lesion calcification
   B Severe mitral regurgitation
   C Cardiogenic shock
   D Serum Creatinine ≥2 mg/dl
   E All of the above

References

1. Cohen MV, Cohn PF, Herman MV, *et al.* Diagnosis and prognosis of main left coronary artery obstruction. Circulation 1972; **45** (1 Suppl): I57–165.
2. Herrick JB. Landmark article (JAMA 1912). Clinical features of sudden obstruction of the coronary arteries. By James B. Herrick. JAMA 1983; **250**(13): 1757–1765.
3. Arnett EN, Isner JM, Redwood DR, *et al.* Coronary artery narrowing in coronary heart disease: comparison of cineangiographic and necropsy findings. Ann Intern Med 1979; **91**(3): 350–356.
4. Jasti V, Ivan E, Yalamanchili V, *et al.* Correlations between fractional flow reserve and intravascular ultrasound in patients with an ambiguous left main coronary artery stenosis. Circulation 2004; **110**(18): 2831–2836.
5. Ellis SG, Tamai H, Nobuyoshi M, *et al.* Contemporary percutaneous treatment of unprotected left main coronary stenoses: initial results from a multicenter registry analysis 1994–1996. Circulation 1997; **96**(11): 3867–3872.
6. Marso SP, Steg G, Plokker T, *et al.* Catheter-based reperfusion of unprotected left main stenosis during an acute myocardial infarction (the ULTIMA experience). Unprotected Left Main Trunk Intervention Multi-center Assessment. The American Journal of Cardiology. 1999; **83**(11): 1513–1517.
7. Park SJ, Hong MK, Lee CW, *et al.* Elective stenting of unprotected left main coronary artery stenosis: effect of debulking before stenting and intravascular ultrasound guidance. Journal of the American College of Cardiology 2001; **38**(4): 1054–1060.
8. Silvestri M, Barragan P, Sainsous J, *et al.* Unprotected left main coronary artery stenting: immediate and medium-term outcomes of 140 elective procedures. Journal of the American College of Cardiology 2000; **35**(6): 1543–1550.
9. Takagi T, Stankovic G, Finci L, *et al.* Results and long-term predictors of adverse clinical events after elective percutaneous interventions on unprotected left main coronary artery. Circulation 2002; **106**(6): 698–702.
10. Park SJ, Park SW, Hong MK, *et al.* Long-term (three-year) outcomes after stenting of unprotected left main coronary artery stenosis in patients with normal left ventricular function. American Journal of Cardiology 2003; **91**(1): 12–16.
11. Silber S, Albertsson P, Aviles FF, *et al.* Guidelines for percutaneous coronary interventions. The Task Force for Percutaneous Coronary Interventions of the European Society of Cardiology. Eur Heart J 2005; **26**(8): 804–847.
12. Smith SC, Jr., Feldman TE, Hirshfeld JW, Jr., *et al.* ACC/AHA/SCAI 2005 Guideline Update for Percutaneous Coronary Intervention—summary article: A report of the American College of Cardiology/American Heart Association Task Force on Practice Guidelines (ACC/AHA/SCAI Writing Committee to Update the 2001 Guidelines for Percutaneous Coronary Intervention). Circulation 2006; **113**(1): 156–175.
13. de Lezo JS, Medina A, Pan M, *et al.* Rapamycin-eluting stents for the treatment of unprotected left main coronary disease. American Heart Journal 2004; **148**(3): 481–485.
14. Park SJ, Kim YH, Lee BK, *et al.* Sirolimus-eluting stent implantation for unprotected left main coronary artery stenosis: comparison with bare metal stent implantation. Journal of the American College of Cardiology 2005; **45**(3): 351–356.
15. Chieffo A, Stankovic G, Bonizzoni E, *et al.* Early and mid-term results of drug-eluting stent implantation in unprotected left main. Circulation 2005; **111**(6): 791–795.
16. Lee MS, Kapoor N, Jamal F, *et al.* Comparison of coronary artery bypass surgery with percutaneous coronary intervention with drug-eluting stents for unprotected left main coronary artery disease. Journal of the American College of Cardiology 2006; **47**(4): 864–870.

17. Price MJ, Cristea E, Sawhney N, *et al.* Serial angiographic follow-up of sirolimus-eluting stents for unprotected left main coronary artery revascularization. Journal of the American College of Cardiology 2006; **47**(4): 871–877.

18. Beauford RB, Saunders CR, Lunceford TA, *et al.* Multivessel off-pump revascularization in patients with significant left main coronary artery stenosis: early and midterm outcome analysis. J Card Surg 2005; **20**(2): 112–118.

19. d'Allonnes FR, Corbineau H, Le Breton H, *et al.* Isolated left main coronary artery stenosis: long term follow up in 106 patients after surgery. Heart 2002; **87**(6): 544–548.

20. Holm F, Lubanda JC, Semrad M, *et al.* Main clinical and surgical determinants of in-hospital mortality after surgical revascularization of left main coronary artery stenosis: 2 year retrospective study (1998–1999)]. J Mal Vasc 2004; **29**(2): 89–93.

21. Lu JC, Grayson AD, Pullan DM. On-pump versus off-pump surgical revascularization for left main stem stenosis: risk adjusted outcomes. Ann Thorac Surg 2005; **80**(1): 136–142.

22. Sabik JF, III, Blackstone EH, Firstenberg M, *et al.* A benchmark for evaluating innovative treatment of left main coronary disease. Circulation 2007; **116**(11 Suppl): I232–1239.

23. Buzman PE, Buzman PP, Kiesz RS, *et al.* Early and long-term results of unprotected left main coronary artery stenting: the LE MANS (Left Main Coronary Artery Stenting) registry. J Am Coll Cardiol 2009; **54**: 1500–1511.

24. Valgimigli M, Malagutti P, Rodriguez-Granillo GA, *et al.* Distal left main coronary disease is a major predictor of outcome in patients undergoing percutaneous intervention in the drug-eluting stent era: an integrated clinical and angiographic analysis based on the Rapamycin-Eluting Stent Evaluated At Rotterdam Cardiology Hospital (RESEARCH) and Taxus-Stent Evaluated At Rotterdam Cardiology Hospital (T-SEARCH) registries. Journal of the American College of Cardiology 2006; **47**(8): 1530–1537.

25. Lefèvre T, Vaquerizo B, Darremont O, *et al.* Long-term predictors of cardiac death after unprotected left main stenting using a provisional T stenting strategy and paclitaxel-eluting stents: insights from the French left main Taxus registry. Catheter Cardiovasc Interv 2008; **71**(4).

26. Valgimigli M, van Mieghem CAG, Ong ATL, *et al.* Short- and Long-term Clinical Outcome after Drug-Eluting Stent Implantation for the Percutaneous Treatment of Left Main Coronary Artery Disease. Circulation 2005; **111**: 1383–1389.

27. Kim YH, Park DW, Lee SW, *et al.* Long-term safety and effectiveness of unprotected left main coronary stenting with drug-eluting stents compared with bare-metal stents. Circulation 2009; **120**: 400–407.

28. Valgimigli M, Malagutti P, Rodriguez Granillo GA, *et al.* Single-vessel versus bifurcation stenting for the treatment of distal left main coronary artery disease in the drug-eluting stenting era: Clinical and angiographic insights into the Rapamycin-Eluting Stent Evaluated at Rotterdam Cardiology Hospital (RESEARCH) and Taxus-Stent Evaluated at Rotterdam Cardiology Hospital (T-SEARCH) registries. American Heart Journal 2006; **152**(5): 896–902.

29. Magni V, Chieffo A, Ielasi A, *et al.* A. Long Term (4 Years) Outcome in Patients with Unprotected Left Main Coronary Artery Stenosis Treated with Drug-Eluting Stent Implantation. The American Journal of Cardiology 2008; **102**(8): TCT-68.

30. Sheiban I, Meliga E, Moretti C, *et al.* Long-term clinical and angiographic outcomes of treatment of unprotected left main coronary artery stenosis with sirolimus-eluting stents. The American Journal of Cardiology 2007; **100**(3): 431–435.

31. Nashef SA, Roques F, Michel P, *et al.* European system for cardiac operative risk evaluation (EuroSCORE). Eur J Cardiothorac Surg1999; **16**(1): 9–13.

32. Kim YH, Dangas GD, Solinas E, *et al.* Effectiveness of drug-eluting stent implantation for patients with unprotected left main coronary artery stenosis. American Journal of Cardiology. 2008; **101**(6): 801–806.

33. Mehilli J, Kastrati A, Byrne RA, *et al.* For the ISAR-LEFT MAIN (Intracoronary Stenting and Angiographic Results: Drug-Eluting Stents for Unprotected Coronary Left Main Lesions) Study Investigators. Paclitaxel-versus sirolimus-eluting stents for unprotected left main coronary artery disease. J Am Coll Cardiol 2009; **53**(19): 1760–1768.

34. Chieffo A, Park SJ, Valgimigli M, *et al.* Favorable long-term outcome after drug-eluting stent implantation in nonbifurcation lesions that involve unprotected left main coronary artery: a multicenter registry. Circulation 2007; **116**(2): 158–162.

35. Parsonnet V, Dean D, Bernstein AD. A method of uniform stratification of risk for evaluating the results of surgery in acquired adult heart disease. Circulation 1989; **79**(6 Pt 2): I3–12.

36. Agostoni P, Valgimigli M, Van Mieghem CA, *et al.* Comparison of early outcome of percutaneous coronary intervention for unprotected left main coronary artery disease in the drug-eluting stent era with versus without intravascular ultrasonic guidance. American Journal of Cardiology 2005; **95**(5): 644–647.

37. Hong M-K, Park D-W, Kim Y-H, *et al.* Impact of Intravascular Ultrasound Guidance on Long-Term Clinical Outcomes in Patients Undergoing Percutaneous Coronary Intervention for Unprotected Left Main Disease. Journal of the American College of Cardiology 2008; **51**(Suppl 2): B7.

38. Meliga E, Garcia-Garcia HM, Valgimigli M, *et al.* DELFT (Drug Eluting stent for LeFT main) Registry. Longest available clinical outcomes after drug-eluting stent implantation for unprotected left main coronary artery disease: The DELFT (Drug Eluting stent for LeFT main) Registry. J Am Coll Cardiol 2008; **51**(23): 2212–2219.

39. Chieffo A, Mehran R, Fischella D, *et al.* Two Year Outcome in Patients with Unprotected Left Main Coronary Artery Stenosis Treated with Drug-Eluting Stent Implantation: Milan and New York Experience. American Journal of Cardiology 2008; **102**(8) (TCT-67).

40. Toyofuku M, Kimura T, Morimoto T, *et al.* Three-year outcomes after sirolimus-eluting stent implantation for unprotected left main coronary artery disease: insights from the j-Cypher registry. Circulation 2009; **120**: 1866–1874.

41. Chieffo A, Morici N, Maisano F, *et al.* Percutaneous treatment with drug-eluting stent implantation versus bypass surgery for unprotected left main stenosis: a single-center experience. Circulation 2006; **113**(21): 2542–2547.

42. Palmerini T, Marzocchi A, Marrozzini C, *et al.* Comparison between coronary angioplasty and coronary artery bypass surgery for the treatment of unprotected left main coronary artery stenosis (the Bologna Registry). The American Journal of cardiology 2006; **98**(1): 54–59.

43. Brener SJ, Galla JM, Bryant R, III, *et al.* Comparison of percutaneous versus surgical revascularization of severe unprotected left main coronary stenosis in matched patients. The American Journal of Cardiology 2008; **101**(2): 169–172.

44. Seung KB, Park DW, Kim YH, *et al.* Stents versus coronary-artery bypass grafting for left main coronary artery disease. The New England journal of medicine. Apr 24 2008; **358**(17): 1781–1792.

45. Buszman PE, Kiesz SR, Bochenek A, *et al.* Acute and late outcomes of unprotected left main stenting in comparison with surgical revascularization. Journal of the American College of Cardiology 2008; **51**(5): 538–545.

46. Serruys PW, Morice MC, Kappetein AP, *et al.* SYNTAX Investigators. Percutaneous coronary intervention versus coronary-artery bypass grafting for severe coronary artery disease. N Engl J Med 2009; **360**(10): 961–972.

47. Serruys PW. The Synergy between Percutaneous Coronary Intervention with TAXUS and Cardiac Surgery: The SYNTAX Study. Primary Endpoint Results at One Year in Subset of Patients With Left Main Disease Accessed November 27, 2008 at: http://www.tctmd.com/txshow.aspx?tid=2432&id=69976&trid=2380.

48. Kim YH, Park DW, Suh IW, *et al.* Long-term outcome of simultaneous kissing stenting technique with sirolimus-eluting stent for large bifurcation coronary lesions. Catheter Cardiovasc Interv 2007; **70**(6): 840–846.

49. Steigen TK, Maeng M, Wiseth R, *et al.* Randomized study on simple versus complex stenting of coronary artery bifurcation lesions: the Nordic bifurcation study. Circulation 2006; **114**(18): 1955–1961.

50. Koo BK, Kang HJ, Youn TJ, *et al.* Physiologic assessment of jailed side branch lesions using fractional flow reserve. Journal of the American College of Cardiology 2005; **46**(4): 633–637.

51. Chieffo A, Kim YH, Meliga E, *et al.* Late and very late stent thrombosis following elective drug eluting stent implantation in unprotected left main coronary artery: a multicenter registry. Circulation 2007; **116**(16): II-666.

52. Kandzari DE, Colombo A, Park SJ, *et al.* American College of Cardiology Interventional Scientific Council. Revascularization for unprotected left main disease: evolution of the evidence basis to redefine treatment standards. J Am Coll Cardiol. 2009 Oct 20; **54**: 1576–1588.

Answers

1. C
2. D
3. E

CHAPTER 19

Bifurcation Lesions

Leif Thuesen

Aarhus University Hospital, Skejby, Denmark

Introduction

Good short- and long-term results in percutaneous coronary intervention (PCI) depend on factors related to the patient and to the coronary artery lesion. Factors related to the patient include age, co-morbidity (diabetes, heart failure, renal failure or general arteriosclerosis) and a clinical condition of an acute coronary syndrome. Such factors should be taken into account when a PCI is planned.

Bifurcation lesions are frequent and account for about 15% of all PCI cases [1]). Bifurcations are a challenging lesion subset involving a main vessel and its side branch. A bifurcation lesion may be looked upon as the proximal main vessel, the distal main vessel, the side branch and the area of bifurcation. Short- and long-term results depend on optimal handling of all parts of the bifurcation. Coronary bifurcation lesions can often be treated in a number of different ways. The choice of treatment will depend on the condition of the patient and the experience of the operator. Here, it will often be an advantage to select a simple approach for the bifurcation treatment and focus treatment on major vessels.

Interventional Cardiology, First Edition. Edited by Carlo Di Mario, George D. Dangas, Peter Barlis. © 2010 Blackwell Publishing Ltd. Published 2010 by Blackwell Publishing Ltd.

Balloon Angioplasty (POBA) and Bare Metal Stents (BMS)

Initial results with balloon angioplasty in bifurcation lesions were poor with high risk of acute closure of the main vessel or side branch and with a high restenosis rate [2]. Today, coronary stenting has become routine praxis in these lesions and problems with acute main vessel closure have been eliminated. However, bifurcation stenting is still associated with a high rate of restenosis, and acute side branch closure is not uncommon [3]. The restenosis problem is especially pronounced, when multiple stents are used [4]. Therefore, in many centers, presence of a bifurcation lesion may favor recommendation of coronary bypass surgery.

Drug Eluting Stents (DES)

The use of DESs in both main vessel and side branch has reduced the problems of acute side branch closure and high restenosis rates in these lesions. At present there are no randomized studies comparing DES and BMS in bifurcation lesions. However, data from the bifurcation subgroup of the SCANDSTENT study (DES vs. BMS in complex coronary lesions) demonstrated that the use of DES was associated with a low restenosis rate as compared to BMS treated patients [5]. Other studies on the use of DES in bifurcation lesions showed that a technically correct use of these stents resulted in very low restenosis rates, both of the main vessel and of the side branch [6,7].

The Bifurcation Lesion

The Medina Classification

The Medina bifurcation classification is now the generally accepted bifurcation classification [8,9]. It is a simple classification using the three components of a bifurcation; the main branch proximal, the main branch distal and the side branch. Respecting that sequence, the value of "1" (compromised flow) or "0" '(uncompromised flow) is given to each of the segments. Figure 19.1 shows the seven possible bifurcation morphologies.

Type 1,1,1

Bifurcation lesion involving the main vessel proximal and distal to the side branch and the ostium of the side branch.

Type 1,1,0

Bifurcation lesion involving the main vessel proximal and distal to the side branch, but not the ostium of the side branch.

Type 1,0,1

Bifurcation lesion involving the main vessel proximal and the side branch, but not the main vessel distal to the side branch.

Type 0,1,1

Bifurcation lesion involving the distal part of the main vessel and the side branch, but not the proximal part of the main vessel.

Type 1,0,0

Bifurcation lesion involving the proximal part of the main vessel, but not the distal main vessel and the side branch.

Type 0,1,0

Bifurcation lesion involving the distal part of the main vessel, but not the proximal part of the main vessel and the side branch.

Type 0,0,1

Bifurcation lesion involving only the side branch.

Analysis of Types

Type 1,1,1 is a true bifurcation lesion since all branches are involved. Approximately 15% of

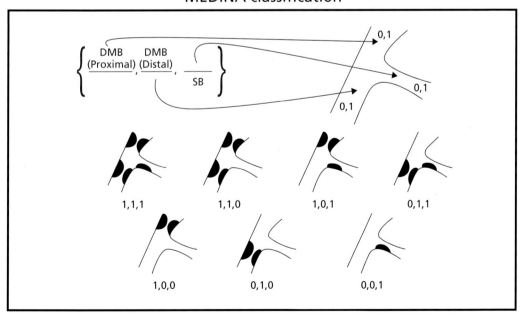

Figure 19.1. The MEDINA bifurcation classification.

bifurcation lesions are of this type. Types 1,1,1 and 1,0,1 and 0,1,1 are true bifurcation lesions in the sense that there are lesions in both main vessel and side branch [8].

Although the type 0,0,1 lesion involves only the side branch, the treatment of this lesion often needs considerable consideration, as stenting of the side branch may result in plaque shift to the main vessel or stent protrusion into the main vessel, so that a simple lesion in a vessel supplying a minor myocardial territory may end up with a disproportionately complex intervention.

Important Lesion-related Characteristics
Y- and T-shaped Bifurcations
In the Y-shape lesion, the angle between side branch and main vessel is <70°. Side branch access is usually easy, but plaque shift may be pronounced with this bifurcation morphology. In the T-shape lesion, the main vessel-bifurcation angle is >70°. Here side branch access may be difficult, but plaque shift usually less pronounced.

Side Branch Size
The absolute size of the side branch or its size in relation to the main vessel is an important factor, when the interventional strategy is planned. Whilst occlusion of a small side branch may not be clinically important, it is a major concern to keep a large side branch open and preferably free from significant stenosis on short- and long-term basis. Bifurcations, where the side branch is considerably smaller than the main vessel may be a problem in culotte stenting technique.

Large plaque burden, plaque eccentricity and high degree of obstruction
These lesion characteristics are associated with procedural problems in wiring, dilatation and stenting of the lesion. However, after successful DES implantation the long-term results seem to be excellent. Debulking by directional- or rotational atherectomy and ostial cutting balloon side branch dilatation have also been advocated, but so far there is no hard evidence on these recommendations.

Calcification
Severe calcification is associated with difficulties in dilatation and stenting. Also, calcification is associated with increased risk of stent thrombosis. Use of rotational atherectomy may be the only way to treat these very difficult lesions, and prophylactic rotational atherectomy has been advocated by some interventionalists to facilitate and optimize stent implantation.

Tortuosity of the Bifurcation Region and the Vessel Proximal to the Bifurcation
Vessel tortuosity is a general problem in PCI and the problems are especially pronounced in bifurcation lesions with involvement of multiple wires, balloons and stents. With optimal predilatation, use of flexible stents, buddy wire technique and selection of a simple bifurcation approach these difficulties can usually be overcome.

Lesion Length
A long lesion located in the main vessel does not constitute a major problem after the introduction of DES. However, the option of leaving the side branch without a stent may not be possible in bifurcations with a long lesion located in the side branch.

Thrombus
Thrombotic lesions are primarily seen in the setting of acute myocardial infarction. In case of excessive thrombus located in both main vessel and side branch we usually perform thrombectomy and balloon dilatation after GPIIb/IIIa loading trying to minimize the use of stents. A special and potentially severe clinical problem may be seen with heavy thrombus burden at the ostium of the LAD or the Cx. Dilatation or stenting of this type of lesion may result in disastrous thrombus embolization to the adjacent artery. In these cases we recommend insertion of a guidewire or even a filter in the adjacent artery before treating the culprit lesion.

Bifurcation Treatment Strategies

In clinical practice, it has been difficult to choose a treatment strategy based on the lesion types mentioned above because of difficulties in assessing the true plaque burden and localization by angiography alone, and because plaque shift during the PCI procedure may be pronounced and unpredictable. Also, side branch angulation may be modified by the procedure.

A number of different treatment strategies have been recommended by different centers or by opinion leaders in the field of PCI. The different treatment strategies may be divided in two basic strategies:

1. The simple one stent strategy of stenting main vessel and optional treatment of side branch.
2. The complex two stent strategy of stenting both main vessel and side branch.

Although it is usually not problematic to switch from a one stent to a two stent technique, the operator should decide on which technique to be used before the procedure, so that adequate guiding and access site may be used from the beginning of the procedure. Also, the conventional crush technique cannot be used, if the procedure is initiated with stenting of the main vessel.

Randomized Studies on the Treatment of Bifurcation Lesions

Whilst there are no randomized trials from the bare metal stent era assessing different stent strategies in bifurcation lesions, there are randomized studies on the use of DES and different stent techniques [6,7,10], with the large British BBC I study, also recently presented [11]. The Sirius bifurcation study compared optional side branch stenting with a two stent approach. Unfortunately, the crossover rate in this study was high and the results were not analysed according to the intention to treat principle [7]. A 3.5% risk of stent thrombosis in patients, who had been stented in both branches, raised a concern for this strategy [7]. In a study by Pan *et al.* [6] patients were randomized to a simple vs. a complex strategy of bifurcation treatment using a Sirolimus-eluting stent. In this study the main branch was stented and the side branch dilated with balloon. According to randomization the side branch was subsequently stented or not stented. MACE rates were low in both groups, and the overall conclusion from this study was that both strategies were effective in reducing restenosis rate, with no differences in terms of clinical outcome.

In the Nordic Bifurcation Study, 413 patients with a bifurcation lesion were randomized to DES implantation in the main vessel or to DES implantation both in the main vessel and the side branch. The primary end point MACE (cardiac death, myocardial infarction, target vessel revascularization or stent thrombosis) after six months showed no significant differences between the two groups; MV+SB 3.4%, MV 2.9%. However, in the MV+SB group there were significantly longer procedure and fluoroscopy times, higher contrast volumes and higher rates of procedure related increase in biomarkers of myocardial injury. In a subgroup of 307 patients a quantitative coronary assessment was performed at the index procedure and after eight months. The combined angiographic end point of diameter stenosis >50% of main vessel and occlusion of the side branch after eight months was found in 5.3% in the MV and in 5.1% in the MV+SB group. The authors concluded that independent of stenting strategy, excellent clinical and angiographic results were obtained, and that the simple stenting strategy of stenting the MV could be recommended as the routine bifurcation stenting technique. In the BBC I study [11], provisional T-stenting using the Taxus stent, instead of the crush or culotte techniques, was associated with a lower rate of death, MI, and target-vessel failure (TVF) at nine months (8.0% versus 15.2%, p = 0.009 for the combined end-point).

Stenting of Main Vessel and Optional Treatment of Side Branch
The Step By Step Approach

This is the standard bifurcation strategy at many centres, often referred to as the step by step approach. It may be carried out in different ways. The strategy described here was used in the Nordic Bifurcation Study. It is shown as a cartoon in Figure 19.2 and may be described step by step as follows:

1. Wiring of main vessel and side branch.
2. Balloon pre-dilatation of main vessel and/or side branch.
3. Stenting of main vessel with both wires in place.
4. Optional post-dilatation of the proximal part of the main vessel.
5. If the flow in the side branch is normal (TIMI 3 flow) after stenting the main vessel, the procedure is completed.

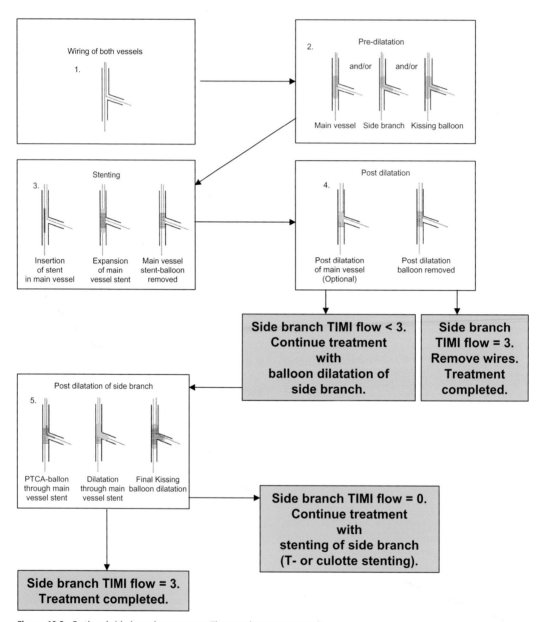

Figure 19.2. Optional side branch treatment. The step by step approach.

6. If the side branch TIMI flow rate is <3, the side branch is dilated through the main vessel stent struts.

7. The side branch is stented, if the side branch TIMI flow rate is 0 after dilatation. Thus, side branch stenting is not indicated merely because of residual stenosis or dissection. T or culotte techniques may be applied. We do not recommend internal crush in this situation or in general.

Some interventionalists may find these recommendations for side branch treatment after main vessel stenting too conservative. However, this approach was used in the Nordic Bifurcation Study with excellent clinical and angiographic results [10]. Other investigators use wider and not always quite clear indications for stenting of the side branch. Using the simple technique described, there may be significant residual stenosis of the side branch ostium at the end of the procedure. However, a post-procedure side branch stenosis seems to be associated with few long-term clinical problems and seems to decrease over time, probably due to elements of post-stenting side branch spasm and plaque shift, which may diminish over time.

Stenting of Both Main Vessel and Side Branch

This technique has gained increasing popularity in the DES era, as the restenosis problems by the use of multiple BMS in bifurcations seems to have been solved with the advent of DES. However, none of the techniques have been subject of randomized studies and long-term data are not available.

In the two stent strategy, both vessels are wired and usually pre-dilated. Thereafter, there are a number of treatment options:

Stent Crush Technique

The side branch is stented with a non-expanded stent in the main vessel (Figure 19.3). The side branch stent is implanted with its proximal end protruding more than half of the main vessel diameter into the main vessel. The side branch wire is removed and the side branch stent crushed during expansion of the main vessel stent [12]. Initially the crushed part of the side branch stent was rather long. Now, most operators try to minimize the length of the crush in order to avoid larger areas with multiple layers of stent (minimal crush technique).

A variant of this technique is the inverted crush technique. Here the main vessel stent is crushed by the side branch stent. Another variant is the internal crush technique. Here the side branch stent is crushed within the main vessel stent.

Problems with the crush technique include difficulties in re-wiring of the side branch through the main vessel stent and the crushed side branch stent. If rewiring is unsuccessful by a conventional soft wire, a hydrophilic wire will almost always do the job. It may be necessary to use 1.5 or 1.25 mm low profile balloons to get access to the side branch for final side branch dilatation. A final kissing balloon dilatation is strongly recommended. The crush technique necessitates a 7 or 8Fr guiding catheter.

Balloon Crush Technique

The balloon crush technique is identical to the stent crush technique with the exception that the side branch stent is crushed with a dilatation balloon. Thereafter, the main vessel stent is implanted, usually without problems. This technique can be performed through a 6Fr guiding catheter.

Culotte Technique

Here the side branch or the main vessel is stented (Figure 19.4). The non-stented vessel is wired, dilated and stented through the implanted stent, so that a varying part of the proximal main vessel lesion is covered by two stents, one inside the other. Then the first vessel is re-wired and re-dilated through the second stent [13]. It is advisable to stent the main vessel first. If re-wiring is unsuccessful by a conventional soft wire, a hydrophilic wire will usually be successful. It may be necessary to use 1.5 or 1.25 mm low profile balloons to get access to the side branch through the main vessel stent. We have found this technique safe and very promising concerning long-term results and use this technique in large vessel bifurcations with less than 1.5 mm diameter size between main vessel and side branch. The culotte technique should probably not be used when there is large

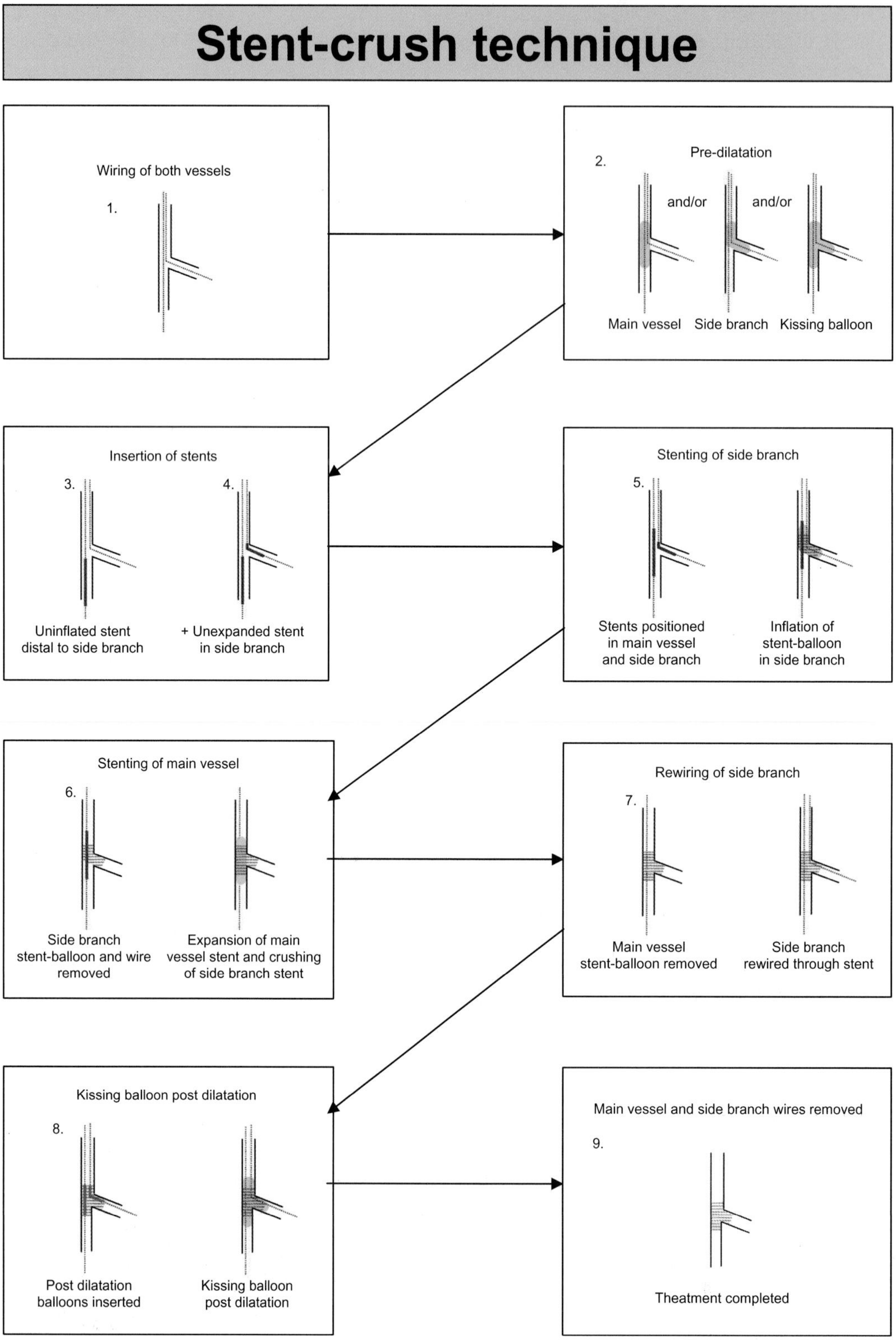

Stent-crush technique

Figure 19.3. The stent crush technique.

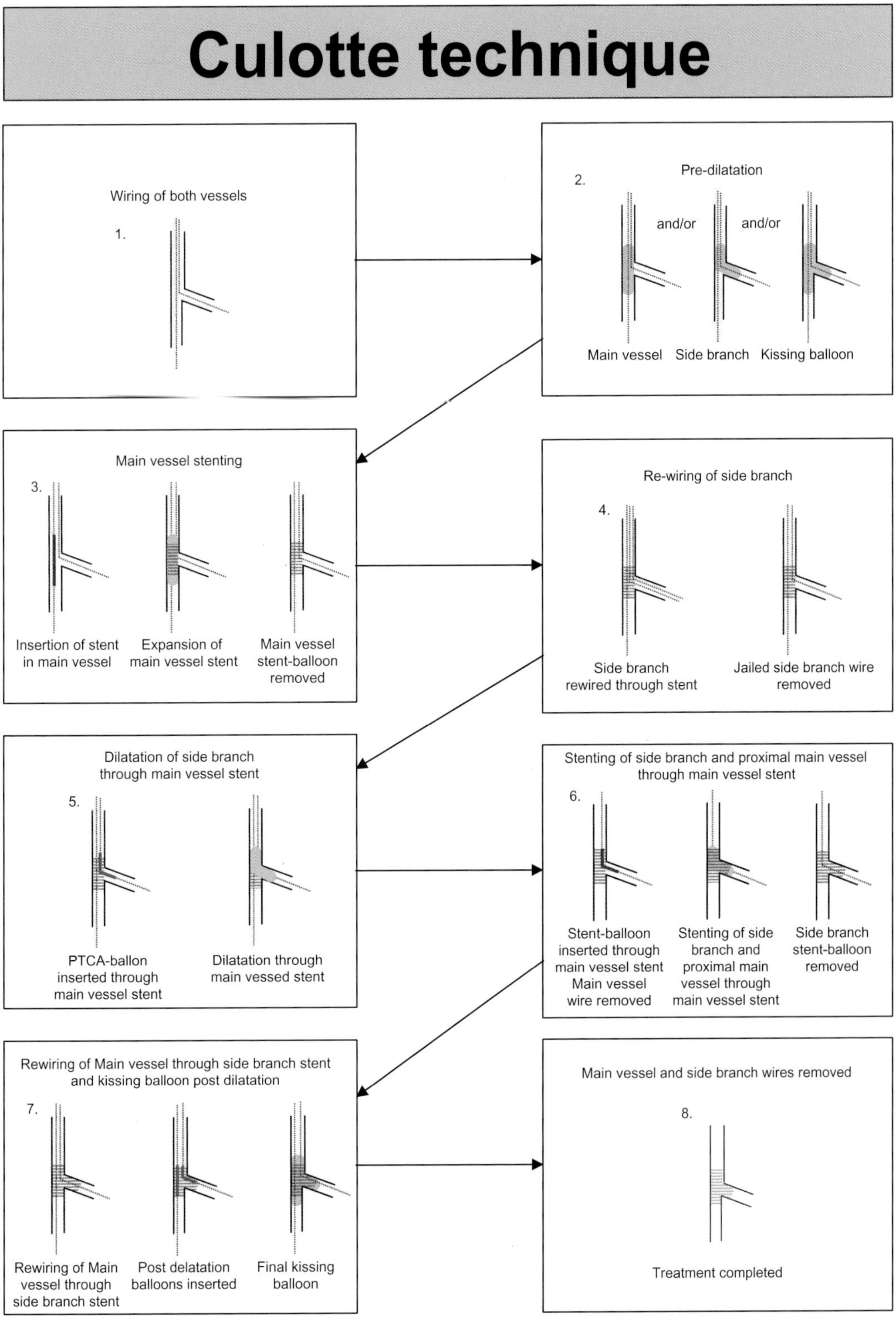

Culotte technique

1. Wiring of both vessels

2. Pre-dilatation
and/or   and/or
Main vessel   Side branch   Kissing balloon

3. Main vessel stenting
Insertion of stent in main vessel   Expansion of main vessel stent   Main vessel stent-balloon removed

4. Re-wiring of side branch
Side branch rewired through stent   Jailed side branch wire removed

5. Dilatation of side branch through main vessel stent
PTCA-ballon inserted through main vessel stent   Dilatation through main vessed stent

6. Stenting of side branch and proximal main vessel through main vessel stent
Stent-balloon inserted through main vessel stent Main vessel wire removed   Stenting of side branch and proximal main vessel through main vessel stent   Side branch stent-balloon removed

7. Rewiring of Main vessel through side branch stent and kissing balloon post dilatation
Rewiring of Main vessel through side branch stent   Post delatation balloons inserted   Final kissing balloon

8. Main vessel and side branch wires removed
Treatment completed

Figure 19.4. The culotte technique.

difference between main vessel and side branch diameter.

T-technique

The main vessel is stented, and the side branch stented through the stent struts of the main vessel stent (Figure 19.5). Alternatively, the side branch may be stented first with the side branch stent not protruding into the main vessel. This can be obtained by inflating a balloon in the main vessel and pulling the side branch stent against the main vessel balloon before deployment. Problems with this technique include a high re-stenosis rate of the side branch ostium, because it may be difficult to get full stent coverage of the bifurcation area with this technique. The technique has been very popular in procedures when the side branch needs to be stented after main vessel stent implantation.

V-technique

Both side branch and main vessel are stented with the stents side by side and with the formation of a very short stent carina. In cases with a rather long carina, this technique may be called double barrel technique or Y-technique. If the V-stenting is preceded with stenting of the main vessel just proximal to the bifurcation, the technique has been referred to as the skirt technique, triple stenting technique or extended Y-technique [14]. The V-techniques all have a stent carina in common. The V-techniques will need a 7 or 8Fr guiding catheter. In principle, the V-techniques differ from other techniques in the creation of a stent carina in the distal bifurcation area. Crush, culotte and T-techniques aim at reconstructing a bifurcation with full stent cover. Presence of an intraluminal stent carina may rise to concern regarding late stent thrombosis in V-stented patients, especially after stopping antiplatelet therapy. Therefore, long-term safety data are needed, before V-stent technique with a long carina can be generally recommended.

Jailing of Guidewires

Jailing of a side branch guidewire between the vessel wall and the proximal part of the main vessel stent is an important precaution in keeping the side branch open after expansion of the main vessel

stent, and removal of a jailed wire is usually unproblematic. However, a wire with damaged wire tip should not be jailed as the deformed tip may get trapped in the stents. Likewise, in two stent procedures a guidewire should never be jailed between two stents.

Kissing Balloon Dilatation

Although there are no randomized data on this issue, register data and sub group analyses concurrently indicate that the above mentioned bifurcation techniques should be finalized by a kissing balloon dilatation [15]. Although there is a constant vessel size relation between the proximal main vessel diameter (PMVD) and the diameter of the distal main vessel (DMVD) and the side branch diameter (SBD), such as PMVD = $0.678 \times (DMVD + SBD)$, we usually use the size of the stent balloons for the final kissing balloon dilatation.

General Treatment Principles
Geographical Miss Using DES

Based on data from the Sirius and the TAXUS studies [16,17] it is recommended to avoid pretreatment of segments, which will not be covered by DES. Also, all parts of the lesion should be completely covered by DES. These recommendations are not always easy to meet in complex bifurcation lesions subsets.

Access Site

The radial or the femoral approach can be used. The most common used size of guiding is 6Fr, but 7 or 8Fr is used in crush- and V-technique procedures.

Anti-thrombotic Treatment

A bifurcation lesion does not by itself indicate special anti-thrombotic treatment strategies. Thus, unfractionated heparin or low-molecular weight heparin, angiox and GPIIb/IIIa inhibitors may be used according to local hospital routine. We recommend life long Acetylsalicylic Acid (ASA) treatment and 12 months clopidogrel treatment for all DES treated patients. Further, we have a low threshold for recommending life long double platelet therapy in left main bifurcation scenarios.

T-stent technique

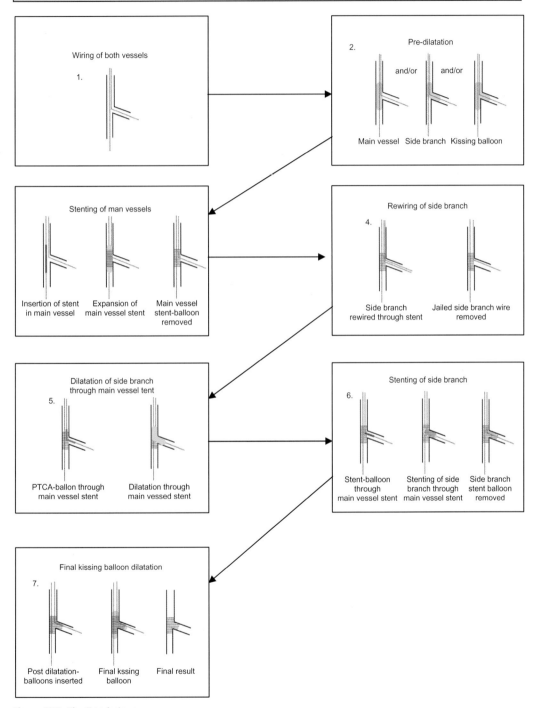

Figure 19.5. The T technique.

Biomarkers

Biomarkers will be increased in 8–18% of bifurcation treated patients and most prevalent when complex bifurcation techniques are used [10]. However, the long-term clinical significance of procedure related biomarker increase is probably small.

Stents

DES or BMS?

Use of DES in bifurcation lesions is not recommended by the FDA, because bifurcation lesion was a contraindication in the first DES vs. BMS studies. Iakovou *et al.* [18] suggested increased risk of late stent thrombosis after DES in bifurcation lesions. However, recent studies [19,20] does not indicate a safety problem with these stents. Also, the 14 months follow-up data of the Nordic Bifurcation study, presented at the ESC 2007, showed rates of angiographic proven stent thrombosis combined with sudden cardiac death of 2.0% in the main vessel stented group vs. 0.5% in the both main vessel and side branch stented group. Therefore, we recommend the use of DES in bifurcation lesions. BMS may be used in one stent treatment situations, but should be avoided in lesions, where both main vessel and side branch are stented.

Dedicated Bifurcation Stents

Dedicated bifurcation stents have been under investigation for years with no proven superiority to the currently used techniques. The diversity of bifurcation lesions is a major difficulty in the development of dedicated bifurcation devices.

Summary

In PCI, bifurcations are a challenging lesion subset. It is recommended to use the step by step approach (stenting of main vessel and optional treatment of side branch). This is a simple approach that keeps the main vessel treatment in focus. In experienced hands results of the complex two stent strategies are equally good and may be preferred in large side branch bifurcations. Treatment with DES combined with at least 12 months of dual antiplatelet therapy seems to especially efficient in bifurcation lesions. A two stent procedure should always be finalized with kissing balloon dilatation.

Questions

1. **With regard to bifurcation stenting which statement is true?**

   A T-shaped lesions (angle between side branch and main branch >70 degrees) are easier to wire and plaque shifting is more common than Y-shaped lesions (SB – MB angle <70 degrees)

   B Wiring of the side branch in a T-shaped lesion results in a more favorable angle for subsequent access

   C Initial access to side branch of T-shaped lesions is easier than Y-shaped lesions

   D The jailed wire technique is contraindicated for T lesions

2. **With regard to bifurcation PCI:**

   A Overall restenosis rates are reduced when two stents are used rather than one

   B Stent thrombosis occurs more frequently if one stent is used rather than 2

   C The use of the kissing balloon post dilatation technique improves event free survival when the crush technique is used

   D The V or SKS technique is most suitable for true bifurcation lesions involving the proximal main branch (French classification Type 1 lesions)

3. **Application of kissing stenting in the crush technique:**

   A Is successful in <80% of lesions

   B Leads to a reduction in restenosis and TLR

   C Leads to a better initial angiographic result with no long term clinical advantages

   D Requires at least 8Fr guiding catheters

   E Is indicated only with acute angles between the daughter vessels

4. **Which of these techniques is the operator committed to stent both branches:**

   A Culotte

   B V-Stenting (simultaneous kissing stenting)

   C Inverted Crush Stenting

   D T-stenting

   E Cross-over stenting

5. **Which is the technique of bifurcational stenting which forces the operator to alternatively loose access to both the SB and the MV during the procedure?**

   A Culotte

   B V-Stenting (simultaneous kissing stenting)

   C Crush Stenting

   D T-stenting

   E Inverted Crush Stenting

References

1. Meier B, Gruentzig AR, King SB III, et al. Risk of side branch occlusion during coronary angioplasty. Am J Cardiol 1984; **53**: 10–104.

2. Pinkerton CA, Slack JD, Van Tassel JW, et al. Angioplasty for dilatation of complex coronary artery bifurcation stenoses. Am J Cardiol 1985; **55**: 1626-1628.

3. Al Suwaidi J, Yeh W, Cohen HA, et al. Immediate and one-year outcome in patients with coronary bifurcation lesions in the modern era (NHLBI dynamic registry). Am J Cardiol 2001; **87**: 1139–1144.

4. Yamashita T, Nishida T, Adamian MG, et al. Bifurcation lesions: two stents vs. one stent—immediate and follow-up results. J Am Coll Cardiol 2000; **35**: 1145–1151.

5. Thuesen L, Kelbaek H, Klovgaard L, et al. SCANDSTENT Investigators. Comparison of sirolimus-eluting and bare metal stents in coronary bifurcation lesions: subgroup analysis of the Stenting Coronary Arteries in Non-Stress/Benestent Disease Trial (SCANDSTENT). Am Heart J 2006; **152**: 1140–1145.

6. Pan M, de Lezo JS, Medina A, et al. Rapamycin-eluting stents for the treatment of bifurcated coronary lesions: a randomized comparison of a simple vs. complex strategy. Am Heart J 2004; **148**: 857–864.

7. Colombo A, Moses JW, Morice MC, et al. Randomized study to evaluate sirolimus-eluting stents implanted at coronary bifurcation lesions. Circulation 2004; **109**: 1244–1249.

8. Legrand V, Thomas M, Zelisko M, et al. Percutaneous coronary intervention of bifurcationlesions: state-of-the-art. Insight from the second meeting of the European Bifurcation Club. Eurointerv 2007; **3**: 44–49.

9. Medina A, Suarez de Lezo J, et al. A new classification of coronary bifurcation lesions. Rev Esp Cardiol 2006; **59**: 183.

10. Steigen TK, Maeng M, Wiseth R, et al. Nordic PCI Study Group. Randomized study on simple versus. complex stenting of coronary artery bifurcation lesions: the Nordic bifurcation study. Circulation 2006; **114**: 1955–1961.

11. Hildick-Smith DJ. British Bifurcation Coronary Study. *TCT. Washington* 2008.

12. Colombo A, Stankovic G, Orlic D, et al. Modified T-stenting technique with crushing for bifurcation

lesions: immediate results and 30-day outcome. Catheter Cardiovasc Interv 2003; **60**: 145–151.

13. Chevalier B, Glatt B, Royer T, *et al.* Placement of coronary stents in bifurcation lesions by the "culotte" technique. Am J Cardiol 1998; **82**(8): 943–949.

14. Helqvist S, Jorgensen E, Kelbaek H, *et al.* Percutaneous treatment of coronary bifurcation lesions: a novel "extended Y" technique with complete lesion stent coverage. Heart 2006; **92**: 981–982.

15. Ge L, Airoldi F, Iakovou I, *et al.* Clinical and angiographic outcome after implantation of drug-eluting stents in bifurcation lesions with the crush stent technique: importance of final kissing balloon post-dilation. J Am Coll Cardiol 2005; **46**: 613–620.

16. Stone GW, Ellis SG, Cox DA, *et al.* TAXUS-IV Investigators. A polymer-based, paclitaxel-eluting stent in patients with coronary artery disease. N Engl J Med 2004; **350**: 221–231.

17. Moses JW, Leon MB, Popma JJ, *et al.* SIRIUS Investigators. Sirolimus-eluting stents versus standard stents in patients with stenosis in a native coronary artery. N Engl J Med 2003; **349**: 1315–1323.

18. Iakovou I, Schmidt T, Bonizzoni E, *et al.* Incidence, predictors, and outcome of thrombosis after successful implantation of drug-eluting stents. JAMA 2005; **293**: 2126–2130.

19. Tsuchida K, Colombo A, Lefevre T, *et al.* The clinical outcome of percutaneous treatment of bifurcation lesions in multivessel coronary artery disease with the sirolimus-eluting stent: insights from the Arterial Revascularization Therapies Study part II (ARTS II). Eur Heart J 2007; **28**: 433–442.

20. Kelbaek H, Thuesen L, Helqvist S, *et al.* SCANDSTENT Investigators. The Stenting Coronary Arteries in Non-stress/benestent Disease (SCANDSTENT) trial. J Am Coll Cardiol 2006; **47**: 449–455.

Answers

1. B
2. C
3. B
4. B
5. A

CHAPTER 20

Approach to Multivessel Coronary Artery Disease

Bryan P. Yan[1], Andrew E. Ajani[2], & David J. Clark[3]

[1] Prince of Wales Hospital and Department of Medicine and Therapeutics, The Chinese University of Hong Kong, Hong Kong, China
[2] Royal Melbourne Hospital, Melbourne, VIC, Australia
[3] Austin Hospital, Melbourne, VIC, Australia

Introduction

Myocardial revascularization in patients with multivessel coronary artery disease (MVD) may be accomplished by percutaneous coronary interventions (PCI) or coronary artery bypass grafting (CABG). Approximately two thirds of patients who require revascularization have MVD and two thirds of these have anatomy that is amenable to treatment by percutaneous or open heart surgery. Large trials in the 1990s have shown that PCI can be equally successful compared to the "gold standard" CABG for patients with MVD [1,2]. Today, more complex lesions and sicker patients are being taken for multivessel PCI, the success rates have increased and complication rates have remained the same or improved [3,4]. This has been brought about by increasing operator experience, technological advances such as the availability of drug-eluting stents (DES) and more potent antiplatelet therapy with glycoprotein 2b3a receptor antagonists and clopidogrel. As a result, the frequency of multivessel PCI is expected to increase.

Many factors should be considered when approaching a patient with MVD. First, these patients have a less favorable long-term outcome. They are more likely to have adverse clinical fea-

tures including diabetes mellitus, prior myocardial infarction, and reduced left ventricular function. Secondly, the functional significance and complexity of each lesion need to be assessed to determine the appropriate percutaneous strategy. Procedural complexity and the risk of multivessel intervention is increased when unfavorable anatomy such as chronic total occlusions, calcified bifurcation lesions, and diffusely diseased small vessels are present. Thirdly, the impact of restenosis needs to be considered. (See Figure 20.1.) The decision to choose PCI as a revascularization strategy should be based not only on whether it can be done safely and successfully but also on its short- and long-term benefit when compared to the alternative of medical or surgical treatment (Table 20.1).

Revascularization Strategy

The extent of planned revascularization, on all diseased lesions or directed to selectively targeted coronary segments, is a major determinant of treatment strategy.

Complete Revascularization

The concept of complete revascularization initiated from early studies on CABG which demonstrated that patients who were completely revascularized derived symptomatic and survival benefits over those who were incompletely revascularized [5,6]. Patients with diabetes mellitus,

Interventional Cardiology, First Edition. Edited by Carlo Di Mario, George D. Dangas, Peter Barlis.
© 2010 Blackwell Publishing Ltd. Published 2010 by Blackwell Publishing Ltd.

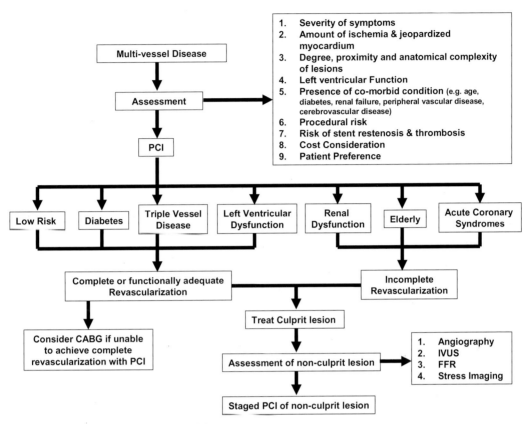

Figure 20.1. Approach to PCI for multivessel disease.

Table 20.1. High risk MVD patient sub-sets to consider CABG.

High Risk Features
Diabetes mellitus
Renal failure
Impaired left ventricular function
Inability to achieve complete revascularization with PCI
Multiple chronic total occlusions
Left main disease
Three vessel disease
Diffuse disease

extensive coronary artery disease, large ischemic burden and left ventricular dysfunction, required the most complete revascularization to achieve long-term event-free survival.

There is large variability in the definition of completeness of myocardial revascularization adopted by different studies. We propose a simple definition that takes into account the size of the vessel, the severity of the lesion and the viability of the myocardial territory (Table 20.2). An anatomically complete revascularization is accomplished when all vessels with clinically significant stenosis (≥50% stenosis in vessel >1.5 mm diameter) are treated irrespective of the underlying myocardial function. A functionally complete revascularization refers to cases in which only lesions supplying viable myocardium are treated. Therefore, revascularization may be anatomically incomplete but functionally adequate.

Although complete revascularization is the goal in most patients undergoing multivessel intervention, incomplete revascularization is common in clinical practice. The ability to achieve complete revascularization depends on the selection of patients. In early angioplasty series, only 40–60% patients with MVD undergoing PCI had complete revascularization [6–8]. Reasons for not attempting to treat all diseased vessels may include the

Table 20.2. Revascularization strategies in patients with multivessel coronary artery disease.

Strategy		Definition
Anatomic	Functional	
Complete	Complete	Treatment of all coronary segments >1.5 mm in diameter with ≥50% stenosis
Incomplete	Adequate	Treatment of all coronary segments ≥50% stenosis supplying viable myocardium
Incomplete	Incomplete	Inability to treat all coronary segments with ≥50% stenosis supplying viable myocardium

presence of chronic total occlusions, the presence of serious medical conditions such as severe left ventricular dysfunction, or the decision to treat only the "culprit lesion" that is thought to be responsible for the patient's symptoms. Functionally adequate revascularization aims to treat all significant stenoses in vessels that supply viable myocardium. Lesions in small or diffusely diseased vessels and lesions serving infarcted territories may be safely left alone.

Culprit Lesion Strategy

Culprit lesion refers to the lesion responsible for the acute coronary syndrome or the stenosis most likely responsible for the patient's symptoms. In most cases of MVD, target or culprit lesion can be identified by a combination of historical data, electrocardiographic findings, angiography supplemented by radionucletide studies, intravascular ultrasonography or Doppler wire. Morphological characteristics that are associated with an unstable or culprit lesion include scalloped edges, irregular borders and the presence of thrombus. In patients in whom a culprit lesion or lesions can be determined, PCI can be directed to treat that lesion alone without exposing the patient to the risks of dilating other lesions not responsible for the patient's symptoms. If the patient continues to have angina or a subsequent stress test shows ischemia in that territory, a second procedure can be performed to revascularize the vessel that was previously not attempted.

The safety, efficacy, and costs of complete versus culprit vessel PCI was assessed in patients with MVD with an identifiable culprit vessel randomly assigned to complete revascularization of all vessels ≥50% stenoses (n = 108) versus revascularization limited to the culprit vessel (n = 111). Complete revascularization was associated with a lower strategy success rate (81.5% vs 93.7%, p = .007), similar 4-years MACE rates (40.4% vs. 34.6%), and initially higher costs. However, over the long term, more repeat PCI were conducted in patients treated by culprit revascularization only, mostly because of the need to treat lesions initially left untreated. As a consequence, costs had equalized within one year [9]. Therefore, the decision of whether to perform culprit vessel or complete revascularization needs to be individualized.

Staged PCI

The decision to perform multivessel PCI in the same procedure or planned staged procedures include the desire to diminish procedural risk, avoid excessive contrast use, lessen patient discomfort, and reduce physician fatigue. Whereas it is reasonable to attempt two simple lesions during the same procedure, the presence of complex lesion should deter the operator from attempting more than one lesion at a time.

Staging potentially limits the amount of myocardium at risk in the event of acute closure. However, the incidence of acute closure is rare with the advent of stents and dual-antiplatelet therapy. Although techniques for PCI have improved, multivessel PCI is still associated with increased peri-procedural risk. A prospective observational study evaluating multivessel and single-vessel procedures showed multivessel PCI was a predictor of postprocedural troponin T rise (OR 1.90, 95% CI 1.17–3.06) and a higher incidence of cardiac events during follow-up [10]. In patients who presented with acute coronary syndrome, multivessel PCI was more often associated with peri-procedural myocardial infarction than single-vessel intervention, although this did not translate into higher one-year mortality [11].

Multivessel PCI during the same setting has several inherent advantages. It expedites patient care, avoids a second invasive procedure with its associated morbidity, and reduces total radiation exposure and potentially cost. However, multivessel intervention is associated with a higher procedural contrast use and should be avoided in situations where the risk of contrast induced nephropathy is high.

The order in which diseased vessels are treated needs to planned. In acute coronary syndrome, the culprit lesion is treated first. In elective PCI for stable angina, the artery either supplying the largest amount of myocardium or involving the technically most difficult lesion is usually approached first. Chronic total occlusions are often the most technically demanding lesions to treat and are usually approached first in multivessel PCI. In the event of failed PCI to the CTO, the patient could be referred for CABG. Before attempting to open a CTO, it is important to determine the viability of the myocardium supplied by the occluded artery. The hypothesis that late mechanical reperfusion in patients with asymptomatic occluded infarct-related artery will improve long-term clinical outcomes remains to be proved.

The time interval for planning the second procedure varies from days to few months according to the operator's discretion. One approach is to stage at an interval of 4–8 weeks to allow the first lesion to stabilize with complete endothelialization (when bare-metal stents are used). However, with advances in PCI, the safety and long-term outcomes of multivessel PCI has improved. Recently, patients who underwent staged PCI within seven days after an AMI had satisfactory outcomes [12].

Assessment of Non-culprit or Intermediate Lesion

Assessment of a coronary lesion of intermediate severity continues to be a challenge. There can be significant observer variability in interpretation of the severity of an intermediate coronary lesion defined as luminal stenosis >40% but <70%. Intravascular ultrasound (IVUS) has become a more accurate standard for defining the severity of atherosclerosis and luminal dimensions compared to angiography. In the cardiac catheterization laboratory, coronary pressure wire-derived fractional flow reserve (FFR) can be used to determine the

physiologic significance of a coronary stenosis that is distinct from the anatomic visualization provided by IVUS. This method relies on the decrease in intra-arterial pressure induced by a functionally significant stenosis to determine whether an intermediate lesion is producing ischemia.

High Risk Patients

The risk-benefit ratio must be assessed carefully for each patient with MVD. The risks of complications from PCI depend on several factors, including specific anatomic features of the artery and lesion, the overall cardiac and non-cardiac condition of the patients, and the clinical setting.

Risk models can be used to help predict the likelihood of procedural complication. For example, the Mayo Clinic risk score using seven variables (age, myocardial infarction less than or equal to 24 hours, pre-procedural shock, serum creatinine level, left ventricular ejection fraction, congestive heart failure, and peripheral artery disease) has been validated to predict MACE and procedural death with excellent discrimination [13]. The model was robust across many subgroups, including those undergoing elective PCI, those with diabetes mellitus, and in elderly patients.

Acute Coronary Syndrome

Patients with acute coronary syndrome (ACS) frequently presents with multiple complex coronary plaques. About 40–60% of patients who presented with acute myocardial infarction have evidence of ulcerated plaques or thrombus in other than the infarct-related artery (IRA) [14]. Patients with intermediate-to-high risk non-ST elevation ACS, based on clinical, biomarker and angiographic assessment, should undergo early revascularization. In this scenario, initial incomplete revascularization with PCI of the culprit lesion/s is preferred with subsequent staged PCI to non-culprit lesions if required. Whether the patient will ultimately need surgical bypass or staged PCI should be determined at time of initial angiography. If the patient is a surgical candidate, balloon angioplasty alone or bare-metal stents should be used to avoid delay to surgery due to the need for prolonged dual-antiplatelet therapy after drug-eluting stent implantation.

In patients with MVD and ST elevation myocardial infarction (STEMI), the conventional strategy for primary PCI is recanalization of the IRA with decisions about PCI of non-culprit lesions at later follow-up guided by objective evidence of residual ischemia. The current ACC/AHA guideline gives a class III indication for elective PCI on non infarct related lesion/vessel at time of primary PCI for acute STEMI [15]. The decision to defer non-culprit lesion PCI is supported by evidence of possible overestimation of non-culprit lesion severity in the setting of acute MI due to enhanced vascular tone often resistant to nitrate administration [16,17].

With the improvement of PCI outcomes, recent studies have shown multivessel PCI during acute myocardial infarction may be safe in selected patients compared with treating only the IRA [18,19]. Multivessel PCI during STEMI should be considered when the patient remains hemodynamically unstable after PCI of the IRA. This can occur if there is more than one IRA or critical stenoses in non-IRA that supply a significant amount of myocardium not collateralized by the IRA. Potential advantages of multivessel PCI during STEMI include decrease in ischemic burden and improvement of LV function.

Diabetes Mellitus

Diabetic patients with MVD typically have smaller vessel size, longer lesion length and greater plaque burden compared to non-diabetic patients. These adverse characteristics are associated with accelerated atherosclerosis, high restenosis rates and less favorable long-term survival following PCI compared to non-diabetic patients. Most trials comparing CABG with PCI in diabetic patients have shown increased long-term survival with CABG [20]. Based on long-term outcomes from large randomized trials comparing bare-metal stents and CABG [20–23], CABG remains the preferred treatment for diabetic patients with MVD (Table 20.3). Recent advent of DES may narrow the gap between PCI and CABG in MVD in terms of the need for repeat revascularization. Currently, two prospective randomized trials (FREEDOM, CARDIA) specifically designed to compare the outcomes of diabetic patients treated with either

Table 20.3. Summary of major trials comparing PCI vs. CABG for MVD in the stent era.

	ARTS (21)	ERACI II (23)	SoS (22)	AWESOME (24)	ARTS II (31)	ERACI III (32)
Number of Patients	1205	450	988	454	607	225
Primary Endpoint	MACCE-free survival at 1 yr	MACCE at 30-days	Rate of revascularization	Survival	MACCE-free survival at 1 yr	MACCE-free survival at 3 yr
Trial Design	Randomized PCI vs. CABG	Randomized PCI vs. CABG	Randomized PCI vs. CABG	Randomized PCI vs. CABG	PCI registry with same inclusion criteria ARTS	PCI registry with same inclusion criteria ERACI II
Diabetics, %	17	17	14	31	26	20.4
3-vessel disease, %	31	56	42	45	54	38
Ejection fraction, %	61	N/A	57	45	60	N/A
Stent type	BMS	BMS	BMS	BMS	DES	DES
GP IIb/IIIa use, %	N/A	28	8	11	33	N/A
MACCE at 1–3 year follow-up (PCI vs. CABG, %)	26.2 vs. 12.2	29.8 vs. 22.7	22.5 vs. 12.4	52 vs. 39	10.4	22.7

MACCE = Major adverse cardiac and cerebral events.

Table 20.4. Current trials comparing PCI vs. CABG for MVD.

	CARDIA	*SYNTAX*	*FREEDOM*
Trial Design	Randomized with associated registries	Randomized with nested registries	Randomized with nested registries
Inclusion Criteria	Diabetics with MVD or complex single vessel disease	3-vessel disease, LM disease or LM equivalent	Diabetics with MVD
Number of Patients	600	1500	2400
Study Stent	Sirolimus-eluting stent	Paclitaxel-eluting stent	Sirolimus- or paclitaxel-eluting stent
Primary Endpoints	12-month MACCE	12-month MACCE	5-year mortality

MACCE = Major adverse cardiac and cerebral events.

CABG or PCI with DES are ongoing (Table 20.4, see below).

Elderly

Elderly patients have a higher risk profile compared to younger patients and mandate thorough clinical evaluation before acceptance for PCI. The long-term benefit of PCI in the elderly remains controversial. Culprit lesion PCI for symptom relief may be adequate in most patients rather than aiming for complete revascularization despite more extensive coronary disease than younger patients.

Left Ventricular Dysfunction

Left ventricular dysfunction is a major determinant of peri-procedural risk. Complete revascularization of viable myocardium in patients with MVD and left ventricular dysfunction is a strong independent predictor for improved survival [24]. Currently available non-invasive techniques to assess myocardial viability include thallium single photon emission computed tomography (SPECT), dobutamine echocardiography, positron emission tomography with ^{18}F-fluoro-deoxyglucose and contrast-enhanced magnetic resonance imaging. A study by Sciagra *et al.* demonstrated that survival of patients with preserved viability treated with complete revascularization (PCI or CABG) was significantly better than patients treated with either medical therapy (p < 0.0002) or incomplete revascularization (p < 0.03) [25].

Renal Dysfunction

Patients with renal dysfunction are at increased risk of developing contrast-induced nephropathy (CIN) and long-term mortality after PCI [26,27]. The cornerstone of CIN prevention is adequate pre-hydration. In patient at increased risk for CIN, nephrotoxic medications should be withheld, N-acetylcysteine should be considered for prophylaxis, and low or iso-osmolar contrast agents should be utilized. A strategy of staging the PCI initially targeting the culprit lesion is preferable to minimize contrast volume.

Three Vessel Disease

Triple vessel PCI is more likely to result in incomplete revascularization and less favorable outcomes compared to CABG. A study of 59,000 patients with MVD from the New York registries of CABG and PCI demonstrated survival benefit for surgery in patients with three-vessel disease [28]. However, triple vessel disease can be highly heterogeneous. Patients with multifocal discrete stenoses are generally amendable to PCI whereas CABG is preferable for those with diffuse disease and multiple chronic total occlusions.

Restenosis and Drug-eluting Stents

Restenosis has remained one of the main limitations of coronary balloon angioplasty and stenting since its introduction 25 years ago, particularly for patients with multivessel disease. Diabetes, lesion length, vessel size, total occlusion, and number of lesions all influence the incidence of restenosis. The risk of restenosis in a patient increases with each additional lesion that is dilated. This increased restenosis rate may negate the positive features complete revascularization. Nobuyoshi *et al.* [29] found that patients with MVD and complete revascularization had significantly higher restenosis rates per patient (15.4%) than patients with MVD and incomplete revascularization (11.7%). The incidence of multilesion restenosis was significantly greater in patients with three-vessel disease than in those with two-vessel disease.

Multiple randomized trials have consistently demonstrated that DES reduce restenosis compared to BMS in single lesions. A number of single center registries have reported the efficacy of DES for multivessel disease [30,31] (Table 20.3). The first major trial in the era of DES for the treatment of MVD was the ARTS II trial, which enrolled 607 patients with MVD treated with sirolimus-eluting stents, and the outcomes of these patients were compared with those of the CABG arm (n = 605) and the BMS arm (n = 600) in the earlier, randomized ARTS I trial. Despite more patients with diabetes and more complex lesions enrolled in ARTS II trial, there was no difference in MACE at one year between patients treated with DES and CABG (10.4 vs. 11.6%). These findings indicate that the use of DES may be a promising alternative to CABG in the treatment of patients with MVD. In the ERACI III registry, patients with MVD treated with DES (n = 225) were compared with the matched BMS (n = 225) and CABG (n = 225) arms of the ERACI II study. Patients treated with DES were older, higher risk by euroSCORE and incidence of type C lesions [31]. Three-year MACCE was lower in ERACI III-DES (22.7%) than in ERACI II-BMS (29.8%, P = 0.015), mainly reflecting less target vessel revascularization (14.2 vs. 24.4%, P = 0.009). MACCE rates at three years were similar in DES and CABG-treated patients (22.7%, P = 1.0). However, MACCE rates in ERACI III-DES were higher in diabetics (RR 0.81, 0.66–0.99; P = 0.018). There are three large ongoing randomized trials (FREEDOM, SYNTAX and CARDIA) comparing DES against CABG (see below). Given the recent concern regarding late stent thrombosis with DES, the long-term outcomes of these three studies will be critical in determining the safety and effectiveness of these devices in MVD (Table 20.4).

The SYNTAX Trial

The SYNTAX trial is the first randomized controlled trial to compare PCI using a DES to CABG in patients with left main disease and three vessel disease [32]. Eighteen hundred patients were randomized in a 1:1 fashion to PCI or CABG. One-year follow-up indicates that DES was statistically inferior to CABG for the primary composite end point of all-cause death, cerebrovascular event, MI, and repeat revascularization (17.8% vs. 12.1%, p = 0.0015). But the combined rate of "hard" end points (death, MI, and stroke) were no different between the two trial groups (7.6% vs. 7.7%, p = 0.98). Secondary-end-point findings showed a statistically lower risk of stroke among PCI-treated patients (0.6% vs. 2.2 %, p = 0.003) and higher risk of revascularization (5.9% vs. 13.7%, p < 0.0001). The SYNTAX trial suggested that, although the need for reintervention remains the main limitation of PCI, complex anatomy and advance disease which has traditionally been in the domain of CABG, can be safely revascularized by PCI.

The CARDIA Trial

The CARDIA (Coronary Artery Revascularisation in Diabetes) trial was designed to demonstrate non-inferiority of PCI to CABG in diabetic patients with MVD. The trial fell short of its planned recruitment, enrolling only 510 patients out of the intended 600, meaning that the non-inferiority parameters set for the trial were not reached due to insufficient power. Preliminary 12-month results showed no apparent difference between CABG and PCI in terms of the composite endpoints of death, non-fatal MI and non-fatal stroke (10.2% vs. 11.6%, p = 0.63). This suggests that PCI may be a safe alternative to CABG in selected patients with diabetes and MVD. Repeat revascularization was higher in the PCI group as expected with a rate of 9.9% vs. 2.0% for CABG. Comparing CABG and a subgroup of 179 PCI patients who received DES rather than BMS, the composite endpoint of death, non-fatal MI and non-fatal stroke was 10.2% vs. 10.1% (p = 0.98) again showing no difference in this composite endpoint.

Medical Therapy

Patients with MVD have diffuse disease and progression of untreated plaques. Multiple stents only treat focal areas of most significant stenosis. Untreated vulnerable plaques could potentially develop into culprit lesions over time. Aggressive medical therapy with risk factor modification and lipid lowering is essential. This fact was underscored in the recently reported COURAGE trial, where patients with stable CAD treated medically had similar rates of long-term death and MI compared to PCI [33].

Conclusion

Patients with multivessel disease comprise the majority of patients undergoing PCI today and will likely remain so. With improved techniques, stents, and adjunctive drugs, short- and medium-term outcomes after PCI have improved significantly. If long-term outcomes after DES are comparable with CABG, PCI may become the preferred revascularization strategy for many patients. The role of PCI in patients with multivessel disease will depend—both on the patient's anatomy and the clinical setting in which the revascularization is planned. For each patient, the risk-benefit ratio should be examined. The procedure should be performed only after considering all therapeutic options and their short- and long-term outcomes.

References

1. Comparison of coronary bypass surgery with angioplasty in patients with multivessel disease. The Bypass Angioplasty Revascularization Investigation (BARI) Investigators. N Engl J Med 1996; **335**(4): 217–225.

2. First-year results of CABRI (Coronary Angioplasty versus Bypass Revascularisation Investigation). CABRI Trial Participants. Lancet 1995; **346**(8984): 1179–1184.

3. Singh M, Rihal CS, Gersh BJ, et al. Twenty-five-year trends in in-hospital and long-term outcome after percutaneous coronary intervention: a single-institution experience. Circulation 2007; **115**(22): 2835–2841.

4. Jones EL, Craver JM, Guyton RA, et al. Importance of complete revascularization in performance of the coronary bypass operation. Am J Cardiol 1983; **51**(1): 7–12.

5. Buda AJ, Macdonald IL, Anderson MJ, et al. Long-term results following coronary bypass operation. Importance of preoperative actors and complete revascularization. J Thorac Cardiovasc Surg 1981; **82**(3): 383–390.

6. Bell MR, Bailey KR, Reeder GS, et al. Percutaneous transluminal angioplasty in patients with multivessel coronary disease: How important is complete revascularization for cardiac event-free survival? J Am Coll Cardiol 1990; **16**(3): 553–562.

7. Vandormael MG, Chaitman BR, Ischinger T, et al. Immediate and short-term benefit of multilesion coronary angioplasty: influence of degree of revascularization. J Am Coll Cardiol 1985; **6**(5): 983–991.

8. Hasdai D, Berger PB, Bell MR, et al. The changing face of coronary interventional practice: The Mayo Clinic experience. Arch Intern Med 1997; **157**(6): 677–682.

9. Ijsselmuiden AJ, Ezechiels J, Westendorp IC, et al. Complete versus culprit vessel percutaneous coronary intervention in multivessel disease: a randomized comparison. Am Heart J 2004; **148**(3): 467–474.

10. Nienhuis MB, Ottervanger JP, Dambrink JH, et al. Troponin T elevation and prognosis after multivessel compared with single-vessel elective percutaneous coronary intervention. Neth Heart J 2007; **15**(5): 178–183.

11. Shishehbor MH, Topol EJ, Mukherjee D, et al. TARGET Investigators. Outcome of multivessel coronary intervention in the contemporary percutaneous revascularization era. Am J Cardiol 2006; **97**(11): 1585–1590.

12. Chen LY, Lennon RJ, Grantham JA, et al. In-hospital and long-term outcomes of multivessel percutaneous coronary revascularization after acute myocardial infarction. Am J Cardiol 2005; **95**(3): 349–354.

13. Singh M, Rihal CS, Lennon RJ, et al. Bedside estimation of risk from percutaneous coronary intervention: the new Mayo Clinic risk scores. Mayo Clin Proc 2007 June; **82**(6): 701–708.

14. Goldstein JA, Demetriou D, Grines CL, et al. Multiple complex coronary plaques in patients with acute myocardial infarction. N Engl J Med 2000; **343**(13): 915–922.

15. Smith SC Jr, Feldman TE, Hirshfeld JW Jr, et al. American College of Cardiology/American Heart Association Task Force on Practice Guidelines; American College of Cardiology/American Heart Association/Society for Cardiovascular Angiography and Interventions Writing Committee to Update the 2001 Guidelines for Percutaneous Coronary Intervention. ACC/AHA/SCAI 2005 Guideline Update for Percutaneous Coronary Intervention—summary article: A report of the American College of Cardiology/American Heart Association Task Force on Practice Guidelines (ACC/AHA/SCAI Writing Committee to Update the 2001 Guidelines for Percutaneous Coronary Intervention). Circulation 2006; **113**(1): 156–175.

16. Hanratty CG, Koyama Y, Rasmussen HH, et al. Exaggeration of nonculprit stenosis severity during acute myocardial infarction: Implications for immediate multivessel revascularization. J Am Coll Cardiol 2002; **40**(5): 911–916.

17. Gibson CM, Ryan KA, Murphy SA, et al. Impaired coronary blood flow in nonculprit arteries in the setting of acute myocardial infarction: The TIMI Study Group. Thrombolysis in myocardial infarction. J Am Coll Cardiol 1999; **34**(4): 974–982.

18. Di Mario C, Mara S, Flavio A, et al. Single vs multivessel treatment during primary angioplasty: results of the multicentre randomised HEpacoat for cuLPrit or multivessel stenting for Acute Myocardial Infarction (HELP AMI) Study. Int J Cardiovasc Intervent 2004; **6**(3–4): 128–133.

19. Kong JA, Chou ET, Minutello RM, et al. Safety of single versus multi-vessel angioplasty for patients with acute myocardial infarction and multi-vessel coronary artery disease: report from the New York State Angioplasty Registry. Coron Artery Dis 2006; **17**(1): 71–75.

20. Serruys PW, Unger F, Sousa JE, et al. Arterial Revascularization Therapies Study Group. Comparison of coronary-artery bypass surgery and stenting for the treatment of multivessel disease. N Engl J Med 2001; **344**(15): 1117–1124.

21. SoS Investigators. Coronary artery bypass surgery versus percutaneous coronary intervention with stent implantation in patients with multivessel coronary artery disease (the Stent or Surgery trial): A randomised controlled trial. Lancet 2002, September 28; **360**(9338): 965–970.

22. Rodriguez A, Bernardi V, Navia J, et al. Argentine Randomized Study: Coronary Angioplasty with Stenting

versus Coronary Bypass Surgery in patients with Multiple-Vessel Disease (ERACI II): 30-day and one-year follow-up results. ERACI II Investigators. J Am Coll Cardiol 2001; **37**(1): 51–58.

23. Morrison DA, Sethi G, Sacks J, *et al.* Angina With Extremely Serious Operative Mortality Evaluation (AWESOME). Percutaneous coronary intervention versus coronary artery bypass graft surgery for patients with medically refractory myocardial ischemia and risk factors for adverse outcomes with bypass: a multicenter, randomized trial. Investigators of the Department of Veterans Affairs Cooperative Study #385, the Angina With Extremely Serious Operative Mortality Evaluation (AWESOME). J Am Coll Cardiol 2001; **38**(1): 143–149.

24. Trachiotis GD, Weintraub WS, Johnston TS, *et al.* Coronary artery bypass grafting in patients with advanced left ventricular dysfunction. Ann Thorac Surg 1998; **66**(5): 1632–1639.

25. Sciagra R, Pellegri M, Pupi A, *et al.* Prognostic implications of Tc-99m sestamibi viability imaging and subsequent therapeutic strategy in patients with chronic coronary artery disease and left ventricular dysfunction. J Am Coll Cardiol 2000; **36**(3): 739–745.

26. Papafaklis MI, Naka KK, Papamichael ND, *et al.* The impact of renal function on the long-term clinical course of patients who underwent percutaneous coronary intervention. Catheter Cardiovasc Interv 2007; **69**(2): 189–197.

27. Schweiger MJ, Chambers CE, Davidson CJ, *et al.* Prevention of contrast induced nephropathy: recommendations for the high risk patient undergoing cardiovascular procedures. Catheter Cardiovasc Interv 2007; **69**(1): 135–140.

28. Hannan EL, Racz MJ, Walford G, *et al.* Long-term outcomes of coronary-artery bypass grafting versus stent implantation. N Engl J Med 2005; **352**(21): 2174–2183.

29. Nobuyoshi M, Kimura T, Nosaka H, *et al.* Restenosis after successful percutaneous transluminal coronary angioplasty: serial angiographic follow-up of 229 patients. J Am Coll Cardiol 1988; **12**(3): 616–623.

30. Serruys PW. ARTS II. Arterial Revascularization Therapies Study Part II of the sirolimus-eluting stent in the treatment of patients with multivessel de novo coronary artery lesions. EuroInterventions 2005; **1**: 147–156.

31. Rodriguez AE, Maree AO, Mieres J, *et al.* Late loss of early benefit from drug-eluting stents when compared with bare-metal stents and coronary artery bypass surgery: 3 years follow-up of the ERACI III registry. Eur Heart J 2007; **28**(17): 2118–2125.

32. Serruys PW, Morice MC, Kappetein, *et al.* Percutaneous coronary intervention versus coronary-artery bypass grafting for severe coronary artery disease. N Engl J Med 2009; **360**(10): 961–972.

33. Boden WE, O'Rourke RA, Teo KK, *et al.* COURAGE Trial Research Group. Optimal medical therapy with or without PCI for stable coronary disease. N Engl J Med 2007; **356**(15): 1503–1516.

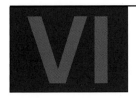

PART VI

Interventional Techniques

CHAPTER 21

Rotational Atherectomy

Saidi A. Mohiddin, & Martin T. Rothman

Barts and The London NHS Trust, The London Chest Hospital, London, UK

Introduction

Rotational atherectomy (RA) belongs to a group of techniques designed to restore vessel patency through the ablation of atherosclerotic material in stenosed coronary arteries. These techniques, that also include directional atherectomy and laser atherectomy, were intended as alternatives to plain old balloon angioplasty (POBA) in an era preceding the routine-stenting and drug eluting stent (DES) revolutions. RA is the best studied of these and its continued use seems assured by its role as an enabling and optimizing therapy adjunctive to stenting, particularly in patients with complex coronary lesions.

This chapter will begin with a summary of how RA's role in contemporary percutaneous coronary intervention (PCI) has developed; this may be considered sufficient for the needs of those readers that seek only to have an overview of RA. We then describe certain procedural details and complications, following which we present some of the details of the evidence responsible for the evolution of RA's role in PCI.

Summary: Vessel Patency Achieved Through Ablation

Arterial dissection, early vessel elastic recoil and later restenosis due to cell proliferation often lead

Interventional Cardiology, First Edition. Edited by Carlo Di Mario, George D. Dangas, Peter Barlis.

to a failure to maintain vessel patency after plain old balloon angioplasty (POBA). Long and calcified lesions are particularly non-compliant and high balloon inflation pressures may be needed. Shearing forces, persistence of the shifted atheromatous mass (containing cells capable of proliferation), and a stimulus to proliferation resulting from balloon injury are important features in determining POBA failures. An ablative technique that can restore vessel patency by selectively removing atheromatous bulk without injuring more normal vessel components has the potential to overcome some of POBA's shortcomings. In this context, RA was developed in the late 1980s in as an alternative percutaneous method for lumen enlargement [1,2]. Randomized trials demonstrated some advantages of RA over POBA in either procedural success but not in reducing rates of restenosis, and routine stent use very effectively solved the problems of vessel dissection and elastic recoil [3–11].

Problems with cell proliferation and in-stent restenosis (ISR) remained major determinants of target lesion revascularization (TLR), affecting as many as one third of stented lesions. Balloon treatment of ISR is frequently complicated by recurrent restenosis, particularly when restenosis is diffuse along the length of the stent. Again, the persistence and elasticity of the obstructing proliferating cell mass are responsible for balloon failure and recurrent restenosis. RA's role in the solution of this problem remains equivocal after the publication of two randomized trials with contrary findings [3–5]. Again, stent development, with the introduction of DES, has significantly reduced rates of ISR as a reason for TLR. However, a major contemporary challenge to PCI is the accessibility of some lesions, particularly calcified lesions, to balloon or stent placement, or to balloon dilatation. In complex lesions, even high inflation pressures may not achieve satisfactory stent expansion in as many as half of the cases. Restenosis and acute in-stent thrombosis occur more frequently following such procedures.

RA alters the physical characteristics of the obstructing lesion, reducing its physical bulk and rigidity, and increasing the accessibility of the debulked coronary segment to balloon and stent devices. As such, RA improves lesion access and may optimize minimum lumen diameter (MLD) gains as an adjunctive technique to enable and/or optimize stenting. Furthermore, with increasing numbers of elderly and diabetic patients with diffuse and calcific coronary disease being considered for PCI, RA's role as a useful adjunctive tool to 'prepare' the lesion will continue to be developed in most advanced cardiac centers. The capability for RA to enable lesion access and optimize MLD gain as an adjunct to stenting now comprise the major indications for rotational atherectomy. Thus, paradoxically, DES have reinvigorated interest in RA as ever more complex coronary disease is managed percutaneously.

Technical Considerations

The business end of rotational atherectomy (Rotablator, Boston Scientific) is a nickel-plated brass elliptical burr coated with diamond microchips on the front or crossing surface of the burr, the rear half of the burr having no diamond chips and therefore no abrading surface. (Figure 21.1—Rotablator system with burrs, console, Rotalink system). Rotational speeds up to 190,000 RPM are transmitted via a flexible drive shaft enclosed within a Teflon sheath (4.3 Fr) connected to a gas-driven turbine. Femoral arterial access with an 8 Fr (check) sheath is typical and supports the use of burr sizes up to 2.5 mm. A radial approach through a 6 or 7 Fr catheter restricts the maximum burr size (6 Fr—1.25 mm, 1.5 mm, 1.75 mm; 7 Fr—2.0 mm, 2.15 mm) but may be satisfactory for suitable patients/lesions. Following passage of a proprietary spring-tipped steel guidewire (Boston

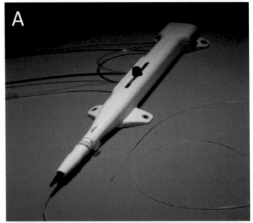

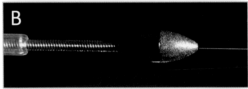

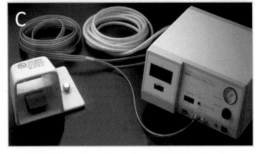

Figure 21.1. Rotablation set-up. (A) A single advancer can be used for multiple burr exchanges. (B) The diamond coated burr is advanced on the guidewire and torque transmitted via the Teflon-coated 4.3 French sheath. (C) Control console and foot pedal. Images courtesy of Boston Scientific.

Scientific, RotaWire, 0.009 inches) into the distal vessel beyond the target lesion, the shaft-mounted burr is advanced into position proximal to the lesion. In some of the early RA studies, a failure to pass the RotaWire into the distal vessel accounted for most procedural failures. A variety of RotaWires with different characteristics are now available although handling of these is said by many operators to be inferior to many coronary guidewires. Although only the RotaWire may be used for RA, an over-the-wire balloon configuration may facilitate location of the RotaWire having once crossed the lesion with a regular guidewire using guidewire exchange for troublesome lesions such as chronic total occlusions.

A saline-based infusion cocktail delivered through the Teflon coated sheath provides lubrication for the drive shaft. Heparin anticoagulation (typically 5000 iu in 500 ml normal saline) and vasodilators (verapamil 5 mg and isosorbide dinitrate 5 mg) are frequently added to the cocktail and are delivered directly into the coronary artery. Systemic anticoagulation aims for an activated clotting time of about 300 seconds. A temporary transvenous pacemaker is often positioned either in the right atrium, ready for advancement to the right ventricle if required, or to the right ventricle when right coronary lesions are being treated as RA may be complicated by transient complete heart block.

Once an appropriately sized burr is in position proximal to the lesion and it is confirmed that cocktail is reliably being delivered, the drive is switched on and engaged. Rotational speeds are typically between 130,000 and 150,000 RPM [7,8]. More rapid rotational speeds may generate excessive heat, and lower speeds may result in ablative behavior less selective for atheroma, but also in fewer complications. More rapid rotational speeds may also result in greater platelet activation [12]. The burr is advanced into and beyond the target lesion slowly and with caution taken to maintain rotational speed as the burr encounters friction; it is necessary to maintain rotational speed, so retreat from the target lesion may be necessary. Significant decrements in rotational speed (>5000 RPM) must be avoided as these are associated with excessive heat production through friction and are associated with poorer immediate and chronic outcomes [13,14]. Sudden drop in burr speed may also be associated with burr trapping in the lesion, hence the cautious advancement and attention to burr speed. Burr advancement is best accomplished in a piecemeal 'pecking' fashion rather than through a steady constant movement. The recommended movement comprises short (about 20 seconds), slow, smooth advances of the burr into the lesion. It is not desirable to force the burr through the lesion; as the rear of burr does not have an abrading surface, in such circumstances the burr may become trapped by the lesion and the device have

difficulty retreating. Used carefully, the operator retreats from the lesion between "pecks" and this maintains rotational speed and enables coronary flow to flush ablative debris beyond the lesion. After the lesion is crossed, the burr is withdrawn with the drive engaged so the burr is spinning and the sequence repeated until the operator feels or sees no further resistance to that burr. Larger burrs may then be selected and the procedure repeated, typically until a maximum burr size of 60–80% of the reference vessel diameter has successfully crossed the lesion. More modest degrees of ablation may be associated with fewer short and long-term complications [14,15], and in any case may be considered satisfactory if the principal indication for RA has been to debulk rather than abolish the lesion (as an adjunct to stenting) or to facilitate tracking of balloons or stents across the target lesion. A strategy using a single 1.5 mm or 1.75 mm burr may be satisfactory for the majority of cases [8].

The rotating burr abrades atherosclerotic material, selectively removing non compliant tissue to improve vessel patency. Intravascular ultrasound (IVUS) examination following RA typically demonstrates a circular lumen with a smooth distinct luminal-vessel wall interface distinct from that seen following balloon barotrauma (Figure 21.2) [16]. The diameter of the newly created lumen tends usually to exceed that of the largest burr used, perhaps due to non axial movement of the burr about its long axis, or as a consequence of vessel spasm during ablation [2,16].

In-vitro studies suggest that normal (compliant, soft) vascular tissue is relatively unharmed and therefore not easily abraded, but that more rigid, calcified structures are more accessible to abrasion [2,16]. Burr abrasion generates minute particles (5–10 microns) that are propagated distally into and through the coronary microcirculation. Consequences of distal micro-embolization of these atheromatous particles and of platelet activation by the rotating burr are believed to contribute to vessel spasm and no-reflow complications observed during RA. In vitro, glycoprotein IIb/IIIa inhibitors attenuate platelet activation resulting from RA, and may be associated with fewer ischaemic complications [12,17]. Routine IIb/IIIa inhibitor use in some laboratories is justified by

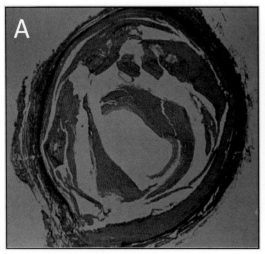 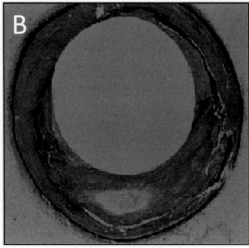

Figure 21.2. Histological samples comparing the disruptive effects on the arterial wall from POBA (A) and RA (B). Images obtained from Ahn *et al.* J Vasc Surg 1988; **7**: 292–300. POBA—plain old balloon angioplasty. RA—rotational atherectomy.

significantly lower increases in serum cardiac enzyme concentrations following abciximab in a small randomized study [18].

Complications

Complications associated with interventional coronary techniques such as RA are minimized by good technique. Inexperienced operators, prolonged burring, excessive decrements in rotational speed, oversized burrs and inappropriate vessel selection all increase complication rates. Serious complications following RA are no commoner than those associated with POBA in the randomized trials [6,7,9,10,19].

Coronary vasospasm was a prominent feature in the initial RA experience. The routine addition of vasodilators to the heparinised saline device flush may prevent vasospasm, and prompt delivery of additional intracoronary nitrate resolves most cases. Contemporary series report vasospasm in 1.6–6.6% of cases. The slow flow/no flow phenomenon is occasionally seen and may result from vasospasm, platelet activation or distal embolization of atheromatous debris and complicates approximately 1.2–7.6% of RA procedures. Treatment with adenosine, verapamil or nitroglycerine may promote reflow, but careful burr technique is advised in its prevention. Coronary

dissection (10–13%) following RA is less common than following POBA as described above. Risks of coronary perforation (0–1.5%) are reduced if oversized burrs, aggressive burr advancement and treatment of angulated lesions is avoided.

Non Q-wave myocardial infarction detected as increases in serum cardiac enzyme concentrations occur as a result of no-reflow, dissection and distal embolization are seen in 4–6% of cases, Q-wave infarcts (1.2–1.3%) and the need for emergency CABG (1.0–2.5%) occur less commonly. Death may complicate RA in 1% of cases.

Rotational Atherectomy

Following the development of RA in the late 1980s [1,2], several hundred publications have reported on the use of RA in coronary disease. Whilst many of these studies have been important for the dissemination and development of the technique, few have adequately examined RA's role relative to other PCI techniques. In a systematic evaluation of the few randomized trials of RA in the treatment of coronary disease recently published by the Cochrane Collaboration, only nine studies met the reviewers' selection criteria for quality, two of which were published in abstract form only (see Table 21.1, the nine randomized

Table 21.1. The nine studies.

DART [10]	Dilation vs. Ablation Revascularization Trial targeting restenosis.
ARTIST [4]	Angioplasty versus Rotational Atherectomy for Treatment of Diffuse In-Stent Restenosis Trial.
ROSTER [5]	Rotational Atherectomy versus Balloon Angioplasty for Diffuse In-Stent Restenosis.
SPORT [49]	Stenting Post Rotational Atherectomy Trial.
EDRES [50]	Effects of Debulking on Restenosis.
COBRA [7]	COmparison of Balloon angioplasty versus Rotational Atherectomy.
ERBAC [6]	Excimer Laser, Rotational Atherectomy and Balloon Angioplasty Comparison.
Eltchaninoff et al. [9]	
Guerin et al. [19]	

studies) [3]. Broadly speaking, these trials examined: (1) the relative roles of POBA and RA in treating native coronary disease, and (2) the relative roles of POBA and RA in treating in-stent restenosis. No randomized trials specifically address the capabilities of adjunctive RA in either enabling or optimizing stenting in complex lesions. However, data from these and other studies support the notion that RA is well suited to this latter role.

Rotational Atherectomy as the Sole Revascularization Modality

Lesions with characteristics (particularly calcification) that define them as complex have been a principal focus of RA studies. In fact, there is little evidence comparing RA with POBA in non-complex lesions. Treatment of complex lesions with POBA has relatively high procedural failure rates, acute complications and restenosis [20–22]. Vessel compliance (leading to recoil and dissection) and residual plaque burden (a determinant of restenosis rates) are two important determinants of POBA failure.

Calcified lesions are associated with a higher incidence of dissection and restenosis rates following POBA [20,23]. As many as 30% of lesions had

angiographically evident (longitudinal) dissection following POBA in one study, and these were considered major in nearly 9% [20]. Dissections are more likely in calcified longer lesions in arteries with more than one stenosis [20], and that RA is associated with a lower incidence of coronary dissection [9,10]. Residual plaque burden manifest as residual stenosis or as residual volume of (displaced) atherosclerotic material after intervention are potential determinants of restenosis risk [24]. A post POBA stenosis greater than 30% predicts restenosis [22], and similar relationships between restenosis and post treatment MLD are seen following rotablation [11]. In addition to the greater prevalence of dissection following POBA, non-compliant lesions limit MLD gains.

For these reasons, RA was investigated as a promising technique for the subset of non-compliant complex lesions. The RA Multicenter Registry [11] demonstrated a high procedural success rate with RA (94%), but with restenosis rates (38%) similar to or higher than that following POBA. That RA tended to be associated with enhanced acute procedural success [25] but greater restenosis rates compared with POBA was also demonstrated in other non-randomized studies; restenosis rates as high as 59% [10,12], and as low as 31% [26–28] are reported in some early non-randomized studies of RA. Finally, several randomized trials of RA and POBA were published in the late 1990s [6,7,9,10,19]. These trials included either a strong preponderance of complex lesions [6,9,10] or studied only complex lesions [7,19]. About 20% of all patients in the studies included in the systematic review had unstable angina [3] The results of these trials and the emergence of routine stenting effectively ended interest in RA as the sole revascularization modality. The larger of these studies are discussed here.

The Excimer Laser, Rotational Atherectomy and Balloon Angioplasty Comparison (ERBAC) study randomized 685 patients with complex lesions to POBA, RA or excimer laser ablation [6]. Mean maximal burr to reference lumen ratio was 0.58, and adjunctive POBA followed RA in 93% of the cases. Procedural complications were similar in the three groups, and RA was superior to the other two modalities in achieving acute procedural success. In fact, success was achieved after cross-over to RA in 9 of 15 patients in whom POBA was not possible. Additionally, the advantages of RA over POBA (and laser ablation) in procedural success were more striking in more complex B2 and C lesions than in B1 lesions. Post-procedural MLDs were similar for RA and POBA, as were restenosis (57% vs. 47%, p = 0.14) and mortality rates after six months. However, TLR tended to occur more commonly following RA than POBA (42.4% vs. 36.6%, p = 0.13 for the two-way comparison).

The multicenter randomized COmparison of Balloon angioplasty versus Rotational Atherectomy (COBRA) study compared POBA with RA in the treatment of complex coronary lesions in 502 patients [7]. Stents were used only for bailout or if there were unsatisfactory acute results, and relatively long lesions (approximately 12.8 mm) in small caliber (approximately 2.7 mm) vessels were treated. Stenoses were severe with TIMI II or III flow prior to intervention in nearly 90% of patients. Mean maximal burr to reference lumen ratio was 0.71 and most patients (91%) randomized to the RA group had adjunctive balloon angioplasty. The primary endpoints were both procedural and six-month outcomes. By intention to treat analysis, procedural success (<50% diameter stenosis and >20% stenosis reduction) was more frequently observed in the RA group (84 vs. 71%; p < 0.01) including the less frequent use of bailout stents (6.4% vs. 14.9%; p < 0.001). Additionally, cross-over from RA to POBA occurred more frequently than the converse (10% vs. 4%), in most cases following difficulty in positioning of balloon across the stenosis. Cross-over from RA to POBA occurred when the Rotablator guidewire could not be positioned through and distal to the lesion. In-hospital complications were infrequent and did not statistically differ between groups with no trend favoring either technique. Post procedural MLDs were also similar. Restenosis rates after six months (≥50% diameter stenosis) for RA and POBA were statistically inseparable at 48.9% and 51.1% respectively. This difference remained insignificant if stented lesions were excluded.

The Dilation vs. Ablation Revascularization Trial targeting restenosis (DART) compared balloon angioplasty with RA in slightly smaller arteries with shorter lesions (mean diameter 2.5 mm, length 10 mm) in 446 patients [10]. Target burr: artery ratios were 0.7–0.85, very low pressure POBA (not exceeding 1 ATM) could be used if RA results were considered suboptimal. Actual burr size and balloon pressure data are not presented. Outcome measurements for RA and POBA were similar for acute procedural success rates (91.6 % and 94.1% respectively), MLD gains, and for 8 month outcomes including target vessel revascularization (30.5% and 31.2%), percent diameter restenosis (28% and 29%) and binary restenosis rate (50.5% for each). Non q-wave MIs with elevation in creatinine kinase were slightly, though not significantly, commoner in the RA group (2.2% vs. 1.4%). Although dissection occurred less commonly following RA (12% vs. 26%, p < 0.001), the occurrence of higher-grade dissections and rates of bailout stenting were similar.

The systematic overview of these and other studies reports similar restenosis rates at six months and a trend toward greater restenosis rates at 12 months following RA [3]. These studies demonstrate that RA has a similar safety profile to POBA in treating complex lesions. Fundamentally, however, although procedural success rates with RA were higher [6], RA did not have any benefits compared with POBA in its effects on restenosis. However, RA was followed by adjunctive balloon angioplasty in many patients in these studies, and restenosis rates were rather similar following RA+POBA or POBA alone. ERBAC and COBRA methods both specify that a low balloon pressure <4 atmospheres was to be used if RA was to be followed by balloon inflation, but information on comparative balloon inflation pressures is not presented [6,7]. Stents were used infrequently in these studies, and only provisionally to unsatisfactory RA or POBA results.

Thus, the utility of RA in optimizing post procedural MLD or longer term outcome in adjunctive procedures is not adequately examined. This issue is of relevance to the contemporary use of RA in optimizing stent expansion; how does the risk of restenosis following RA plus POBA/stenting relate to risks attributable to either alone? Are the potential benefits of RA in maximizing MLD through lesion modification and atheromatous debulking realized in 'rotastenting'? Whilst MLD gains and their relation to restenosis might appear less important following DES use, suboptimal stent expansion predisposes to in-stent thrombosis [29,30], the *bête noir* of the DES era.

Rotational Atherectomy for Diffuse In-stent Restenosis

Following bare metal stenting (BMS), neointimal cellular proliferation is responsible for late luminal loss and high TLR rates for in-stent restenosis (ISR). TLR frequency is greater following BMS in smaller vessels with complex lesions [31–33] and following inadequate stent expansion. ISR, particularly when diffuse is associated with recurrent restenosis rates up to 85% following re-intervention with balloon angioplasty [34,35]. Where suboptimal stent expansion has contributed to restenosis, balloon intervention may correct this. Otherwise, the hyperplastic intimal cells remain in situ, at best simply extruded to the adluminal vessel through stent struts. Removal of this tissue with RA was associated with high procedural success rates, and with lower restenosis rates than POBA in several registry and non-randomized studies [36–41]. Two randomized trials have reported apparently discrepant results. The single-center US Rotational Atherectomy versus Balloon Angioplasty for Diffuse In-Stent Restenosis (ROSTER) study [5] reports that RA was associated with a much lower rate of repeat stenting than POBA (10% vs. 31%%; P < 0.001) and a lower TLR incidence (32% vs. 45%; P = 0.042). Importantly, one third of patients evaluated for inclusion in ROSTER were excluded from the study if prior intravascular ultrasound (IVUS) demonstrated evidence of inadequate stent expansion. Balloon treatment was considered to be the treatment of choice for these patients. The multicenter European Angioplasty versus Rotational Atherectomy for Treatment of Diffuse In-Stent Resenosis Trial (ARTIST) [4] did not evaluate adequacy of stent expansion with IVUS prior to randomization. Balloon treatment was associated with better outcome; six-month event-free survival was significantly better after POBA compared with RA (91% vs. 80%, p < 0.01). IVUS results at follow-up are consistent with the interpretation that a factor favoring POBA was the resulting stent over-expansion. As registry data suggest that as many as 50% of stents may be incompletely deployed [42], and ROSTER detected this in third of their ISR patients, ARTIST results may be heavily biased by results of balloon treatment of inadequate stent expansion. ARTIST should therefore not be considered to have evaluated the efficacy of RA for treating ISR occurring in optimally deployed BMS.

Rotational Atherectomy as an Adjunct to Stenting in Complex Percutaneous Coronary Intervention

Two developments are relevant to the re-emergence of interest in RA. Low restenosis rates following DES have encouraged us to consider treatment of lesions and patients previously considered at unacceptably high risk of restenosis following POBA or BMS. These lesions include those that are long, ostial and calcified and chronic total occlusions. There appears to be an increasing relative prevalence of more elderly, diabetic patients with relative or absolute contraindications to bypass surgery, and typical characteristics of coronary lesions in these patients include more diffuse coronary disease, calcified lesions and chronic total or subtotal occlusions [43]. Challenges to successful stent revascularization in such lesions include resistance to passage of balloons and stents, undilatable lesions, inadequate stent deployment and increased frequencies of stent thrombosis and restenosis. In such lesions, RA may both enable and optimize stenting [42,44–47].

Contemporary indications for RA therefore include facilitating stent delivery and expansion in calcified lesions and in undilatable lesions (Figure 21.3) [8]. RA may also be considered when plaque displacement following ballooning and stenting is felt likely to complicate interventions involving ostia and sidebranches, and also for in-stent restenosis in adequately deployed stents. Few studies have specifically examined this enabling and/or optimizing role for RA as an adjunct to stenting. A recently published Japanese study reports that patients with chronic total occlusions randomized to have a debulking procedure (rotational or directional atherectomy) had lower TLR rates than those that did not receive debulking [48]. Additionally, most of the other trials provide evidence that RA is associated

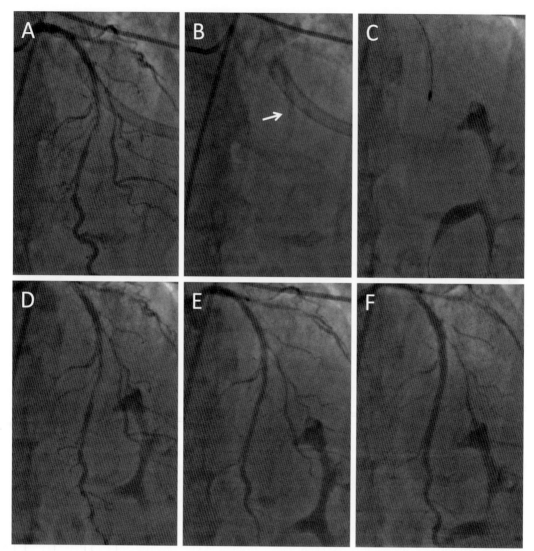

Figure 21.3. A heavily calcified coronary lesion in the left anterior descending artery is treated in a 77 year old female patient. The initial angiographic appearances from a cranial view show a lengthy lesion in the mid LAD (A). The calcified nature of this lesion (arrow) is better appreciated in the absence of contrast (B). A 1.5 mm burr is slowly advanced through the lesion (C). Angiographic appearances are shown following RA only (D), balloon angioplasty with a 2.5 mm balloon (E) and the final result following deployment of a 3 mm stent (F). Images courtesy of Dr Ajay Jain.

with increased procedural success, and restenosis rates following RA and barotrauma are, at worst, similar to that following barotrauma alone [6,7,9,10,19]. In the DES era, restoring vessel patency with minimum residual stenosis and adequate stent expansion in an effort to reduce risks of sub-acute thrombosis may prove particularly important.

Questions

1. **True statements regarding rotational atherectomy are all of the following, except:**
   A The burr speed should be 140–160,000 rpm.
   B Wire bias should be avoided because it may lead to perforation.
   C Late restenosis is superior to balloon angioplasty.
   D The burr speed should not drop by more than 5000 rpm.
   E The burr-to-artery ratio should not exceed 0.7.

2. **Deceleration during rotablation is associated with:**
   A Heat generation
   B Platelet aggregation
   C Major acute adverse clinical events
   D All of the above
   E None of the above

3. **Rotational atherectomy in bifurcation lesions has been shown to:**
   A Improve short and long term outcomes compared to POBA
   B Improve long term but not short term outcomes compared to POBA
   C Improve short and long term outcomes when combined with stenting
   D Not improve long term outcomes when compared with stenting

References

1. Ritchie JL, Hansen DD, Intlekofer MJ, *et al.* Rotational approaches to atherectomy and thrombectomy. Z Kardiol 1987; **76** Suppl 6: 59–65.

2. Ahn SS, Auth D, Marcus DR, *et al.* Removal of focal atheromatous lesions by angioscopically guided high-speed rotary atherectomy. Preliminary experimental observations. J Vasc Surg 1988; **7**: 292–300.

3. Villanueva EV, Wasiak J, Petherick ES. Percutaneous transluminal rotational atherectomy for coronary artery disease. Cochrane Database Syst Rev 2003: CD003334.

4. vom Dahl J, Dietz U, Haager PK, *et al.* Rotational atherectomy does not reduce recurrent in-stent restenosis: results of the angioplasty versus rotational atherectomy for treatment of diffuse in-stent restenosis trial (ARTIST). Circulation 2002; **105**: 583–588.

5. Sharma SK, Kini A, Mehran R, *et al.* Randomized trial of Rotational Atherectomy Versus Balloon Angioplasty for Diffuse In-stent Restenosis (ROSTER). Am Heart J 2004; **147**: 16–22.

6. Reifart N, Vandormael M, Krajcar M, *et al.* Randomized comparison of angioplasty of complex coronary lesions at a single center. Excimer Laser, Rotational Atherectomy, and Balloon Angioplasty Comparison (ERBAC) Study. Circulation 1997; **96**: 91–98.

7. Dill T, Dietz U, Hamm CW, *et al.* A randomized comparison of balloon angioplasty versus rotational atherectomy in complex coronary lesions (COBRA study). Eur Heart J 2000; **21**: 1759–1766.

8. Cavusoglu E, Kini AS, Marmur JD, *et al.* Current status of rotational atherectomy. Catheter Cardiovasc Interv 2004; **62**. 485–498.

9. Eltchaninoff H, Cribier A, Koning R, *et al.* Angioscopic evaluation of rotational atherectomy followed by additional balloon angioplasty versus balloon angioplasty alone in coronary artery disease: a prospective, randomized study. J Am Coll Cardiol 1997; **30**: 888–893.

10. Mauri L, Reisman M, Buchbinder M, *et al.* Comparison of rotational atherectomy with conventional balloon angioplasty in the prevention of restenosis of small coronary arteries: results of the Dilatation vs Ablation Revascularization Trial Targeting Restenosis (DART). Am Heart J 2003; **145**: 847–854.

11. Warth DC, Leon MB, O'Neill W, *et al.* Rotational atherectomy multicenter registry: acute results, complications and 6-month angiographic follow-up in 709 patients. J Am Coll Cardiol 1994; **24**: 641–648.

12. Williams MS, Coller BS, Vaananen HJ, Scudder LE, Sharma SK, Marmur JD. Activation of platelets in platelet-rich plasma by rotablation is speed-dependent and can be inhibited by abciximab (c7E3 Fab; ReoPro). Circulation 1998; **98**: 742–748.

13. Reisman M, Shuman BJ, Harms V. Analysis of heat generation during rotational atherectomy using different operational techniques. Cathet Cardiovasc Diagn 1998; **44**: 453–455.

14. Whitlow PL, Bass TA, Kipperman RM, *et al.* Results of the study to determine rotablator and transluminal angioplasty strategy (STRATAS). Am J Cardiol 2001; **87**: 699–705.

15. Safian RD, Feldman T, Muller DW, *et al.* Coronary angioplasty and Rotablator atherectomy trial (CARAT): immediate and late results of a prospective multicenter randomized trial. Catheter Cardiovasc Interv 2001; **53**: 213–220.

16. Mintz GS, Potkin BN, Keren G, *et al.* Intravascular ultrasound evaluation of the effect of rotational atherectomy in obstructive atherosclerotic coronary artery disease. Circulation 1992; **86**: 1383–1393.

17. Koch KC, vom Dahl J, Kleinhans E, *et al.* Influence of a platelet GPIIb/IIIa receptor antagonist on myocardial hypoperfusion during rotational atherectomy as assessed by myocardial Tc-99m sestamibi scintigraphy. J Am Coll Cardiol 1999; **33**: 998–1004.

18. Kini A, Reich D, Marmur JD, *et al.* Reduction in periprocedural enzyme elevation by abciximab after rotational atherectomy of type B2 lesions: Results of the Rota ReoPro randomized trial. Am Heart J 2001; **142**: 965–969.

19. Guerin Y, Spaulding C, Desnos M, *et al.* Rotational atherectomy with adjunctive balloon angioplasty versus conventional percutaneous transluminal coronary angioplasty in type B2 lesions: results of a randomized study. Am Heart J 1996; **131**: 879–883.

20. Sharma SK, Israel DH, Kamean JL, *et al.* Clinical, angiographic, and procedural determinants of major and minor coronary dissection during angioplasty. Am Heart J 1993; **126**: 39–47.

21. Myler RK, Shaw RE, Stertzer SH, *et al.* Lesion morphology and coronary angioplasty: current experience and analysis. J Am Coll Cardiol 1992; **19**: 1641–1652.

22. Ellis SG, Roubin GS, King SB III, *et al.* Importance of stenosis morphology in the estimation of restenosis risk after elective percutaneous transluminal coronary angioplasty. Am J Cardiol 1989; **63**: 30–34.

23. Alfonso F, Macaya C, Goicolea J, *et al.* Determinants of coronary compliance in patients with coronary artery disease: an intravascular ultrasound study. J Am Coll Cardiol 1994; **23**: 879–884.

24. Honda Y, Yock PG, Fitzgerald PJ. Impact of residual plaque burden on clinical outcomes of coronary interventions. Catheter Cardiovasc Interv 1999; **46**: 265–276.

25. Ellis SG, Popma JJ, Buchbinder M, *et al.* Relation of clinical presentation, stenosis morphology, and operator technique to the procedural results of rotational atherectomy and rotational atherectomy-facilitated angioplasty. Circulation 1994; **89**: 882–892.

26. Safian RD, Niazi KA, Strzelecki M, *et al.* Detailed angiographic analysis of high-speed mechanical rotational atherectomy in human coronary arteries. Circulation 1993; **88**: 961–968.

27. Teirstein PS, Warth DC, Haq N, *et al.* High speed rotational coronary atherectomy for patients with diffuse coronary artery disease. J Am Coll Cardiol 1991; **18**: 1694–1701.

28. Bertrand ME, Lablanche JM, Leroy F, *et al.* Percutaneous transluminal coronary rotary ablation with Rotablator (European experience). Am J Cardiol 1992; **69**: 470–474.

29. Moussa I, Di Mario C, Reimers B, *et al.* Subacute stent thrombosis in the era of intravascular ultrasound-guided coronary stenting without anticoagulation: frequency, predictors and clinical outcome. J Am Coll Cardiol 1997; **29**: 6–12.

30. Colombo A, Hall P, Nakamura S, *et al.* Intracoronary stenting without anticoagulation accomplished with intravascular ultrasound guidance. Circulation 1995; **91**: 1676–1688.

31. Barlis P, Tanigawa J, Kaplan S, *et al.* Complex coronary interventions: unprotected left main and bifurcation lesions. J Interv Cardiol 2006; **19**: 510–524.

32. Ardissino D, Cavallini C, Bramucci E, *et al.* Sirolimus-eluting vs uncoated stents for prevention of restenosis in small coronary arteries: a randomized trial. Jama 2004; **292**: 2727–2734.

33. Agostoni P, Biondi-Zoccai GG, *et al.* Is bare-metal stenting superior to balloon angioplasty for small vessel coronary artery disease? Evidence from a meta-analysis of randomized trials. Eur Heart J 2005; **26**: 881–889.

34. Mehran R, Dangas G, Abizaid AS, Mintz GS, Lansky AJ, Satler LF, Pichard AD, Kent KM, Stone GW, Leon MB. Angiographic patterns of in-stent restenosis: classification and implications for long-term outcome. Circulation 1999; **100**: 1872–1878.

35. Kini A, Marmur JD, Dangas G, *et al.* Angiographic patterns of in-stent restenosis and implications on subsequent revascularization. Catheter Cardiovasc Interv 2000; **49**: 23–29.

36. Sharma SK, Duvvuri S, Dangas G, *et al.* Rotational atherectomy for in-stent restenosis: acute and long-term results of the first 100 cases. J Am Coll Cardiol 1998; **32**: 1358–1365.

37. vom Dahl J, Radke PW, Haager PK, *et al.* Clinical and angiographic predictors of recurrent restenosis after percutaneous transluminal rotational atherectomy for treatment of diffuse in-stent restenosis. Am J Cardiol 1999; **83**: 862–867.

38. Mehran R, Dangas G, Mintz GS, *et al.* Treatment of in-stent restenosis with excimer laser coronary angioplasty versus rotational atherectomy: comparative mechanisms and results. Circulation 2000; **101**: 2484–2489.

39. Goldberg SL, Berger P, Cohen DJ, *et al.* Rotational atherectomy or balloon angioplasty in the treatment of intra-stent restenosis: BARASTER multicenter registry. Catheter Cardiovasc Interv 2000; **51**: 407–413.

40. Radke PW, Blindt R, Haager PK, *et al.* Minerva Cardioangiol 2002; **50**: 555–563.

41. Radke PW, vom Dahl J, Hoffmann R, *et al.* Three-year follow-up after rotational atherectomy for the treatment of diffuse in-stent restenosis: predictors of major adverse cardiac events. Catheter Cardiovasc Interv 2001; **53**: 334–340.

42. Moussa I, Di Mario C, Moses J, *et al.* Coronary stenting after rotational atherectomy in calcified and complex lesions. Angiographic and clinical follow-up results. Circulation 1997; **96**: 128–136.

43. Cannon CP. Elderly patients with acute coronary syndromes: Higher risk and greater benefit from antiplatelet therapy and/or interventional therapies. Am J Geriatr Cardiol 2003; **12**: 259–262.

44. Hong MK, Mintz GS, Popma JJ, *et al.* Safety and efficacy of elective stent implantation following rotational atherectomy in large calcified coronary arteries. Cathet Cardiovasc Diagn 1996; Suppl 3: 50–54.

45. Hoffmann R, Mintz GS, Kent KM, *et al.* Comparative early and nine-month results of rotational atherectomy, stents, and the combination of both for calcified lesions in large coronary arteries. Am J Cardiol 1998; **81**: 552–557.

46. Lee SW, Hong MK, Lee CW, *et al.* Early and late clinical outcomes after rotational atherectomy with stenting versus rotational atherectomy with balloon angioplasty for complex coronary lesions. J Invasive Cardiol 2004; **16**: 406–409.

47. Hong MK, Mintz GS, Popma JJ, *et al.* Angiographic Results and Late Clinical Outcomes Utilizing a Stent Synergy (Pre-Stent Atheroablation) Approach in Complex Lesion Subsets. J Invasive Cardiol 1996; **8**: 15–22.

48. Tsuchikane E, Suzuki T, Asakura Y, *et al.* Debulking of chronic coronary total occlusions with rotational or directional atherectomy before stenting: Final results of DOCTORS study. Int J Cardiol 2007; **125**(3): 397–403.

49. Buchbinder M, Fortuna R, Sharma S, *et al.* Debulking prior to stenting improves acute outcomes: early results from the SPORT trial. J Am Coll Cardiol 2000; **35**(supp A): 8A.

50. Niazi K, Patel A, Nohza F, *et al.* A prospective randomized study of the effects of debulking on restenosis (EDRES Trial). Circulation 1997; **98**: I–709.

Answers

1. C—Late restenosis is superior to balloon angioplasty—No trial has shown superiority of rotational atherectomy in reducing clinical or angiographic restenosis compared to PTCA. Reifart N *et al.* Circulation 1997; **96**: 91–98.

2. D—All of the above—Multiple bench and in vivo studies have demonstrated the deleterious effect of deceleration and heat generation during rotational atherectomy. A subset analysis of the STRATAS data indicated the deceleration >5000 rpm correlated with increased major procedural complications.

3. D

CHAPTER 22

Thrombectomy and Embolic Protection

William J. van Gaal[1], & Adrian P. Banning[2]

[1] The Northern Hospital, Epping, VIC, Australia
[2] John Radcliffe Hospital, Oxford, UK

Introduction

Angiographic thrombus and effective protection of the distal vascular bed remain significant challenges in percutaneous coronary intervention (PCI). Thrombus mechanically obstructs antegrade flow, impairs visualization of coronary anatomy and acts as a substrate for further thrombotic events, either occlusive or embolic. For these reasons, removal of thrombus during PCI is theoretically sound, yet thrombectomy devices remain an unproven technology for routine use in any setting. However, there is little doubt that the select application of thrombectomy devices is useful in the management of large, bulky thrombi which may otherwise overwhelm pharmacologic measures.

Distal embolization can occur in the presence, or absence, of thrombus. Thrombectomy alone may be insufficient to prevent distal embolization, as the devices themselves may dislodge thrombi into the distal vascular bed. Protection of the microvasculature (and thus myocardium) includes the use of pharmacologic agents such as glycoprotein IIb/IIIa inhibitors and coronary vasodilators, however mechanical protection is mandated in

Interventional Cardiology, First Edition. Edited by Carlo Di Mario, George D. Dangas, Peter Barlis.
© 2010 Blackwell Publishing Ltd. Published 2010 by Blackwell Publishing Ltd.

some settings to prevent embolization of thrombus and/or plaque material. This is particularly true in PCI of degenerative saphenous vein graft (SVG) disease due to the bulky and friable nature of SVG atheroma.

Thrombectomy

Thrombus usually appears as a mobile filling defect on coronary angiography in the setting of PCI for acute coronary syndromes, but may also occur as a procedural complication, usually in the setting of inadequate anti-thrombin and/or antiplatelet therapy, which may occur with longer, more complicated procedures. In managing thrombus, the age and therefore amount of cross-linking and thrombus organization will influence the choice of device. Typically, simpler techniques such as aspiration/rinspiration are more likely to be successful in the setting of acute, fresh thrombus, whilst more aggressive removal techniques are required for older, more organized thrombus.

Aspiration Thrombectomy

Simple aspiration of thrombus relies on manual suction of clot through a catheter. Whilst large amounts of proximal thrombus can be aspirated via the guide catheter, this carries a risk of vessel trauma and necessitates guide catheter exchange to prevent embolization of thrombotic debris. Specific, over the wire, small bore devices are available to extract intracoronary thrombus by applying suction via a syringe. Fresh thrombus may successfully be aspirated using this technique, however more organized thrombus may simply occlude the catheter tip and prevent aspiration. Several devices are available and most now employ a beveled opening and/or side holes to minimize the chances of this occurring (Figure 22.1).

The Pronto V3 (Vascular Solutions Inc., Minneapolis, Minnesota) and Diver (Invatec, Brescia, Italy) thrombus extraction systems are manual, over-the-wire devices which connect to a syringe. Manual suction on the syringe is performed whilst the tip of the catheter is engaged in the thrombus. The catheter can be gently passed distally as clot is evacuated. The Export (Medtronic, Santa Rosa, California) and QuickCat (Kensey Nash, Exton, Pennsylvania) systems are semi-automated thrombus extraction systems which employ a vacuum system. The vacuum assembly consists of extension tubing with a one way stopcock attached to a syringe with a self-locking plunger. The vacuum is prepared by connecting the syringe via tubing to the catheter. The tubing is locked off using the stopcock, and negative pressure created within the syringe by drawing back the plunger which is then locked in position. The catheter tip is then placed just proximal to the thrombus. The stopcock is turned to transmit the negative pressure to the catheter lumen, and thrombus aspirated whilst gently passing the catheter tip distally.

Two small randomized studies of the Diver extraction catheter, in which patients were randomized to thrombus extraction prior to primary PCI for acute ST elevation myocardial infarction (STEMI) have been conducted [1,2]. Both demonstrated improvement in the surrogate marker of myocardial blush grade in the aspiration groups compared with control; however, no differences in 30-day major adverse cardiac events (MACE) were noted.

The Dethrombosis to Enhance Acute Reperfusion in Myocardial Infarction (DEAR-MI) trial was designed to assess the impact of the Pronto aspiration device on acute reperfusion in STEMI patients. Use of the device resulted in improved thrombolysis in myocardial infarction (TIMI) flow, myocardial blush grade and ST segment resolution [3]. Clinical events at six month follow-up, however, were very low in both groups, and again, no clinical benefit with adjunctive aspiration was seen. In a small (n = 50) randomized study of the export catheter, thrombus aspiration prior to primary PCI reduced the incidence of no-reflow and improved ST segment resolution. There was a non-significant trend toward better clinical outcomes in the aspiration group [4]. Aspiration devices have subsequently been shown to improve clinical out-

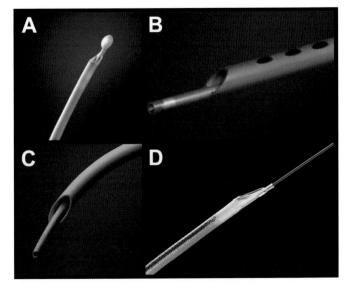

Figure 22.1. Simple aspiration devices. The Pronto V3 (A) and Diver extraction catheter (B) are simple aspiration devices employing manual suction to remove intracoronary thrombus. The QuickCat (C) and Export catheter (D) are semi-automated thrombus extraction systems which employ a vacuum system. The Export catheter is a 6 Fr compatible aspiration system attached to a 20 ml locking syringe (not shown). The over-the-wire catheter has an oblique aspiration tip with a radiopaque marker 2 mm from the distal tip.

comes and reduce infarct size following primary angioplasty for acute ST elevation myocardial infarction. The large (n = 1071) randomized Thrombus Aspiration during Primary Percutaneous Coronary Intervention in Acute Myocardial Infarction Study (TAPAS) using the Export catheter, thrombus aspiration prior to direct stenting for primary PCI was shown to improve myocardial blush post-procedure and ST segment resolution compared with standard pre-dilatation and stenting [5], and at one year follow-up there was a significant reduction in cardiac death and myocardial infarction [6]. As such, thrombus aspiration prior to stenting in primary PCI is now routine care in many centers performing primary PCI.

Rinspiration

The Rinspiration System *(Kerberos Proximal Solutions Inc., Sunnyvale, California)* employs simultaneous irrigation and aspiration of the vessel to remove thrombus. The Rinspiration catheter has three lumens. One 25 cm monorail wire lumen allows passage over a standard 0.014-inch coronary guidewire, a second lumen for aspiration, and a third lumen for injection of saline through perforations located proximal to the aspiration lumen. The hand-activated Rinspiration device allows for simultaneous irrigation and aspiration at the treatment site by activating two syringes, one for infusion and one for aspiration. No randomized controlled trials of rinspiration compared with other devices or control in any setting have been published to date.

Rheolytic Thrombectomy

Rheolytic thrombectomy devices are generally more effective than simpler aspiration devices at removing thrombus, but are more complicated to use and have a higher incidence of complications. The X-Sizer thrombectomy device (ev3 Inc., Plymouth, Minnesota) is an over-the-wire dual-channeled catheter with a spinning helical tip in the first channel which fragments thrombus. At the same time, a miniature vacuum system in the second channel removes the debris created (Figure 22.2). The AngioJet rheolytic thrombectomy System (Possis Medical Inc., Minneapolis, Minnesota) makes use of the Venturi effect to effectively remove thrombus. Saline is injected at high pressure through small steel tubing by an external pump, creating an area of low pressure around the jet, which pulls surrounding blood, including thrombus, into the catheter (Figure 22.3). The latest generation device is smaller (4Fr), and available in both over-the-wire and rapid-exchange formats that can be delivered through 6 Fr guiding catheters over 0.014-inch guidewires. The larger 5 Fr XVG catheter is better suited to achieve complete thrombus removal in large coronary arteries and saphenous vein bypass grafts.

Three randomized studies of the X-Sizer thrombectomy device have produced similar findings when used as an adjunct to primary PCI. The X-Sizer device effectively reduces thrombus burden, improves myocardial perfusion assessed by corrected TIMI frame count and/or myocardial blush grade, and hastens ST segment resolution [7–9]. Whilst none of these studies were able to demonstrate any clinical benefit, there was no harm associated with use of the device.

In an early small randomized study (n = 100) of the AngioJet rheolytic thrombectomy device, thrombectomy resulted in earlier ST segment resolution, improved corrected TIMI frame counts and a reduction in infarct size [10]. The AngioJet Rheolytic Thrombectomy in Patients Undergoing Primary Angioplasty for Acute Myocardial Infarction (AIMI) trial was the largest (n = 480) randomized study of thrombectomy in primary PCI to date, which failed to demonstrate any reduction in the primary end-point of myocardial infarct size in the AngioJet arm [11]. In this study, thrombectomy actually increased infarct size, resulted in worse TIMI flow post-PCI (97% vs. 92% for the AngioJet group; p < 0.02) and caused an increase in 30 day MACE (6.7% vs. 1.7%), including an increase in 30-day mortality.

Clinical Applications

The major potential clinical utility of thrombectomy devices is in the management of patients with acute coronary syndromes, particularly STEMI where thrombus is likely to be present. Primary PCI for acute STEMI has proven to be a very effective treatment, achieving TIMI 3 flow in the great majority of patients. Some patients, however, do not achieve normal restoration of epicardial flow following primary PCI, and thus represents a

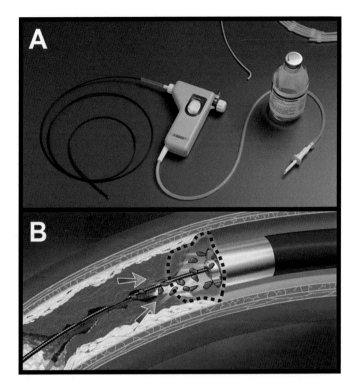

Figure 22.2. The X-Sizer thrombectomy device consists of a double barrel catheter, hand held battery driven motor module and vacuum bottle (A). A helical rotational cutter is housed within the tip of the dual lumen catheter. One lumen is for over-the-wire use, and one for debris aspiration (B).

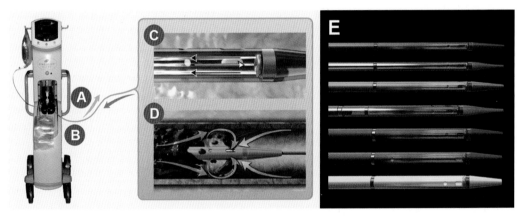

Figure 22.3. The AngioJet console delivers pressurized saline to the catheter tip (A). The high velocity saline creates a vacuum (B), and the inflow and outflow ports allow removal of thrombus (C) into a disposal bag (D). Several catheters are available including 4 Fr and 5 Fr systems (E).

subset of patients who could benefit from the use of aspiration devices.

Despite the association of distal embolization during primary PCI with larger infarct size and worse prognosis, studies of thrombectomy devices aimed at reducing the amount of embolic debris reaching the microvasculature have proved disappointing. Why aspiration thrombectomy has failed to result in clinical benefits for patients with acute STEMI in randomized trials is uncertain. Increased procedural time as a result of device deployment may delay restoration of coronary flow in acute

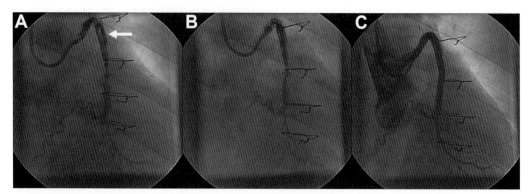

Figure 22.4. Diffuse instent restenosis with a large thrombotic burden is present (white arrow) (A). Following glycoprotein IIb/IIIa administration, an X-Sizer (ev3) thrombus extraction device was used achieving a significant reduction in thrombus burden (B). A SpiderRx (ev3) distal protection device was then deployed distally in the graft which was stented from the filter basket back to the ostium using four overlapping 5.0 mm TAXUS stents (Boston Scientific, Natick, MA) with a total length of 104 mm, achieving an excellent angiographic result, with TIMI III flow and good distal run off (C).

STEMI, and it is also likely that some devices may cause distal embolization during initial lesion crossing. Furthermore, some devices may not adequately aspirate thrombus and/or may allow release of vasoactive material into the microvasculature. Clearly the routine use of thrombectomy devices in patients with acute STEMI is the wrong strategy. A recent non-randomized study does suggest a role for the select use of such devices in patients undergoing primary PCI who have a significant thrombus burden [12].

There is no randomized data available for the use of aspiration or thrombectomy devices for the prevention of no-reflow in SVG PCI. However, despite the lack of evidence, these devices can prove useful in cases of significant thrombotic burden, particularly when combined with other pharmacologic agents and/or protection devices. (See Figure 22.4.)

Embolic Protection

Distal embolization of thrombotic material is particularly problematic during SVG PCI and PCI for acute coronary syndromes. The occurrence of distal embolization may be clinically and angiographically silent, or may present as a subtle reduction in coronary flow as measured by the corrected TIMI frame count and/or myocardial perfusion blush grade. When significant amounts of embolic debris reach the microvasculature, slow flow, or no-reflow may occur, defined as inadequate myocardial perfusion of a given coronary segment without angiographic evidence of mechanical vessel obstruction [13]. In the cardiac catheterization laboratory, coronary no-reflow is visualized angiographically as a reduction in TIMI flow grade, and is typically accompanied by chest pain, electrocardiographic changes with ST segment shift, and possible hemodynamic compromise.

Prevention of distal embolization is challenging and requires careful operator technique, particularly when crossing plaque with coronary guidewires or other devices. In particular high risk settings, embolic protection devices are effective at reducing the amount of embolic debris reaching the microvasculature. Several devices are approved for use which employ distal or proximal balloon occlusion and aspiration, or filter based protection.

Distal Balloon Occlusive Devices

The PercuSurge Guardwire device (Medtronic, Santa Rosa, California) is a balloon occlusive distal protection system designed to arrest antegrade flow and allow for aspiration of liberated plaque debris during PCI (Figure 22.5). The device consists of a 0.014-inch wire with a pentatetrafluoroethane balloon at its tip. The wire is advanced across the lesion and then the compliant balloon

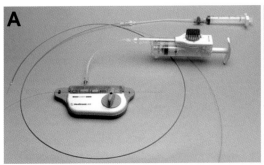
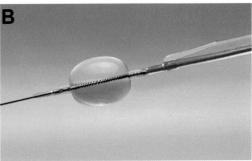

Figure 22.5. The GuardWire embolic protection system consists of four major components: the Export aspiration catheter (A), an inflation system consisting of the EZ Adaptor device and EZ Flator inflation device (A), and the GuardWire balloon occlusion wire (B). Once the GuardWire balloon occlusion wire tip is properly positioned distal to the lesion, the balloon is inflated.

After confirming that the vessel is occluded by injecting a small amount of contrast, the intervention is performed with the occlusion balloon inflated. Prior to deflating the balloon, any debris that may have been created during the intervention is aspirated using the Export aspiration catheter. It is recommended to aspirate the vessel twice to ensure complete debris removal.

inflated to arrest flow. Following lesion treatment, the vessel is aspirated using the Export aspiration catheter to retrieve debris liberated during the intervention. The Guardwire balloon is then deflated to restore antegrade flow. The TriActiv system (Kensey Nash, Exton, Pennsylvania) is another balloon occlusive distal protection system which works using a similar principle. The TriActiv system differs slightly in that it employs the use of a flush catheter to infuse saline following intervention, with effluent, blood and debris extracted through the guiding catheter.

Small studies using the Guardwire distal embolic protection system as adjunctive treatment during rescue or primary PCI for acute STEMI have demonstrated improved coronary perfusion postprocedure [14,15]. However, these findings were not supported by the large randomized EMERALD study, which was unable to demonstrate any improvement in coronary microvascular flow, reperfusion success, infarct size or event-free survival in patients undergoing primary PCI with distal balloon protection despite capture of embolic debris in 73% of patients in the treatment group [16]. Furthermore, the potential for harm was present, with fluoroscopy and procedural times significantly increased by 5 and 25 minutes respectively, and a delay in door to first balloon inflation of 21 minutes in the Guardwire group.

Early studies of the Guardwire device demonstrated that considerable amounts of debris were retrieved following SVG PCI, including cholesterol crystals, fibrin and lipid-rich macrophages [17]. The first randomized study of embolic protection vs. no embolic protection for SVG PCI was the SAFER study [18]. This large study demonstrated a 42% relative risk reduction in 30 day major adverse cardiac events (MACE) using the Guardwire device, driven mainly by a reduction in no-reflow (3% vs. 9%) and myocardial infarction (8.6% vs. 14.7%). The TriActiv system has demonstrated non-inferiority to both the Guardwire and FilterWire devices (see below) in the setting of SVG PCI [19].

Distal Filter Based Devices

Distal filter based embolic protection devices employ the use of a fenestrated basket deployed distal to the treated lesion prior to intervention. Due to the porous nature of filter based distal protection devices, they offer certain advantages over occlusive balloon devices, including better visualization of the lesion during PCI, and allowing for perfusion of the distal vascular bed during the period of embolic protection. Among their disadvantages, the most significant may be incomplete protection of the vascular bed, not only from embolic debris, but also soluble vasoactive substances released during PCI which may pass through the filter into the microcirculation [20].

The FilterWire EX device (Boston Scientific, Natick, MA) was the first such device available. The latest generation device (FilterWire EZ) contains a nitinol loop supporting the filter which floats free from the shaft allowing for better apposition to the vessel wall and thus the potential for better myocardial protection (Figure 22.6). It has a 3.2 Fr crossing profile, and comes in lengths of 190 cm and 300 cm, and basket sizes of 3.5 and 5.5 mm. Vessels suitable for use of the FilterWire are those that are <5.5 cm in diameter, have at least a one inch gap between the lesion and anastomosis (or branches), and have a relatively straight landing zone of 2 cm for the filter basket (Figure 22.7).

The SpiderRX (ev3 Inc., Plymouth, Minnesota) is another filter-based distal protection device which allows for operator choice of coronary guidewire to cross the lesion. The filter-basket is then delivered using a low-profile monorail exchange system designed to improve deliverability. The newer generation SpiderFX device is more flexible with improved deliverability, and comes in 3, 4, 5 and 6 mm sizes (Figure 22.6).

Data for the efficacy of distal filter-based protection devices comes from the FIRE trial which demonstrated the non-inferiority of the FilterWire EX

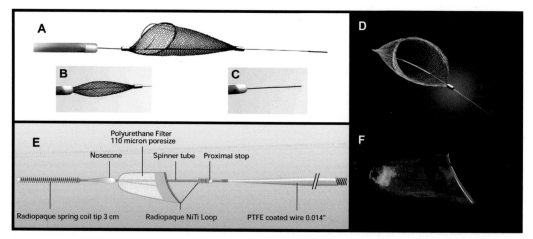

Figure 22.6. The SpiderRX device fully deployed (A). The basket is partially retracted within the recovery sheath, and the device can be withdrawn as is when significant amounts of thrombus are present to avoid "spillage" of contents (B). The basket is fully retracted within the recovery sheath (C). The newer generation SpiderFX has a simplified monorail delivery system and is more flexible allowing for improved deliverability (D). The newer generation FilterWire EZ device contains a nitinol loop which suspends the filter basket free from the spinner tube (E). This allows for better apposition to the vessel wall with improved embolic protection. A photomicrograph of the device is pictured (F) demonstrating embolic debris captured from a saphenous vein graft.

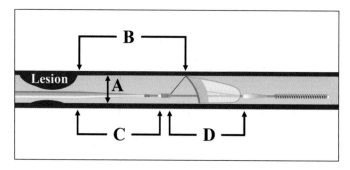

Figure 22.7. Landing zone requirements for the FilterWire EZ device. (A) The radiopaque nitinol loop accommodates 3.5–5.5 mm vessels. (B) There should be at least 2.5 cm from the lesion to the anastomosis for saphenous vein graft applications, and (C) the loop of the filter should be placed ≥1.5 cm distal to the distal edge of the lesion. (D) The nitinol loop requires a 2 cm segment of relatively straight vessel.

device compared with the Guardwire device in a large randomized study of SVG PCI [21]. The SpiderRX device has also proved non-inferior to currently available distal protection systems in the setting of SVG PCI [22].

Initial results with filter based protection in native coronary arteries were encouraging, particularly with the FilterWire EX system which was shown to improve angiographic measures of reperfusion for patients with acute STEMI undergoing primary PCI [23]. The larger randomized PROMISE study of the same device however was unable to demonstrate a benefit in the primary end point of coronary flow reserve. Likewise, no benefit was seen in TIMI flow, myocardial blush grade or 30 day mortality [24]. The FLAME trial examined the ability of the second generation FilterWire EZ device to capture embolic debris compared with either aspiration alone using the Export or Rescue catheter, or in combination with aspiration. It showed that the combined approach of filter protection and aspiration was significantly more efficient at capturing embolic debris (70% vs. 15% for FilterWire EZ only and 11% for aspiration only). Despite the encouraging results seen in the combined group with respect to capture of embolic debris, no effect on infarct size or clinical benefit was demonstrable [25].

The PREMIAR study evaluated the Spider RX filter system in native vessel PCI for high-risk patients with STEMI [26]. The primary end point was ST-segment resolution, whilst secondary end points included MACE, TIMI blush score, corrected TIMI frame count, distal embolization, and no-reflow. No differences in the primary or secondary endpoints were found. Likewise, no differences in MACE were seen at 30 days or six months following the procedure.

Proximal Balloon Occlusive Devices

Proximal protection devices offer theoretical advantages over distal protection including the ability to protect the distal vascular bed without first crossing the lesion with a bulky device which may itself cause distal embolization, and the inclusion of sidebranch protection. Some vessels are also not suitable for distal protection systems due to the lack of an appropriate "landing zone" for the device, either due to tortuosity, plaque disease or

both. The Proxis device (St. Jude Medical, St. Paul, Minnesota) is a proximal balloon occlusive protection system which has also demonstrated similar efficacy to distal protection systems [27] (Figure 22.8). Registry data including over 200 patients treated for acute STEMI with primary PCI has shown that the Proxis embolic protection device appears safe and effective in capturing debris, however no prospective randomized controlled trials have been performed to date [28].

Clinical Applications

During SVG PCI, distal embolization has proven to be virtually universal and can occur regardless of lesion characteristics or procedural technique [29]. Despite the universality of distal embolization during SVG intervention [17,30], only 15–20% of patients experience MACE in the absence of embolic protection [18]. In other words, distal embolization is often clinically silent, presumably when the amount of embolic debris is small. Despite this, even patients with vein grafts considered to be low risk on the bases of minimal degeneracy and lower plaque volume benefit equally from distal embolic protection [31]. This has created much debate on which patients should receive embolic protection during SVG PCI. Unfortunately no clinical, angiographic or procedural variables can predict which patients undergoing SVG PCI are likely to obtain the most benefit from embolic protection, nor which grafts will liberate the greatest amount debris [29]. Even the most benign looking vein grafts have the potential to liberate significant amounts of debris during PCI (Figure 22.9). As such, some form of embolic protection for all SVG procedures is recommend where feasible, regardless of graft age, degeneracy or appearance. There are three exceptions where distal embolization during SVG PCI is less likely to occur and do not mandate embolic protection. Firstly, PCI of vein grafts <3 years old are associated with less bulky disease and a reduced incidence of distal embolization and no-reflow [32,33]. Ostial SVG lesions are subject to sheer stress which creates more fibrotic lesions [34], and likewise, the hyperplastic lesions of in-stent restenosis are relatively stable and less prone to cause distal embolization and subsequent no-reflow [35,36].

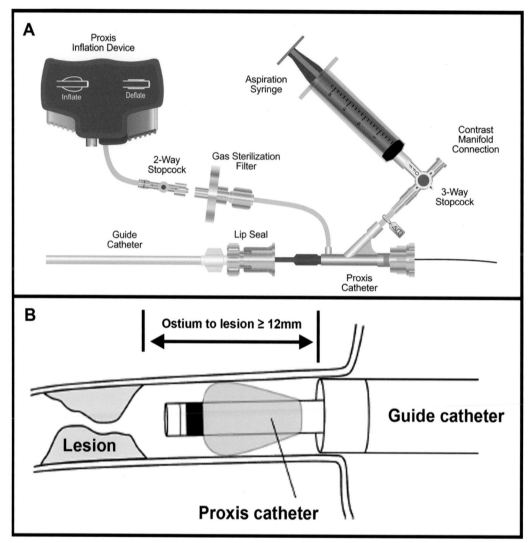

Figure 22.8. The Proxis device. The proximal end of the Proxis catheter has a built-in standard Y-adapter configuration (hemostasis valve for device entry and a luer connection for aspiration) and an additional luer connection for the inflation device. The catheter is connected to an automated carbon dioxide inflation device. A 20 cc evacuation syringe with a 3-way stopcock is provided for the removal of blood, thrombus and embolic debris (A). Landing zone requirements for the Proxis catheter include at least 12 mm from the tip of the guiding catheter to the lesion (B). Once deployed, PCI is undertaken through the the Proxis catheter with the balloon inflated.

The incidence of no-reflow during native vessel PCI is 0.6–2.0% for all comers [37]. This is higher for patients with acute STEMI than non-infarct patients (11.5% vs. 1.5%) [38], although it may be as high as 30% [39,40]. Certain angiographic criteria predictive of no-reflow suggest distal embolization as a causative factor. Thrombus rich lesions predict no-reflow in the setting of primary PCI [41,42], which probably reflects an increased risk of distal embolization resulting in microvascular plugging. Studies have also documented that the majority of patients undergoing primary PCI for acute STEMI sustain distal emboli to the vascular bed subtended by the infarct related artery [43,44]. Indeed approximately 15% of patients undergoing primary PCI for acute STEMI have angiographi-

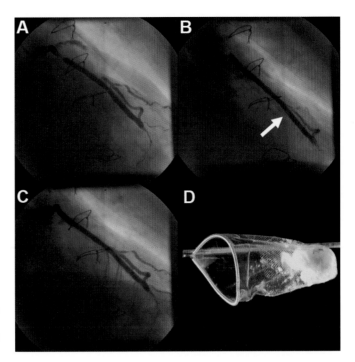

Figure 22.9. An innocuous appearing lesion in the proximal portion of a saphenous vein graft (A). Following placement of a FilterWire EX, the lesion is direct stented. Embolized material can be seen as a mobile filling defect in the filter basket (white arrow) (B). After removal of the FilterWire, there is TIMI III flow with good distal run off (C). The FilterWire contains a significant amount of embolized material (D).

cally visible emboli, which are associated with larger infarct size and a significant increase in five year mortality (44% vs. 9%) [43]. Patients with acute coronary syndromes involving the right coronary artery (RCA) may be at higher risk of distal embolization during PCI [44]. It is likely that distal embolization contributes to no-reflow and poor blush following primary PCI, and may be the predominant mechanism in some patients, particularly when significant amounts of thrombus are present [41,42].

Conclusions

Preventing the occurrence of distal embolization is important, as patients who experience a transient reduction in TIMI flow during primary PCI have significantly higher 6 month mortality compared with those who do not (31% vs. 3%) [45]. Despite the rationale, like thrombectomy devices, no randomized study of embolic protection in native coronary arteries has demonstrated a clinical benefit for their use. A recent meta-analysis has confirmed that whilst adjunctive devices for primary PCI reduce distal embolization and improve final myocardial blush grade, they have no impact on clinical outcomes [46]. It may be that blanket use of embolic protection and/or thrombectomy devices for all patients undergoing native vessel PCI for acute STEMI is the wrong approach, and reserving these devices for patients with significant thrombotic burden seems more appropriate.

Questions

1. A 56 year-old man presents 5 hours after symptom onset with a STEMI. Emergency catheterization shows near total occlusion of the LAD with 3 cm length thrombus just distal to the 1st septal perforator. What is the most reasonable course of action?
   A Direct stenting over a filter wire
   B Aspiration thrombectomy in conjunction with stenting
   C Direct stenting over a distal balloon occlusion aspiration system
   D Intracoronary TPA infusion followed by a bare metal stent

2. The optimal therapy for a patient with an 80% ulcerated lesion in a 12 year old saphenous vein graft located 1.5 cm from the distal anastomosis to a 2.5 mm LCX/OM2 vessel is:
   A A stent directly delivered over a BMW wire
   B A stent delivered over a FilterWire
   C A stent with the use of a balloon/aspiration distal protection system
   D A stent used in conjunction with a proximal balloon occlusion/aspiration system

3. All of the following have been shown to be of no benefit in SVG interventions, except:
   A Intra-graft abciximab bolus followed by 12 hr infusion
   B Intravenous integrilin followed by 12–18 hr infusion
   C Excisional atherectomy of bulky lesions
   D Use of balloon occlusion/aspiration distal protection system

4. With regards to no-reflow phenomenon during SVG intervention, which of the following is true?
   A It is effectively treated by intra-graft infusion of sodium nitroprusside
   B Its incidence is reduced by intravenous glycoprotein administration
   C Its incidence is reduced to a greater degree by distal filters as compared with balloon occlusion systems
   D Its incidence is reduced to a greater degree by balloon occlusion systems as compared with distal filters

5. With respect to the pathophysiology of no-reflow, which of the following is false?

   A In SVG intervention, no-reflow results primarily from vasospasm
   B In-situ acute platelet aggregation as well as thrombotic embolization may contribute
   C Compared to non-vein graft intervention, SVG-intervention is associated with a higher frequency of atheroembolization
   D Atherectomy, in comparison to PTCA, is associated with a higher frequency of clinically significant atheroemboli as measured by CKMB release

References

1. Burzotta F, Trani C, Romagnoli E, et al. Manual Thrombus-Aspiration Improves Myocardial Reperfusion: The Randomized Evaluation of the Effect of Mechanical Reduction of Distal Embolization by Thrombus-Aspiration in Primary and Rescue Angioplasty (REMEDIA) Trial. J Am Coll Cardiol 2005; 46(2): 371–376.

2. De Luca L, Sardella G, Davidson CJ, et al. Impact of intracoronary aspiration thrombectomy during primary angioplasty on left ventricular remodelling in patients with anterior ST elevation myocardial infarction. Heart 2006; 92(7): 951–957.

3. Colombo P. Dethrombosis to Enhance Acute Reperfusion in Myocardial Infarction; DEAR-MI. Presented at the European Paris Course on Revascularization; May 16–19, 2006, Paris.

4. Noel B. The Export Study: Thromboaspiration in Acute ST-Elevation MI Improves Myocardial Reperfusion. Presented at the European Paris Course on Revascularization; May 24–27, 2005, Paris.

5. Svilaas T, Vlaar PJ, van der Horst IC, Diercks GF, de Smet BJ, van den Heuvel AF, et al. Thrombus aspiration during primary percutaneous coronary intervention. N Engl J Med 2008 Feb 7; 358(6): 557–567.

6. Vlaar PJ, Svilaas T, van der Horst IC, Diercks GF, Fokkema ML, de Smet BJ, et al. Cardiac death and reinfarction after 1 year in the Thrombus Aspiration during Percutaneous coronary intervention in Acute myocardial infarction Study (TAPAS): a 1-year follow-up study. Lancet 2008 Jun 7; 371(9628): 1915–1920.

7. Napodano M, Pasquetto G, Sacca S, et al. Intracoronary thrombectomy improves myocardial reperfusion in patients undergoing direct angioplasty for acute myocardial infarction. J Am Coll Cardiol 2003; 42(8): 1395–1402.

8. Beran G, Lang I, Schreiber W, et al. Intracoronary Thrombectomy With the X-Sizer Catheter System Improves Epicardial Flow and Accelerates ST-Segment

Resolution in Patients With Acute Coronary Syndrome: A Prospective, Randomized, Controlled Study. Circulation 2002; 105(20): 2355–2360.

9. Lefevre T, Garcia E, Reimers B, et al. X-Sizer for Thrombectomy in Acute Myocardial Infarction Improves ST-Segment Resolution: Results of the X-Sizer in AMI for Negligible Embolization and Optimal ST Resolution (X AMINE ST) Trial. J Am Coll Cardiol 2005; 46(2): 246–252.

10. Antoniucci D, Valenti R, Migliorini A, et al. Comparison of rheolytic thrombectomy before direct infarct artery stenting vs. direct stenting alone in patients undergoing percutaneous coronary intervention for acute myocardial infarction. Am J Cardiol 2004; 93(8): 1033–1035.

11. Arshad A. Angiojet rheolytic thrombectomy in patients undergoing primary angioplasty for acute myocardial infarction: The AIMI study. Presented at the 15th Annual Transcatheter Cardiovascular Therapeutics. September 27–October 1, 2004, Washington, DC.

12. Arshad A, Cox D, Dib N, et al. Rheolytic Thrombectomy With Percutaneous Coronary Intervention for Infarct Size Reduction in Acute Myocardial Infarction: 30-Day Results From a Multicenter Randomized Study. J Am Coll Cardiol 2006; 48: 244–252.

13. Kloner RA, Ganote CE, Jennings RB. The "no-reflow" phenomenon after temporary coronary occlusion in the dog. J Clin Invest 1974; 54(6): 1496–1508.

14. Nakamura T, Kubo N, Seki Y, et al. Effects of a distal protection device during primary stenting in patients with acute anterior myocardial infarction. Circ J 2004; 68(8): 763–768.

15. Yip H-K, Wu C-J, Chang H-W, et al. Effect of the PercuSurge GuardWire device on the integrity of microvasculature and clinical outcomes during primary transradial coronary intervention in acute myocardial infarction. Am J Cardiol 2003; 92(11): 1331–1335.

16. Stone GW, Webb J, Cox DA, et al. Distal Microcirculatory Protection During Percutaneous Coronary Intervention in Acute ST-Segment Elevation Myocardial Infarction: A Randomized Controlled Trial. JAMA 2005; 293(9): 1063–1072.

17. Webb JG, Carere RG, Virmani R, et al. Retrieval and analysis of particulate debris after saphenous vein graft intervention. J Am Coll Cardiol 1999; 34(2): 468–475.

18. Baim DS, Wahr D, George B, et al. Randomized Trial of a Distal Embolic Protection Device During Percutaneous Intervention of Saphenous Vein Aorto-Coronary Bypass Grafts. Circulation 2002; 105(11): 1285–1290.

19. Carrozza J, Joseph P, Mumma M, Breall JA, et al. Randomized Evaluation of the TriActiv Balloon-Protection Flush and Extraction System for the Treatment of Saphenous Vein Graft Disease. J Am Coll Cardiol 2005; 46(9): 1677–1683.

20. Leineweber K, Bose D, Vogelsang M, et al. Intense Vasoconstriction in Response to Aspirate From Stented Saphenous Vein Aortocoronary Bypass Grafts. J Am Coll Cardiol 2006; 47(5): 981–986.

21. Stone GW, Rogers C, Hermiller J, et al. Randomized comparison of distal protection with a filter-based catheter and a balloon occlusion and aspiration system during percutaneous intervention of diseased saphenous vein aorto-coronary bypass grafts. Circulation 2003; 108(5): 548–553.

22. Dixon R. SPIDER: Saphenous Vein Protection In a Distal Embolic Protection Randomized Trial. Presented at the 16th Annual Transcatheter Cardiovascular Therapeutics; October 16–21, 2005, Washington, DC.

23. Limbruno U, Micheli A, De Carlo M, et al. Mechanical Prevention of Distal Embolization During Primary Angioplasty: Safety, Feasibility, and Impact on Myocardial Reperfusion. Circulation 2003; 108(2): 171–176.

24. Gick M, Jander N, Bestehorn H-P, et al. Randomized Evaluation of the Effects of Filter-Based Distal Protection on Myocardial Perfusion and Infarct Size After Primary Percutaneous Catheter Intervention in Myocardial Infarction With and Without ST-Segment Elevation. Circulation 2005; 112(10): 1462–1469.

25. Hermiller J, Cox D, Barbeau G, et al. Distal Filter Embolic Protection in AMI—The FLAME Registry. Presented at the 16th Annual Transcatheter Cardiovascular Therapeutics; October 16–21, 2005, Washington, DC.

26. Cura FA, Escudero AG, Berrocal D, et al. Protection of Distal Embolization in High-Risk Patients with Acute ST-Segment Elevation Myocardial Infarction (PREMIAR). Am J Cardiol 2007; 99(3): 357–363.

27. Rogers C. A prospective randomized comparison of proximal and distal protection in patients with diseased saphenous vein grafts. Presented at the 16th Annual Transcatheter Cardiovascular Therapeutics; October 16–21, 2005, Washington, DC.

28. Koch K. Proximal Aspiration in AMI Introduced: The Proxis Registry. Presented at the 16th Annual Transcatheter Cardiovascular Therapeutics; October 16–21, 2005, Washington, DC.

29. van Gaal WJ, Choudhury RP, Porto I, et al. Prediction of distal embolization during percutaneous coronary intervention in saphenous vein grafts. Am J Cardiol 2007; 99(5): 603–606.

30. Popma JJ, Cox N, Hauptmann KE, et al. Initial clinical experience with distal protection using the FilterWire in patients undergoing coronary artery and saphenous vein graft percutaneous intervention. Catheter Cardiovasc Interv 2002; 57(2): 125–134.

31. Giugliano GR, Kuntz RE, Popma JJ, *et al.* Determinants of 30-day adverse events following saphenous vein graft intervention with and without a distal occlusion embolic protection device. Am J Cardiol 2005; **95**(2): 173–177.

32. Kalan JM, Roberts WC. Morphologic findings in saphenous veins used as coronary arterial bypass conduits for longer than 1 year: necropsy analysis of 53 patients, 123 saphenous veins, and 1865 five-millimeter segments of veins. Am Heart J 1990; **119**(5): 1164–1184.

33. Neitzel GF, Barboriak JJ, Pintar K, *et al.* Atherosclerosis in aortocoronary bypass grafts. Morphologic study and risk factor analysis 6 to 12 years after surgery. Arteriosclerosis 1986; **6**(6): 594–600.

34. Saltissi S, Webb-Peploe MM, Coltart DJ. Effect of variation in coronary artery anatomy on distribution of stenotic lesions. Br Heart J 1979; **42**(2): 186–191.

35. Assali AR, Sdringola S, Moustapha A, *et al.* Percutaneous intervention in saphenous venous grafts: in-stent restenosis lesions are safer than de novo lesions. J Invasive Cardiol 2001; **13**(6): 446–450.

36. Ashby DT, Dangas G, Aymong EA, *et al.* Effect of percutaneous coronary interventions for in-stent restenosis in degenerated saphenous vein grafts without distal embolic protection. J Am Coll Cardiol 2003; **41**(5): 749–752.

37. Abbo KM, Dooris M, Glazier S, *et al.* Features and outcome of no-reflow after percutaneous coronary intervention. Am J Cardiol 1995; **75**(12): 778–782.

38. Piana RN, Paik GY, Moscucci M, *et al.* Incidence and treatment of "no-reflow" after percutaneous coronary intervention. Circulation 1994; **89**(6): 2514–2518.

39. Ito H, Tomooka T, Sakai N, *et al.* Lack of myocardial perfusion immediately after successful thrombolysis. A predictor of poor recovery of left ventricular function in anterior myocardial infarction. Circulation 1992; **85**(5): 1699–1705.

40. Ito H, Maruyama A, Iwakura K, *et al.* Clinical implications of the 'no reflow' phenomenon. A predictor of complications and left ventricular remodeling in reperfused anterior wall myocardial infarction. Circulation 1996; **93**(2): 223–228.

41. Yip HK, Chen MC, Chang HW, *et al.* Angiographic morphologic features of infarct-related arteries and timely reperfusion in acute myocardial infarction: predictors of slow-flow and no-reflow phenomenon. Chest 2002; **122**(4): 1322–1332.

42. Hara M, Saikawa T, Tsunematsu Y, *et al.* Predicting no-reflow based on angiographic features of lesions in patients with acute myocardial infarction. J Atheroscler Thromb 2005; **12**(6): 315–321.

43. Henriques JPS, Zijlstra F, Ottervanger JP, *et al.* Incidence and clinical significance of distal embolization during primary angioplasty for acute myocardial infarction. Eur Heart J 2002; **23**(14): 1112–1117.

44. Napodano M. Predictors of Distal Embolization during Direct Angioplasty for Acute Myocardial Infarction. Presented at the 16th Annual Transcatheter Cardiovascular Therapeutics; October 16–21, 2005, Washington, DC.

45. Mehta RH, Harjai KJ, Boura J, *et al.* Prognostic significance of transient no-reflow during primary percutaneous coronary intervention for ST-elevation acute myocardial infarction. Am J Cardiol 2003; **92**(12): 1445–1447.

46. Burzotta F, Testa L, Giannico F, *et al.* Adjunctive devices in primary or rescue PCI: A meta-analysis of randomized trials. Int J Cardiol. March 23, 2007 (Epub ahead of print).

Answers

1. B
2. D
3. D
4. A
5. A

CHAPTER 23

Carotid Artery Angioplasty and Stenting

Alberto Cremonesi, Shane Gieowarsingh, Estêvão C. de Campos Martins, & Fausto Castriota

GVM Hospitals of Care and Research, Cotignola (RA), Italy

Stroke has been acknowledged as the third leading cause of death, subsequent to heart disease and cancer, in the industrialized nations [1]. In the last decade, there has been unprecedented investment at national levels to develop the quality of services for heart disease and cancer leading to an improvement in patient-survival. The focus now is on advancing the management of stroke patients, as it is recognized with an ageing population the burden of this disease due to its high mortality, major disability and dependence, is truly substantial [2]. For this reason, it is vital that the more mature approach to the prevention and treatment at different levels in the pathogenesis and manifestation of this disease is pursued further by all concerned.

The single most common cause of ischemic stroke is atherosclerotic carotid artery disease. Carotid endarterectomy (CEA) has been shown to be efficacious in the long-term prevention of stroke for both symptomatic and asymptomatic patients with severe obstructive carotid disease [3–6]. Presently, carotid angioplasty and stenting (CAS) is a promising field due to its potential as complimentary therapy for patients who are considered high-risk for CEA; and as an alternative less-invasive and effective revascularization procedure for a large subset of patients.

Interventional Cardiology, First Edition. Edited by Carlo Di Mario, George D. Dangas, Peter Barlis.

Background

The main goal of carotid intervention is the prevention of stroke, in particular, disabling stroke in both the short and long term. Following the application of surgical endarterectomy for treating carotid bifurcation disease in the 1950s, it was not until 40 years later that Level-1 evidence from large randomized trials for its efficacy was established. Although there has been significant development of pharmacotherapy for vascular disease over the last 20 years, the stroke-prevention benefit has not been established specifically for patients with high-grade carotid stenosis [7,8]. CAS was developed due to a need to provide a less-invasive revascularization strategy for patients considered high-risk for surgical revascularization. The rapid advancement in endovascular technologies and techniques has resulted in the evolution of CAS to a refined technique with great potential to be applied to routine carotid revascularization practice.

Currently, controversy exists whether CAS should be accepted as an alternative to CEA. To answer this question there have been a few randomized trials comparing both therapies [9–12]; however, some have been hampered by difficulties with enrolment, results have been conflicting, many criticisms have been levied against trial designs, and hence a clear consensus cannot be established. Ongoing large randomized trials will hopefully address this uncertainty. Over the last decade there have been publications of single-center and multicenter case series and registry data providing valuable evidence for the effectiveness of this therapy in both the short- and mid-term. Nonetheless, arising from the discussions and debates one thing is clear; to move forward towards our goal of stroke prevention, these procedures must be performed by high-level and well-trained operators.

Important Concepts and Considerations

Tailored Approach Concept

To achieve high procedural-success the multifactorial CAS strategy involves a *"tailored approach"* in the application of endovascular techniques to a specific-patient with a specific-lesion and vascular anatomy. This requires an in-depth knowledge of neuro-assessment, carotid plaque characteristics, vascular anatomy, and technical features of endovascular materials: guiding-catheters and sheaths, guidewires, embolic protection devices (EPDs), balloons and stents. Following the experience gained in this field since 1997, with over 2000 procedures, our group strongly believes that each device has special characteristics and should be used following pre-defined logic indications.

Stent Intrinsic Anti-Embolic Property Concept

The major source of complications is distal embolization, either intraprocedural or postprocedural. For effective reduction of intraprocedural risk great emphasis is placed on the use of EPDs. An important concept to consider is the view that in the presence of an EPD, the type of stent implanted may not significantly impact on the risk of intraprocedural complications but may subsequently play a vital part in preventing neurological events due to plaque-prolapse. It is appreciated, that, whereas in the open surgical techniques the atheroma and thrombus burden are excised; the stent-protected angioplasty technique compacts this material to the wall, retaining it with its supporting scaffolding and wall-coverage properties. The stent-cell geometry may thus have an *"intrinsic anti-embolic property"* influencing the risk of plaque-prolapse and distal embolization during the 24-hour postprocedural and recuperative periods until re-endothelializaton is completed.

Safe CAS and Protected-Procedure Concept

The interventionalist *"safe CAS and protected-procedure"* concept should encompass the idea that two protection-positions should be implemented in practice. In addition to the use of high-tech devices to contain plaque (stents) or capture and remove embolic debris (EPDs), the implementation of the tailored approach to the entire management strategy from appropriate patient/lesion selection to meticulous device choice and interventional techniques is essential. An important element of this concept is the recognition of high-risk cases for CAS dependent primarily on the skill of the interventional vascular specialist. This is considerably more relevant in this field than other areas of percutaneous interventions.

Clinical Governance and Regulation

Establishment of standard operating procedures is critical to a successful CAS program. This is based on informed consent and patient choice, and effective clinical governance including consideration of setting up a prospective registry as a measure of quality assurance. This approach should be performed as part of a local institutional review board approved-protocol with dispassionate oversight and assessment by an independent neurologist. This *"regulation"* must be emphasized because of the need to always be critical of our management to improve patient care.

Measurement of Early Outcomes and Complications

In order to determine the safety of what we do in our clinical practice, *"early outcomes and complications"* should be analyzed in a focused manner. Several factors influence the 30-day risk of transient ischemic attack (TIA), stroke and death: among these are patient characteristics such as age and neurological symptom-status; and operational variables such as operator experience, aortic arch and carotid anatomy, plaque characteristics, stent technology and type of EPD employed. If complications are recorded with no discrimination of time-distribution, analysis on this cumulative data may not be useful to determine in detail the relevance of specified variables and may be misleading due to the heavy weight of confounding variables. Hence, we recommend documentation and analysis of adverse events within specified time-periods: the intraprocedural period, the 24-hour postprocedural period and the subsequent recuperative period up to 30 days.

Indications and Contra-indications

The indication for carotid intervention includes a symptomatic patient with an angiographic stenosis of ≥50% (that is, a lesion-related neurological event in the preceding six months); and an asymptomatic patient with an angiographic stenosis of ≥80%. The specific absolute contraindication for elective CAS is floating thrombus in the carotid artery. Standard relative contraindications to endovascular techniques would apply. The potential factors for considering a patient high-risk for CEA, due to medical co-morbidities and anatomic factors, thus indicating an endovascular approach are shown in Table 23.1; and Table 23.2 provides some insight into the issues that may prove a challenge or increase the risk of the stenting procedure.

Table 23.1. High surgical risk criteria.

Clinical Criteria	Anatomical Criteria
1. Age >75 years	1. High cervical lesion
2. CCS Class 3–4 or unstable angina	2. Tandem lesions >70%
3. NYHA Class III–IV	3. CEA restenosis
4. LVEF <35%	4. Contralateral ICA occlusion
5. MI <6 weeks	5. Hostile neck (prior irradiation, tracheostomy, radical neck dissection)
6. Multivessel coronary artery disease	6. Cervical immobility
7. Severe pulmonary disease	
8. Severe renal impairment	
9. Contralateral cranial nerve injury	

Table 23.2. Challenges for CAS.

1. Tortuous iliac vessels
2. Bovine or type III aortic arch
3. Calcified and irregular aortic arch
4. Tortuous supra-aortic vessels
5. Long irregular dishomogeneous plaque
6. Highly-calcified carotid lesions

Carotid Plaque Characteristics and Vascular Anatomy

The evaluation of carotid plaque profile should describe in addition to degree stenosis and vessel dimensions; both the length of disease and the morphologic features that predict plaque complexity and embolization-risk ("vulnerable plaque").

Both long lesions and clinically unstable plaques (i.e. recurrent TIAs) define a high-risk lesion subset, because of high plaque-burden and inflammatory activation respectively. Indeed, Krapf et al. [13] reported, using diffusion-weighted MRI, that the risk of new cerebral ischemic lesions after CAS was related to the length of the lesion; and Aronow et al. [14] described preprocedural leucocyte count to be associated with increased microembolization during CAS.

A study analyzing 200 CEA specimens showed that plaque-phenotype correlated with embolization-risk, where "vulnerable plaques" characterized by a large lipid pool covered by a thin fibrous cap were more prone to perioperative microem-

bolization as compared to fibrous plaques [15]. These vulnerable plaques are less echogenic, described as "soft-lesions," and this pattern can be quantified by the Grey Scale Median (GSM) method. In the ICAROS study [16], the risk of CAS-related stroke was 7.1% in lesions with GSM <25 and 1.5% in lesions with GSM > 25.

Therefore clinical, biochemical and morphological data should be assessed and integrated to predict the embolic-risk of a specific carotid lesion in order to plan the tailored approach to intervention.

Assessment of vascular profile includes defining the configuration of the aortic arch (Figure 23.1), angulation and tortuosity of supra-aortic trunks, lesion-site characteristics, intracranial segment of the internal carotid artery (ICA), and ipsilateral/contralateral cerebral circulation (Figure 23.2).

Cerebral Protection Devices

Carotid lesions contain friable, ulcerated plaque and thrombotic material that can embolize during

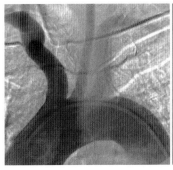
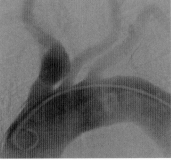
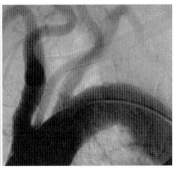

Figure 23.1 Aortic arch anatomy classified as type I, II and III with increasing levels of complexity for catheter engagement and provision of support for intervention.

A bovine configuration is where the left CCA originates from the brachiocephalic trunk.

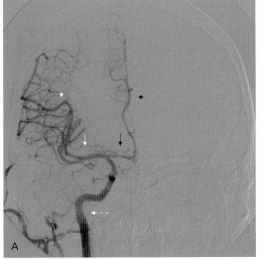
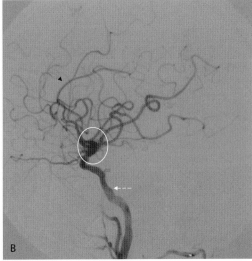

Figure 23.2 (A) Right AP intracranial angiogram. The outlined arrow shows the right ICA. The black arrow points to the anterior cerebral artery leading to the pericallosal artery (black arrow-head). The middle cerebral artery is showed by the white arrow and its branches (white arrow-head). (B) Right lateral intracranial angiogram. The outlined arrow shows the right ICA. The black arrow-head shows the pericallosal artery. The middle cerebral and anterior cerebral arteries are not well separated in this projection.

an intervention as shown in histopathologic analysis [17] and transcranial Doppler studies [18]. Embolic particles can be classified as either macroemboli (>100 μm) or microemboli (<100 μm). Macroemboli, especially >200 μm, are usually associated with clinical events, however, the effects of microembolization are not well known and may include subtle changes in neurocognitive function. Despite advanced stenting techniques and dual antiplatelet therapy embolization occurs invariably. A reduction of the Doppler-defined embolic load by an EPD has been shown [19]; and preliminary results indicate that with the routine use of such devices the results of CAS are comparable with the best surgical series [20,21].

Protected-CAS: Clinical Results

There is no randomized trial comparing the efficacy of protected- with unprotected-CAS and it is difficult to imagine that such a study will ever be conducted on a significant number of patients. Recent literature data shed some light:

- visible debris was documented in 60% of cases of filter protected-CAS by Sprouse [22], and in 66.8% by our group [23];
- in the German registry [24] protected-CAS was associated with a significantly lower rate of ipsilateral stroke (1.7% vs 4.1%, p = 0.007);
- our group reported a 79% reduction in the rate of embolic complications with protected-CAS [25];
- in the early phase of the EVA-3S study unprotected-CAS was associated with a 3.9 times higher stroke rate at 30 days as compared to protected-CAS [26];
- a 2003 review of the global registry found that the rates of stroke and death were 5.2% for unprotected-CAS and 2.2% for protected-CAS [27];
- Kastrup *et al.* [20] in a systematic review of the literature regarding the early outcome of CAS with and without EPD analyzed studies published between 1990 and 2002 (2537 unprotected-CAS and 896 protected-CAS procedures); and the combined 30-day stroke and death rates were 5.5% and 1.8% respectively (P < 0.001).

On the basis of this review EPDs appear to reduce thromboembolic complications during CAS.

Distal Protection Devices

Distal protection devices work by interrupting or filtering blood flow by positioning the device distal to the lesion in a straight portion of the ICA (landing-zone). The first system utilized an occlusion balloon, but today filters are usually employed because they are less complex and perhaps they are intuitive to use. Filters entrap debris from medium to large size, generally particles >100 μm. Filter performance can be summed up in crossing profile and capturing capability. Crossing profile is an important characteristic justified by the fact that the wire and the filter, constrained in the delivery system, must pass the lesion without detaching friable material. Capturing capability is dependent on membrane pore size and adequate wall apposition of the filter.

Limitations of Distal Protection Devices

The distal occlusion balloon shares with filters, especially in tight stenoses, the limitation of unprotected crossing of the lesion in order to deploy the device. Filters are not effective in trapping microemboli, limited by pore size. In tortuous or large distal ICA anatomy incomplete wall apposition may allow even macroemboli to bypass the system. In addition debris may be dislodged during the recapture phase (squeezing effect) of the procedure. The distal occlusion balloon, despite being able to block microemboli by occluding the ICA, can lead to embolization via collaterals from the external carotid artery (ECA) to the middle cerebral artery. Moreover, about 5% to 8% of patients develop clamping intolerance to the interruption of cerebral perfusion [28]. Additionally, both systems may be an embolic source themselves due to intimal damage at the landing-zone.

Proximal Protection Devices

Proximal protection devices work by interrupting or reversing blood flow in the ICA. They offer the advantage of crossing the lesion under protection and blocking both macro- and microemboli. Moreover, navigation of the device in the distal ICA is not required, thus reducing the risk of intimal damage, spasm or dissection. There are two such devices:

Mo.Ma™ (Invatec)

The Mo.Ma system consists of a 9 Fr sheath (8F in the new system) with an effective working channel of 6 Fr and 5 Fr respectively; and two independently inflatable balloons placed at a distance of 7.2 cm. The distal balloon occludes the ECA up to a diameter of 6 mm and the proximal balloon occludes the common carotid artery (CCA) up to a diameter of 13 mm, thus preventing antegrade flow from the CCA and retrograde flow from the ECA. Then the lesion can be crossed and treated under protection; and following post-dilatation three 20 ml syringes of blood are actively aspirated and checked for debris before deflating the balloons.

NeuroProtection System™ (NPS) (Gore)

The NeuroProtection System, derived from the Parodi anti-embolic system (PAES) (ArteriA), allows continuous passive ICA flow-reversal through endovascular clamping of the CCA by inflating a balloon located at the tip of an 11F sheath (9 Fr in the new system) and of the ECA by inflating an independent balloon-catheter advanced into the ECA via the sheath. The system is connected to the contralateral femoral vein which allows flow-reversal of blood from the contralateral cerebral circulation via the circle of Willis, down the ICA and through the sheath into the venous system. A filter (pore size 180 μm) collects debris before the blood re-enters the venous system. Then the lesion can be crossed and treated under protection. After each stage, particularly those associated with the greatest risk of embolization, 10 ml of blood are actively aspirated and at the end balloons are deflated while active suction is applied to retrieve any particle contiguous to the balloon-occluder. The effective working channel of the assembled system is 6 Fr.

Proximal Protection During CAS: Clinical Outcomes

Most of the clinical data on the NPS was obtained with the first version, i.e. the PAES. In 2005, Parodi *et al.* [29] reported on the first 200 patients treated, with a technical success rate of 98.5%, 30-day stroke and death rate of 1.5% and clamping intolerance of 3%. Other small, non-randomized studies confirmed the efficacy of the PAES in preventing embolic complications [30].

The efficacy of the Mo.Ma device in preventing microembolization was assessed in a comparative study with a distal filter system by observing microembolic signals (MES) with transcranial Doppler during the CAS procedure [31]. Five procedural steps were analyzed: (1) positioning the protection system; (2) crossing the stenosis; (3) stent deployment; (4) post-dilatation; (5) retrieving the system. The Mo.Ma system was associated with significantly lower counts during Steps 2 to 4. MES detection is a surrogate marker of microembolization which can be hampered by technical limitations, such as the inability to differentiate between solid and gaseous emboli; nevertheless, the association of a high MES count with neurological complications was established in the Antonius CAS registry [20]. In the PRIAMUS multicenter registry [32], 416 patients underwent CAS with the Mo.Ma device. Technical success was achieved in 99% of cases, mean clamping time was

4.9 ± 1.1 minutes, transient clamping intolerance was observed in 5.8% and macroscopic debris was retrieved in about 60% of patients. At 30-day follow-up, the cumulative incidence of adverse events was 4.6%; with a 0.7% rate of major stroke and death.

Limitations of Proximal Protection Devices

The drawbacks of proximal protection devices include their large size, clamping intolerance and the impossibility of their use with severe disease of the ECA or CCA. Contralateral ICA occlusion is not necessarily a contraindication in the presence of a functional circle of Willis with adequate flow from the vertebral system.

The need for large femoral sheaths may preclude use in patients with severe peripheral disease and could be associated with an increase in access site complications. Nevertheless, with the first version of the Mo.Ma device (10 Fr), in the PRIAMUS registry, the rate of local complications was 4.1%, none requiring surgical repair or blood transfusions. Higher complication rates were reported by Rabe *et al.* [33] with the PAES, but, given the current availability of 8–9 Fr size for the Mo.Ma and 9 Fr for the NPS device, it is reasonable to expect a low rate of clinically-significant access site complications.

Clamping intolerance may occur in up to 8% of patients and is generally associated with severe contralateral disease or poorly developed cerebral collateral circulation. An intraprocedural parameter predictive of tolerance is represented by a backpressure >30 mmHg. Another key factor is overall clamping time, which has progressively shortened with increased experience (for the Mo.Ma system from ten minutes in the study of Diederich *et al.* [34] to five minutes in the PRIAMUS registry, with a parallel decline in the rate of clamping intolerance from 12% to about 6%). The same holds true for the PAES/NPS device, since the rate of clamping intolerance dropped from 8% in 2001 to 3% in 2005 [29]. However, clamping intolerance does not represent an absolute contraindication to carry on the procedure. Indeed, three strategies can be adopted: hurry up in order to restore perfusion as soon as possible; positioning under protection a distal filter and then deflating the balloons ("seatbelt and air-bag" technique); perform a step-by-step procedure in which the balloons are inflated and deflated at each procedural-step.

When to Use Proximal or Distal Protection and Potential Complications

Large studies comparing proximal with distal protection are lacking, so device selection should be based on the tailored approach. In challenging anatomies, with angulated ICA-CCA take-off and/ or lack of a suitable ICA landing-zone, proximal protection should be strongly recommended. The same holds true for lesions with high embolic-risk, since proximal protection devices seem to be more effective than filter systems in avoiding distal embolization. The most frequent complications with distal protection devices are spasm and slow-flow with an incidence of up to 3.6% and 7.2% respectively [35]. In our experience a gentle approach as well as the use of a soft-tipped filter-wire minimized the frequency of this problem. Slow-flow may occur when the filter-pores are partially or completely occluded with debris and disappears following removal of the filter. Dissections at the landing-zone have been described in 0.5% to 0.9% of cases [21,36]. Device retrieval occasionally poses a problem and it is here that the torqueability of a guiding-catheter can help change the attitude of the system allowing the retrieval sheath to cross the stent. Other manoeuvres include turning the patient's head or using a buddy wire. Complications related to proximal protection devices are mostly related to intolerance. In the recently completed Mo.Ma registry [37] intolerance was observed in 7.1% of patients (in 1.9% intermittent balloon deflation was necessary to complete the procedure, and in 0.6% a distal filter was positioned). All patients completed the procedure without in-hospital and 30-day neurological complications.

Self-expanding Carotid Stents

Structural and Functional Characteristics

The first self-expanding stent dedicated to carotid application was the cobalt-alloy braided-mesh frame that is highly flexible with acceptable radial strength. The frame is compressible and con-strained within a sheath: a spring-like action allows it to expand as the sheath is withdrawn during deployment. Advantages include a small and flexible delivery system, a small free-cell area with high scaffolding and wall-coverage properties (plaque-covering) and adaptability to the changing diameter across the bifurcation. However, it tends to straighten the vessel and has an unpredictable foreshortening during deployment.

The second group of self-expanding stents is represented by a nitinol structure (nickel-titanium alloy). The thermal expansion properties of nitinol characterize these devices and when exposed to body temperature they expand to the predetermined shape and size. Most are obtained from a tube of nitinol which is laser-cut to create a frame comprised of sequential aligned annular rings interconnected in a helical fashion. Another frame is the flat-sheet nitinol-roll closed-cell design. An advantage of the nitinol stents is minimal foreshortening on deployment.

Nitinol stents, for simplicity, can be categorized as an open-cell or closed-cell design, with either a cylindrical- or tapered-shape. The open-cell designs tend to have a larger free-cell area compared to the closed-cell designs. The advantages of open-cell stents include high conformability and flexibility, and high vessel-wall adaptability. Disadvantages include moderate scaffolding and wall-coverage properties, and stent-strut malalignment in complex carotid lesions. The closed-cell stents have high scaffolding and wall-coverage properties but are disadvantaged by stiffness with poor conformability and flexibility. The semi-quantitative comparison of functional differences among stent designs are shown in Table 23.3.

New Developments

The Cristallo Ideale™ stent (Invatec) is a nitinol self-expanding stent loaded on a 5F delivery system, characterized by a hybrid solution of open-cells in the distal and proximal segments in order to enhance flexibility and adaptability; and a closed-cell design in the middle to obtain the appropriate scaffolding and wall-coverage to prevent plaque-prolapse (Figure 23.3). Safety and performance for the treatment of ICA stenosis have been recently evaluated in an international multi-center prospective registry (Cristallo

Table 23.3. Semi-quantitative comparison of functional differences amongst stents.

Stent technical features	Braided mesh	Nitinol OCG*	Nitinol CCG**
a) Foreshortening	TS	TI	TI
b) Conformability/flexibility	+	++	−
c) Vessel wall adaptability	+	++	+
d) Scaffolding	++	+	++
e) Radial strength	+	++	++
f) Radial stiffness	+	+	+
g) Wall coverage	++	−	++

Technically Insignificant (TI): <15%
Technically Significant (TS): >15%
Worse than others (−)
Comparable with others (+)
Better than others (++)
*OCD: Segmented crown, Open Cell Geometry
**CCD: Closed Cell Geometry (including flat rolled sheath frame)

	Distal	Middle	Proximal
Flexibility	High	Appropriate	High
Radial Force	Low	Appropriate	Low
Scaffolding	Low	High	Low
M/A Ratio	Low	Appropriate	Low

A

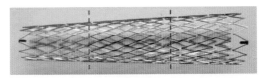

Open cell Ø1.94   Closed cell Ø1.02   Open cell Ø2.00

B

Figure 23.3. (A) Functional characteristics of the hybrid carotid stent. The closed-cell mid portion and two open-cell portions at both edges provide adequate scaffolding to the plaque while assuring high flexibility and vessel wall adaptability respectively. (B) Comparison of free cell area (mm²) in the three segments of the hybrid carotid stent.

Registry) [38]. The primary endpoint was the 30-day incidence of device or procedure-related major or minor stroke and death. The results are very encouraging with no major neurological events reported; and two episodes of TIAs (1.6%) both occurring in the postprocedural period were documented. Secondary end-points were technical success (ability to deploy the stent in the target lesion with the residual diameter stenosis <30%) and procedural-success (technical success free of procedural-major neurological events). Technical and procedural-success were achieved in all the enrolled patients (100%). Three patients (2.5%) died from non-neurological death during the study period (two pulmonary-related and one cardiac-related). All these fatal events were neither device- nor procedure-related complications.

Another 5 Fr delivery system is the recent Vivexx™ (Bard) family of nitinol self-expanding open-cell stent design that offers a broad range of sizes including a 12 mm option for dealing with very large CCAs.

Is There A Logical Scheme for Stent Selection?
Different stent designs demonstrate functional equivalence when used in uncomplicated scenar- ios: simple supra-aortic anatomies, straight carotid bifurcations, stable fibrous plaques. However, fre- quently the operator has to face challenging situa- tions requiring a move toward a tailored approach. Table 23.4 shows a functional categorization where cobalt-alloy braided-mesh stents are the first choice when the greatest need is to achieve reliable plaque-coverage and long-acting plaque-prolapse prevention due to the constant radial force prop- erty (soft and long dishomogeneous lesions are very prone to distal embolization). Bosiers *et al* [39] demonstrated a clear benefit in favor of stent

Table 23.4. Functional categorization of stents.

Carotid lesion/bifurcation profile	Type of stent
1. medium to long lesions (15 to 25 mm)	Cobalt-alloy braided mesh stent
2. soft dishomogeneous lesions	
3. straight carotid bifurcations	
4. carotid bifurcation lesions with ICA/CCA diameter mismatch	Nitinol open cell stents
5. angled carotid bifurcation	
6. short lesions (<15 mm)	Nitinol closed cell stents
7. highly calcified lesions	
8. straight carotid bifurcation	

scaffolding and wall-coverage for reducing post- procedural neurological complications for symp- tomatic patients (unstable risky plaque). When the main technical challenge is represented by the carotid bifurcation and plaque complexity (severely-angled lesions, plaque ulceration), or the main goal is to maintain the original anatomy/ course of a very tortuous vessel; the in-vessel flex- ibility and the wall/plaque conformability of nitinol open-cell stents are unmatched. Nitinol closed-cell stents represent a great technical solution for focal concentric lesions, especially if resistant or calci- fied: in such a clinical subset the functional key point is the outward radial force exerted by the stent over time.

Step-by-Step Technique of Carotid Stenting

Clinical Protocol
Pre-medication
- Dual antiplatelet therapy with aspirin and clopidogrel, ideally, initiated five days before the procedure; and continued for at least 30 days at which time clopidogrel is usually discontinued.

Pre-procedure investigations
- Carotid duplex scan, CTA/MRA scan
- Independent neurological evaluation

General procedural measures
- Head-restrain and no sedation, with neuro- evaluation during procedure by simple com- munication and movement parameters
- Standard monitoring of vital parameters
- Heparin iv 70 U/Kg (ACT 250–300 seconds)

Technique
Vascular Access
Femoral access is recommended, but in the pres- ence of extreme tortuosity or occlusion of the iliac arteries the radial/brachial approach is feasible; however, consideration needs to be given to the compatibility of the materials in planning the intervention. Generally, the right CCA is approached from the left arm and vice versa, but in the reality is determined by the distance between the origins of the supra-aortic trunks.

Baseline Angiographic Evaluation

In the absence of a CTA/MRA scan aortic arch angiography is undertaken with a pigtail catheter (30° to 45° LAO) to visualize the origin of the supra-aortic vessels. Selective cannulation of the target vessel is performed to evaluate the carotid bifurcation in at least two orthogonal projections, demonstrating the maximum severity of the lesion and adequate separation of the ICA from the ECA, in both digitally subtracted and regular formats. The RAO view is helpful to separate the division of the brachiocephalic trunk into the subclavian artery and CCA. It is mandatory to perform an intracranial angiogram which may reveal an unexpected arteriovenous malformation or for comparative assessment with the postintervention angiogram in the event of embolization. Four-vessel angiography is indicated only where the complexity of the case recommends it as mandatory; such as establishing the adequacy of the collateral circulation and the function of the circle of Willis when considering endovascular clamping in the presence of contralateral ICA occlusion.

Common Carotid Engagement

Obtaining a safe and stable engagement of the CCA is one of the most important technical aspects to the CAS procedure. Two standard techniques are described outlining the most commonly used materials in our laboratory.

Guiding-Catheter Engagement
- A 90–100 cm 8 Fr guiding-catheter is chosen according to the aortic arch configuration:
- For simple anatomy a 40° angled soft-tip catheter is advanced to the mid-CCA over a soft-angled 0.035″ standard hydrophilic wire positioned just below the bifurcation.
  - For complex anatomy an angulated guide such as a Hockey-stick curve catheter is advanced into the proximal CCA.
- The introduction of two, or possibly three, 0.035″ wires in order to advance the catheter in the presence of an unstable situation is feasible. Another option is the placement of a 0.014″ wire in the ECA for increased stability during the intervention.

- The great advantage of this technique is steerability but it is critical to be cognizant of the risk of scraping the aortic arch during manipulation with the attendant risk of embolization. This can be avoided by meticulous technique, executed by gentle, small and slow movements; always advancing under rotation and with the right orientation of the catheter using the wire to engage the artery. Of course, a drawback of this strategy is the large femoral access with the attendant risk of complications.

Sheath Placement
- A 100 cm 5 Fr JR4 guiding-catheter is advanced over a soft-angled 0.035″ standard hydrophilic wire into the CCA. The use of a guiding-catheter allows contrast injection with a 0.035" wire.
- Following an angiogram delineating the bifurcation the hydrophilic wire is advanced into the ECA and positioned in a distal branch avoiding the lingual artery. The guiding-catheter is then advanced deeply into the ECA in a stable position, and if added support is needed a 0.018″ wire may also be accommodated. The standard 0.035″ wire is exchanged for a long 260–300 cm 0.035″ support-wire.
- The guiding-catheter is then withdrawn and a guiding-sheath is advanced to the mid-CCA over the support wire. In our practice the Mo.Ma device, which incorporates the functional aspect of a proximal protection device into a shuttle sheath, is applied and its respective aspects are advanced into the ECA and CCA.
- The advantage of this technique is its safety but it is less steerable and with a tortuous CCA kinks can result or existing tortuous loops can be exaggerated and displaced cephalad. In addition, with significant disease in the proximal CCA or an occluded ECA this technique is not feasible.

EPD management

Managing the EPD in a safe and expeditious manner is one of the key points to successful CAS and several issues were discussed in the relevant section.

Pre-dilatation

Pre-dilatation is reserved for very tight lesions, heavily calcified lesions or stenoses with a high tendency to recoil such as long fibrotic lesions. This is usually undertaken with a low profile coronary balloon in the range of 2.5–3.5 mm diameter and 20–30 mm length, and inflated at nominal pressure to minimize the risk of embolization. Consideration should be given to using a cutting balloon for heavily calcified lesions usually with a diameter of 3.5–4.0 mm and inflated at moderate pressure (8 atm). Our group reported on the use of this application in 111 patients with severe highly calcific *de novo* disease with a procedural-technical success rate of 100% [40]. The combined all stroke and death rate at 30 days follow-up was 0.9%, one major stroke. Pretreatment with 0.5 to 1 mg of intravenous atropine is required at this stage and/or post-dilatation phase. Large doses of atropine are avoided in the elderly, as this can result in confusion and make accurate neurological assessment difficult.

Stent Deployment

The unconstrained diameter of the self-expanding stent should be 1–2 mm larger than the reference vessel diameter in order to obtain a stable position and a reliable wall apposition. Usually, we recommend to stent from "angiographically normal-to-normal" vessel. In the presence of challenging anatomy it is helpful when bringing up materials across the arch is to view the stability of the guide in an LAO view. When deploying the stent, release at least 5 mm of the stent distally and wait for it to expand and stabilize against the wall before releasing the remainder of the stent. If the distal edge lands into a tortuous segment injury may result. It is prudent to be aware that tortuous segments are not straightened by a stent but are simply displaced cephalad and may be exaggerated. Speed and minimum use of devices across the lesion are not negligible keys for successful CAS.

Post-dilatation

Post-dilatation is always a critical step as the greatest amounts of emboli are released in this phase. To minimize the embolic load we recommend:

- balloons no larger than 5.5 mm in diameter
- inflating to nominal pressure
- accepting a 10–15% residual stenosis
- persistent flow via the struts into an ulcer does not require further dilatation
- if the ECA becomes occluded recanalization should be attempted only if the patient is symptomatic (jaw or facial pain) and in such a case it may be sufficient to restore only TIMI II flow.

Final Angiographic Evaluation

Following EPD removal, final angiograms are acquired in the same baseline projections. If a distal protection device was used the landing-zone has to checked carefully, particularly if the ICA is tortuous, to exclude any spasm or dissection. Ipsilateral intracranial angiography should be routinely acquired.

Vascular Access Site Management

General access site management should apply and we must take into account that an early ambulation and discharge can counteract the activated carotid sinus reflex and the occasionally observed post-procedural hypotension.

Case Histories

The following cases were selected to illustrate the tailored approach to CAS.

Case 1: Short and Soft Plaque Associated with Complex Anatomy (Figure 23.4)

Technical Issues

- Vessel tortuosity is challenging for distal EPDs and necessitates a stent with good conformability to respect the original vessel anatomy; and the mismatch between the ICA and CCA requires a tapered design.
- Soft highly-embologenic plaque needs a stent with high scaffolding properties.

"Tailored" CAS Strategy

- Proximal EPDs avoid the risk of un-protected crossing of the lesion and tortuous segment with a distal device.
- The Cristallo Ideale stent provides good conformability because of the open-cells at the

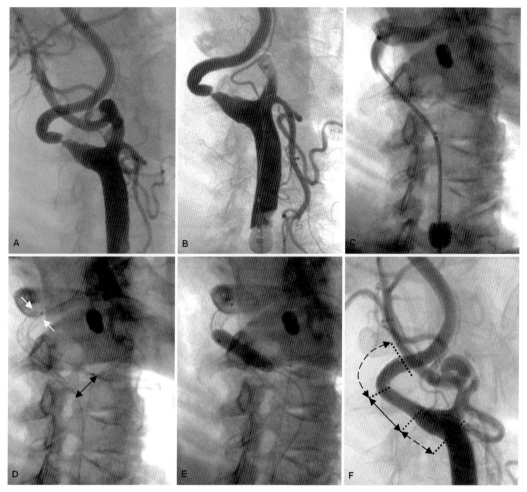

Figure 23.4. (A) Short and high-grade lesion in right ICA with significant "soft" component identified by duplex scan. (B) Contrast injection through the Mo.Ma device after flow blockage "roadmap." (C) Stent 7/10 x 40 mm positioning; (D) Stent deployed: distal edge diameter showed by white arrows, proximal edge diameter showed by black arrow. (E) Post-dilatation with a 5.5/20 mm balloon. (F) Final result: The closed-cell segment is showed by the full arrow and the outline arrows show the open-cell segments.

distal and proximal parts; the closed-cells in the middle part afford adequate scaffolding and the tapered design suitably adjusts to the vessel mismatch.

Case 2: Challenging Supra-aortic Anatomy (Figure 23.5)
Technical Issues
- Marked tortuosity of the brachiocephalic trunk and CCA, in addition to posing a challenge to engagement makes it difficult to establish good support to complete the intervention.

"Tailored" CAS Strategy
- Use of multiple wires to engage the CCA and maintain stability; in addition to the use of a soft-tip guiding-catheter are key strategies.
- Also, the choice of a highly deliverable stent is crucial.

Case 3: Long Ulcerated Lesion (Figure 23.6)
Technical Issues
- A long irregular lesion with severe ulcerations poses a high-embologenic risk. In addition,

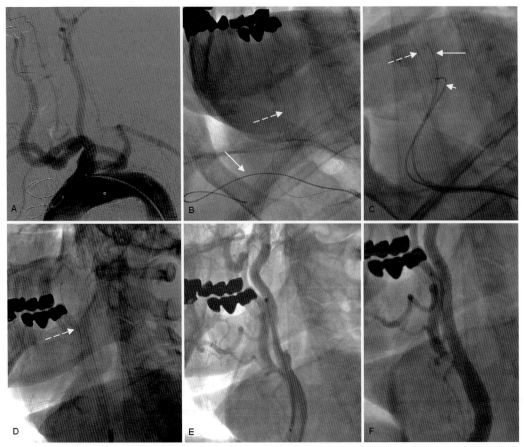

Figure 23.5. (A) Arch angiogram shows marked tortuosity of the supra-aortic vessels. (B) A 0.035″ hydrophilic wire placed in the right subclavian artery (full arrow) stabilizes the 40° 8 Fr guide in order to advance a 0.014″ wire to the ECA (outline arrow). (C) Then the 0.035″ wire is brought up into the CCA followed by another 0.035″ wire (head arrow). With this support the guide can be safely advanced into the CCA. (D) A filter is positioned in the distal ICA with the 0.014″ wire in the ECA providing extra support. (E) Carotid Wallstent (Boston Scientific) positioning, (F) Final result after post-dilatation.

crossing of the lesion with a wire affixed to a filter is risky.

"Tailored" CAS Strategy

- The Spider filter (eV3) allows the choice of an independent 0.014″ wire to gently cross the lesion.
- Carotid Wallstent provides high scaffolding and long-acting plaque-prolapse prevention until the ulcerations are obliterated. As the ICA is aligned to the CCA the tendency of the Wallstent to

straighten the vessel does not pose a problem in this case.

Case 4: Very Large CCA > 10 mm and Consequent Vessel Mismatch (Figure 23.7)

Technical Issues and "Tailored" CAS Strategy

The very large CCA and vessel mismatch requires the right stent, and currently the Vivexx family of stents include a 12 mm size. In addition it is an open-cell design and available in a tapered shape which is suitable for the mismatch.

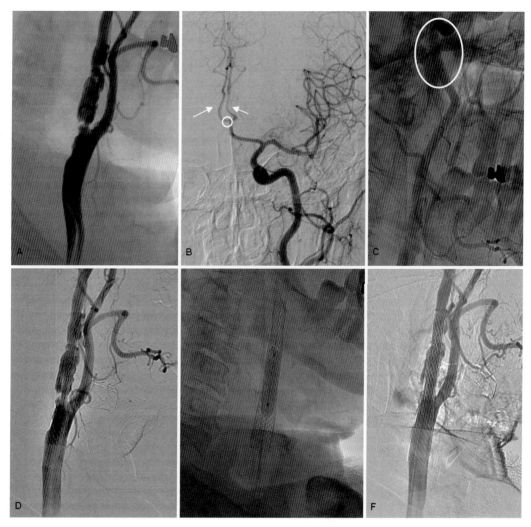

Figure 23.6. (A) Long ulcerated lesion involving the left ICA and distal CCA. (B) Cerebral angiogram shows a dominant left hemisphere with visualization of both anterior cerebral arteries (full arrows) and the anterior communicating artery (circle). (C) Confirmation of good wall apposition of filter (circle); (D) Suboptimal wall apposition of 9/40 mm stent. (E) Post-dilatation with a 5.5/20 mm balloon. (F) Final result showing good stent expansion. The concept to cover from angiographically normal-to-normal segments is illustrated. The persistent ulcerations will be excluded by in two to three weeks.

Case 5: Unexpected Findings (Figure 23.8)

- A patient awaiting aortic valve surgery attended for intervention to an asymptomatic right ICA stenosis. Unexpectedly, intracranial angiography revealed an arteriovenous malformation (AVM) feeding off from the right anterior cerebral circulation. Our neurosurgical colleagues were consulted and based on the possibility that stenting will increase the perfusion pressure to the AVM thus risking a hemorrhagic complication; a decision was made to manage the patient conservatively until further assessment and treatment of the AVM. This case illustrates the value of obtaining an intracranial angiogram when planning CAS; and emphasizes the importance of teamwork and consultation of colleagues in a safe CAS practice.

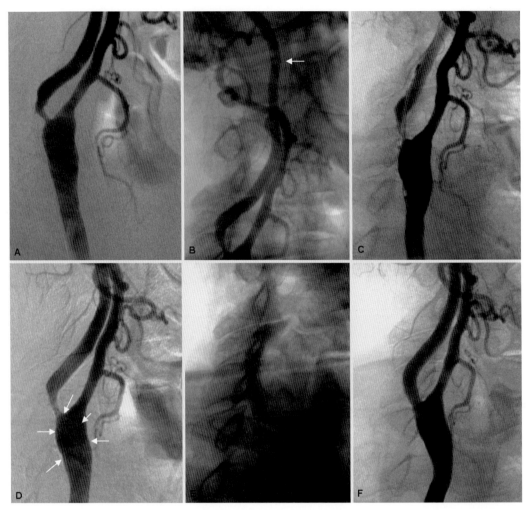

Figure 23.7. (A) Short and severe lesion of right ICA with an enormous CCA. (B) Confirmation of good filter wall apposition. (C) Stent positioning 8/12 x 40 mm. (D) Stent aspect after deployment, noting the struts in the CCA. (E) Post-dilatation with 5.5/20 mm balloon. (F) Final result.

Carotid Stenting Complications

Bradycardia and Hypotension

Transient sinus bradycardia or asystole are relatively common responses during balloon dilatation at the carotid bifurcation and pretreatment with atropine is preventative. This is less commonly observed in treating restenosis after CEA where the receptors may have been denervated by surgical dissection. Hypotension due to stimulation of the baroreceptors from both balloon dilatation and the persisting stretch of the self-expanding stent is not uncommon and is usually managed by adequate intravascular volume expansion; but with heavily-calcified lesions may be more pronounced and may require small doses of intravenous vasopressors such as 0.5 mg metaraminol. Continued hemodynamic monitoring in the 24-hour postprocedural period is crucial. Severe sustained hypotension may require dopamine infusion, but it is important not to overlook other potential causes of hypotension such as retroperitoneal hemorrhage. Hypotension should be corrected expeditiously in the presence of contralateral ICA occlusion, intracranial stenoses, vertebrobasilar disease and periprocedural cerebral ischemia secondary to an embolic event.

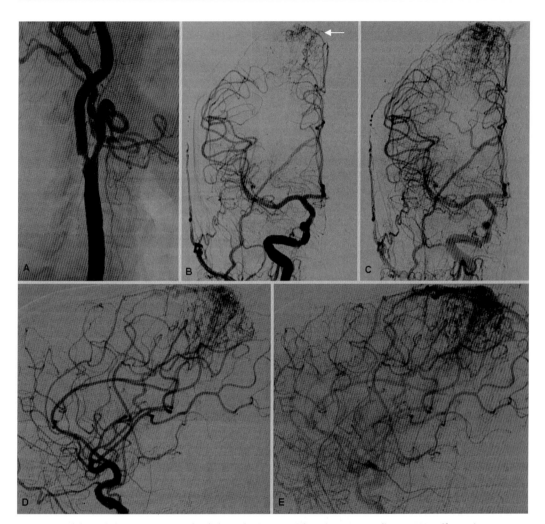

Figure 23.8. (A) Focal right ICA stenosis. (B–E) show the intracranial angiogram revealing an AV malformation.

Carotid Artery Spasm

Spasm of the distal ICA following filter deployment usually resolves spontaneously within several minutes after removal. A flow-limiting spasm could be a potential hazard in the presence of contralateral ICA occlusion and/or incomplete circle of Willis. Intra-arterial administration of 100 to 400 μg of nitroglycerin, once blood pressure allows, through the guiding-catheter generally aids in resolution of the spasm. Recalcitrant spasm usually responds to low-pressure balloon-angioplasty (≤2 atm).

Distal Embolization

Symptomatic distal embolization is the most important complication and the extensive use of

EPDs has reduced this to a rare event (0.4 to 1.5%). The predisposing factors are shown in Table 23.5. It is essential to monitor the patient's neurological status after every step of the procedure. If a significant change appears and persist, general patient care should be instituted with emphasis on maintaining normal blood pressure and intravascular volume status, stabilizing heart rate, and maintaining a viable airway with oxygen administration. If the patient becomes agitated and especially if the airway is compromised, the assistance of an anesthesiologist should be utilized. Whenever possible the procedure should be concluded quickly and intracranial angiography undertaken. The most likely sites are the distal ICA and the middle cerebral artery including its branches. Large vessel

Table 23.5. Considered factors increasing risk of embolization.

1. Inadequate pre-treatment with antiplatelet therapy
2. Inadequate anti-coagulation
3. Prolonged attempts to engage CCA in challenging anatomies
4. Soft plaque
5. Aggressive guidewire manipulation
6. Aggressive balloon dilatation pre- or post-stent implantation
7. Forceful crossing of a heavily-calcified plaque with a high-profile stent

occlusion is easy to detect, but embolism in the smaller branches requires careful scrutiny utilizing the preprocedural angiogram. An attempt should be made to recanalize an occluded large vessel as soon as possible (balloon angioplasty, thrombolytic agents, IIb/IIIa inhibitors). For a symptomatic small branch occlusion adequate hydration, blood pressure and anti-coagulation should be ensured.

Intracranial Hemorrhage

Cerebral hemorrhage is a life-threatening complication, though rare. Sudden loss of consciousness preceded by severe headache in the absence of vessel occlusion should alert the operator. A more subtle feature may be signs of a localized expanding phenomenon on angiography. Once suspected, anti-coagulation should be reversed and an emergency CT scan performed. Cerebral hemorrhage has been associated with a combination of excessive anti-coagulation, poorly controlled hypertension, aggressive attempts at intracranial neurovascular rescue, presence of a vulnerable berry aneurysm, or CAS in the presence of a recent ischemic stroke (less than three weeks).

Hyperperfusion Syndrome

The hyperperfusion syndrome is related to long-standing hypoperfusion that results in impaired autoregulation of the microcirculation; thus following revascularization the increased perfusion pressure overwhelms the ability of the dilated arterioles to constrict. This is a rare complication manifested as ipsilateral headache, nausea, confusion, neurological deficits, focal seizures and intracranial hemorrhage; typically occurring in patients with severe carotid stenosis and poor collateral circulation, such as with occlusion of the contralateral ICA or underdeveloped circle of Willis. In addition, bilateral carotid stenting during the same sitting may contribute. Contrary to the surgical hyperperfusion syndrome where symptoms develop within a few days, the endovascular hyperperfusion syndrome develops during or in the immediate postprocedural period. This is likely related to heparin administration, dual antiplatelet agents and the previous use of glycoprotein IIB/IIIA antagonists which is no longer recommended. Meticulous control of anti-coagulation and blood pressure in predisposed patients is critical to prevention.

Contrast Encephalopathy

Contrast encephalopathy is very rare and is a transient neurological syndrome mostly related to a prolonged procedure where a large volume of contrast is used. Neurological deficit with marked contrast enhancement "staining" in the basal ganglion and the cortex can develop, but without brain abnormalities on CT. No abnormalities on intracranial angiography are detected. Because the contrast medium does not cross the blood-brain barrier, this phenomenon may be caused by both a fine particulate embolization and excessive local contrast. Patients typically recover completely within 24 hours without permanent neurological deficit.

Carotid Dissection

Carotid dissection is a rare complication, predisposed by severe tortuosity and poor control of filter position or use of a distal balloon occlusion device. Post-dilatation of the distal stent edge within the ICA and aggressive manipulation of the guiding-catheter in the CCA are also risky. Management options include balloon-angioplasty, additional stent implantation, or a conservative strategy dependent on severity and flow.

Carotid Perforation

Carotid perforation is an extremely rare event predisposed by oversizing the post-dilatation balloon or aggressive dilatation. Prolonged balloon inflation or a covered stent may be considered to manage the situation.

Acute Stent Thrombosis

Acute stent thrombosis is a remarkably rare event. Dual antiplatelet therapy has demonstrated to lower the rate of stent thrombosis and the periprocedural embolic events. In addition, good stenting techniques can play a positive role. As a general rule, based mostly on common sense, we treat patients referred for non-atherosclerotic lesions or with sub-optimal results with dual antiplatelet agents indefinitely.

Restenosis

The restenosis rate after CAS is remarkably low and recently Setacci *et al.* [41] reported on one of the largest assessments undertaken which showed an intrastent restenosis (>70%) rate of 2.7%.

Tailored Approach to CAS: Scientific Evidence

Only a few published data are available regarding the potential impact of technical features of stents and EPDs on CAS clinical outcome. Our group published an analysis of 377 consecutive patients, prospectively studied from 2001 to 2004, to evaluate the feasibility of lesion-related treatment strategies for severe ICA stenosis with protected-CAS [23]. A wide rage of stents and EPDs were used. The primary endpoint was the combined death and stroke rate at discharge. Secondary endpoints

were to test the feasibility and safety of the tailored approach to CAS (procedural-technical success, complication rates between discharge and 30 days and death at 30 days). Procedural-technical success was achieved in all cases with two intraprocedural TIAs, 0.5%. All adverse-events rate at discharge was 2.9%; combined stroke and death rate at discharge was 1.1%. At 30 days follow-up overall procedure-related stroke and death rate was 1.3%.

No significant correlation was observed between materials and embolic complications. In addition, embolic events were analyzed in depth with regard to their temporal-distribution during and after the procedure (Figure 23.9). It is clear that with a tailored approach procedural-embolic complications were limited to two TIAs, and embolic neurological events (minor and major strokes) occurred invariably within the 24-hour postprocedural and recuperative periods up to 30 days follow-up. It is a reasonable hypothesis that there was a partial stent-frame failure: despite the routine application of selected stents, advanced protection techniques, and combined antiplatelet therapy, we were able to protect the procedure but not the patient over time.

Future Directions

Carotid artery stenting has become an increasingly important procedure in the optimal management

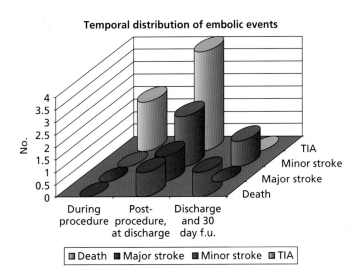

Figure 23.9. Temporal-distribution of CAS adverse embolic events.

of patients with atherosclerotic disease. The need for highly-trained operators is clear. The *tailored approach* has been emphasized as the key to achieving a safe practice; and emerging technologies and further innovation applied in this way may allow us to achieve the aim of stroke prevention. It is, however, necessary to recognize when we are making important technical advances; to determine if what we do are working in the long term, and consider ways of continuously improving on the management of patient care.

Acknowledgments

We thank the entire organization of Villa Maria Cecilia Hospital and Gruppo Villa Maria for their support in the development of the carotid stenting program. Special thanks to Dr Shane Gieowarsingh Master in Endovascular Techniques Fellow, and Dr Estevao C. de Campos Martins EuroPCR Peripheral Fellow for their contribution and dedication in helping prepare this chapter.

References

1. AHA Statistical Update. Heart Disease and Stroke Statistics—2008 Update. Circulation 2008; **117**: e25–e146.
2. Department of Health/Vascular Programme/Stroke. National Stroke Strategy. Department of Health, London, 2007.
3. Beneficial effect of carotid endarterectomy in symptomatic patients with high-grade carotid stenosis. North American Symptomatic Carotid Endarterectomy Trial Collaborators. N Engl J Med 1991; **325**(7): 445–453.
4. European Carotid Surgery Trialists' Collaborative Group. MRC European Carotid Surgery Trial: interim results for symptomatic patients with severe (70–99%) or with mild (0–29%) carotid stenosis. Lancet 1991; **337**: 1235–1243.
5. Endarterectomy for asymptomatic carotid artery stenosis. Executive Committee for the Asymptomatic Carotid Atherosclerosis Study. JAMA 1995; **273**(18): 1421–1428.
6. Halliday A, Mansfield A, Marro J, *et al.* Prevention of disabling and fatal strokes by successful carotid endarterectomy in patients without recent neurological symptoms: randomised controlled trial. Lancet 2004; **363**(9420): 1491–14502.
7. The Heart Outcomes Prevention Evaluation Study Investigators. Effects of an Angiotensin-Converting-Enzyme Inhibitor, Ramipril, on Cardiovascular Events in High-Risk Patients. N Engl J Med 2000; **342**: 145–153.
8. Heart Protection Study Collaborative Group: Effects of cholesterol-lowering with simvastastin on stroke and other major vascular events in 20,536 people with cerebrovascular disease or other high-risk conditions. Lancet 2004; **363**: 757.
9. Endovascular versus surgical treatment in patients with carotid stenosis in the Carotid and Vertebral Artery Transluminal Angioplasty Study (CAVATAS): a randomised trial. Lancet 2001; **357**(9270): 1729–1737.
10. Yadav JS, Wholey MH, Kuntz RE, *et al.* Protected carotid-artery stenting versus endarterectomy in high-risk patients. N Engl J Med 2004; **351**(15): 1493–1501.
11. Mas JL, Chatellier G, Beyssen B, *et al.* Endarterectomy versus stenting in patients with symptomatic severe carotid stenosis. N Engl J Med 2006; **355**(16): 1660–1571.
12. SPACE Collaborative Group. 30 day results from the SPACE trial of stent-protected angioplasty versus carotid endarterectomy in symptomatic patients: a randomised non-inferiority trial. Lancet 2006; **368**: 1239–1247.
13. Krapf H, Nagele T, Kastrup A, *et al.* Risk factors for periprocedural complications in carotid artery stenting without filter protection: A serial diffusion-weighted MRI study. J Neurol 2006; **253**(3): 364–371.
14. Aronow HD, Shishehbor M, Davis DA, *et al.* Leukocyte count predicts microembolic Doppler signals during carotid stenting: a link between inflammation and embolization. Stroke 2005; **36**(9): 1910–1914.
15. Verhoeven BA, de Vries JP, Pasterkamp G, *et al.* Carotid atherosclerotic plaque characteristics are associated with microembolization during carotid endarterectomy and procedural outcome. Stroke 2005; **36**(8):1735–1740.
16. Biasi GM, Froio A, Diethrich EB, *et al.* Carotid plaque echolucency increases the risk of stroke in carotid stenting: the Imaging in Carotid Angioplasty and Risk of Stroke (ICAROS) study. Circulation 2004; **110**(6): 756–762.
17. Angelini A, Reimers B, Della Barbera M, Sacca S, Pasquetto G, Cernetti C, et al. Cerebral protection during carotid artery stenting: Collection and histopathologic analysis of embolized debris. Stroke 2002; **33**(2): 456–461.
18. Crawley F, Clifton A, Buckenham T, *et al.* Comparison of hemodynamic cerebral ischemia and microembolic signals detected during carotid endarterectomy and carotid angioplasty. Stroke 1997; **28**(12):2460–2464.

19. Al-Mubarak N, Roubin GS, Vitek JJ, *et al.* Effect of the distal-balloon protection system on microembolization during carotid stenting. Circulation 2001; **104**(17): 1999–2002.

20. Kastrup A, Groschel K, Krapf H, *et al.* Early outcome of carotid angioplasty and stenting with and without cerebral protection devices: a systematic review of the literature. Stroke 2003; **34**(3): 813–619.

21. Reimers B, Schluter M, Castriota F, *et al.* Routine use of cerebral protection during carotid artery stenting: results of a multicenter registry of 753 patients. Am J Med 2004; **116**(4): 217–222.

22. Sprouse LR II, Peeters P, Bosiers M. The capture of visible debris by distal cerebral protection filters during carotid artery stenting: Is it predictable? J Vasc Surg 2005; **41**(6): 950–955.

23. Cremonesi A, Setacci C, Manetti R, *et al.* Carotid angioplasty and stenting: lesion related treatment strategies. EuroIntervention 2005; 289–295.

24. Zahn R, Mark B, Niedermaier N, Zeymer U, Limbourg P, Ischinger T, et al. Embolic protection devices for carotid artery stenting: better results than stenting without protection? Eur Heart J 2004; **25**(17): 1550–1558.

25. Castriota F, Cremonesi A, Manetti R, *et al.* Impact of cerebral protection devices on early outcome of carotid stenting. J Endovasc Ther 2002; **9**(6): 786–792.

26. Mas JL, Chatellier G, Beyssen B. Carotid angioplasty and stenting with and without cerebral protection: clinical alert from the Endarterectomy Versus Angioplasty in Patients With Symptomatic Severe Carotid Stenosis (EVA-3S) trial. Stroke 2004; **35**(1): e18–20.

27. Wholey MH, Al-Mubarek N. Updated review of the global carotid artery stent registry. Catheter Cardiovasc Interv 2003; **60**(2): 259–266.

28. Whitlow PL, Lylyk P, Londero H, *et al.* Carotid artery stenting protected with an emboli containment system. Stroke 2002; **33**(5): 1308–1314.

29. Parodi JC, Ferriera LM, Lamura R, *et al.* Results of the first 200 cases of carotid stents using the ArteriA device. Presented at International Congress of Endovascular Interventions XVII; February 13–17, 2005; Scottsdale, AZ.

30. Adami CA, Scuro A, Spinamano L, *et al.* Use of the Parodi anti-embolism system in carotid stenting: Italian trial results. J Endovasc Ther 2002; **9**(2): 147–154.

31. Schmidt A, Diederich KW, Scheinert S, *et al.* Effect of two different neuroprotection systems on microembolization during carotid artery stenting. J Am Coll Cardiol 2004; **44**(10): 1966–1969.

32. Coppi G, Moratto R, Silingardi R, *et al.* PRIAMUS— proximal flow blockage cerebral protection during carotid stenting: results from a multicenter Italian registry. J Cardiovasc Surg (Torino) 2005; **46**(3): 219–227.

33. Rabe K, Sugita J, Godel H, Sievert H. Flow-reversal device for cerebral protection during carotid artery stenting—acute and long-term results. J Interv Cardiol 2006; **19**(1): 55–62.

34. Diederich KW, Scheinert D, Schmidt A, *et al.* First clinical experiences with an endovascular clamping system for neuroprotection during carotid stenting. Eur J Vasc Endovasc Surg 2004; **28**(6): 629–633.

35. Reimers B, Corvaja N, Moshiri S, *et al.* Cerebral protection with filter devices during carotid artery stenting. Circulation 2001; **104**(1): 12–15.

36. Cremonesi A, Manetti R, Setacci F, *et al.* Protected carotid stenting: clinical advantages and complications of embolic protection devices in 442 consecutive patients. Stroke 2003; **34**(8): 1936–1941.

37. Reimers B, Sievert H, Schuler GC, *et al.* Proximal endovascular flow blockage for cerebral protection during carotid artery stenting: results from a prospective multicenter registry. J Endovasc Ther 2005; **12**(2): 156–165.

38. Cremonesi A, Rubino P, Grattoni C, *et al.* Multicenter Experience With a New "Hybrid" Carotid Stent. J Endovasc Ther 2008; **15**: 186–192.

39. Bosiers M, de Donato G, Deloose K, *et al.* Does free cell area influence the outcome in carotid artery stenting? Eur J Vasc Endovasc Surg 2007; **33**(2): 135–141; discussion 142–143.

40. Gieowarsingh S, Castriota F, Spagnolo B, *et al.* Carotid Percutaneous Interventions for Both Restenosis and Calcified Lesions: Success and Safety with Cutting Balloon Angioplasty. Presented at Cardiovascular Revascularization Therapies; February 11–13, 2008; Washington, DC.

41. Setacci C, Chisci E, Setacci F, *et al.* Grading Carotid Intrastent Restenosis. A 6-Year Follow-up Study. Stroke 2008; **39**(4):1189–1196.

CHAPTER 24

Aortic Valve Disease Interventions

Srinivas Iyengar, & Martin B. Leon
Columbia University Medical Center, New York, NY, USA

Introduction

The genesis of percutaneous aortic valve disease therapies has grown dramatically over the last five years. Whereas treatment options for aortic valve disease has been historically confined to the surgical realm, given the bleak options availed by medical therapy alone, the emergence of percutaneous transcatheter therapies has opened a new chapter in the treatment paradigm of this entity. Given the advent of percutaneously deliverable valve therapies, treatment of aortic valve disease, specifically aortic stenosis (AS), has recently become the focus of intense clinical research. Though initial transcatheter therapies for aortic stenosis (i.e. aortic balloon valvuloplasty) has had poor long-term results, the potential of replacing a diseased valve with a bio-prosthesis via this minimally invasive approach truly represents an exciting step forward in our approach to this disease process.

Current Standard of Therapy

The prevalence of AS has sharply increased in the USA over the past few decades given our increas-

ingly aging population [1]. Given the limited available medical options, the definitive treatment of patients with severe, symptomatic AS has been largely made up of surgical therapy for well over four decades.

Surgical aortic valve replacement (AVR) for patients with severe AS has had a strong clinical track record, improving both morbidity and mortality in this cohort [2–4]. The current American College of Cardiology/American Heart Association (ACC/AHA) guidelines for the management of patients with valvular heart disease lists severe AS with symptoms, concomitant coronary artery bypass surgery (CABG) and/or surgery on the aorta or other heart valves, and severe AS with a decreased ejection fraction (EF) of less than 50% as all Class I indications for surgery [1].

Although surgical intervention has been the mainstay of therapy for patients with AS, it is not applicable to every patient with this condition given the significant morbidity and mortality associated with operating on patients who possess high-risk surgical features. When an AVR is combined with coronary artery bypass surgery (CABG), the average perioperative mortality can increase to between 5.5% and 6.8%, according to recent reporting from the Society of Thoracic Surgeons (STS) database [5]. In low-volume centers, surgical mortality can increase by 33% and >10% in octogenarians [6–9]. Additionally, "traditional"

Interventional Cardiology, First Edition. Edited by
Carlo Di Mario, George D. Dangas, Peter Barlis.
© 2010 Blackwell Publishing Ltd. Published 2010 by
Blackwell Publishing Ltd.

surgical risk factors, such as female gender, prior cardiac surgical procedures, pulmonary hypertension, chronic renal insufficiency, and New York Heart Association Class II–IV heart failure (especially with an ejection fraction of <30%) also increase the morbidity and mortality of surgical AVR [10,11].

Although not considered as being "traditional" surgical risk factors, the presence of issues such as previous chest wall radiation exposure, traumatic or congenital chest wall deformities, and a heavily calcified thoracic aorta ("porcelain aorta"), can all contribute to increased surgical morbidity/mortality as well. When these previously mentioned factors are all taken into account, the resultant mortality curve from surgical AVR can dramatically rise, especially patients >80 years old [12], thus limiting the effective use of this treatment modality. Given the USA's aging population, the quest for alternative methods to treat this patient group has become a vital issue in cardiology, as the only options for patients with severe AS who are deemed "inoperable" have been palliative at best.

Initial Transcatheter Methods of Treatment

Medical therapy, as previously discussed, has had a dismal track record in effectively treating patients with severe AS. The use of balloon aortic valvuloplasty (BAV) was hailed initially as a minimally-invasive method to address this specific disease entity. BAV has been available for nearly two decades and unfortunately, has proven to be quite fruitless in providing a long-term cure for patients with severe AS. Although BAV can provide initial improvements in valve area (approx. $1.0\,cm^2$) and cardiac symptoms, major procedural complications can occur in nearly 10% of patients and restenosis with concurrent clinical deterioration can be seen in >75% of patients within one year of the initial procedure [13,14]. The current ACC/AHA guidelines have bestowed a Class IIb recommendation for BAV in severe AS, with the proviso that this therapy only be employed as a bridge to surgery in hemodynamically unstable patients or as a palliative measure in patients who are not candidates for surgical AVR [1].

Evolution of Therapy: Percutaneously Delivered Aortic Valves

Spurned by the earlier successes of the Andersen and Bonhoeffer groups [15,16], the dawn of percutaneous AVR (pAVR) officially began with the implantation of a stent-mounted bioprosthetic aortic valve by Cribier and colleagues [17]. The sentinel valve was delivered without complications and hemodynamic improvement was quickly realized. Since this initial event, the design and make-up of transcatheter-delivered aortic valves has gone under significant renovations.

The use of biological tri-leaflet tissue valves, with the valve material being made up of pericardium (bovine, porcine, or equine), is currently considered the preferred working standard. The valve is then sewn or affixed to a circular balloon-expanding or self-expanding stent (or cage) and positioned on a catheter-based system for delivery. Initially, the first percutaneous aortic valves were quite bulky and stiff (24 Fr to 26 Fr in diameter), but continued innovations with valve design have reduced some working valves to as small as 18 Fr. The stent valve is deployed by either balloon expansion or after withdrawal of a sheath that releases a self-expanding stent. It is imperative that the deployed valve remain secure in its position, displacing the native aortic valve, in order to function properly. Once deployed properly, the hemodynamic profile of the new percutaneous valve should mirror its surgically implanted counterparts, with only a minimal transvalvular gradient (<10 mm Hg) and valve areas of 1.5 to $2.0\,cm^2$.

Major issues to be considered with the process of deployment include careful avoidance of obstructing either coronary ostia or any negative interactions with the functionality of the mitral valve apparatus. Circumferential apposition of the deployed valve to the aortic annulus is critical as well, as this can prevent the occurrence of paravalvular aortic regurgitation (AI). Additionally, since all catheter-based aortic valve stent procedures begin with a standard BAV to increase the insertion site for a stent-valve device, careful vascular screening of all patients is mandatory. Given the heightened complications rates associated with the antegrade method of stent-valve delivery, the trans-arterial retrograde approach is now viewed as the preferred and safer technique.

In order to utilize this form of delivery, the femoral artery must be accessed. Generally, a surgical form of closure will be necessary at the conclusion of the procedure due to the large delivery catheters. Manipulation of the catheters through the femoral, iliac, and aortic anatomy re-emphasizes the need for proper vascular screening prior to attempting this approach. Retrograde crossing of the aortic valve is inherent in this approach and can be assisted by a low-friction covered sheath or a tip-deflecting catheter to better position the stent-valve in a central orientation. Generally, the implanted stent-valve is relatively over-sized to the aortic annulus to ensure maximum stability and minimal paravalvular leak. During the actual deployment, in order to ensure minimal valve movement due to altering waves of cardiac/aortic blood flow, the use of temporary rapid right ventricular pacing (at rates >200 beats per minute) can be utilized. After deployment, the presence of paravalvular regurgitation (as evidenced by either angiography or continuous trans-esophageal echocardiographic monitoring), may necessitate the use of a slightly larger balloon-catheter to further dilate the stent-valve and reduce the regurgitation.

The Cribier-Edwards Valve

The Cribier-Edwards Aortic Bioprosthesis (Edwards Lifesciences Inc., Orange, CA) has been undergoing continuous renovations over the last decade since its introduction [18]. The leaflet material is made up of thin, equine pericardium. The tri-leaflets are hand-sewn to a stainless steel, tubular, slotted balloon expandable stent (Figure 24.1). Current stent-valve models include 23-mm and 26-mm diameter versions that can accommodate aortic annulus sizes between 18 mm and 24 mm. Prior to implantation, the sterile stent-valve is carefully mounted and crimped onto conventionally balloon dilatation catheters (Figure 24.2).

At the present time for retrograde procedures, both balloon catheter and stent valve assembly are placed within a tip-deflecting catheter, which can then be inserted into a 22 Fr to 24 Fr flexible arterial sheath [19]. The active flexion enabled by this tip-deflecting catheter can assist in navigating aortic

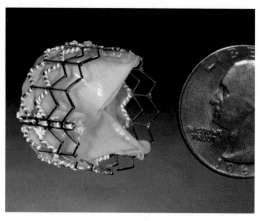

Figure 24.1. The Cribier-Edwards Aortic Bioprosthesis™ consisting of a stainless steel, tubular slotted, balloon-expandable stent within which is a suture mounted trileaflet equine pericardial valve.

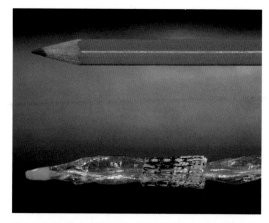

Figure 24.2. The Cribier-Edwards Aortic Bioprosthesis™: size and appearance after crimping prior to deployment.

tortuosity and in crossing the native valve. After successful BAV and retrograde positioning of the aortic stent-valve, rapid ventricular pacing can be initiated. Focused stent-valve deployment, via balloon inflation, should occur in the sub-annular position.

An alternative method to deploy this specific bioprosthesis is via the trans-apical approach [20]. After a left anterolateral intercostal incision is performed to expose the left ventricular apex, a direct needle puncture is followed by insertion of a 33 Fr sheath into the left ventricle. The bioprosthesis, which is identical to the stent-valve delivered via the trans-femoral route, is mounted on a shorter catheter in the antegrade direction. This procedure can be done either in a catheterization lab or operating room with fluoroscopic/angiographic capabilities. This approach generally requires a strong collaborative effort between interventional cardiologists and cardio-thoracic surgeons, and requires that additional ancillary staff be present for assistance, given the dual aspects of this procedure.

Clinical Studies: Cribier-Edwards Valve

As previously mentioned, the first successful percutaneous AVR (pAVR) was performed by Cribier and colleagues in 2002 [17]. The valve-recipient presented in cardiogenic shock with critical AS, and was deemed as "inoperable" due to multiple co-morbidities. The antegrade approach was undertaken and a 23-mm bovine pericardial stent-valve was deployed without incidence. The patient survived 17 weeks, passing away at that time due to complications from lower limb amputation secondary to severe peripheral vascular disease. Bolstered by this success, Cribier followed up this initial case with additional patients, although initially on a "compassionate" use only basis [21].

At this time, a European registry was initiated for patients with severe AS and no surgical options: Initial Registry of EndoVascular Implantation of Valves in Europe (I-REVIVE). This was followed by another single-center registry in Rouen, France that used the antegrade approach in high-risk patients who had been refused surgical AVR (Registry of Endovascular Critical Aortic Stenosis Treatment (RECAST). The results of these registries were published by Cribier and associates in 2006, which included 27 "inoperable" patients with severe AS who had successfully undergone pAVR (23 antegrade, 4 retrograde) [22]. The authors reported significant improvements in valve area ($0.60 +/- 0.11\,cm^2$ to $1.70 +/- 0.10\,cm^2$, $p < 0.0001$) and transvalvular gradient ($37 +/- 13\,mmHg$ to $9 +/- 2\,mmHg$, $p < 0.0001$) with implantation of the pAVR. One week post-procedure, improvement in ventricular function was most apparent in patients with a baseline left ventricular ejection fraction (LVEF) <50% ($35 +/- 10\%$ to $50 +/- 16\%$, $p < 0.0001$). Additionally, eleven patients were alive at nine month follow-up,

with nearly complete resolution of symptoms (>90% NYHA Class I or II).

Although encouraging, the actual make-up and deployment of the device required major adjustments, in particular, the cumbersome and complication-laden antegrade method of delivery. Webb *et al.* refined the technique of transcatheter AVR by utilizing a retrograde approach via the femoral artery in 18 patients, in which fourteen had successful valve deployment [23]. Additionally, the availability of a 26-mm valve prosthesis reduced the likelihood of valve embolization and the severity of paravalvular regurgitation. The use of a supportive tip-deflecting loading catheter assisted with catheter navigation and native valve crossing.

Webb and colleagues recently published their data on a larger series of 50 "high-risk" surgical patients with severe AS who underwent pAVR [24]. The authors reported successful valve implantation in 86% of patients with an intra-procedural mortality rate of 2%. Patients were discharged home at a median of five days and mortality at one month was 12% in patients in whom the logistic European System for Cardiac Operative Risk Evaluation risk score was 28%. Additionally, after insertion of the pAVR, significant improvement in LVEF ($P < 0.0001$) and functional class ($P < 0.0001$) was observed and maintained at one year.

In the United States, the PARTNER trial (Placement of AoRTic traNscathetER valves) is currently enrolling patients. The study, funded by Edward Lifesciences, plans to enroll 1040 total patients. The study population will be made up of 690 high risk patients with severe AS who are eligible for surgery that will then be randomized to either conventional open-heart valve surgery or minimally-invasive implantation of Edwards' Sapien pAVR (modified from the original Cribier-Edwards pAVR). The Sapien pAVR will be delivered either by the transapical or transfemoral route depending on patient anatomy. The other trial arm will randomize 350 patients considered to be surgically inoperable to either standard medical management or pAVR treatment (via the transfemoral route) (Figure 24.3). The primary endpoint for the study will be one-year mortality. The two-arm study is designed to show that the Sapien pAVR is noninferior to open-heart valve surgery and superior to medical management with secondary end-

Randomized Trials Total = 600 Patients

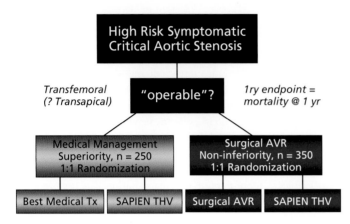

High Risk Symptomatic
Critical Aortic Stenosis

Transfemoral
(? Transapical)

"operable"?

1ry endpoint =
mortality @ 1 yr

Medical Management
Superiority, n = 250
1:1 Randomization

Surgical AVR
Non-inferiority, n = 350
1:1 Randomization

Best Medical Tx   SAPIEN THV   Surgical AVR   SAPIEN THV

Figure 24.3. PARTNER trial (Placement of AoRTic traNscathetER valves): The study population will be made up of 350 high-risk patients with severe AS who are eligible for surgery who will then be randomized to either conventional open-heart valve surgery or minimally-invasive implantation of Edwards' Sapien pAVR. The other trial arm will randomize 250 patients considered to be surgically inoperable to either standard medical management or pAVR treatment. The primary endpoint for the study will be one-year mortality.

points to include quality of life and a number of valve performance measures.

Although both antegrade and retrograde delivery methods have been utilized for the Edwards pAVR, additional methods of implantation have also been researched. In 2006, Lichenstein *et al.* reported the successful deployment of a pAVR via a transapical route in seven "high-risk" patients with severe AS [20]. The authors reported that this method of delivery did not require cardiopulmonary bypass nor a sternotomy. Improvements in valve area were immediately identified, and at a follow-up of 87 +/− 56 days, six of seven patients were still alive and free of symptoms. This study was followed up with a six-month evaluation of these same patients [25]. Four of the seven patients were alive at six months. The aortic valve area in the four patients increased from 0.7 +/− 0.3 cm^2 to 1.8 +/− 0.7 cm^2 and 1.5 +/− 0.5 cm^2 at one and six months respectively. The mean transaortic gradient was reduced from 32 +/− 8 mmHg to 10 +/− 5 mmHg and 11 +/− 8 mmHg at one and six months, respectively. Although limited in size, the results from this study reveal a potential alternate approach for transcatheter valvular implantation.

The CoreValve System

The ReValving System™ (CoreValve, Paris, France) is made up of three major components: a self-expanding frame with trileaflet porcine pericardial valve, a newly reduced delivery catheter of 18 Fr

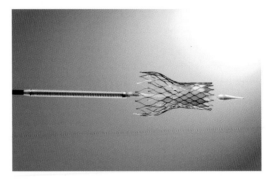

Figure 24.4. The new 18 Fr CoreValve platform with mounted porcine pericardial tissue valve and delivery catheter.

(previously 25 Fr), and a loading system [26] (Figure 24.4). The self-expanding nitinol support frame, which has a total length of 45 mm, has a diamond-cell configuration and utilizes three different areas of radial force (Figure 24.5). The upper frame portion anchors in the aorta above the coronary sinuses with low radial force, the middle portion contains the valve leaflets, and the lower portion has high radial force and implants in the sub-annular area. Despite actually crossing the coronary ostia, the frame geometry is narrowed and unapposed in the mid-portion, thus allowing normal coronary flow and free access to the coronary ostia via the stent struts.

Polytetrafluoroethylene (PTFE) sutures anchor the single-layer porcine pericardial tissue valve to the frame. The CoreValve nitinol frame-tissue

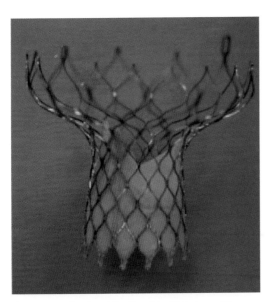

Figure 24.5. The CoreValve Revalving™ System with a self-expanding nitinol frame extending from the sub-annular implantation zone to the supra-coronary sinus aorta zone for fixation with a porcine pericardial trileaflet valve sewn to the frame with PTFE sutures.

valve assembly is loaded onto a flexible sheath-based delivery catheter by compressing the frame uniformly using an atraumatic loading system. Currently, the CoreValve system can be utilized in patients with distal aortas <45 mm and with aortic annulus sizes less than 23 mm in diameter.

After BAV, the CoreValve ReValving™ system is positioned in a transaortic valve location and the overriding sheath is slowly withdrawn over several minutes to expose and anchor the frame-valve unit. It is during this critical juncture that external hemodynamic support is most likely to be used to maintain clinical stability. Due to the self-expanding nature of the device, continuous expansion of the system can occur over 30 to 60 minutes. This further expansion provides more thorough apposition at both proximal and distal implantation zones, which results in minimal paravalvular regurgitation. At the conclusion of the procedure, surgically mediated repair of the femoral artery is required.

Clinical Studies: CoreValve

The CoreValve ReValving™ System was first successfully implanted in a human in 2005 [27].

Grube and colleagues followed up their initial implantation with a study of 25 patients with symptomatic AS (mean gradient before implantation- 44.2 +/− 10.8 mmHg) and multiple co-morbidities (median logistic EuroScore, 11.0%) [28]. Procedural success and device success were achieved in 84% and 88% of patients, respectively. Successful device implantation resulted in significant reduction in the mean aortic valve gradient (mean gradient after implantation, 12.4 +/− 3.0 mmHg, P < 0.0001). Among patients with device success surviving to discharge (n = 18), no adverse events occurred within one month after discharge.

Grube *et al.* recently published data on second- and third- generation CoreValve utilization [29]. The second-generation (21 Fr) and third-generation (18 Fr) prostheses were studied in 86 "high-risk" patients with severe, symptomatic AS. Acute device success was 88% and acute procedural success was 74% (21 Fr—78%; 18 Fr—69%). Successful device implantation resulted in significant reduction of mean aortic gradients (mean pre 43.7 mmHg vs. post 9.0 mmHg, p < 0.001). Procedural mortality was 6% with an overall 30-day mortality rate of 12%. Additionally, the combined rate of death, stroke, and myocardial infarction was 22%. Given the high-risk nature of the patients being enrolled in the study, the authors concluded that the CoreValve pAVR can potentially be a suitable therapeutic option in this specific population.

Recently, Grube and associates reported the use of the CoreValve pAVR as a replacement valve for a patient who had severe aortic regurgitation from a previously placed bioprosthetic valve [30]. This usage of pAVR technology could represent another leap forward in the management of patients with deteriorated bioprosthetic aortic valves who are deemed too "high-risk" for re-operation.

Promising Technologies

Currently, there are several new transcatheter AVR technologies that are actively being developed. The aims of these new devices lay primarily in addressing the weaknesses of the first-generations technologies. These new devices mainly incorporate

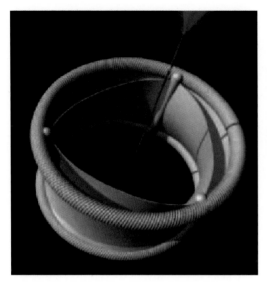

Figure 24.6. The DirectFlow percutaneous "stentless" inflatable fabric cuff equine pericardial aortic valve.

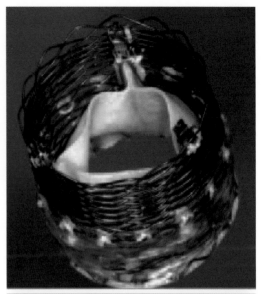

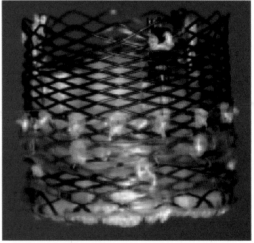

Figure 24.7. The Sadra Medical Lotus™ percutaneous aortic valve with a nitinol continuous braid frame surrounded by a conforming membrane and incorporating a bovine pericardial trileaflet tissue valve.

retrograde valve crossing, reduced system profiles, pericardial tissue valve leaflets, and probably most ground-breaking feature—the ability to retrieve and reposition the device before final deployment and release.

The DirectFlow percutaneous aortic valve (Santa Rosa, CA) is a stentless, inflatable, fabric-cuff, equine pericardial tissue valve (Figure 24.6). Once the native valve is traversed, the distal ring is positioned in a suitable sub-annular location and inflated with contrast to secure fixation. Tethers are utilized to align the valve properly and the proximal ring is deployed in a similar fashion. When valve position, function, and sealing are all confirmed, a permanent polymer medium is infused to replace the contrast, followed by detachment of the control tethers and the inflation ports.

The Lotus™ percutaneous aortic valve by Sadra Medical (Saratoga, CA) is primarily comprised of a nitinol continuous braid frame with a bovine pericardial trileaflet tissue valve (Figure 24.7). The 19 Fr outer diameter catheter is delivered across the aortic valve and unsheathed. The self-expanding nitinol prosthesis shortens passively and self-center with low radial force, which has the dual purpose of allowing the valve to begin functioning as well as providing the opportunity for correct position-

ing. Once optimal location is achieved, the nitinol frame is actively shortened and locked to its final height (19 mm), which then subsequently increases the radial force and secures its position. The assembly of the frame-valve is unique in that it is attached to the catheter deployment system by fifteen arms thereby enabling the device to be retrieved and repositioned at any time before final release from the catheter.

Conclusions

The development of percutaneous transcatheter therapies for aortic valve disease is rapidly evolving. Whereas once thought a purely surgical issue, the entity of aortic stenosis is one which can potentially be cured via a minimally invasive technique. Obviously, before any therapy can be completely embraced by the medical community, rigorous multi-center trials must occur. Given the rapid pace of technology, and our ever-aging population it behooves us as clinicians to tread carefully toward the future, as this therapy represents an extremely exciting, albeit immature, treatment modality.

References

1. Bonow RO, Carabella BA, Chatterjee K, *et al.* ACC/AHA guidelines for the management of patients with valvular heart disease: A report of the American College of Cardiology/American Heart Association Task Force on Practice Guidelines. American Heart Association Web Site. Available at: http://www.americanheart.org.

2. Schwarz F, Baumann P, Manthey J, *et al.* The effects of aortic valve replacement on survival. Circulation 1982; **66**: 1105–1110.

3. Smith N, McAnulty JH, Rahimtoola SH, *et al.* Severe aortic stenosis with impaired left ventricular function and clinical heart failure: results of valve replacement. Circulation 1978; **58**: 255–264.

4. Kvidal P, Bergstrom R, Horte LG, *et al.* Observed and relative survival after aortic valve replacement. J Am Coll Cardiol 2000; **35**: 747–756.

5. Society of Thoracic Surgeons National Cardiac Surgery Database. Available at: http://www.sts.org/documents.

6. Birkmeyer JD, Siewers AE, Finlayson EV, *et al.* Hospital volume and surgical mortality in the United States. N Engl J Med 2002; **346**: 1128–1137.

7. Goodney PP, O'Connor GT, Wennberg DE, *et al.* Do hospitals with low mortality rates in coronary artery bypass also perform well in valve replacement? Ann Thorac Surg 2003; **76**: 1131–1136.

8. Levinson JR, Akins CW, Buckley MJ, *et al.* Octogenarians with aortic stenosis. Outcome after aortic valve replacement. Circulation 1989; 80: I49–I56.

9. Kolh P, Kerzmann A, Lahaye L, *et al.* Cardiac surgery in octogenarians; peri-operative outcomes and long-term results. Eur Heart J 2001; **22**: 1235–1243.

10. Powell DE, Tunick PA, Rosenzweig BP, *et al.* Aortic valve replacement in patients with aortic stenosis and severe left ventricular dysfunction. Arch Intern Med 2000; **160**: 1337–1341.

11. Connolly HM, Oh JK, Schaff HV, *et al.* Severe aortic stenosis with low-transvalvular gradient and severe left ventricular dysfunction: result of aortic valve replacement in 52 patients. Circulation 2000; **101**: 1940–1946.

12. Sundt TM, Bailey MS, Moon MR, *et al.* Quality of life after aortic valve replacement at the age of >80 years. Circulation 2000; **102**: II170–II174.

13. Otto CM, Mickel MC, Kennedy JW, *et al.* Three-year outcome after balloon aortic valvuloplasty: insights into prognosis of valvular aortic stenosis. Circulation 1994; **89**: 642–650.

14. Lieberman EB, Bashore TM, Hermiller JB, *et al.* Balloon aortic valvuloplasty in adults: failure of procedure to improve long-term survival. J Am Coll Cardiol 1995; **26**: 1522–1528.

15. Andersen HR, Knudsen LL, Hasenkam JM. Transluminal implantation of artificial heart valves. Description of a new expandable aortic valve and initial results with implantation by catheter technique in closed chest pigs. Eur Heart J 1992; **13**: 704–708

16. Bonhoeffer P, Boudjemline Y, Saliba Z, *et al.* Percutaneous replacement of pulmonary valve in a right-ventricle to pulmonary-artery prosthetic conduit with valve dysfunction. Lancet 2000; **356**: 1403–1405.

17. Cribier A, Eltchaninoff H, Bash A, *et al.* Percutaneous transcatheter implantation of an aortic valve prosthesis for calcific aortic stenosis: first human case description. Circulation 2002; **106**: 3006–3008.

18. Eltchaninoff H, Tron C, Cribier A. Percutaneous implantation of aortic valve prosthesis in patients with calcific aortic stenosis: technical aspects. J Interv Cardiol 2003; **16**: 515–521.

19. Webb JG, Chandavimol M, Thompson CR, *et al.* Percutaneous aortic valve implantation retrograde from the femoral artery. Circulation 2006; **113**: 842–850.

20. Lichtenstein SV, Cheung A, Ye J, *et al.* Transapical transcatheter aortic valve implantation in humans: initial clinical experience. Circulation 2006; **114**: 591–596.

21. Cribier A, Eltchaninoff H, Tron C, *et al.* Early experience with percutaneous transcatheter implantation of heart valve prosthesis for the treatment of end-stage inoperable patients with calcific aortic stenosis. J Am Coll Cardiol 2004; **43**: 698–703.

22. Cribier A, Eltchaninoff H, Tron C, *et al.* Treatment of calcific aortic stenosis with the percutaneous heart valve: mid-term follow-up from the initial feasibility studies: the French experience. J Am Coll Cardiol 2006; **47**: 1214–1223.

23. Webb JG, Chandavimol M, Thompson CR, *et al.* Percutaneous aortic valve implantation retrograde from the femoral artery. Circulation 2006; **113**: 842–850.

24. Webb JG, Pasupati S, Humphries K, *et al.* Percutaneous transarterial aortic valve replacement in selected high-risk patients with aortic stenosis. Circulation 2007; July 23 (Epub ahead of print).

25. Ye J, Cheung A, Lichtenstein SV, *et al.* Six-month outcome of transapical transcatheter aortic valve implantation in the initial seven patients. Eur J Cardiothorac Surg 2007; **31**: 16–21.

26. Laborde JC, Borenstein N, Behr L, *et al.* Percutaneous implantation of the Corevalve aortic valve prosthesis for patients presenting high-risk for high-risk surgical valve intervention. Eurointervention 2006; **1**: 472–474.

27. Grube E, Laborde JC, Zickmann B, *et al.* First report on a human percutaneous transluminal implantation of a self-expanding valve prosthesis for interventional treatment of aortic valve stenosis. Catheter Cardiovasc Interv 2005; **66**: 465–469.

28. Grube E, Laborde JC, Gerkens U, *et al.* Percutaneous implantation of the CoreValve self-expanding valve prosthesis in high-risk patients with aortic valve disease: the Siegburg first-in-man study. Circulation 2006; **114**: 1616–1624.

29. Grube E, Schuler G, Buelledfeld L, *et al.* Percutaneous aortic valve replacement for severe aortic stenosis in high-risk patients using the second- and current third-generation self expanding CoreValve prosthesis: device success and 30-day clinical outcome. J Am Coll Cardiol 2007; **50**: 69–76.

30. Wenaweser P, Buellesfeld L, Gerckens U, *et al.* Percutaneous aortic valve replacement for severe aortic regurgitation in degenerated bioprosthesis: the first valve in valve procedure using the Corevalve Revalving system. Catheter Cardiovasc Interv 2007; **70**: 760–764.

CHAPTER 25

Transseptal Puncture

Alec Vahanian, Dominique Himbert, & Eric Brochet
Bichat Hospital, Paris, France

Introduction

Transseptal catheterization remains an integral yet specialized technique for interventional cardiologists and electrophysiologists. It was introduced in the late 1950s [1]. Initially seldom used, mostly due to lack of experience and fear, this relatively complex technique has had a revival with the introduction of the new percutaneous electrophysiological and valvular interventions (Table 25.1). New percutaneous mitral valve repair techniques may also further increase its usage [2–5].

This chapter will describe the technical aspects of the procedure, in particular as the first step of percutaneous mitral valve interventions. This same technique applies for electrophysiological interventions.

Contra-indications

Before considering transseptal catheterization, the possibility of any contra-indications must be eliminated.

The performance of transesophageal echocardiography is recommended before transseptal catheterization to disclose left atrial thrombosis as the technique is contraindicated in patients with a thrombus floating in the left atrial cavity or on the

Interventional Cardiology, First Edition. Edited by Carlo Di Mario, George D. Dangas, Peter Barlis.
© 2010 Blackwell Publishing Ltd. Published 2010 by Blackwell Publishing Ltd.

atrial septum. No consensus has been reached regarding patients with thrombosis in the left atrial appendage. In such cases, transseptal catheterization can only be indicated in patients who are candidates for intervention but not surgery, or if intervention is not required urgently and when oral anticoagulation can be given for at least two and up to six months, and new transesophageal echocardiography shows the thrombus has disappeared. Left atrial myxoma also constitutes a contra-indication [6].

Transseptal catheterization should not be performed in patients with bleeding disorders, especially due to too high anticoagulation (INR > 1.2 in particular in patients who have not undergone previous cardiac operation). When intravenous heparin is necessary, it should be discontinued four hours before and can be restarted two hours after the procedure.

Thoracic deformity, such as cyphoscoliosis, is a contra-indication if severe. In practice, the level of acceptable deformity depends on operator experience and the availability of echocardiographic guidance.

Complex congenital diseases are also considered contra-indicative due to the altered anatomic landmarks.

Obstruction of the vena cava is a classic contra-indication for femoral access but membranous obstruction of the vena cava can be dilated [7].

Another contra-indication is agenesis of the vena cava associated with azygos return. This latter condition should be diagnosed by X-ray before the

Table 25.1. Indications for the technique.

Diagnostic measurements

- Quantification of mitral gradient
  - Unreliable capillary wedge pressure and inconclusive echocardiographic findings
  - Mechanical aortic/mitral valve prosthesis
- Quantification of aortic gradient
  - Mechanical aortic prosthesis when echocardiography is not conclusive
  - Severe aortic stenosis when valve cannot be crossed
  - Hypertrophic obstructive cardiomyopathy
- Interventional procedures
  - Percutaneous mitral balloon valvuloplasty
  - Percutaneous edge-to-edge mitral repair
  - Antegrade aortic balloon valvuloplasty
  - Percutaneous aortic heart valve implantation
  - Transseptal PFO closure
  - Percutaneous occlusion of the left atrial appendage
- Electrophysiology studies and catheter ablation
  - Left sided accessory pathways
  - Pulmonary vein ablation for paroxysmal atrial fibrillation
  - Left atrial tachycardia
  - Atypical left atrial flutters
  - Left ventricular tachycardia
- **Circulatory support**
  - Percutaneous left ventricular assist device

procedure or if during the procedure the catheter has an unusually posterior position behind the heart, confirmed by venous angiography in the right atrium (RA) [8].

The presence of a filter in the vena cava is not an absolute contra-indication if it is permeable [9]. Presence of an inter-atrial patch [10], or even atrial septal occluder, at least during the first few days after implantation [11], is not an absolute contra-indication but may render the crossing difficult. Transseptal catheterization can be performed in dextrocardia by experienced operators using left femoral access, inversion of the X-ray image and echocardiographic guidance [12]. Finally, the increased difficulty engendered by extreme right and or left atrial enlargement restricts the performance of the procedure to experienced operators, possibly under echographic guidance.

Technique

Equipment

The most commonly used transseptal needle is the Brockenbrough needle, which is 70 cm long, has a curved tip and tapers distally. A hub arrow on the proximal part indicates the direction of the needle. The stylet inside the needle should be removed before use.

An 8 Fr Teflon catheter with end holes and a curved tip can be used. The curve ranges from 2 to 3.5 cm in length and is chosen according to the size of the left atrium (LA) [13]. The other option is the Mullins sheath, which comprises a dilator and a sheath, and is also 8 Fr [14]. This latter option has the advantage of a more tapered tip, which facilitates the crossing of the septum. It also allows the introduction of another catheter, such as a floating balloon, in the LA after penetration to catheterize the left ventricle. Its relative disadvantage is the less satisfactory quality of pressure recording and the shorter length of needle that can be extruded from the catheter, possibly problematic when the septum is hypertrophic (Figure 25.1).

Before performing transseptal catheterization, it is necessary to carefully check (1) that the proximal arrow is aligned with the needle tip and (2) to measure the distance (in fingers) between the proximal part of the catheter and the proximal arrow when the tip of needle is advanced to lie just inside of the dilator to avoid inadvertent puncture during the manipulation (Figure 25.2).

Procedure

The following steps should be taken:

Before starting the procedure verify that the patient is lying flat for better anatomic landmarks. This could be difficult in emergency cases such as pulmonary edema, which requires a semi-supine-position. In such cases, the procedure should only be performed by experienced operators.

A 5 Fr pigtail is positioned retrogradely from the femoral artery to the right coronary sinus for identification of the aorta and systemic pressure monitoring. Left heart catheterization can, however, be omitted by experienced operators, but is useful otherwise.

Percutaneous access is via a puncture of the right femoral vein as this offers a direct approach from

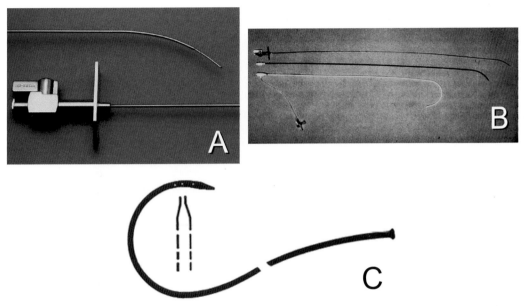

Figure 25.1. Equipment.
A) The needle: Proximal tip with an arrow and a tap; distal tip which is tapered.
B) Transseptal needle, 70 cm long, alongside the Mullins dilator and sheath.

C) Brockenbrough catheter with different curves and presence of side holes.

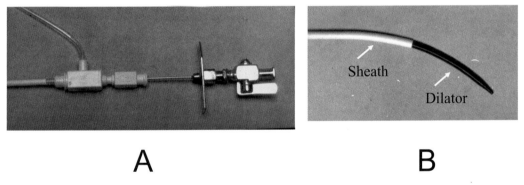

Figure 25.2. Measurements of the landmarks between needle and catheter. Measurement of the distance between the proximal of the needle arrow and the proximal part of the catheter (A) necessary to position the needle just inside the catheter (B).

the inferior vena cava to the inter-atrial septum at the fossa ovalis. If right access is not possible, left femoral access can be attempted but this renders the procedure more difficult, and may be painful for the patient and lead to vagal reaction. In very rare cases, transseptal catheterization has been performed using a trans-jugular or trans-hepatic approach [7].

A 0.032-inch J-tipped guidewire is advanced into the superior vena cava, up to the origin of the left innominate vein, in antero-posterior view. It is important to avoid forcing the guidewire in the right atrial appendage, which is a fragile structure.

The catheter is advanced over the guidewire into the superior vena cava and the guidewire is removed (Figure 25.3).

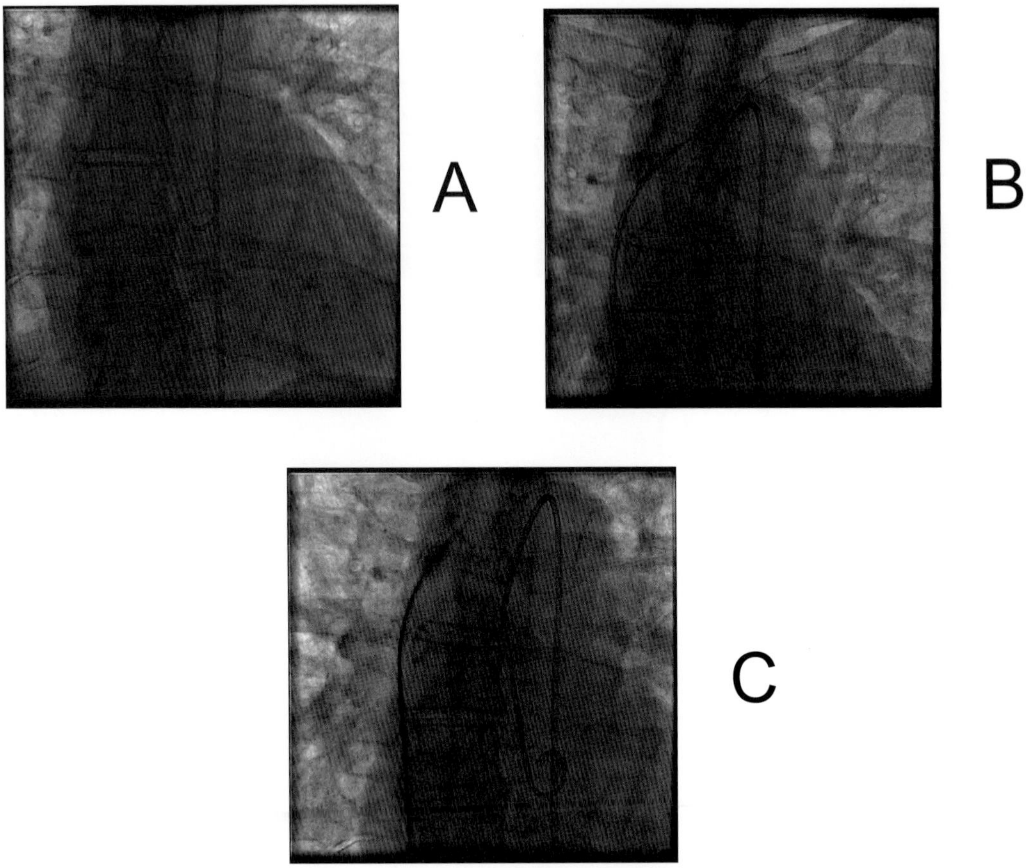

Figure 25.3. Procedure I: Positioning in antero-posterior view.
A) Pigtail catheter placed on the aortic cusps. The dilator is advanced in the superior vena cava.

B) The guidewire is removed.
C) The needle is advanced with the dilator. Courtesy of Professor A. Cribier.

The Brockenbrough needle is connected to a pressure line, which is continuously flushed, and is inserted into the dilator just inside the distal end under fluoroscopic guidance and using the predetermined measurement. The needle is allowed to rotate freely whilst being advanced. If resistance is felt the proximal hub arrow should be gently rotated until the needle can be advanced without resistance. In the very rare cases where difficulties persist, it could be helpful to push the needle over a 0.0014 angioplasty guidewire [10,15]. This latter modification seems more useful than the stylet provided with the needle.

When the needle reaches the desired position inside, the catheter the flush is stopped and pressure is continuously monitored.

From then on, it is necessary to hold the needle and the catheter firmly and to move them as a unit (Figure 25.4).

Initially, the tip of the catheter is orientated toward the right shoulder of the patient in antero-posterior view. Then, under continuous fluoroscopic and pressure monitoring, both the catheter and needle are withdrawn downward and rotated counterclockwise until the contact with the septum is felt.

Others initially orientate the catheter toward the left shoulder (innominate vein) and perform a clockwise rotation. In such cases, when the system is withdrawn three sequential bumps can be felt representing (1) the RA/superior vena cava junction; (2) movement over the ascending aorta of

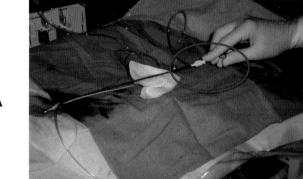

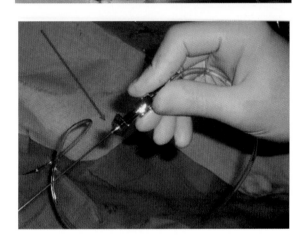

Figure 25.4. Procedure II: Positioning of the needle.

A) The catheter and the needle are moved as a unit keeping in mind the predetermined distance necessary to avoid protrusion of the needle out of the catheter.

B) The needle is rotated so that the arrow is oriented to 5 o'clock.

Courtesy of Professor A Cribier.

which pulsations may be felt; and finally (3) the passage over the limbus to enter the fossa ovalis.

Whatever the method used, the proximal arrow and the tip of the needle have a postero-medial position of 4 to 6 o'clock, looking from bottom to top in antero-posterior view. The angle is chosen according to the size of the LA (4'o clock in normal size; up to 6 in a large atrium).

In antero-posterior view, the correct position of the tip of the needle is usually mid-way between the pigtail and the right atrial border in the horizontal axis and slightly below the horizontal line at the level of the pigtail.

In most cases a sensation of more or less elastic resistance is felt through the catheter.

In patients with enlarged RA and LA the ideal puncture site is lower. In such cases, the convexity of the septum due to LA enlargement may cause catheter slippage and, thus, may impede adequate

contact with the septum. In addition, in patients with severely enlarged RA it is useful to slightly bend the needle at 10 cm from the tip to facilitate contact with the septum (Figure 25.5).

It is recommended to use a complementary view to provide further information on the orientation of the needle in the antero-posterior axis before puncturing the septum (Figure 25.6). This could be a lateral view with a target zone at the mid-part of the line between the pigtail and the spina, or right anterior oblique 30° with a target zone vertically in the middle of the line between the pigtail and the spina and below a horizontal line at the level of the pigtail. In both methods, the puncture site is posterior and inferior to the aortic plane. In these additional views a lower puncture point is also expected in patients with enlarged atria.

If an adequate position cannot be reached, the catheter and needle should not be re-advanced

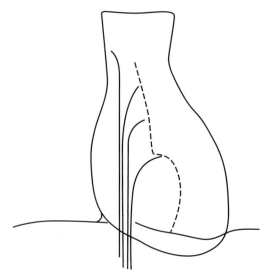

Figure 25.5. Procedure III: Reaching the fossa ovale. The catheter and needle are moved downward to the fossa ovale. Courtesy of Dr S Shaw.

upward, and the maneuver should be restarted. The entire system is withdrawn in the inferior vena cava, the needle is withdrawn, and the J-tipped guidewire is advanced through the catheter and repositioned in the superior vena cava.

If the previous stage is successfully performed, the catheter may pass into the LA through a patent foramen ovale, which is shown by the LA pressure recording. If this is the case, the catheter and the needle are gently pushed without resistance and the needle is withdrawn.

However, in most cases it is necessary to puncture the septum. Before puncturing the septum the following three key parameters should be checked: right atrial pressure tracing, correct position, and tactile feeling of contact with the septum (Figure 25.6).

If these criteria are fulfilled, the needle can be gently advanced. The entry into the LA is indicated by changes in pressure tracing. If no changes are perceived this may be due to: (1) problems with pressure recording, or problems with the permeability of the needle. In the latter case, as opposed to forceful flushing, it is recommended to gently aspirate blood, which will be red if the positioning is correct. (2) If the position seems adequate, but, there is still resistance to penetra-

tion, it may be due to a thick or fibrous septum, such as in children or in patients with previous cardiac surgery, or a "receding septum" feeling, which may be due to aneurysm of the septum requiring the application of additional pressure. Finally, if this happens when using a Mullins sheath, it may be due to the insufficient length of the needle protruding from the catheter to cross the thickness of the septum, necessitating the repetition of the maneuver with a Brockenbrough catheter. (3) Incorrect positioning requires repuncture at another site.

If transseptal puncture is not possible after a few attempts, it is recommended to perform it under echocardiographic guidance.

The catheter should be advanced only when assurance is obtained that the needle has crossed the septum.

It is recommended to return to the anteroposterior view, which provides a better view of the borders of the LA, before advancing the catheter to avoid damage to the vicinous structures, i.e. LA wall, left atrial appendage, or pulmonary veins.

Before moving forward it is necessary to be sure that the table is fixed and will not move during the following maneuvers.

It is now even more important to move the needle and the catheter as a unit because the needle is protruding into the LA. Continuous pressure is applied with the right hand at the proximal part of the needle whilst the left hand holds the catheter at the groin and provides counter-resistance if necessary.

In most cases the catheter advances easily but resistance may occur. In such cases, pressure must be continuously applied until crossing. If resistance persists when using a Brockenbrough catheter, it is necessary to check that the needle is not in a side hole, which is visible on fluoroscopy. If this is not the case, it is preferable to withdraw the catheter and needle and to redo the procedure using a Mullins catheter, which has a more tapered tip. If there is still resistance, it may be necessary to redo the puncture at another site as the first attempt was likely not at the fossa but at a thicker part of the septum. In the very rare cases where crossing with the catheter is still not possible, it may be useful to introduce an exchange angioplasty 0.014 guidewire into the needle and to withdraw both the needle

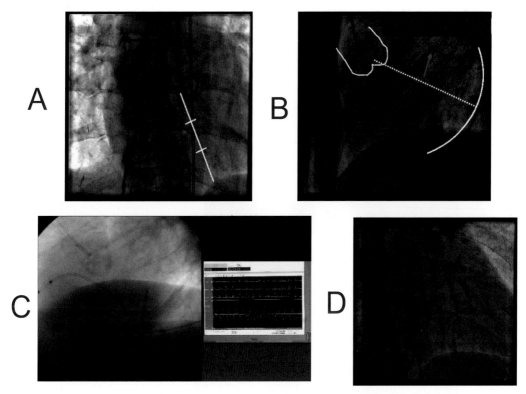

Figure 25.6. Procedure IV: Transseptal puncture.
A) Antero-posterior view. The catheter and needle are at the level of the fossa ovale, below and lateral to the pigtail.
B) Lateral view. The catheter and needle are below and posterior to the pigtail catheter.

C) The needle is advanced and left atrial pressure is obtained. Courtesy of Professor A Cribier.
D) The position of the puncture in right anterior oblique 30° is also inferior and posterior to the aortic cusps.

and catheter and insert an angioplasty balloon to dilate the septum before re-advancing the transseptal catheter [15].

When both the needle and the catheter have crossed the septum, the needle is withdrawn while applying a counter-clockwise rotation to the proximal part in order to orientate the catheter toward the mitral valve. Then the LA pressure is recorded. It is necessary to ensure that both the needle and the catheter have crossed the septum before removing the needle since a too early removal of the needle may lead to a backward movement of the catheter into the RA. When using the Mullins catheter after crossing of the septum, the needle is withdrawn into the dilator. The sheath is then advanced into the LA. The needle and the dilator are removed and the sheath is carefully flushed before connection to the pressure line.

Heparin, usually 3000 to 5000 IU, is given when the catheter is securely positioned in the LA.

Guidance of the Procedure

The procedure is most often performed under fluoroscopic guidance with several views, ideally using biplane fluoroscopy.

It has been proposed to use additional right atrial angiography to better locate the puncture site. However, today, this has been largely replaced by echographic monitoring using either transesophageal [16] or intra-cardiac [17] approaches (Figure 25.7).

Both echocardiographic techniques provide an excellent imaging of the inter-atrial septum, which is useful to guide the orientation of the needle in the fossa ovale, show proper positioning and monitor the crossing of the septum and its tenting.

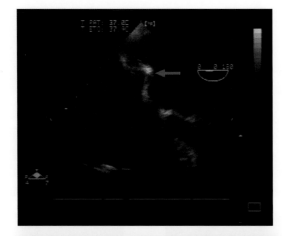

A

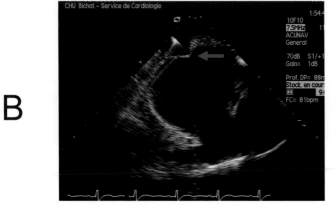

B

Figure 25.7. Guidance of transseptal puncture by echocardiography. A) Transesophageal echocardiography showing the Tenting of the inter-atrial septum during the septal puncture. B) Intra-cardiac echocardiography showing the tenting of the inter-atrial septum.

Echocardiography is a useful adjunct in the early part of the operator's experience. The drawbacks are the need for anesthesia, or at least analgesia, in most patients when transesophageal echocardiography is performed and the cost of the devices as regards intra-cardiac echocardiography. The recent introduction of real time 3D transesophageal echocardiography further improves imaging of the septum.

In experienced teams, echocardiographic guidance is restricted to cases where there are known difficulties, such as severe thoracic deformity, or when unexpected difficulties occur.

Effective echocardiographic guidance also requires specific training of the echocardiographer, without which it may result in a false impression of security.

Finally, transthoracic echographic guidance [18] is seldom used because it is difficult to perform at the same time as fluoroscopic imaging. However, it could be helpful in experienced hands.

Isolated case reports have described the feasibility of transseptal puncture on echocardiographic guidance alone, without fluoroscopy, in emergency cases. However, this approach cannot be recommended at the present time.

Complications

Although generally safe, transseptal catheterization is associated with an incidence of complications, albeit low if it is performed carefully following the rules described above [2,5,13,14,19–24] (Table 25.2).

The failure rate is usually of 1% to 2% and fatality is the exception.

Heart perforation related to the transseptal puncture may concern the free wall of the RA,

Table 25.2. Complications of transseptal catheterization.

	N =	Death (%)	Tamponade (%)	Embolism (%)
Roelke [5]	1279	0.08	1.2	0.08
Fagundes [21]	1150	0	1	0.4
De Ponti [2]	5520	0.008	0.1	0.008

LA, left atrial appendage, or be a puncture going from the RA to the LA via the pericardium, or finally the aorta. It mostly occurs when the operator is less experienced. Unfavorable patient characteristics such as severe atrial enlargement or thoracic deformity also increase risk. The perforation of the heart may result in mild pericardial effusion without clinical consequences but hemopericardium usually has immediate clinical consequences resulting in tamponade. Its incidence is around 1% but may be as high as 4% in centers with limited experience [24]. It should always be suspected when hypotension occurs during transseptal catheterization. Puncture of the aorta by the needle is usually without consequences when it is recognized immediately by pressure monitoring. It requires close monitoring and avoidance of heparin administration. On the other hand, advancement of the catheter in such cases may lead to hemopericardium.

If hemopericardium is suspected, echocardiography should be performed urgently before deterioration occurs.

Hemopericardium requires immediate pericardiocentesis ideally performed under echocardiographic guidance after reversal of anticoagulation if already given. If this is successful, the planned procedure can be then performed and the patient should be closely monitored. In most cases, hemopericardium due to transseptal catheterization can be managed by pericardiocentesis, especially when it results from a puncture by the transseptal needle only.

Embolism may be due to a thrombus that was pre-existing, mostly in the left atrial appendage, or developed during the procedure. Cerebral embolism usually results in a stroke. Less frequently coronary embolism leads to transient ST segment elevation [20].

The treatment of cerebral embolism should be in collaboration with a stroke center. Cerebral imaging should be performed on an emergency basis to rule out hemorrhage, then intra-arterial fibrinolytic therapy should be administered early in the absence of contra-indication.

In the case of persistent ST segment elevation coronary angiography should be performed. If a coronary occlusion is present, coronary angioplasty can be performed, whilst thrombo-aspiration could be an appealing alternative.

ST segment elevation in the inferior leads accompanied by diaphoresis, hypotension, and chest discomfort with normal coronary angiogram has been occasionally observed after transseptal catheterization as is also the case after other intracardiac manipulation. They may be neurally mediated as Bezold-Jarish-like reflex and are responsive to atropine [19].

Inferior vena cava perforation and retroperitoneal hematoma could be the consequences of pushing the needle extruded from the catheter during its positioning in the vena cava.

Atrial tachyarrhythmias could occur but are rare and usually transient.

Persistent inter-atrial shunts are not observed after the performance of transseptal catheterization in isolation.

Specificities According to the Subsequent Mitral Interventional Procedure

For percutaneous mitral commissurotomy, the Inoue technique is now almost exclusively used. The preferred site for the transseptal puncture is usually slightly lower than the fossa ovale if the LA is severely enlarged. However, if the crossing of the mitral valve is not possible using this puncture location, it may be necessary to redo the transseptal puncture in a slightly higher position and more posteriorly [3].

The experience of the new mitral valve repair techniques using the edge-to-edge technique is limited to a few hundred cases today. The transseptal puncture is performed under echo guidance, which is subsequently necessary for the performance of the procedure. The puncture site is usually higher than in percutaneous mitral commissurotomy [4].

Training

The presence of a learning curve has been well described [2,5], thus the training in the performance of transseptal catheterizations requires acquisition of special skills [25]. However, currently there are not specific data regarding the minimum numbers needed for initial training and maintenance of competency.

Physicians performing transseptal catheterization must have a good knowledge of the patho-anatomy of the heart, hemodynamics, and preferably echocardiography.

The interventionist must be able to recognize and manage complications such as tamponade and stroke. Echocardiography should be immediately available when performing the procedure. Proper training in transseptal catheterization will no doubt derive benefit from simulator training before clinical training during specific courses on the technique.

In the Future

Further refinements in the technique may well result from the evaluation of new technologies such as use of radiofrequency, which does not require mechanical force [26], better guidance by catheter remote control systems [27] or non-fluoroscopic mapping using multi-detector row computed tomography [28], electrical and three dimensional recording systems [29], or, in a far distant future direct, trans-blood visualization.

Conclusions

Transseptal catheterization has had a revival since it is the first and an obligatory step for several interventions in valve disease and even more so in interventional electrophysiology. It remains a demanding procedure, which requires specific expertise. The performance of the procedure will no doubt be facilitated in the future by better education and imaging technique development.

References

1. Ross J Jr, Braunwald E, Morrow AG. Transseptal left atrial puncture; new technique for the measurement of left atrial pressure in man. Am J Cardiol 1959; **3**: 653–655.
2. De Ponti R, Cappato R, Curnis A, et al. Trans-septal catheterization in the electrophysiology laboratory: data from a multicenter survey spanning 12 years. J Am Coll Cardiol. 2006; **47**(5): 1037–1042.
3. Vahanian A, Palacios IF. Percutaneous approaches to valvular disease. Circulation 2004; **109**: 1572–1579.
4. Feldman T, Wasserman HS, Herrmann HC, et al. Percutaneous mitral valve repair using the edge-to-edge technique: six-month results of the EVEREST Phase I Clinical Trial. J Am Coll Cardiol 2005; **46**: 2134–2140.
5. Roelke M, Smith AJ, Palacios IF. The technique and safety of transseptal left heart catheterization: the Massachusetts General Hospital experience with 1,279 procedures. Cathet Cardiovasc Diagn 1994; **32**: 332–339.
6. Vahanian A, Baumgartner H, Bax J, et al. Task Force on the Management of Valvular Hearth Disease of the European Society of Cardiology; ESC Committee for Practice Guidelines. Guidelines on the management of valvular heart disease: The Task Force on the Management of Valvular Heart Disease of the European Society of Cardiology. Eur Heart J 2007; **28**: 230–268.
7. Cheng TO. All roads lead to Rome: transjugular or transfemoral approach to percutaneous transseptal balloon mitral valvuloplasty? Catheter Cardiovasc Interv 2003; **59**: 266–267.
8. Attias D, Himbert D, Redheuil A, et al. Piège du cathétérisme trans-septal pour commissurotomie mitral percutanée: l'interruption de la veine cave inférieure avec continuation azygos. A propos d'un cas et revue littérature. Arch Mal Coeur Vaiss. 2007; **100**: 64–67.
9. Schoeffler M, Ringewald J, Schechter E. Transfemoral venous access through inferior vena cava filters for interventions requiring large sheaths. Catheter Cardiovasc Interv 2007; **69**: 47–51.
10. Triantafyllou K, Brochet E, Himbert D, et al. Coronary angioplasty tools to facilitate percutaneous mitral commissurotomy following surgical closure of ostium secundum atrial septal defect. Eurointervention 2007; 10: Case 2. http://www.europcronline.com/eurointervention/10th_issue/case2/.
11. Cook S, Meier B, Windecker S. Transseptal Tandem Heart implantation through an Amplatzer atrial septal occluder. J Invasive Cardiol 2007; **19**: 198–199.

12. Nallet O, Lung B, Cormier B, *et al.* Specifics of technique in percutaneous mitral commissurotomy in a case of dextrocardia and situs inversus with mitral stenosis. Cathet Cardiovasc Diagn 1996; **39**: 85–88.

13. Brockenbrough EC, Braunwald E, Ross J Jr. Transseptal left heart catheterization. A review of 450 studies and description of an improved technic. Circulation 1962; **25**: 15–21.

14. Mullins CE. Transseptal left heart catheterization: experience with a new technique in 520 pediatric and adult patients. Pediatr Cardiol 1983; **4**: 239–245.

15. Hildick-Smith D, McCready J, de Giovanni J. Transseptal puncture: use of an angioplasty guidewire for enhanced safety. Catheter Cardiovasc Interv 2007; **69**: 519–521.

16. Tucker KJ, Curtis AB, Murphy J, *et al.* Transesophageal echocardiographic guidance of transseptal left heart catheterization during radiofrequency ablation of left-sided accessory pathways in humans. Pacing Clin Electrophysiol 1996; **19**: 272–281.

17. Hanaoka T, Suyama K, Taguchi A, *et al.* Shifting of puncture site in the fossa ovalis during radiofrequency catheter ablation: intracardiac echocardiography-guided transseptal left heart catheterization. Jpn Heart J 2003; **44**: 673–680.

18. Trehan VK, Nigam A, Mukhopadhyay S, *et al.* Bedside percutaneous transseptal mitral commissurotomy under sole transthoracic echocardiographic guidance in a critically ill patient. Echocardiography 2006; **23**: 312–314.

19. Hildick-Smith DJ, Ludman PF, Shapiro LM. Inferior ST-segment elevation following transseptal puncture for balloon mitral valvuloplasty is atropine-responsive. J Invasive Cardiol 2004; **16**: 1–2.

20. Hernandez R, Macaya C, Benuelos C, *et al.* Predictors, mechanisms and outcome of severe mitral regurgitation complicating percutaneous mitral valvotomy with the Inoue balloon. Am J Cardiol 1992; **70**(13): 1169–1174.

21. Fagundes RL, Mantica M, De Luca L, *et al.* Safety of Single Transseptal Puncture for Ablation of Atrial Fibrillation: Retrospective Study from a Large Cohort of Patients. J Cardiovasc Electrophysiol; September 19, 2007 (Epub ahead of print).

22. Liu TJ, Lai HC, Lee WL, *et al.* Immediate and late outcomes of patients undergoing transseptal left-sided heart catheterization for symptomatic valvular and arrhythmic diseases. Am Heart J 2006; **151**: 235–241.

23. O'Keefe JH Jr, Vlietstra RE, Hanley PC, *et al.* Revival of the transseptal approach for catheterization of the left atrium and ventricle. Mayo Clin Proc 1985; **60**(11): 790–795.

24. Lew AS, Harper RW, Federman J, Anderson ST, Pitt A. Recent experience with transeptal catheterization. Cathet Cardiovasc Diagn 1983; **9**: 601–609.

25. King SB III, Aversano T, Ballard WL, *et al.* American College of Cardiology Foundation; American Heart Association; American College of Physicians Task Force on Clinical Competence and Training (Writing Committee to Update the 1998 Clinical Competence Statement on Recommendations for the Assessment and Maintenance of Proficiency in Coronary Interventional Procedures). ACCF/AHA/SCAI 2007 Update of the Clinical Competence Statement on Cardiac Interventional Procedures: A report of the American College of Cardiology Foundation/American Heart Association/American College of Physicians Task Force on Clinical Competence and Training (Writing Committee to Update the 1998 Clinical Competence Statement on Recommendations for the Assessment and Maintenance of Proficiency in Coronary Interventional Procedures). J Am Coll Cardiol 2007; **50**: 82–108.

26. Sherman W, Lee P, Hartley A, *et al.* Transatrial septal catheterization using a new radiofrequency probe. Catheter Cardiovasc Interv 2005; **66**: 14–17.

27. Saliba W, Cummings JE, Oh S, *et al.* Novel robotic catheter remote control system: Feasibility and safety of transseptal puncture and endocardial catheter navigation. J Cardiovasc Electrophysiol 2006; **17**(10): 1102–1115.

28. Graham LN, Melton IC, MacDonald S, *et al.* Value of CT localization of the fossa ovalis prior to transseptal left heart catheterization for left atrial ablation. Europace 2007; **9**: 417–423.

29. Verma S, Borganelli M. Real-time, three-dimensional localization of a Brockenbrough needle during transseptal catheterization using a nonfluoroscopic mapping system. J Invasive Cardiol 2006; **18**: 324–327.

CHAPTER 26

Alcohol Septal Ablation for Hypertrophic Obstructive Cardiomyopathy

Amir-Ali Fassa, & Ulrich Sigwart
Geneva University Hospitals, Geneva, Switzerland

Introduction

Left-ventricular outflow tract obstruction is seen in approximately 25% of patients with hypertrophic cardiomyopathy under resting conditions, and is an independent predictor of poor prognosis [1,2]. Although negative inotropic drugs can efficiently alleviate symptoms in many cases, 5–10% of patients with hypertrophic obstructive cardiomyopathy (HOCM) remain refractory to drug therapy [3]. Surgical myectomy (also known as the Morrow operation) has been performed since the 1960s, and has been shown to reduce outflow gradients. Nevertheless, some patients are not regarded as favorable candidates for this major intervention because of factors such as advanced age, concomitant medical conditions or previous cardiac surgery [4,5]. In 1994, a catheter treatment (known under a variety of abbreviations listed in Table 26.1) using absolute alcohol to induce a localized myocardial infarction to the interventricular septum was introduced as an alternative to surgery [6]. Alcohol-induced septal branch ablation had been previously described for therapy of ventricular tachycardia [7]. This technique was applied to HOCM after clinical observations of improvement

Interventional Cardiology, First Edition. Edited by Carlo Di Mario, George D. Dangas, Peter Barlis.

in a patient with septal hypertrophy who suffered an anterior myocardial infarction and also the transient reduction in left-ventricular outflow pressure gradients observed with temporary septal artery balloon occlusion. Since its introduction, there has been growing enthusiasm for this technique. Indeed, over 800 procedures were performed during the first five years [8], and the number to date is probably more than 5000 [9,10]. Although initially confined to Europe and North America, this technique is now being performed worldwide [11].

Selection of Patients

Patient selection for alcohol septal ablation (ASA) should be based on a careful individual evaluation of the clinical symptoms, associated comorbidities, and echocardiographic and angiographic parameters [5,9,12]. The primary indications for the procedure are NYHA (New York Heart Association) or CCS (Canadian Cardiovascular Score) Class III or IV symptoms despite adequately tolerated drug therapy with a documented left ventricular outflow tract (LVOT) gradient variably defined as ≥50 mm Hg at rest or after exercise, or >30 mm Hg at rest or ≥60 mm Hg under stress. Likewise, selected patients with advanced NYHA or CCS Class II symptoms (for example those with syncope and severe pre-syncope) and a resting gradient >50 mm Hg or >30 mm Hg at rest and

Table 26.1. Common abbreviations for alcohol septal ablation.

ASA	Alcohol septal ablation.
ASR	Alcohol septal reduction.
NSMR	Nonsurgical myocardial reduction.
NSRT	Nonsurgical septal reduction therapy.
PTSMA	Percutaneous transluminal septal myocardial ablation.
TAA	Transcoronary alcohol ablation.
TASH	Transcoronary ablation of septal hypertrophy.

Table 26.2. Criteria for selection of patients for alcohol septal ablation.

- Symptoms refractory to adequate tolerated drug therapy.
- NYHA or CCS Class III or IV with a resting gradient of >30 mm Hg or ≥60 mm Hg under stress or ≥50 mm Hg at rest and/or with provocation.
- NYHA or CCS Class II in selected patients (for example those with syncope or severe pre-syncope) with a resting gradient >50 mm Hg or >30 mm Hg at rest and ≥100 mm Hg with stress.
- Basal septal wall thickness ≥18 mm.
- Adequately sized septal perforator supplying the area of the systolic anterior motion-septum contact.
- High risk of surgical morbidity and mortality.
- Absence of concomitant cardiac disease requiring surgery (such as extensive coronary artery disease that would be treated surgically, organic valvular disease, morphological abnormalities of the mitral valve and papillary muscles).

NYHA = New York Heart Association; CCS = Canadian Cardiovascular Society.

≥100 mm Hg with stress may also be considered for the procedure (Table 26.2). Furthermore, a septal wall thickness <18 mm should be taken as a contraindication for ASA because of the risk of septal perforation.

Mechanisms of Treatment Efficacy

In HOCM, obstruction is caused by protrusion of the hypertrophied interventricular septum into the outflow tract and by systolic anterior movement of the mitral valve due to a Venturi phenomenon and a drag effect [5,13].

ASA induces a well-demarcated subaortic necrosis, corresponding to approximately 10% of the post-ablation total left ventricle mass (or 31% of the septal myocardial mass), as assessed by various imaging techniques (such as single-photon emission computed tomography, positron emission tomography and contrast-enhanced magnetic resonance imaging) [14–18]. However, with the use of smaller ethanol doses nowadays, septal necrosis is probably less.

The hemodynamic response to the induced reduction of septal myocardium is usually triphasic [5,19]. Immediately after ASA, there is a marked reduction of the LVOT gradient. Proposed mechanisms involved in the acute benefit are improvement in left ventricular relaxation and compliance via a reduction in regional asynchrony, resulting in an increase in left ventricular passive filling and a reduction in left atrial size and left ventricular ejection force [20–23]. This initial relief is usually followed during the following days by a rise of the LVOT gradient to about 50% of the pre-procedure level, possibly in relation to some degree of recovery from stunning or to edema caused by the infarct, which subsequently disappears [19,24]. Finally, within the following weeks to months, there is a new decrease in LVOT gradient back to the post-ablation level. It is believed that long-term benefit results from the creation of localized septal infarction and scarring, which increase LVOT diameter as a result of septal thinning and "therapeutic remodeling" [14,20,25,26]. The overall effect is an increase in left ventricular size, a decrease in left ventricular mass and hypertrophy [15,25,26], and alteration of septal activation, resulting in incoordination of contraction [27]. The regression of hypertrophy in areas remote from the basal septum after ASA indicates that myocardial hypertrophy in HOCM is in part afterload dependent and is not entirely due to the genetic defect [25,26]. Furthermore, changes in diastolic function resulting from ASA also seem to contribute to long-term improvement in hemodynamics [28]. This effect might be due to more favorable relaxation as well as a reduction in left-ventricular stiffness secondary to regression of hypertrophy [22,23,25,29,30], decrease in interstitial collagen and expression of tumor-necrosis factor [31].

The Technique

Assessment of Outflow Gradient

Although some centers only measure the gradient non-invasively using echocardiography, most operators use hemodynamic measurement of outflow gradient during the procedure to confirm the gradient. A 5 Fr pigtail or multipurpose catheter with side holes situated close to the tip can be used to measure pre-stenotic pressure. Many operators prefer to introduce the catheter retrogradely via a controlateral femoral arterial puncture, rather than perform trans-septal puncture with a Brockenbrough catheter as described initially [6]. It is essential to place the catheter close to the apex particularly in cases with mid-ventricular hypertrophy. A J-wire may sometimes be useful to advance the catheter further toward the apex. Attention should be paid to avoid entrapment in the myocardium, as this may exaggerate the gradient. This may be achieved by injecting a small volume of contrast via the catheter, and checking for proper clearance of the dye.

A 7 Fr or 8 Fr guiding catheter (example.g. short tip Judkins type that allows deep intubation of the vessel if necessary) is placed in the ascending aorta to measure the post-stenotic pressure. A 6 Fr catheter can cause excessive pressure damping with concomitant use of a balloon catheter required for alcohol injection later during the procedure, and should therefore not be used. After exclusion of a valvular gradient, the peak-to-peak intraventricular gradient should be measured at rest, during isoproterenol infusion, and after extra systoles (Figure 26.1). Isoproterenol infusion may be particularly useful to reveal a gradient in sedated patients and may be administered by diluting 200 mcg in 50 cc of saline, with injection of a bolus of 1–3 cc followed by additional boluses until a heart rate of 100–120 bpm is reached.

In order to ensure backup pacing in the advent of complete atrioventricular (AV) block, a temporary pacing wire should be placed in the right ventricle. If extrasystoles are not observed spontaneously, the pacing wire may also serve to measure the post-extrasystolic gradient by programmed stimulation (with coupling intervals of approximately 370 ms). Any beta-blocker therapy should be discontinued because of the increased risk of heart block and also in order to optimally assess the underlying outflow gradient.

Placement and Testing of the Balloon Catheter

An angiogram of the left coronary artery is performed (Figure 26.2A). Milking of the septal perforators that supply the hypertrophied segments, which is often observed, may be a good indicator for identifying the target vessel. Placing the guidewire in the septal branch may occasionally be challenging due to a steep take-off angle. It may be helpful to pre-shape the guidewire with two angles through a needle as shown in Figure 26.3 (rather than a curve). A floppy guidewire should be tried first, and advanced distally into the septal perforator in order to ensure stability. Stiffer guide wires (intermediate, or in rare cases a standard wire) may be needed to make the balloon go through steep angles. Exceptionally, a 4 Fr catheter with a sharp angle (for example an internal mammary catheter) may be used as an inner catheter to preselect septal branches with extremely steep takeoffs for placing the 0.014-inch guidewire. Nonetheless, catheters should be manipulated with extreme caution to avoid dissection. Ultimately, another balloon catheter can also be briefly inflated just distally to the septal branch, and the 0.014-inch guidewire bounced off into the targeted vessel.

The targeted septal branch should have a diameter of at least 1.5 mm. After administration of intravenous heparin, the shortest available balloon catheter (a 10 × 2 mm balloon is suitable for most cases) is placed as proximally as possible in a stable position. The balloon should be adapted to the dimension of the vessel and slightly oversized (usually 2–3 mm). Although balloons dedicated to this procedure have been developed, standard angioplasty balloons may be used. If there is early proximal branching of the septal perforator, a very short balloon (5 mm) may be used. Consequently, the guiding catheter may have to be positioned more deeply to give more support for the balloon catheter and avoid recoil during injection. The balloon should be inflated with a pressure of 4–6 bar, and proper positioning should be verified by injection of contrast agent into the left coronary artery (Figure 26.2B), and then distally via the lumen of the balloon catheter using about 1 cc of

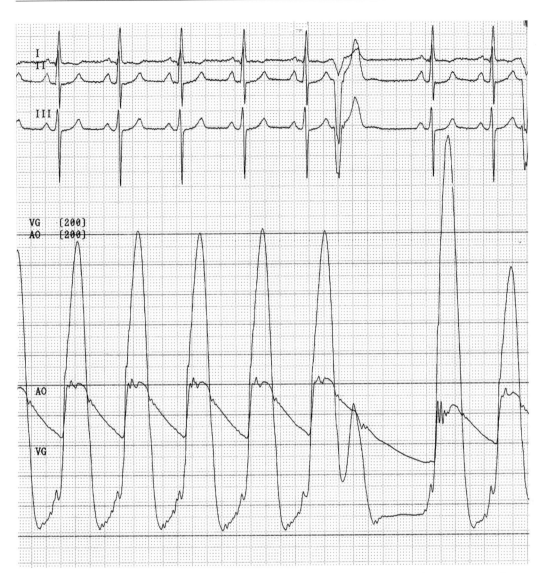

Figure 26.1. Hemodynamic monitoring with a resting peak-to-peak gradient of 100 mm Hg and a post extra-systolic gradient of approximately 170 mm Hg.

dye (Figure 26.2C). Absence of retrograde leakage and stability of balloon position (especially with shorter balloons) should be verified cautiously. A key point is to inject the contrast *forcefully* via the inflated balloon catheter when testing for stability. In addition, the extent of myocardium supplied by the septal branch and shunting of flow to non-targeted regions can also be analyzed, preferably using two different projections. The injection of contrast agent also increases ischemia to the territory of the septal branch. The outflow gradient should be monitored constantly, and within five minutes of balloon occlusion, a drop in the resting gradient by >30 mm Hg or the post-extrasystolic gradient by >50 mm Hg should be observed. In a significant proportion of patients, these criteria are not met [30]. Nowadays most operators prefer echocardiographic criteria using echo-contrast to delineate the target area (see below). If necessary, the balloon catheter may be positioned in another septal branch. The target vessel may occasionally originate from an intermediate or diagonal branch

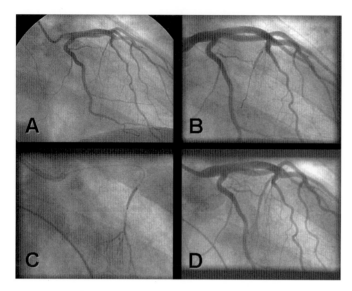

Figure 26.2. Angiography of the left coronary artery (A). Right anterior oblique view (B). Balloon catheter inflated and placed in the first septal branch over a 0.014-inch guidewire (C). Contrast medium is injected via the balloon catheter to confirm the absence of retrograde leakage (D) Angiogram after alcohol injection. Note that the first septal branch is patent.

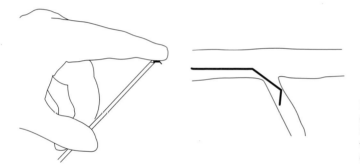

Figure 26.3. Pre-shaping the 0.014-inch guidewire with two angles through a blunt needle (left) and positioning of the guidewire in a septal branch (right).

[32], or from the posterior descending artery in case of a dominant right coronary artery [12].

Guidance by myocardial contrast echocardiography (MCE) has proved to be particularly useful, and may influence the interventional strategy in 15–20% of cases either by changing the target vessel or aborting the procedure. In addition, MCE allows increased success rates despite reduced infarct size, which in turn reduces complications [20,32]. Before injecting alcohol, 1–2 ml of echo contrast (for example, Sonovue®, Levovist®, Optison®, Albunex® etc.) is injected via the inflated balloon catheter under transthoracic echocardiography in the apical 4- and 5-chamber views (Figure 26.4A). This will ascertain whether the opacified myocardium is adjacent to the region where the anterior mitral leaflet comes into contact with the septum, and allow to withhold alcohol administra-

tion in case of a sub-optimal perfusion pattern, such as for example if the right side of the interventricular septum is predominantly opacified [33]. This technique also allows to delineate the infarct zone and rule out any retrograde leakage or involvement of myocardium distant from the expected target region such as the ventricular free wall or papillary muscles [16,32,34]. With echocontrast volumes of more than 1 ml, transcapillary leakage of the contrast medium into the ventricles may occur, more often the right than the left (Figure 26.4B). In the case echo contrast is not available, echocardiography may also be performed by using agitated regular contrast dye injection in the septal perforator via the occluded balloon catheter. Furthermore, contrast dye injections through the inflated balloon should not be done before echographic imaging (e.g. when testing for balloon

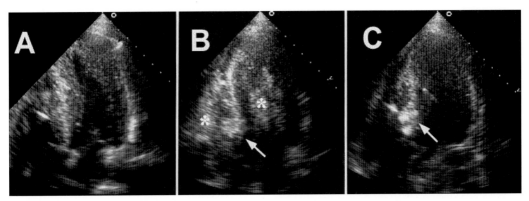

Figure 26.4. (A) Apical four-chamber echocardiogram showing the hypertrophied septum (B). Injection of echo contrast via the occluded balloon catheter positioned in the first septal perforator, with opacification of the basal septum (arrow). Note the presence of echo contrast (asterisks) within both ventricles due to transcapillary passage (C). After alcohol injection, the area of necrosis becomes echodense (arrow).

stability), as this may opacify the myocardium and make interpretation of the images more difficult during subsequent injections.

Alcohol Injection

Once the septal perforator is deemed suitable and the balloon position is stable without any retrograde spilling, 0.7–3 ml of 96% alcohol may be injected through the inflated balloon catheter. Before this, analgesia could be administered for pain control. The volume injected will depend on the dimension of the vessel and the volume of the targeted myocardium. The speed of delivery is subject to debate, as the alcohol may be either injected slowly over 1–5 min or as a bolus. We prefer the latter technique, as this may allow more efficient dissipation of the alcohol over a larger volume of myocardium and avoid preferential streaming to a single region. However, it may be argued that slow injection may allow for longer contact of the alcohol with the myocardium (for instance, by initially inducing capillary leakage which may subsequently allow more alcohol extravasations into the interstitial tissue). Nonetheless, recent animal studies have shown that it is not the speed of alcohol injection but the amount of alcohol injected that determines the resultant infarct size [35,36]. Therefore, during the past years, there has been a tendency to reduce the volume of alcohol injected to a maximum of 2 ml [14,30,37] which may reduce complications.

During the injection, the electrocardiogram should be closely monitored, and the injection aborted if AV block develops. The balloon should remain inflated during at least 5 min in order to enhance contact of alcohol with the tissue and avoid reflux into the left anterior descending artery. Angiography of the left coronary artery should be repeated following balloon deflation in order to confirm patency of the left anterior descending artery (Figure 26.2D). The target septal vessel may not necessarily be occluded, although flow usually appears sluggish. It is not known whether this has any impact on treatment efficacy. Echocardiographically, the injection of alcohol results in a marked contrast effect, which is much stronger than currently available echo contrast agents (Figure 26.4C).

The hemodynamic objective should be a decrease of the gradient to <10 mm Hg at rest in patients with resting gradients >30 mm Hg, or a decrease by >50% of a significant provokable gradient [12]. If there is a significant residual gradient after a period of 5–10 min following the last injection, a new alcohol injection may be attempted by placing the balloon more proximally inside the same septal branch, or using a shorter balloon if branches of the septal perforator were occluded by the balloon inflation during the first injection. Alternatively, a second septal perforator may be targeted using the same procedure as for the first branch. The majority of patients will require one target perforator branch only, especially since the advent of MCE.

Furthermore, a residual gradient of <30 mm Hg is often acceptable, as it has been shown that outflow gradient may further decrease over time [19]. Some operators therefore prefer a "one vessel per session" approach, and it is still unclear whether more than a single septal perforator should be targeted initially.

Post-procedural Management

Vascular sheaths may be removed after normalization of coagulation parameters. Heparin at therapeutic levels does not need to be pursued after the procedure. Furthermore, all patients should receive Aspirin (e.g. 100 mg/d) before the procedure, which should be continued during one month due to the risk of mural thrombosis resulting from the infarct. Creatinine kinase (CK) levels should be dosed every 4 hours in order to measure peak values. Peak rises are commonly in the range of 750–1500 U/l. Patients should be observed in the coronary care unit for 48 hours, with removal of the transvenous pacemaker at the end of this period in the absence of AV block. The patient may then be transferred to a monitored step-down unit for the remainder of the hospital stay (which is usually one day). Inotropic and chronotropic therapy, especially beta-blockers, can be resumed—possibly at lower doses—if there are no significant bradyarrhythmias [12].

Treatment Efficacy

Although no randomized controlled trial comparing ASA to surgical myectomy has ever been performed, the general consensus is that in centers with appropriate expertise, operative risks, hemodynamic benefits, and initial symptomatic benefits are broadly comparable with either technique [38]. Evidence from non-randomized trials also indicate that ASA is similar to myectomy with respect to hemodynamic and functional improvement [39–41]. Pooled results of published studies on ASA show acute reductions in mean resting LVOT gradients from 65 to 17 mm Hg and mean post-extrasystolic gradients from 125 to 53 mm Hg, with persistence of the reduction after 12 months (16 and 32 mm Hg, respectively) [42]. In addition, there is a significant improvement at 12 months of functional class (NYHA Class 2.9 to 1.2, CCS 1.9

to 0.4), peak oxygen consumption (17.8 to 23.6 mL/kg/min) and exercise capacity (86.2 to 122.8 Watts). Procedure success is achieved in 89% of cases. Repeat procedures despite initial success are required because of recurring gradient and symptoms in 7% of patients. Reported predictors of procedural failure are total peak CK < 1300 U/L and immediate residual LVOT gradient ≥25 mm Hg [43].

Adverse Events

Early mortality (occurring during or up to 30 days after the procedure) is low, with a mean value of 1.5% reported [42], which is similar to that for surgical myectomy. Causes of early mortality include LAD dissection, ventricular fibrillation, cardiac tamponade, cardiogenic shock and pulmonary embolism. Late all-cause mortality is reported at 0.5%, the most frequent causes being sudden cardiac death, pulmonary embolism, congestive heart failure and other non-cardiac causes. Other reported adverse events include coronary dissection and spasm (1.8% and 1.4%, respectively), stroke (1.1%) and pericardial effusion (0.6%).

Spontaneous ventricular fibrillation in the immediate periprocedural period is not frequent (2.2%), and sustained ventricular tachycardia is extremely rare (only three cases reported in current literature) [42,44].

The most frequent complication of ASA is complete AV block requiring permanent pacemaker implantation. Occurrence of acute complete AV block during the procedure varies between 21% and 70% of patients [45–49]. Yet, there is recovery of AV conduction in most cases (41%–100%) before leaving the catheterization laboratory, and in two-thirds of patients within the first 3 days [46,47]. Disappearance of procedural complete AV block has been reported as late as 13 days after the procedure [46]. Delayed complete AV block may also develop later during hospitalization in patients without previous procedural complete AV block or as a recurrence after recovery from acute complete AV block. Depending on the definition used, delayed complete AV block occurs in 1–25% of cases, after a mean period of 36 hours post procedure, and usually requires permanent pacemaker implantation due to persistence of the conduction defect [47,49]. The block can appear unexpectedly as late as 96 hours after the procedure [50]. It is thought that transient procedural conduction abnormalities are likely due to the acute effects of alcohol on the myocardium and conduction system (ischemia, edema and inflammation), while permanent conduction abnormalities are probably due to necrosis, scarring and possibly remodeling [47]. Ultimately, around 10% of patients require permanent pacemaker implantation after ASA [42]. Several studies have sought to determine predictors of development of delayed complete AV block, with conflicting results [43,47,49,51]. Overall, the most consistent predictors of subsequent permanent pacing implantation appear to be baseline left bundle branch block (LBBB), baseline first-degree AV block and procedural complete AV block [43,47–49,51]. Some authors suggest elective permanent pacemaker implantation prior to ASA in patients with baseline LBBB [48]. Furthermore, an earlier study showed that use of MCE limits infarct size and reduces the need for permanent pacemaker implantation from 17% to 7%, subsequently leading to widespread use of MCE during ASA [45]. Other parameters reported as significant predictors of complete AV block development are new intraventricular conduction defects, pre- or post- procedure prolongation of QRS duration, retrograde AV nodal block (assessed by simultaneous electrophysiological investigation), advanced age, female gender, bolus injection of alcohol and injection of more than one septal artery. However, none of these parameters were systematically confirmed across different studies [43,47–49,51]. Based on several of these predictors, some groups have elaborated specific management strategies based on risk of complete AV block occurrence [48,49]. We and others implant a pacemaker if the block persists for >48–72 hours, although as mentioned above, AV conduction may recover in many patients with longer observation [43].

New right-bundle-branch block (RBBB) is seen approximately in one half of patients [42]. This finding is not surprising, since the right bundle is a discrete structure that is vascularized by septal branches from the left anterior coronary artery in 90% of patients, whereas the left bundle is fan-like and receives a dual blood supply from perforator branches of both the left anterior descending and posterior descending arteries. The left conduction system may nevertheless be involved, and new left anterior fascicular block is reported in 6% of procedures [42].

Furthermore, one cardiac magnetic resonance study reported a greater left ventricular mass reduction following ASA in patients who developed new RBBB compared to those without RBB [52].

Despite the creation of a septal infarct, new Q-waves in the septal leads are rarely seen after ASA. Baseline Q waves even tend to disappear following the procedure [53].

In patients with permanent pacemakers undergoing ASA, loss of capture may occur if the ventricular lead is placed near the septum [54]. Increasing pacing to maximum output during the first days following the procedure might therefore be prudent in these patients.

Finally, although concern has been raised about creation of an arrhythmogenic substrate by ASA [10,55] there is currently no evidence that indicates an increase in incidence of ventricular arrhythmias or sudden death during follow-up, as assessed by serial electrophysiologic studies before and after the procedure [30,56] or by analysis of implantable cardioverter-defibrillator intervention rate [57].

Future Directions

Since the original description in 1995, the procedure has undergone several modifications and improvements that have led to optimization of the results and minimization of complications, most importantly through the reduction of the effective dose of alcohol and the use of MCE. Recently, use of intracardiac echocardiography has been described as a way to provide continuous imaging of the treated segment of the septum during the whole procedure [58,59]. Facilitation of septal artery cannulation by magnetic navigation has also been reported [60]. Other novelties include use of polyvinyl alcohol foam particles, absorbable gelatin sponge or septal coil embolization as alternatives to alcohol, which may further reduce the incidence of complete heart block [61–63]. Finally, reduction of septum by radiofrequency catheter ablation and cryoablation are currently under investigation [64,65].

Conclusion

Although surgical myectomy has set the standard of therapy for drug-resistant HOCM, ASA is an alternative that may be considered in many patients. Data indicate that functional and hemodynamic success is high and similar to that of surgery, with the advantage that it may be performed in patients in whom major surgery may be considered unsuitable. Benefits in comparison to myectomy also include shorter hospital stay, minimum pain, and avoidance of complications associated with surgery and cardiopulmonary bypass. Nevertheless, ASA has an important learning curve, with potentially serious complications, the most frequent of which is complete AV block requiring permanent pacemaker implantation in approximately 10% of patients. Although these rates are declining with continuing experience, the advent of imaging techniques such as MCE and use of lower alcohol doses, the procedure should be performed only by experienced operators and on carefully selected patients.

References

1. Maron BJ, Olivotto I, Spirito P, et al. Epidemiology of hypertrophic cardiomyopathy-related death: revisited in a large non-referral-based patient population. Circulation 2000; **102**: 858–864.
2. Maron MS, Olivotto I, Betocchi S, et al. Effect of left ventricular outflow tract obstruction on clinical outcome in hypertrophic cardiomyopathy. N Engl J Med 2003; **348**: 295–303.
3. Maron BJ, Bonow RO, Cannon RO III, et al. Hypertrophic cardiomyopathy. Interrelations of clinical manifestations, pathophysiology, and therapy (1). N Engl J Med 1987; **316**: 780–789.
4. Maron BJ. Hypertrophic cardiomyopathy: a systematic review. JAMA 2002;. **287**: 1308–1320.
5. Maron BJ, McKenna WJ, Danielson GK, et al. American College of Cardiology/European Society of Cardiology clinical expert consensus document on hypertrophic cardiomyopathy. A report of the American College of Cardiology Foundation Task Force on Clinical Expert Consensus Documents and the European Society of Cardiology Committee for Practice Guidelines. Eur Heart J 2003; **24**: 1965–1991.
6. Sigwart U. Non-surgical myocardial reduction for hypertrophic obstructive cardiomyopathy. Lancet 1995; **346**: 211–214.
7. Brugada P, de Swart H, Smeets JL, et al. Transcoronary chemical ablation of ventricular tachycardia. Circulation 1989; **79**: 475–482.
8. Spencer WH III, Roberts R. Alcohol septal ablation in hypertrophicobstructive cardiomyopathy: the need for a registry. Circulation 2000; **102**: 600–601.
9. Roberts R, Sigwart U. Current concepts of the pathogenesis and treatment of hypertrophic cardiomyopathy. Circulation 2005; **112**: 293–296.
10. Marron B. Controversies in cardiovascular medicine: surgical myectomy remains the primary treatment option for severely symptomatic patients with obstructive hypertrophic cardiomyopathy. Circulation 2007; **116**: 196–206.
11. Li ZQ, Cheng TO, Zhang WW, et al. Percutaneous transluminal septal myocardial ablation for hypertrophic obstructive cardiomyopathy. The Chinese experience in 119 patients from a single center. Int Journal Cardiol 2004; **93**: 197–202.
12. Holmes DR Jr., Valeti US, Nishimura RA. Alcohol septal ablation for hypertrophic cardiomyopathy: indications and technique. Catheter Cardiovasc Interv 2005; **66**: 375–389.
13. Jiang L, Levine RA, King ME, et al. An integrated mechanism for systolic anterior motion of the mitral valve in hypertrophic cardiomyopathy based on echocardiographic observations. Am Heart J 1987; **113**: 633–644.
14. Kuhn H, Gietzen FH, Schafers M, et al. Changes in the left ventricular outflow tract after transcoronary ablation of septal hypertrophy (TASH) for hypertrophic obstructive cardiomyopathy as assessed by transoesophageal echocardiography and by measuring myocardial glucose utilization and perfusion. Eur Heart J 1999; **20**: 1808–1817.
15. Lakkis NM, Nagueh SF, Kleiman NS, et al. Echocardiography-guided ethanol septal reduction for hypertrophic obstructive cardiomyopathy. Circulation 1998; **98**: 1750–1755.
16. Nagueh SF, Lakkis NM, He ZX, et al. Role of myocardial contrast echocardiography during nonsurgical septal reduction therapy for hypertrophic obstructive cardiomyopathy. J Am Coll Cardiol 1998; **32**: 225–229.
17. van Dockum WG, ten Cate FJ, ten Berg JM, et al. Myocardial infarction after percutaneous transluminal septal myocardial ablation in hypertrophic obstructive cardiomyopathy: evaluation by contrast-enhanced magnetic resonance imaging. J Am Coll Cardiol 2004; **43**: 27–34.
18. Valeti US, Nishimura RA, Holmes DR Jr, et al. Comparison of surgical septal myectomy and alcohol septal ablation with cardiac magnetic resonance imaging

in patients with hypertrophic obstructive cardiomyopathy. J Am Coll Cardiol 2007; **49**: 350–357.

19. Yoerger DM, Picard MH, Palacios IF, *et al.* Time course of pressure gradient response after first alcohol septal ablation for obstructive hypertrophic cardiomyopathy. Am J Cardiol 2006; **97**: 1511–1514.

20. Flores-Ramirez R, Lakkis NM, Middleton KJ, *et al.* Echocardiographic insights into the mechanisms of relief of left ventricular outflow tract obstruction after nonsurgical septal reduction therapy in patients with hypertrophic obstructive cardiomyopathy. J Am Coll Cardiol 2001; **37**: 208–214.

21. Park TH, Lakkis NM, Middleton KJ, *et al.* Acute effect of nonsurgical septal reduction therapy on regional left ventricular asynchrony in patients with hypertrophic obstructive cardiomyopathy. Circulation 2002; **106**: 412–415.

22. Nagueh SF, Lakkis NM, Middleton KJ, *et al.* Changes in left ventricular diastolic function 6 months after nonsurgical septal reduction therapy for hypertrophic obstructive cardiomyopathy. Circulation 1999; **99**: 344–347.

23. Nagueh SF, Lakkis NM, Middleton KJ, *et al.* Changes in left ventricular filling and left atrial function six months after nonsurgical septal reduction therapy for hypertrophic obstructive cardiomyopathy. J Am Coll Cardiol 1999; **34**: 1123–1128.

24. Daggish AL, Smith RN, Palacios I, *et al.* Pathological effects of alcohol septal ablation for hypertrophic obstructive cardiomyopathy. Heart 2006; **92**: 1773–1778.

25. Mazur W, Nagueh SF, Lakkis NM, *et al.* Regression of left ventricular hypertrophy after nonsurgical septal reduction therapy for hypertrophic obstructive cardiomyopathy. Circulation 2001; **103**: 1492–1496.

26. van Dockum WG, Beek AM, ten Cate FJ, *et al.* Early onset and progression of left ventricular remodeling after alcohol septal ablation in hypertrophic obstructive cardiomyopathy. Circulation 2005; **111**: 2503–2508.

27. Henein MY, O'Sullivan CA, Ramzy IS, *et al.* Electromechanical left ventricular behavior after nonsurgical septal reduction in patients with hypertrophic obstructive cardiomyopathy. J Am Coll Cardiol 1999; **34**: 1117–1122.

28. Jassal DS, Neilan TG, Fifer MA, *et al.* Sustained improvement in left ventricular diastolic function after alcohol septal ablation for hypertrophic obstructive cardiomyopathy. Eur Heart J 2006; **27**: 1805–1810.

29. Sitges M, Shiota T, Lever HM, *et al.* Comparison of left ventricular diastolic function in obstructive hypertrophic cardiomyopathy in patients undergoing percutaneous septal alcohol ablation versus surgical myotomy/myectomy. Am J Cardiol 2003; **91**: 817–821.

30. Boekstegers P, Steinbigler P, Molnar A, *et al.* Pressure-guided nonsurgical myocardial reduction induced by small septal infarctions in hypertrophic obstructive cardiomyopathy. J Am Coll Cardiol 2001; **38**: 846–853.

31. Nagueh SF, Stetson SJ, Lakkis NM, *et al.* Decreased expression of tumor necrosis factor-alpha and regression of hypertrophy after nonsurgical septal reduction therapy for patients with hypertrophic obstructive cardiomyopathy. Circulation 2001; **103**: 1844–1850.

32. Faber L, Seggewiss H, Welge D, *et al.* Echo-guided percutaneous septal ablation for symptomatic hypertrophic obstructive cardiomyopathy: 7 years of experience. Eur J Echocardiography 2004; **5**: 347–355.

33. Okayama H, Sumimoto T, Morioka N, *et al.* Usefulness of selective myocardial contrast echocardiography in percutaneous transluminal septal myocardial ablation: a case report. Jpn Circ J 2001; **65**: 842–844.

34. Harada T, Ohtaki E, Sumiyoshi T, *et al.* Papillary muscles identified by myocardial contrast echocardiography in preparation for percutaneous transluminal septal myocardial ablation. Acta Cardiol 2002; **57**: 25–27.

35. Li ZQ, Cheng TO, Liu L, *et al.* Experimental study of relationship between intracoronary alcohol injection and the size of resultant myocardial infarct. Int J Cardiol 2003; **91**: 93–96.

36. Cheng TO. In percutaneous transluminal septal myocardial ablation for hypertrophic obstructive cardiomyopathy, it is not the speed of intracoronary alcohol injection but the amount of alcohol injected that determines the resultant infarct size. Circulation 2004; **110**: e23.

37. Veselka J, Prochazkova S, Duchonova R, *et al.* Alcohol septal ablation for hypertrophic obstructive cardiomyopathy: lower alcohol dose reduces size of infarction and has comparable hemodynamic and clinical outcome. Catheter Cardiovasc Interv 2004; **63**: 231–235.

38. Watkins H, McKenna WJ. The prognostic impact of septal myectomy in obstructive hypertrophic cardiomyopathy. J Am Coll Cardiol 2005; **46**: 477–479.

39. Nagueh SF, Ommen, SR, Lakkis, NM, *et al.* Comparison of ethanol septal reduction therapy with surgical myectomy for the treatment of hypertrophic obstructive cardiomyopathy. J Am Coll Cardiol 2001; **38**: 1701–1706.

40. Qin JX, Shiota T, Lever HM, *et al.* Outcome of patients with hypertrophic obstructive cardiomyopathy after percutaneous transluminal septal myocardial ablation and septal myectomy surgery. J Am Coll Cardiol 2001; **38**: 1994–2000.

41. Firoozi S, Elliott PM, Sharma S, *et al.* Septal myotomy–myectomy and transcoronary septal alcohol ablation in hypertrophic obstructive cardiomyopathy. Eur Heart J 2002; **23**: 1617–1624.

42. Alam M, Dokainish H, Lakkis N. Alcohol septal ablation for hypertrophic obstructive cardiomyopathy: A systematic review of published studies. J Interven Cardiol 2006; **19**: 319–327.

43. Chang SM, Lakkis NM, Franklin J, *et al.* Predictors of outcome after alcohol septal ablation therapy in patients with hypertrophic obstructive cardiomyopathy. Circulation 2004; **109**: 824–827.

44. Simon RDB, Crawford FA III, Spencer WH III, *et al.* Sustained Ventricular Tachycardia Following Alcohol Septal Ablation for Hypertrophic Obstructive Cardiomyopathy. Pacing Clin Electrophysiol 2005; **28**: 1354–1356.

45. Faber L, Seggewiss H, Gleichmann U. Percutaneous transluminal septal myocardial ablation in hypertrophic obstructive cardiomyopathy: Results with respect to intraprocedural myocardial contrast echocardiography. Circulation 1998; **98**: 2415–2421.

46. Reinhard W, Ten Cate FJ, Scholten M, *et al.* Permanent pacing for complete atrioventricular block after nonsurgical (alcohol) septal reduction in patients with obstructive hypertrophic cardiomyopathy. Am J Cardiol 2004; **93**: 1064–1066.

47. Chen AA, Palacios IF, Mela T, *et al.* Acute predictors of subacute complete heart block after alcohol septal ablation for obstructive hypertrophic cardiomyopathy. Am J Cardiol 2006; **97**: 264–269.

48. Faber L, Welge D, Fassbender D, *et al.* Percutaneous septal ablation for symptomatic hypertrophic obstructive cardiomyopathy: managing the risk of procedure-related AV conduction disturbances. Int J Cardiol 2007; **119**: 163–167.

49. Lawrenz T, Lieder F, Bartelsmeier M, *et al.* Predictors of complete heart block after transcoronary ablation of septal hypertrophy. Results of a prospective electrophysiological investigation in 172 patients with hypertrophic obstructive cardiomyopathy. J Am Coll Cardiol 2007; **49**: 2356–2363.

50. Wykrzykowska JJ, Kwaku K, Wylie J, *et al.* Delayed occurrence of unheralded phase IV complete heart block after ethanol septal ablation for symmetric hypertrophic obstructive cardiomyopathy. Pacing Clin Electrophysiol 2006; **29**: 674–678.

51. Talreja DR, Nishimura RA, Edwards WD, *et al.* Alcohol septal ablation versus surgical septal myectomy: comparison of effects on atrioventricular conduction tissue. J Am Coll Cardiol 2004; **44**: 2329–2332.

52. McCann GP, Van Dockum WG, Beek AM, *et al.* Extent of myocardial infarction and reverse remodeling assessed by cardiac magnetic resonance in patients with and without right bundle branch block following alcohol septal ablation for obstructive hypertrophic cardiomyopathy. Am J Cardiol 2007; **99**: 563–567.

53. Runquist LH, Nielsen CD, Killip D, *et al.* Electrocardiographic findings after alcohol septal ablation therapy for obstructive hypertrophic cardiomyopathy. Am J Cardiol 2002; **90**: 1020–1022.

54. Valettas N, Rho R, Beshai J, *et al.* Alcohol septal ablation complicated by complete heart block and permanent pacemaker failure. Catheter Cardiovasc Interv 2003; **58**: 189–193.

55. Maron BJ, Dearani JA, Ommen SR, *et al.* The case for surgery in obstructive hypertrophic cardiomyopathy. J Am Coll Cardiol 2004; **44**: 2044–2053.

56. Gietzen FH, Leuner CJ, Raute-Kreinsen U, *et al.* Acute and long-term results after transcoronary ablation of septal hypertrophy (TASH). Catheter interventional treatment for hypertrophic obstructive cardiomyopathy. Eur Heart J 1999 **20**: 1342–1354.

57. Lawrenz T, Obergassel L, Lieder F, *et al.* Transcoronary ablation of septal hypertrophy does not alter ICD intervention rates in high risk patients with hypertrophic obstructive cardiomyopathy. Pacing Clin Electrophysiol 2005; **28**: 295–300.

58. Pedone C, Vijayakumar M, Ligthart JM, *et al.* Intracardiac echocardiography guidance during percutaneous transluminal septal myocardial ablation in patients with obstructive hypertrophic cardiomyopathy. Int J Cardiovasc Intervent 2005; **7**: 134–137.

59. Alfonso F, Martín D, Fernández-Vázquez F, *et al.* Intracardiac echocardiography guidance for alcohol septal ablation in hypertrophic obstructive cardiomyopathy. J Invasive Cardiol 2007; **19**: E134–E136.

60. Bach RG, Leach C, Milov SA, *et al.* Use of magnetic navigation to facilitate transcatheter alcohol septal ablation for hypertrophic obstructive cardiomyopathy. J Invasive Cardiol 2006; **18**: E176–E178.

61. Gross CM, Schulz-Menger J, Kramer J, *et al.* Percutaneous transluminal septal artery ablation using polyvinyl alcohol foam particles for septal hypertrophy in patients with hypertrophic obstructive cardiomyopathy: acute and three-year outcomes. J Endovasc Ther 2004; **11**: 705–711.

62. Llamas-Espero GA, Sandoval-Navarrete S. Percutaneous septal ablation with absorbable gelatin sponge in hypertrophic obstructive cardiomyopathy. Catheter Cardiovasc Interv 2007; **69**: 231–235.

63. Durand E, Mousseaux E, Coste P, *et al.* Non-surgical septal myocardial reduction by coil embolization for

hypertrophic obstructive cardiomyopathy: early and 6 months follw-up. Eur Heart J 2008; **29**: 348–355.

64. Lawrenz T, Kuhn H. Endocardial radiofrequency ablation of septal hypertrophy: a new catheter-based modality of gradient reduction in hypertrophic obstructive cardiomyopathy. Z Kardiol 2004; **93**: 493–499.

65. Keane D, Hynes B, King G, *et al.* Feasibility study of percutaneous transvalvular endomyocardial cryoablation for the treatment of hypertrophic obstructive cardiomyopathy. J Invasive Cardiol 2007; **19**: 247–251.

CHAPTER 27

Cell Therapy

Zoë Astroulakis[1], Alex Sirker[1], & Jonathan M. Hill[2]

[1] Department of Cardiology, King's College London, James Black Centre, London, UK
[2] King's Health Partners, London, UK

Introduction

Over the past decade, stem cell therapy has emerged as a potential therapeutic intervention in ischaemic heart disease, harnessing the interests of basic scientists and cardiologists alike. Despite recent advances in pharmacological and catheter-based interventions for coronary heart disease, myocardial salvage is often incomplete resulting in a process of adverse left ventricular (LV) remodeling leading to symptomatic heart failure. In this chapter, we discuss the relevance of cell therapy to interventional cardiology, outlining the findings of the first wave of clinical trials, and look to future directions for clinical research.

Origin of Concept

The concept of the adult stem cell was born over 30 years ago, following the identification of a bone marrow cell capable of reconstituting hematopoiesis in irradiated mice [1]. However, it is only in the last 10 years that the relevance of this work to cardiology was realized with the description, from the late Jeffrey Isner's lab, of bone marrow derived stem/progenitor cells which could regenerate cells

constituting the cardiovascular system [2]. This challenged the previously held belief that the vascularization of adult ischemic tissue was restricted to the proliferation and migration of mature endothelial cells. Indeed, Isner's group went on to provide evidence that these cells could home to sites of ischemia and participate in new blood vessel formation, a process previously thought to be restricted to embryonic development. Furthermore, work involving animal models of ischemia demonstrated that bone marrow mononuclear cells (BMNCs) and endothelial progenitor cells (EPC) could participate in myocardial neovascularisation with evidence of functional improvement [3–7].

The next key development, and now widely recognized as the landmark paper within the field of cardiovascular cell therapy, was the description by Orlic *et al.* working in Piero Anversa's group, that a bone marrow derived population of cells from one mouse could be transplanted into recipient mice with myocardial infarction and become incorporated into the area of myocardial injury, exhibiting immunohistochemical evidence of transdifferentiation as well as leading to demonstrable changes in left ventricular function [8]. Further work has shown that stem cells are able to transdifferentiate into multiple different cardiovascular cell types including endothelial cells, vascular smooth muscle cells and cardiac myocytes [9–12].

Interventional Cardiology, First Edition. Edited by Carlo Di Mario, George D. Dangas, Peter Barlis.
© 2010 Blackwell Publishing Ltd. Published 2010 by Blackwell Publishing Ltd.

Subsequent controversies notwithstanding, the papers from the Isner and Anversa groups heralded the beginning of intense activity in cardiovascular therapy which continues to this day. However, many key questions remain regarding the putative mechanisms of action.

Myocardial Regeneration

Within cardiology, stem cell therapy has generated huge interest by challenging the long-held paradigm of developmental biology that the heart is a terminally differentiated organ, and as such cannot be repaired. Previously, the extent of myocardial necrosis had been shown to be intimately linked to the duration of coronary artery occlusion [13,14]. Such studies were critical in creating the drive forward in reperfusion therapy, but also led clinicians and scientists alike to think of myocardial injury as an irreversible event. Indeed, any improvement in LV function post-myocardial infarction (MI) was thought to result from a combination of hypertrophy and fibrosis. Such ideas were called into question with the observation that adult hearts contained large numbers of mitotic figures [15–17]. However, the proportion of mitotic cardiomyocytes was extremely small, suggesting they could not function alone as an effective repair system. The possibility that these dividing cells might have arisen from an extra-cardiac source, such as the bone marrow, was postulated by studies performed in sex-mismatched cardiac transplant patients. In males receiving female hearts, cardiac biopsies revealed Y-chromosome-carrying cardiomyocytes [17–19], intimating that cells from an extra-cardiac source could potentially engraft and differentiate into cardiac tissue. This marked the first recognition that the heart could receive cells from an extra-cardiac source. To explain this phenomenon, it was suggested that these cells might have arisen from the bone marrow, being released and engrafting either as a low-level process of continual renewal or in direct response to injury [8,11]. Alternative suggestions included the possibility of a locally resident population of cardiac stem cells, with self-renewing, multi-potent and clonogenic potential [20].

Mobilization of Stem/Progenitor Cells

Studies in humans have confirmed that bone marrow-derived mononuclear stem cells (BMNCs) and EPCs are indeed mobilized from the bone marrow to sites of ischemia at the time of myocardial infarction [21]. This occurs in response to the release of cytokines leading to the chemotactic migration of stem and progenitor cells to the area of injury. Such cytokines include vascular endothelial growth factor (VEGF) and stromal derived factor-1 (SDF-1) [22]. Reduced oxygen tension in ischemic tissue leads to an increase in SDF-1 levels in response to the up regulation of hypoxia-inducible factor-1 (HIF-1) in endothelial cells [23,24]. This hypoxic gradient directs the migration and homing, and increases the adhesion of, CXCR4-expressing progenitor cells to ischemic tissue [25]. It has been shown that impaired CXCR4-mediated cell signaling contributes to the reduced neovascularisation capacity seen in patients with coronary artery disease [26], and modifications of this pathway appear to offer promise for the enhancement of cell homing and retention. In addition, the capture of cells at the site of ischemia has been shown to be aided by the up regulation of integrins and intercellular adhesion molecules [27–30], and by the mediation of platelets [31].

Mechanism of Action

However, it is still unclear as to the exact mechanism by which transplanted cells exert their beneficial effects on cardiac function. Proposed mechanisms include endothelial differentiation (thereby aiding vascular regeneration and improving blood supply to the infarct border zone and so improving regional/global systolic LV function), cellular fusion, trans-differentiation to cardiomyocytes and/or via paracrine effects on the local cellular milieu, and the issue remains controversial.

Several studies have suggested that BMNCs may co-localize with non-myocardial cells such as fibroblasts [32]. However, these observations are so far anecdotal and could be explained by methodological issues such as the release of dye from apoptotic cells in the area of fibrosis or by the use of unfractionated bone marrow, which includes other cell precursor populations. Nonetheless, they are consistent with the basic postulate that stem cells differentiate along milieu-dependent pathways. Damaged adult myocardium is devoid of key embryonic growth factors, meaning an inability to recreate the necessary environment to stimulate myocyte growth or regeneration. This presents a challenge, and accordingly stimulates the search for novel strategies to encourage transplanted cells down the cardiac differentiation pathway prior to transplantation, if not in-situ.

Cell Therapy Following Acute Myocardial Infarction

The first wave of trials examining BM cell therapy in the setting of acute myocardial infarction indicated that autologous unselected BM cell therapy was indeed both safe and feasible (Table 27.1), and the noted improvements in left ventricular function paved the way for larger scale randomized clinical trials which unfortunately sometimes generated conflicting and controversial results (Table 27.2). This has largely arisen as a result of key differences in the cell population used, the time and mode of delivery, and the different methodologies used to assess changes in left ventricular function. For many clinicians, the demonstration of safety alone is insufficient grounds on which to proceed to larger clinical studies. Indeed, many cite that the statistically significant changes in LV function are clinically insignificant, and further studies are not currently justified.

Cell Type

The transfer of autologous BMNCs is attractive as a form of cell therapy because of the relative ease by which it may be obtained, the lack of requirement for ex-vivo expansion, and of course the lack of risk of rejection by the recipient. It also supports the idea that no particular cell type should be omitted, and that functional recovery is dependent upon a balance between the various subpopulations present in the mononuclear fraction. As such, the majority of clinical trials so far have used unfractionated BMNCs [33–36]. The problem with this, however, is that any functionally superior sub-group of cells would have to compete for engraftment along with all the other "non-stem"

cells. CD34$^+$ cells have been shown to mediate cardiac repair by inducing angiogenesis, inhibiting apoptosis and by promoting myocyte recovery in experimental models of myocardial infarction [37]. Indeed, it has been shown that CD34$^+$ enriched BM cells are up to seven times more efficient at engrafting in ischemic myocardium [38]. In addition to the CD34$^+$ marker expressed by stem/progenitor cells, CD133 (a prominin 5 transmembrane glycoprotein 1 marker of currently unknown function) is co-expressed in a substantial number of hematopoietic cells with potent angiogenic capacity [39–41]. The intracoronary injection of CD133$^+$ enriched BM cells has been shown to be feasible, and to be associated with the promotion of cardiac recovery in a small study, albeit with a slightly increased incidence of in-stent restenosis and re-occlusion [42]. CD133$^+$ cells have been shown to enhance functional response in patients following an acute myocardial infarction (MI) [43]. Other cell types which have now reached early phase clinical trials include mesenchymal stem cells and adipose tissue derived stem cells.

Timing of Cell Delivery

The timing of cell delivery is an obvious design difference between trials. The course of the normal healing processes at the time of myocardial infarction seems to coincide with the expression of putative homing signals favoring cell engraftment via transendothelial passage during the early days post-reperfusion. However, when cells were transplanted within 24 hours of optimal reperfusion therapy no benefit was seen in global LVEF [35]. This has led to the suggestion that the early proinflammatory environment required for healing in MI is toxic to stem/progenitor cells either in terms of survival or function or both, given that initial ischemia and reperfusion injury are characterized by the rapid rise of reactive oxygen radicals and inflammatory cytokines, and that this explains the lack of benefit seen when therapy is delivered within the first 24 hours. Consistent with this theory are the findings of the sub analysis of the REPAIR-AMI trial [36] indicating that the greatest benefit is seen when delivery occurs more than four days post-reperfusion. It remains unclear as to how late cells may be delivered and benefits still seen, and future studies are planned to investigate this

Table 27.1. Non-randomized clinical trials of cell therapy in acute myocardial infarction.

Study	Year	No. Participants Control/Treatment	Route of Cell Delivery	Cell Type	Follow-up (months)	Assessment of LVEF	LVEF (%) Treatment Group	LVEF (%) Control Group
Strauer et al. [54]	2002	–/10	IC	BMNC	3	LV angio	57 ± 8 → 62 ± 10 p = NS	60 ± 7 → 64 ± 7 p = NS
TOPCARE-AMI [55]	2002	–/59†	IC	BMNC/CPC	12	LV angio	51.6 ± 9.6 → 60.1 ± 8.6 p = 0.03	51.1 ± 10 → 53.5 ± 7.9 p = NS
Fernandez-Avilés et al. [56]	2004	–/20	IC	BMNC	6	MRI	51.3 ± 6.6 → 57.1 ± 10.4 p = 0.002	* p = NS
Bartunek et al. [42]	2005	16/19	IC	CD133+ BMNC	4	LV angio	45 ± 2.5 → 52.1 ± 3.5 P < 0.05	44.3 ± 3.1 → 48.6 ± 3.6 p = NS

IC = Intra-coronary; BMNC = Bone-marrow mononuclear cells; CPC = Circulating progenitor cells; LV angio = Left ventricular angiography; MRI = Magnetic resonance imaging; p = p-value where significance set at <0.05 and NS = non significant; † = 59 patients of whom 29 received BMNC and 30 CPC; * = raw data not provided.

Table 27.2. Randomized clinical trials of cell therapy in acute myocardial infarction.

Study	Year	No. Participants Control/Treatment	Route of Cell Delivery	Cell Type	Follow-up (months)	Assessment of LVEF	LVEF (%) Treatment Group	LVEF (%) Control Group
Chen et al. [57]	2004	34/35	IC	MSC	6	Echo	49 ± 9 → 67 ± 11 p = 0.01	48 ± 10 → 53 ± 18 p = NS
BOOST [33]	2004	30/30	IC	BMNC	6 18	MRI	50 ± 10 → 56.7 ± 12.5 p = 0.0026 p = NS	51.3 ± 9.3 → 52 ± 12.4 p = NS p = NS
Janssens et al. [35]	2006	34/33	IC	BMNC	4	MRI	48.5 ± 7.2 → 51.8 ± 8.8 p = NS	46.9 ± 8.2 → 49.1 ± 10.7 p = NS
ASTAMI [34]	2006	50/47	IC	BMNC	6	SPECT Echo	41.3 ± 10.4 → 49.3 ± 13.2 p = NS 45.7 ± 9.4 → 48.8 ± 10.7 p = NS	42.6 ± 11.7 → 49.3 ± 11 p = NS 46.9 ± 9.6 → 49 ± 9.5 p = NS
REPAIR-AMI [36]	2006	102/102	IC	BMNC	12	LV angio	48.3 ± 9.2 → 53.8 ± 10.2 p = 0.01	46.9 ± 10.4 → 49.9 ± 13 p = NS

IC = Intra-coronary; MSC = Mesenchymal stem cells; BMNC = Bone-marrow mononuclear cells; Echo = echocardiography; MRI = Magnetic resonance imaging; SPECT = Single photon emission computed tomography; LV angio = Left ventricular angiography.

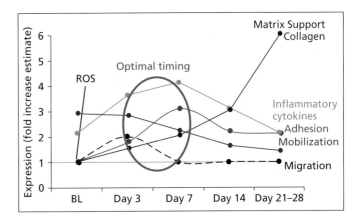

Figure 27.1. Schematic representation of the timing of various factors related to stem cell homing as currently understood. (Reproduced by kind permission of Dr J. Bartunek.)

further [44]. Taking all these factors into account, the optimum time interval for cell delivery post-MI is probably somewhere around days 3–7, when the balance is in favor of cell homing and survival [45] (see Figure 27.1).

Homing and Engraftment

Even the positive reports from randomized clinical trials using autologous BMNC transplantation have showed at best a 6–9% increase in measures of LV function, and it is difficult to understand how such a small increase in global LVEF could be translated into significant clinical improvement. Countering the idea that stem cells transdifferentiate into functioning cardiomyocytes, Hofmann *et al.* used 2-[^{18}F]-fluoro-2-deoxy-D-glucose (18F-FDG) labeling to follow the fate of intra-coronary delivered unselected and CD34$^+$ enriched autologous BMNCs in patients following acute MI. They noted that only 1.3 to 2.6% of unselected BMNCs could be detected in the myocardium following intracoronary delivery, with the majority of detected activity in the liver and spleen [38]. However, when they delivered CD34$^+$ enriched BMNCs they found increased engraftment in the infarct border zone to 14–39% of the total detectable activity. Furthermore, a study examining the one day kinetics of transplanted cells indicated that engraftment is a temporary phenomenon, with myocardial activity dropping off between 2–20 hours post-intracoronary delivery from ~5% to ~1% [46]. Additionally, in patients with a history of MI more than six months prior, myocardial activity disappeared altogether.

This would suggest any positive effects are likely to occur by means other than by direct tissue incorporation. Factors accounting for the transiency of cell retention could be related to a reduced adhesive status of the myocardial microcirculation, and/or the functional performance of delivered cells. Studies are required to investigate this further, and to examine whether pharmacological manipulation of the microcirculation either at the time of, or prior to, cell delivery makes any difference. Further important differences between trials include whether they were randomized/blinded and/or placebo-controlled, the methods used in assessing LV function and duration of follow-up (Table 27.2).

Cell Therapy in Chronic Ischemic Heart Disease

Whilst the majority of trials have examined the effects of cell therapy in acute MI, only a limited number of trials have focused their attention on its use in chronic ischemic heart disease. One of the first studies looked at a small group of patients undergoing elective coronary artery bypass graft surgery (CABG), in whom they found improved myocardial perfusion and metabolism after enriched CD133$^+$ cells were injected into the infarct border zone [47]. Similar observations were noted in an open-label randomized study where patients with LV dysfunction undergoing CABG surgery together with direct intramyocardial injection of BMNCs showed better functional improvement as compared to CABG alone [48].

Perin *et al.* went on to study the electromechanically-mapped guidance of transendomyocardially injected BMNCs in patients with refractory angina and myocardial ischemia. They demonstrated not only that it was procedurally safe, but that it was associated with clinical improvement detectable at 3 months and maintained to 12 months [49].

A randomized, blinded placebo-controlled trial of 26 patients with chronic total arterial occlusions was conducted, where autologous granulocyte-colony stimulating factor (G-CSF) mobilized circulating progenitor cells were injected down percutaneously revascularized coronary arteries. Assessment of LV function by magnetic resonance imaging showed that LV ejection fraction (LVEF) in treated patients had increased by 14% whilst infarct size had been reduced by 16%. Notably, there was a demonstrable improvement in regional wall motion at the target site [50].

The controlled crossover TOPCARE-CHD trial (Transplantation of Progenitor Cells and Regeneration Enhancement–Chronic Heart Disease) enrolled 75 patients with stable chronic ischemic heart disease who had previously sustained an MI [51]. Here, patients were randomly assigned to receive BMNCs, circulating progenitor cells or no cells into the (patent) coronary artery supplying the most dyskinetic LV region. The increase in mean LVEF seen in the BMNC group was modest (2.9%), but significantly greater than in the circulating progenitor and control groups. The crossover phase of the study indicated that BMNC therapy was indeed associated with a greater increase in both global and regional LV function.

Future Research

The European Society of Cardiology has established a task force for the future of stem cell therapy in cardiology which has recommended for the moment that research is confined to using autologous BM stem/progenitor cells, or skeletal myoblasts, in repairing the acute or chronically damaged myocardium [52]. A similar task force has been established by the National Heart, Lung and Blood Institute which has provided a framework to coordinate the resources and funding of cardiovascular cell based therapy in the United States [53]. Both

of these groups offer clear advice, and warn against research proceeding without international consensus, aiming to avoid further small, underpowered studies.

Conclusion

Despite recent technological and pharmacological advances made within the field of interventional cardiology reducing mortality from coronary artery disease, it continues to cause significant morbidity and efforts have been directed to developing ways of improving endothelial and myocardial function in patients in order to prevent future coronary events. The last decade has seen an explosion of interest in the use of autologous stem cell therapy to improve the outcome for patients living with coronary heart disease with several randomized controlled trials suggesting, but not proving conclusively, an improvement in myocardial perfusion, function and a reduced risk of future coronary events. Although the delivery of autologous stem cells to the heart appears to be safe, many unanswered questions remain regarding their mechanism of action, the optimum cell type, method and timing of delivery. It is anticipated that future larger scale randomized controlled trials will provide us with the answers to some of these in due course.

Acknowledgments

We would like to thank Dr J. Bartunek, Alst, Belgium.

References

1. McCulloch EA, Till JE. The radiation sensitivity of normal mouse bone marrow cells, determined by quantitative marrow transplantation into irradiated mice. Radiat Res 1960; **13**: 115–125.
2. Asahara T, Murohara T, Sullivan A, *et al.* Isolation of putative progenitor endothelial cells for angiogenesis. Science 1997; **275**(5302): 964–967.
3. Shi Q, Rafii S, Wu MH, *et al.* Evidence for circulating bone marrow-derived endothelial cells. Blood 1998; **92**(2): 362–367.
4. Takahashi T, Kalka C, Masuda H, *et al.* Ischemia- and cytokine-induced mobilization of bone marrow-derived

endothelial progenitor cells for neovascularization. Nat Med 1999; **5**(4): 434–438.

5. Kawamoto A, Gwon HC, Iwaguro H, *et al.* Therapeutic potential of ex vivo expanded endothelial progenitor cells for myocardial ischemia. Circulation 2001; **103**(5): 634–637.

6. Kocher AA, Schuster MD, Szabolcs MJ, *et al.* Neovascularization of ischemic myocardium by human bone-marrow-derived angioblasts prevents cardiomyocyte apoptosis, reduces remodeling and improves cardiac function. Nat Med 2001; **7**(4): 430–436.

7. Tateishi-Yuyama E, Matsubara H, Murohara T, *et al.* Therapeutic angiogenesis for patients with limb ischaemia by autologous transplantation of bone-marrow cells: a pilot study and a randomised controlled trial. Lancet 2002; **360**(9331): 427–435.

8. Orlic D, Kajstura J, Chimenti S, *et al.* Mobilized bone marrow cells repair the infarcted heart, improving function and survival. Proc Natl Acad Sci USA 2001; **98**(18): 10344–10349.

9. Forbes SJ, Vig P, Poulsom R, *et al.* Adult stem cell plasticity: new pathways of tissue regeneration become visible. Clin Sci (Lond) 2002; **103**(4): 355–369.

10. Eisenberg LM, Burns L, Eisenberg, CA. Hematopoietic cells from bone marrow have the potential to differentiate into cardiomyocytes in vitro. Anat Rec A Discov Mol Cell Evol Biol 2003; **274**(1): 870–882.

11. Jackson KA, Majka SM, Wang H, *et al.* Regeneration of ischemic cardiac muscle and vascular endothelium by adult stem cells. J Clin Invest 2001; **107**(11): 1395–1402.

12. Kajstura J, Rota M, Wang B, *et al.* Bone marrow cells differentiate in cardiac cell lineages after infarction independently of cell fusion. Circ Res 2005; **96**(1): 127–137.

13. Maroko PR, Libby P, Ginks WR, *et al.* Coronary artery reperfusion. I. Early effects on local myocardial function and the extent of myocardial necrosis. J Clin Invest 1972; **51**(10): 2710–2716.

14. Ginks WR, Sybers HD, Maroko PR, *et al.* Coronary artery reperfusion. II. Reduction of myocardial infarct size at 1 week after the coronary occlusion. J Clin Invest 1972; **51**(10): 2717–2723.

15. Kajstura J, Leri A, Finato N, *et al.* Myocyte proliferation in end-stage cardiac failure in humans. Proc Natl Acad Sci USA 1998; **95**(15): 8801–8805.

16. Beltrami AP, Urbanek K, Kajstura J, *et al.* Evidence that human cardiac myocytes divide after myocardial infarction. N Engl J Med 2001; **344**(23): 1750–1757.

17. Quaini F, Urbanek K, Beltrami AP, *et al.* Chimerism of the transplanted heart. N Engl J Med 2002; **346**(1): 5–15.

18. Laflamme MA, Myerson D, Saffitz JE, *et al.* Evidence for cardiomyocyte repopulation by extracardiac progenitors in transplanted human hearts. Circ Res 2002; **90**(6): 634–640.

19. Muller P, Pfeiffer P, Koglin J, *et al.* Cardiomyocytes of noncardiac origin in myocardial biopsies of human transplanted hearts. Circulation 2002; **106**(1): 31–35.

20. Oh H, Bradfute SB, Gallardo TD, *et al.* Cardiac progenitor cells from adult myocardium: homing, differentiation, and fusion after infarction. Proc Natl Acad Sci USA 2003; **100**(21): 12313–12318.

21. Shintani S, Murohara T, Ikeda H, *et al.* Mobilization of endothelial progenitor cells in patients with acute myocardial infarction. Circulation 2001; **103**(23): 2776–2779.

22. Yamaguchi J, Kusano KF, Masuo O, *et al.* Stromal cell-derived factor-1 effects on ex vivo expanded endothelial progenitor cell recruitment for ischemic neovascularization. Circulation 2003; **107**(9): 1322–1328.

23. Ceradini DJ, Kulkarni AR, Callagham MJ, *et al.* Progenitor cell trafficking is regulated by hypoxic gradients through HIF-1 induction of SDF-1. Nat Med 2004; **10**(8): 858–864.

24. De Falco, E, Porcelli D, Torella AR, *et al.* SDF-1 involvement in endothelial phenotype and ischemia-induced recruitment of bone marrow progenitor cells. Blood 2004; **104**(12): 3472–3482.

25. Peled A, Petit I, Collet O, *et al.* Dependence of human stem cell engraftment and repopulation of NOD/SCID mice on CXCR4. Science 1999; **283**(5403): 845–848.

26. Walter DH, Haendeler J, Reinhold J, *et al.* Impaired CXCR4 signaling contributes to the reduced neovascularization capacity of endothelial progenitor cells from patients with coronary artery disease. Circ Res 2005; **97**(11): 1142–1151.

27. Yoon CH, Hur J, Oh IY, *et al.* Intercellular adhesion molecule-1 is upregulated in ischemic muscle, which mediates trafficking of endothelial progenitor cells. Arterioscler Thromb Vasc Biol 2006; **26**(5): 1066–1072.

28. Vajkoczy P, Blum S, Lamparter M, *et al.* Multistep nature of microvascular recruitment of ex vivo-expanded embryonic endothelial progenitor cells during tumor angiogenesis. J Exp Med 2003; **197**(12): 1755–1765.

29. Chavakis E, Aicher A, Heeschen C, *et al.* Role of beta2-integrins for homing and neovascularization capacity of endothelial progenitor cells. J Exp Med 2005; **201**(1): 63–72.

30. Jin H, Aiyer A, Su J, *et al.* A homing mechanism for bone marrow-derived progenitor cell recruitment to the neovasculature. J Clin Invest 2006; **116**(3): 652–662.

31. Massberg S, Konrad I, Schurzinger K, *et al.* Platelets secrete stromal cell-derived factor 1alpha and recruit bone marrow-derived progenitor cells to arterial thrombi in vivo. J Exp Med 2006; **203**(5): 1221–1233.

32. Wang JS, Shum-Tim D, Galipeau J, *et al.* Marrow stromal cells for cellular cardiomyoplasty: feasibility and potential clinical advantages. J Thorac Cardiovasc Surg 2000; **120**(5): 999–1005.

33. Wollert KC, Meyer GP, Lotz J, *et al.* Intracoronary autologous bone-marrow cell transfer after myocardial infarction: the BOOST randomised controlled clinical trial. Lancet 2004; **364**(9429): 141–148.

34. Lunde K, Solheim S, Aakhus S, *et al.* Intracoronary injection of mononuclear bone marrow cells in acute myocardial infarction. N Engl J Med 2006; **355**(12): 1199–1209.

35. Janssens S, Dubois C, Bogaert J, *et al.* Autologous bone marrow-derived stem-cell transfer in patients with ST-segment elevation myocardial infarction: double-blind, randomised controlled trial. Lancet 2006; **367**(9505): 113–121.

36. Schachinger V, Erbs S, Elsasser A, *et al.* Intracoronary bone marrow-derived progenitor cells in acute myocardial infarction. N Engl J Med 2006; **355**(12): 1210–1221.

37. Katritsis DG, Sotiropoulou A, Karvouni E, *et al.* Transcoronary transplantation of autologous mesenchymal stem cells and endothelial progenitors into infarcted human myocardium. Catheter Cardiovasc Interv 2005; **65**(3): 321–329.

38. Hofmann M, Wollert KC, Meyer GP, *et al.* Monitoring of bone marrow cell homing into the infarcted human myocardium. Circulation 2005; **111**(17): 2198–2202.

39. Bhatia M. AC133 expression in human stem cells. Leukemia, 2001; **15**(11): 1685–1688.

40. Quirici N, Soligo D, Caneva L, *et al.* Differentiation and expansion of endothelial cells from human bone marrow CD133(+) cells. Br J Haematol 2001; **115**(1): 186–194.

41. Kuci S, Wessels JT, Buhring HJ, *et al.* Identification of a novel class of human adherent CD34- stem cells that give rise to SCID-repopulating cells. Blood 2003; **101**(3): 869–876.

42. Bartunek J, Vanderheyden M, Vandekerckhove B, *et al.* Intracoronary injection of CD133-positive enriched bone marrow progenitor cells promotes cardiac recovery after recent myocardial infarction: feasibility and safety. Circulation 2005; **112**(9 Suppl): I178–183.

43. Voo S, Eggermann J, Dunaeva M, *et al.* Enhanced functional response of CD133+ circulating progenitor cells in patients early after acute myocardial infarction. Eur Heart J 2008; **29**(2): 241–250.

44. Nyolczas N, Gyongyosi M, Beran G, *et al.* Design and rationale for the Myocardial Stem Cell Administration After Acute Myocardial Infarction (MYSTAR) Study: a multicenter, prospective, randomized, single-blind trial comparing early and late intracoronary or combined (percutaneous intramyocardial and intracoronary) administration of nonselected autologous bone marrow cells to patients after acute myocardial infarction. Am Heart J 2007; **153**(2): 212 e1–7.

45. Bartunek J, Vanderheyden M, Wijns W, *et al.* Bone-marrow-derived cells for cardiac stem cell therapy: safe or still under scrutiny? Nat Clin Pract Cardiovasc Med 2007; **4 Suppl 1**: S100–105.

46. Penicka M, Lang O, Widimsky P, *et al.* One-day kinetics of myocardial engraftment after intracoronary injection of bone marrow mononuclear cells in patients with acute and chronic myocardial infarction. Heart 2007; **93**(7): 837–841.

47. Stamm C, Kleine HD, Choi YH, *et al.* Intramyocardial delivery of CD133+ bone marrow cells and coronary artery bypass grafting for chronic ischemic heart disease: safety and efficacy studies. J Thorac Cardiovasc Surg 2007; **133**(3): 717–725.

48. Patel AN, Geffner L, Vina RF, *et al.* Surgical treatment for congestive heart failure with autologous adult stem cell transplantation: a prospective randomized study. J Thorac Cardiovasc Surg 2005; **130**(6): 1631–1638.

49. Perin EC, Dohmann HF, Borojevic, *et al.* Transendocardial, autologous bone marrow cell transplantation for severe, chronic ischemic heart failure. Circulation 2003; **107**(18): 2294–2302.

50. Erbs S, Linke A, Adams V, *et al.* Transplantation of blood-derived progenitor cells after recanalization of chronic coronary artery occlusion: first randomized and placebo-controlled study. Circ Res 2005; **97**(8): 756–762.

51. Assmus B, Fischer-Rasokat U, Honold J, *et al.* Transcoronary transplantation of functionally competent BMCs is associated with a decrease in natriuretic peptide serum levels and improved survival of patients with chronic postinfarction heart failure: results of the TOPCARE-CHD Registry. Circ Res 2007; **100**(8): 1234–1241.

52. Bartunek J, Dimmeler S, Drexler H, *et al.* The consensus of the task force of the European Society of Cardiology concerning the clinical investigation of the use of autologous adult stem cells for repair of the heart. Eur Heart J 2006; **27**(11): 1338–1340.

53. Thomas JW, National Heart, Lung, and Blood Institute resources and programs for cell-based therapies. Circ Res 2007; **101**(1): 1–6.

54. Strauer BE, Brehm M, Zeus T, *et al.* Repair of infarcted myocardium by autologous intracoronary mononuclear

bone marrow cell transplantation in humans. Circulation 2002; **106**(15): 1913–1918.

55. Assmus B, Schachinger V, Teupe C, *et al.* Transplantation of Progenitor Cells and Regeneration Enhancement in Acute Myocardial Infarction (TOPCARE-AMI). Circulation 2002; **106**(24): 3009–3017.

56. Fernandez-Aviles F, San Roman J, Garcia-Frade J, *et al.* Experimental and clinical regenerative capability of

human bone marrow cells after myocardial infarction. Circ Res 2004; **95**(7): 742–748.

57. Chen SL, Fang WW, Ye F, *et al.* Effect on left ventricular function of intracoronary transplantation of autologous bone marrow mesenchymal stem cell in patients with acute myocardial infarction. Am J Cardiol 2004; **94**(1): 92–95.

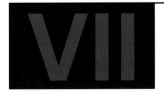

PART VII
Complications

CHAPTER 28

No Reflow

Azeem Latib[1], & Flavio Airoldi[2]

[1] San Raffaele Scientific Institute, Milan, Italy
[2] IRCCS Multimedica, Sesto San Giovanni (MI), Italy

Introduction

No-reflow (or slow-flow) during percutaneous coronary intervention (PCI) refers to a condition of decreased or absent myocardial perfusion without angiographic evidence of mechanical vessel obstruction in the coronary artery supplying that territory [1,2]. Transient occlusion of the coronary artery is usually a prerequisite for no-reflow. Its occurrence is recognized angiographically as reduced Thrombolysis in Myocardial Infarction (TIMI) [3] flow with a column of contrast in the vessel distal to the original target stenosis that does not rapidly clear [4–6]. By definition, no-reflow can be diagnosed only after excluding other causes of reduced antegrade flow such as dissection, spasm, thrombus, or a residual high-grade stenosis. Persistent no-reflow has important prognostic implications as it is associated with higher clinical complication rates [6–9]. Patients who develop no-reflow during PCI have a significantly higher incidence of in-hospital and long-term complications such as myocardial infarction (MI), heart failure, negative ventricular remodelling, ventricular tachycardia, and death [6,7,9–13]. As a result, interventional cardiologists need to be vigilant for this complication and initiate therapy without delay.

Interventional Cardiology, First Edition. Edited by Carlo Di Mario, George D. Dangas, Peter Barlis.
© 2010 Blackwell Publishing Ltd. Published 2010 by Blackwell Publishing Ltd.

Types of No-reflow

The most applicable classification of no-reflow as it applies to the interventional cardiologist is that proposed by Eeckhout and Kern [1] in Table 28.1:
1. Myocardial infarction reperfusion no-reflow.
2. Angiographic no-reflow.

However, a combination of myocardial infarction and angiographic no-reflow can also occur in patients undergoing primary PCI for myocardial infarction.

No-reflow has a tendency to occur more often in certain lesion subtypes and patients. It has been observed more commonly in diabetics; following mechanical debulking (rotational or directional atherectomy); during PCI in saphenous vein grafts (especially in older grafts >7 years and those with diffuse and bulky lesions[5]); during primary PCI for acute myocardial infarction (AMI); in lesions with a large thrombotic burden and in patients without pre-infarction angina [1,4,5,11,12]. Also it is more pronounced with longer periods of coronary occlusions [2]. However, except for thrombus-containing long lesions and degenerative SVGs, it can be difficult to predict the risk of no-reflow based on the angiographic appearance of a lesion. It must always be kept in mind that other causes of impaired coronary flow can simulate no-reflow and need to be excluded (dissection, intracoronary thrombus formation, epicardial coronary spasm, or remaining high-grade stenosis).

Table 28.1. Classification of no-reflow as proposed by Eeckhout and Kern [9]. Reprinted with permission from Eur Heart J 2001; **22**: 729–739

	Myocardial infarction no-reflow	Angiographic no-reflow
Definition	No-reflow after pharmacological and/or mechanical revascularisation	No-reflow during PCI usually during the treatment of SVG, atherectomy, thrombus-containing lesions
Incidence	20–30% [7,8]	0.6–5.0% [4,6]
Mechanisms	Myocardial necrosis and stunning, reperfusion injury from oxygen free radicals, α-mediated vasoconstriction, inflammation	Distal embolization of plaque and/or thrombus, local release of vasoconstrictor substances
Prognosis	Greater risk to have larger infarction, early heart failure and progressive left ventricular dilatation [7,8]	Increased mortality and higher incidence of MI [4,6]

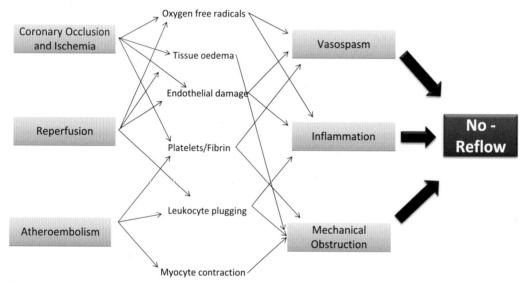

Figure 28.1. Summarizes the multifactorial pathogenesis of no-reflow. Adapted with permission from Am J Cardiol 2007; **99**: 916–920

Pathophysiology

The pathophysiology of no-reflow is complex, multifactorial, and incompletely understood. The mechanism differs depending on the clinical setting and lesion type undergoing PCI. In humans, it appears to be a combination of distal embolization, inflammation and microvascular spasm (see Figure 28.1) [1,11,12,14–16]. Distal microembolization appears to have an important role in certain cases of no-reflow. In fact, aspiration of coronary arteries in patients with thrombotic lesions and no-reflow has shown embolic debris (containing both thrombi and atheromatous gruel) in the majority of cases [14]. Vasospasm appears to have a central role in the pathogenesis of no-reflow irrespective of the clinical scenario in which it occurs. Experimental data suggests that microvascular vasospasm is caused by the release of serotonin, angiotensin II, thromboxane and α-adrenergic agonists [6,17–19]. The local release of these vasoconstrictor substances impairs capillary autoregulation and increases reflex sympathetic activity.

Other mechanisms that have been implicated include oxygen free radical-mediated injury, reperfusion injury with loss of microvascular integrity

[14,15] endothelial dysfunction, neutrophil infiltration, platelet aggregation, plasminogen activator inhibitor-1, tissue factor and inflammatory factors (sCD40L, soluble E-selectin) [1,14,15,20]. In summary, microvascular spasm and dysfunction are likely to play a considerable role in all of these potential mechanisms.

Prevention of No-Reflow

As described above, the dislodgment of thrombus or plaque components during PCI has been postulated to be one of the mechanisms causing slow-flow or no-reflow phenomena. For this reason, preventing the embolization of friable material contained in the target lesion by mechanical aspiration or distal entrapment seems an attractive option. Several studies have been addressed to this issue in two different settings: (1) treatment of diseased SVG; (2) acute coronary syndromes.

Saphenous Vein Grafts (SVG)

The use of distal protection devices has decreased the incidence of no-reflow during PCI in several studies, and confirmed the role of distal embolization in the development of this complication. The PercuSurge (Export, PercuSurge, Sunnyvale, CA, USA) device which allows distal occlusion and aspiration of thrombotic and non-thrombotic debris was the first of these devices to show that no-reflow could be prevented. In the Saphenous vein graft Angioplasty Free of Emboli Randomized (SAFER) trial, the use of the PercuSurge device in patients undergoing stent placement in SVG resulted in a reduction of no-reflow from 9% to 3% (p = 0.026) as well as a reduction in 30-day MI (8.6% vs. 16.4%; p = 0.008) [21]. A number of other embolic protection devices have been developed that have been shown to be equivalent to the PercuSurge (see Table 28.2). As a result of their proven effectiveness in preventing distal embolization, no-reflow and major adverse cardiac events, the AHA/ACC/SCAI have given embolic protection devices a Class 1B recommendation: "*It is recommended that distal embolic protection devices be used when technically feasible in patients undergoing PCI to SVGs*" [22,23].

On the other hand, the effect of glycoprotein IIb/IIIa receptor inhibitors in preventing no-reflow

Table 28.2. Embolic protection device trials in saphenous vein graft intervention.

Type	Trial	N° of patients	30-day MACE		p value	Result
Distal Occlusion Device	SAFER [21]	801	Guard Wire 9.6	No device 16.5	0.0004	GuardWire Superior
	PRIDE[51]	631	TriActive 11.2	Guard Wire 10.1	0.02	TriActive System not inferior
Distal Filter Device	FIRE[52]	651	FilterWireEX 9.9	Guard Wire 11.6	0.0008	FilterWireEX not inferior
	CAPTIVE[53]	652	CardioShield 11.4	Guard Wire 9.1	0.57	CardioShield not inferior
	SPIDER[54]	747	SPIDER/SpideRX 9.1	Guard Wire or FilterWireEX/EZ 8.4	0.012	SPIDER/SpideRX not inferior
Proximal Occlusion Device	PROXIMAL[55]	600	Proxis 9.2	FilterWire or Guard Wire 10	0.006	Proxis not inferior

MACE = major adverse cardiac event.
[51] Carrozza , Mumma, Breall, *et al.* J Am Coll Cardiol 2005; **46**(9): 1677–1683.
[52] Stone, Rogers, Hermiller, *et al.* Circulation 2003; **108**(5): 548–553.

during SVG intervention has been disappointing [24]. Roffi *et al.* have performed a pooled analysis of five randomized intravenous glycoprotein IIb/IIIa inhibitor trials (EPIC, EPILOG, EPISTENT, IMPACT II, and PURSUIT) showing that prophylactic administration of these agents does not improve outcomes during PCI of SVG [25].

Acute Myocardial Infarction (AMI)

Occlusive thrombosis from an unstable atherosclerotic plaque is the substrate of most AMIs. Therefore, macro- and micro-embolization during PCI in AMI may result in obstruction of the microvascular network and subsequently in reduced efficacy of reperfusion and myocardial salvage [26]. Operators performing coronary angioplasty in AMI have many different devices available and the decision about which one should be employed may be intricate. Today's armamentarium includes thrombectomy devices, aspiration systems and distal protection filters. In recent years, investigators have designed and conducted many trials to understand whether the use of embolic-prevention devices provides better outcomes in comparison to standard stent implantation. The recent randomized trials provide evidence against the routine use of embolic protection devices in primary PCI (see Table 28.3). Several explanations can be proposed regarding these negative findings. First of all we should con-

sider that in the setting of AMI distal embolization may induce an additional, although limited myocardial necrosis. This increase plays a minor role against the large background of necrosis due to ischemia/reperfusion. This condition differs from embolization that may occur in SVGs, in which the myocardial area distal to the graft is viable. Also, the type of device used, operator's experience and technique of usage may play a relevant role. Some devices have a significant crossing profile that can itself induce embolization whilst crossing the thrombotic lesion. Moreover, the simple use of an anti-embolic device does not necessarily translate into effective thrombus removal and no embolization. Whatever role embolic protection devices might play, they cannot be employed in all patients, but only in a minority of them with particular clinical or anatomical features. The problem is how to select patients who may benefit from dedicated devices. The indiscriminate utilization of this resource to all patients not only represents an unjustified adjunctive cost, but also may be associated to increased procedural time and reperfusion delay. Finally, serious complications due to thrombectomy devices or distal filters have been sporadically reported (vessel dissection, filter entrapment into the stent). The identification of the lesion that may merit the use of a dedicated device is the key point for the success of impaired flow prevention. Nevertheless, there is no agree-

Table 28.3. Reports: A list of the most recent randomized trials with embolic protection devices in acute myocardial infarction and their outcome.

	N° of pts	Device	Category	Result
Dudek *et al.* [56]	72	Rescue	Aspiration	Positive
Antoniucci *et al.* [57]	100	AngioJet	Thrombectomy	Positive
Napodano *et al.* [58]	92	X-sizer	Thrombectomy	Positive
X AMINE ST [59]	201	X-sizer	Thrombectomy	Positive
REMEDIA Burzotta *et al.* [60]	100	Diver	Aspiration	Positive
De Luca *et al.* [61]	76	Pronto	Aspiration	Positive
DEZR-MI [62]	148	Diver	Aspiration	Positive
AIMI [63]	480	AngioJet	Thrombectomy	Negative
Kaltoft *et al.* [64]	215	Rescue	Aspiration	Negative
TAPAS [65]	1071	Export	Aspiration	Positive
PREMIAR [66]	140	SpideRX	Distal filter	Negative
EMERALD [27]	252	Pecusurge, Guard wire	Distal occlusion	Negative
PROMISE; Glick *et al.* [67]	200	Filter wire	Distal filter	Negative

ment about which clinical or angiographic parameters should be taken into account. In clinical practice, operators are more prone to use a specific device when there is angiographic evidence of a large thrombus burden. However, in the EMERALD trial a subgroup analysis did not identify any subset of patients in whom an advantage of distal protection was occurring [27]. Rather, the infarct size was actually increased by GuardWire in patients with an assumed high thrombus burden (i.e. those with totally occluded vessels or angiographic signs of intracoronary thrombus). Another criterion for adopting an antithrombotic device is the presence of poor left ventricular ejection fraction or a large amount of myocardium at jeopardy. Unfortunately, these two conditions are present only in a small minority of the patients included in the studies listed in Table 28.3.

Treatment of No-reflow

Once no-reflow occurs, every attempt must be made to reverse it in order to reduce the risk of adverse outcome [28]. During PCI procedures, no-reflow may manifest as acute ischemia and may be associated with chest pain, ECG changes, bradycardia, conduction disturbances, and hypotension leading to marked hemodynamic instability and cardiogenic shock. However, there are also rare cases of no-reflow that occur without any clinical sequelae. The initial evaluation and treatment of no-reflow consists of maintaining hemodynamic and electrophysiological stability. In Table 28.4, we have provided a guide to the evaluation and management of no-reflow.

As the predominant abnormality during no-reflow appears to be microvascular constriction, different vasoactive drugs have been employed for the treatment of this phenomenon and their efficacy depends on coronary artery vasodilation and hyperaemia induction especially at the microvascular level [1,5,16,24]. In Table 28.5, we have summarized the most important studies evaluating vasodilators in no-reflow and below some insights into their mechanisms of action.

Nitroglycerin (NTG)

We mention NTG first not due to its efficacy in reversing no-reflow but rather because it is often

Table 28.4. Strategy for evaluating and treating no-reflow.

1. Exclude dissection, epicardial spasm, thrombus at lesion site, distal macroembolism or air embolism
2. Check ACT levels (250–300 seconds)
3. Ensure oxygenation, hemodynamic stability and maintain adequate coronary perfusion pressures
4. Intracoronary nitrates to exclude epicardial coronary artery spasm
5. Administer pharmacological agents selectively into distal arterial bed by infusion catheter or over-the-wire balloon
   a. Nitroprusside 80–200 µg bolus (up to 1000 µg total dose). Consider alternating with boluses of Epinephrine 50–200 µg
   b. Adenosine 10–20 µg high velocity boluses repeated as needed (10–30 doses)
   c. Verapamil 50–200 µg bolus (up to 1000 µg total dose with temporary pacemaker standby)
   d. Second-line agents for which evidence is less strong: Epinephrine 50–200 µg, Nicorandil 2 µg, Papaverine 10–20 µg, Nicardipine 200 µg, Diltiazem 0.5–2.5 mg over 1 min up to 5 mg
6. Consider administering a glycoprotein IIb/IIIa receptor inhibitor intracoronary/intragraft or intravenous

the first-line agent most operators use when faced with no-reflow. In fact, NTG is not effective in reversing no-reflow and is given at the onset of no-reflow in order to exclude epicardial coronary spasm. We have shown that nitroglycerin administration results in an increase in minimum lumen diameter that is not further increased by nitroprusside (see Figure 28.2) [29]. NTG also did not change any of the examined angiographic parameters (TIMI grade, corrected TIMI frame count, and TIMI myocardial blush) compared with baseline values (after stent deployment). This lack of effect on no-reflow has been confirmed in a number of studies [6,10].

Nitropusside (NTP)

NTG and NTP are both donors of nitric oxide, an endothelium-derived compound that has multiple vascular functions, including vasodilation, inhibition of platelet adhesion and anti-inflammatory activity [30]. Nitric oxide is a potent vasodilator in the resistance arteriolar circulation [31] and plays

Table 28.5. A summary of the most important studies assessing vasodilators in the treatment of no-reflow.

Study	Drug	Dose	No of patients	Incidence in specific lesion types	Response to pharmacological Rx as assessed by having TIMI 3 flow at the end of the procedure	Comment
NITROPRUSSIDE						
Airoldi et al[30]	Nitroprusside	80–200 µg bolus (max 1000 µg)	0.9% (21/2212)	11.5% of AMI and 8.2% of SVG lesions	100% in AMI and 56% in SVG lesions	Nitroglycerin had no effect on TIMI flow
Hillegass et al[31]	Nitroprusside	50–1000 µg	20	45% of lesions were SVG and 15% AMI	75%	No adverse effect on blood pressure from nitroprusside
Wang et al[68]	Nitroprusside	100–700 µg	15.7% (11/70)	Only lesions undergoing primary PCI for AMI	82%	Multiple 100 µg boluses injected with 3 ml syringe via guiding catheter
Pasceri et al[69]	Nitroprusside	50–200 µg	11.1% (23/208)	Only lesions undergoing primary PCI for AMI	91%	
ADENOSINE						
Sdringola et al[42]	Adenosine	24 µg/bolus	14% (20/143)	SVG only	82% with ≥5 boluses and 33% with <5 boluses	Prophylactic adenosine does not prevent no-reflow during SVG PCI
Fischell et al[43]	Adenosine	18 µg high-velocity boluses	8 patients with 11 slow flow events	SVG only	91%	High velocity adenosine and saline flushes with a 3 ml syringe
ADENOSINE vs. COMBINATION THERAPY						
Parikh et al[44]	Saline		75 High risk ACS patients with TIMI flow <3 treated with saline or	70% (16/23)	30%	Crossover to combination in 16 patients resulted in TIMI 2 in 12.5% (2) and TIMI 3 in 87.5% (14)
	Adenosine	12 µg/bolus	Adenosine or Adenosine + NTP	31% (8/26)	69%	Crossover to combination in 8 patients resulted in TIMI 2 in 25% (2) and TIMI 3 in 75% (6)
	Adenosine + Nitroprusside	12 µg/bolus + 50 µg bolus		4% (1/26)	94%	

Study	Drug	Dose	Incidence	Setting	Response	Outcome
Barcin et al[40]	Adenosine	98 ± 62μg	2.8% (53/1893)	21	29%	Crossover to combination in 8 patients resulted in TIMI 2 in 25% (2) and TIMI 3 in 75% (6)
	Adenosine + Nitroprusside	71 ± 49μg/ml + 285 ± 195μg		20	60%	
Lim et al. [49]	Adenosine	55 ± 20.6μg	50	Only lesions undergoing primary PCI for AMI	TIMI flow grade: 0.5 ± 0.6 to 2.0 ± 0.9	Grade 3 myocardial blush score: 44%
	Adenosine + Nicorandil	41 ± 17 μg + 3.5 ± 1.3mg			0.4 ± 0.5 to 2.6 ± 0.6	76%
VERAPAMIL						
Abbo et al[4]	Verapamil, Urokinase, Nitroglycerin	Verapamil 50–500μg	0.6% (66/10676)	0.3% in PTCA, 7.7% in Rotablator, 4.5% for extraction atherectomy, 1.7% for DCA	Urokinase 10%, NTG 35%, Verapamil 67%	Resolution in 29% with best response in rotablator cases (63%)
Werner et al[37]	Verapamil	1mg/2min infusion	10.8% (23/212)	Only lesions undergoing primary or rescue PCI for AMI	65%	13% rate of intermittent Grade II atrioventricular block
Kaplan et al[10]	Nitroglycerin	10–300μg	32 patients with 36 SVG lesions	(42%) 15/36 SVG lesions	No improvement in TIMI flow	
	Verapamil	100–500μg			88%	
Piana et al[6]	Verapamil	50–900μg	2% (39/1919)	11.5% in AMI and 4% in SVG	81%	No benefit from Nitroglycerin and improved TIMI flow grade in 89%

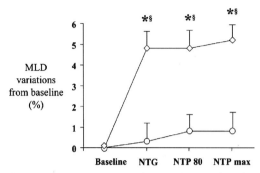

Figure 28.2. Changes in minimal lumen diameter (MLD) after administration of nitroglycerin, and increasing doses of Nitroprusside. Adapted from Airoldi, Briguori, Cianflone, et al. [29].

a significant role in the control of coronary blood flow through the microcirculation [32]. However, there is an important distinction between NTG and NTP. Resistance vessels, which primarily determine coronary blood flow, have a decreased capacity for enzymatic conversion of NTG into nitric oxide. Unlike NTG, NTP is a direct donor of nitric oxide and is reported to require no intracellular metabolism to derive nitric oxide; thus making nitric oxide available to the microcirculation and effectively dilating these distal vessels.

NTP has gained favor with many operators for its rapid and marked vasodilating effect with limited systemic hypotension. However, its dosage and efficacy in different clinical settings are not yet clearly established, because available information is derived from retrospective analysis of angiographic findings in different clinical conditions with different doses, routes of administration, and efficacy assessments [16,29,30]. Thus we performed a prospective study utilizing a standardized protocol of selective intracoronary administration of incremental doses of NTP in consecutive patients who developed slow flow or no reflow after stent placement [29]. In our experience no-reflow occurred in 0.9% of cases undergoing stent implantation at our institution. In 2212 patients undergoing stent implantation over a 10 month period, we observed 21 cases of no-reflow which occurred only in patients treated for AMI (11.5%, 12 of 105) or SVG stenosis

(8.2%, 9 of 109). Intracoronary boluses of NTG did not restore normal TIMI flow in any of the patients. Our standardized NTP protocol is as follows:

1. Insert a multifunction catheter or over-the-wire balloon into the culprit vessel
2. Initial 80-μg bolus of NTP is selectively administered distal to the site of stent implantation or balloon dilatation via the multifunction catheter.
3. If no response, boluses of NTP with an increment of 40 μg each time is repeated every two minutes.
4. NTP boluses are continued until TIMI 3 flow is achieved or systolic blood pressure decreases to <80 mm Hg.

We observed that the initial 80-μg bolus restored normal TIMI flow normal in 58% of patients (7 of 12) with AMI and in 44% of patients (4 of 9) with SVG stenosis. The maximal dose (120/160 μg) restored normal TIMI flow in all remaining patients with AMI but in only one additional patient with SVG stenosis. Thus our standardized protocol for intracoronary NTP administration succeeded in normalizing coronary flow in all patients with AMI but in only 55% of patients with slow flow in SVG. Our study highlights what we believe are two important factors why NTP has not been shown to be effective in some of the previous studies:

1. Local drug delivery: we believe that selectively delivering the drug distal in the coronary bed via a microcatheter is essential and superior to injection via guiding catheter or systemically. This exploits its maximal effect at the target site and allowing, when necessary, the use of higher doses of NTP without detrimental systemic effects on blood pressure. Agents administered via the guiding catheter will preferentially distribute to areas with normal flow.
2. Incremental doses: in a large proportion of patients only large doses of NTP were effective. Due its relatively short half-life (50 to 70 seconds), a greater effect of NTP cannot be obtained by repeated cumulative small boluses but only by single large boluses.

Verapamil

Intracoronary calcium-channel blockers such as Verapamil have been administered for no-reflow during PCI for AMI and have been shown to improve microvascular perfusion and myocardial salvage [19] Although microvascular and macrovascular spasm may be calcium mediated [33], their mechanism of action may go beyond the fact that they act directly on the vascular smooth muscle rather than nitric oxide. In the setting of acute ischemia invoked by balloon inflations during PTCA, Verapamil has been shown to increase the ischemic tolerance significantly. Its cardioprotective effects are ascribed to the reduction of calcium influx into the ischemic myocardial cell, restitution of the calcium homeostasis, and improved myocardial blood flow by relief of microvascular spasm [34,35]. Verapamil may also affect platelet aggregation in the setting of AMI by reducing the effects of catecholamines [34–36].

Verapamil is the most studied drug for the treatment of no-reflow. Piana et al. [6] showed that intracoronary verapmil improved the TIMI flow grade in 89% (33 of 37) no-reflow patients. Abbo et al. [4] showed similar beneficial results from verapamil with resolution of no-reflow in 6 of 9 (67%) patients treated with verapamil only. Similarly Kaplan et al. [10] performed a nonrandomized study comparing verapamil with NTG in 32 separate episodes of no-reflow in 15 SVG interventions. All 32 episodes improved by at least 1 TIMI grade and 28/32 (88%) improved to TIMI 3 after the first dose of verapamil. Pomerantz et al. [37] and Taniyama et al. [19] also showed similar results. Furthermore, verapamil pre-treatment has been shown to be effective in reducing no-reflow during SVG intervention in a small (n = 32) randomized trial [38]. However, the intragraft verapamil failed to reduce the mortality or MI in patients with no-reflow and has not been incorporated into clinical practice.

A major limitation of verapamil and the main reason why many interventionalists are reluctant to use it are due to its adverse effects such as hypotension, prolonged heart block, and a negative inotropic effect. In a patient who is already hypotensive or having conduction disturbances from no-reflow, we would strongly advise not using verapamil. Similarly in patients with severe left ventricular dysfunction, this negative inotropic agent should not be used.

Adenosine

Adenosine has a very short half-life (usually a few seconds) and is well tolerated without significant side-effects. It is capable of dilating the coronary resistance vessels and appears to be more potent than verapamil for relieving microvascular spasm. The vasodilator effect of this drug is mediated by specific adenosine A2A and A2B receptors and related to the opening of ATP-sensitive K+ channels. Furthermore, adenosine has been suggested to have a role in the preservation of endothelium integrity [39–41]. In experimental studies, adenosine has also been shown to inhibit neutrophil accumulation, superoxide generation, and adherence of coronary endothelium as well as cardiac release of endothelin [39]. Although the preventive effect of adenosine against now-reflow may be due to both the vasodilator and anti-inflammatory actions of the drug, the beneficial effect observed after no-reflow is more likely a result of its vasodilator action. Unlike verapamil, adenosine has little potential to cause prolonged detrimental effects upon atrio-ventricular conduction or myocardial contractility.

Both the studies by Sdringola et al. [41] and Fischell et al. [42] have shown that adenosine has a beneficial effect in treating no-reflow during SVG intervention. One of the novel aspects of the study by Fischell and colleagues was the use of repetitive forceful injections of adenosine and saline flushes using a small-volume (3-ml) syringe. In an ex vivo model intended to simulate the conditions of no-reflow, the authors demonstrated the potentially beneficial effects of this approach in generating greater velocity and pressure during saline administration. It is likely that the mechanical advantage afforded by a small syringe allows more effective delivery of the active vasodilator to the target vascular bed, without the need for a drug infusion catheter. It is also possible that these forceful injections may help to mechanically drive debris and/or aggregating platelets through the microvascular bed and into the coronary and then systemic venous circulation. Two studies have compared the combination of adenosine and NTP to adenosine alone. Both agents mediate vasodilatation in the coronary microcirculation in different but potentially additive mechanisms and the combination has been shown to be superior to adenosine alone [39,43].

Other Agents

Several other approaches to the treatment of no-reflow have been published or suggested such as intracoronary or intragraft injections of abciximab, nicorandil, epinephrine, nicardipine, diltiazem, urokinase, abciximab, intra-aortic balloon pumps and papaverine [4,44–47].

Intravenous platelet glycoprotein IIb/IIIa receptor inhibitors are usually administered in cases of no-reflow when distal embolization is considered to be the predominant underlying cause. They resolve any platelet-rich thrombi that may have occurred and prevent platelet plugs from developing. However, only a single case report suggests utility in this setting [45]. There are also anecdotal reports regarding the use of antiplatelet agents (abciximab) to treat no-reflow after failed treatment with intracoronary verapamil in native coronary arteries. In addition, a report by Heitzer *et al.* has found that the GP IIb/IIIa inhibitors (tirofiban and eptifibatide) improve the bioavailability of vascular nitric oxide in patients with coronary artery disease, by blocking platelet–endothelial interactions, which may potentially add vasodilator properties to these agents [48].

Nicorandil is a direct ATP K+ channel opener and as the vasodilatory action of adenosine is mediated by these channels, Nicorandil has been attempted in treating no-reflow either alone or in combination with adenosine. However, data are still limited [49]. Finally, intracoronary epinephrine has been shown to improve flow in 69% of PCI patients with refractory no-reflow [50]. However, the data on all the above agents are still limited to small case series or anecdotal reports and thus these agents have not been incorporated into daily practice.

Prognosis of No-reflow

No-reflow has been associated with an increase in MI of up to 32% and a 5–15% higher incidence of death [4–6]. Also the reversibility of no-flow is an important prognostic factor in that it has been associated with a lower 30-day mortality rate [28]. Although restoration of epicardial flow does not always imply complete reperfusion at the myocardial level, achievement of TIMI 3 flow is extremely important for improvement of myocardial function and outcome [4,7]. No-reflow has also been associated with long-term detrimental effects, including an increased risk for cardiac death, congestive heart failure, malignant arrhythmias and a decrease in ejection fraction. The predictors of death with no-reflow include cardiogenic shock, large amount of jeopardized myocardium, history of congestive heart failure or LVEF < 30%, age ≥65–70 years, multivessel disease (especially with collaterals from the index vessel to another location), female gender, and prolonged time needed to restore flow [4–6].

Conclusions

No-reflow during PCI is an important procedural complication that can result in significant cardiac morbidity and mortality. Although it is a diagnosis of exclusion, it needs to be treated promptly. In our opinion this is best done by selective distal intracoronary injection of Nitroprusside using an over-the-wire angioplasty balloon or coronary infusion catheter. During SVG intervention, an embolic protection device should always be used if technically feasible to prevent no-reflow.

References

1. Eeckhout E, Kern MJ. The coronary no-reflow phenomenon: a review of mechanisms and therapies. Eur Heart J 2001; **22**(9): 729–739.

2. Kloner RA, Ganote CE, Jennings RB. The "no-reflow" phenomenon after temporary coronary occlusion in the dog. J Clin Invest 1974; **54**(6): 1496–1508.

3. TIMI Study Group. The Thrombolysis in Myocardial Infarction (TIMI) trial. Phase I findings. N Engl J Med 1985; **312**(14): 932–936.

4. Abbo KM, Dooris M, Glazier S, et al. Features and outcome of no-reflow after percutaneous coronary intervention. Am J Cardiol 1995; **75**(12): 778–782.

5. Klein LW, Kern MJ, Berger P, et al. Society of cardiac angiography and interventions: Suggested management of the no-reflow phenomenon in the cardiac catheterization laboratory. Catheter Cardiovasc Interv 2003; **60**(2): 194–201.

6. Piana RN, Paik GY, Moscucci M, et al. Incidence and treatment of "no-reflow" after percutaneous coronary intervention. Circulation 1994; **89**(6): 2514–2518.

7. Ito H, Maruyama A, Iwakura K, Takiuchi S, et al. Clinical implications of the "no reflow" phenomenon. A predictor of complications and left ventricular remodeling in reperfused anterior wall myocardial infarction. Circulation 1996; **93**(2): 223–228.

8. Ito H, Tomooka T, Sakai N, Yu H, et al. Lack of myocardial perfusion immediately after successful thrombolysis. A predictor of poor recovery of left ventricular function in anterior myocardial infarction. Circulation 1992; **85**(5): 1699–1705.

9. Resnic FS, Wainstein M, Lee MK, et al. No-reflow is an independent predictor of death and myocardial infarction after percutaneous coronary intervention. Am Heart J 2003; **145**(1): 42–46.

10. Kaplan BM, Benzuly KH, Kinn JW, et al. Treatment of no-reflow in degenerated saphenous vein graft interventions: comparison of intracoronary verapamil and nitroglycerin. Cathet Cardiovasc Diagn 1996; **39**(2): 113–118.

11. Kaul S, Ito H. Microvasculature in Acute Myocardial Ischemia: Part II: Evolving Concepts in Pathophysiology, Diagnosis, and Treatment. Circulation 2004; **109**(3): 310–315.

12. Kaul S, Ito H. Microvasculature in Acute Myocardial Ischemia: Part I: Evolving Concepts in Pathophysiology, Diagnosis, and Treatment. Circulation 2004; **109**(2): 146–149.

13. Morishima I, Sone T, Okumura K, et al. Angiographic no-reflow phenomenon as a predictor of adverse long-term outcome in patients treated with percutaneous transluminal coronary angioplasty for first acute myocardial infarction. J Am Coll Cardiol 2000; **36**(4): 1202–1209.

14. Kotani J-i, Nanto S, Mintz GS, et al. Plaque Gruel of Atheromatous Coronary Lesion May Contribute to the No-Reflow Phenomenon in Patients With Acute Coronary Syndrome. Circulation 2002; **106**(13): 1672–1677.

15. Rezkalla SH, Kloner RA. No-Reflow Phenomenon. Circulation 2002; **105**(5): 656–662.

16. Silva JA, White CJ. Large thrombus burden, slow flow, no-reflow, and distal embolization. In: Martinez EE, Lemos PA, Ong ATL, Serruys PW, eds. Common Clinical Dilemmas in Percutaneous Coronary Interventions: Informa Healthcare, 2007: 261–282.

17. Leosco D, Fineschi M, Pierli C, et al. Intracoronary serotonin release after high-pressure coronary stenting. Am J Cardiol 1999; **84**(11): 1317–1322.

18. Wilson RF, Laxson DD, Lesser JR, et al. Intense microvascular constriction after angioplasty of acute thrombotic coronary arterial lesions. Lancet 1989; **1**(8642): 807–811.

19. Taniyama Y, Ito H, Iwakura K, et al. Beneficial effect of intracoronary verapamil on microvascular and myocardial salvage in patients with acute myocardial infarction. J Am Coll Cardiol 1997; **30**(5): 1193–1199.

20. Salloum J, Tharpe C, Vaughan D, et al. Release and elimination of soluble vasoactive factors during percutaneous coronary intervention of saphenous vein grafts: analysis using the PercuSurge GuardWire distal protection device. J Invasive Cardiol 2005; **17**(11): 575–579.

21. Baim DS, Wahr D, George B, et al. Randomized trial of a distal embolic protection device during percutaneous intervention of saphenous vein aorto-coronary bypass grafts. Circulation 2002; **105**(11): 1285–1290.

22. King SB, III, Smith SC, Jr., Hirshfeld JW, Jr., et al. 2007 Focused Update of the ACC/AHA/SCAI 2005 Guideline Update for Percutaneous Coronary Intervention: A Report of the American College of Cardiology/American Heart Association Task Force on Practice Guidelines. J Am Coll Cardiol 2008; **51**(2): 172–209.

23. Smith SC, Jr., Feldman TE, Hirshfeld JW, Jr., et al. ACC/AHA/SCAI 2005 Guideline Update for Percutaneous Coronary Intervention—summary article: A report of the American College of Cardiology/American Heart Association Task Force on Practice Guidelines (ACC/AHA/SCAI Writing Committee to Update the 2001 Guidelines for Percutaneous Coronary Intervention). Circulation 2006; **113**(1): 156–175.

24. Movahed MR, Butman SM. The pathogenesis and treatment of no-reflow occurring during percutaneous coronary intervention. Cardiovasc Revasc Med 2008; **9**(1): 56–61.

25. Roffi M, Mukherjee D, Chew DP, *et al.* Lack of benefit from intravenous platelet glycoprotein IIb/IIIa receptor inhibition as adjunctive treatment for percutaneous interventions of aortocoronary bypass grafts: a pooled analysis of five randomized clinical trials. Circulation 2002; **106**(24): 3063–3067.

26. Antoniucci D, Valenti R, Migliorini A. Thrombectomy during PCI for acute myocardial infarction: are the randomized controlled trial data relevant to the patients who really need this technique? Catheter Cardiovasc Interv 2008; **71**(7): 863–869.

27. Stone GW, Webb J, Cox DA, *et al.* For the Enhanced Myocardial Efficacy and Recovery by Aspiration of Liberated Debris I. Distal Microcirculatory Protection During Percutaneous Coronary Intervention in Acute ST-Segment Elevation Myocardial Infarction: A Randomized Controlled Trial. JAMA 2005; **293**(9): 1063–1072.

28. Lee CH, Wong HB, Tan HC, Zhang JJ, Teo SG, Ong HY, Low A, Sutandar A, Lim YT. Impact of reversibility of no reflow phenomenon on 30-day mortality following percutaneous revascularization for acute myocardial infarction-insights from a 1,328 patient registry. J Interv Cardiol 2005; **18**(4): 261–266.

29. Airoldi F, Briguori C, Cianflone D, *et al.* Frequency of slow coronary flow following successful stent implantation and effect of Nitroprusside. Am J Cardiol 2007; **99**(7): 916–920.

30. Hillegass WB, Dean NA, Liao L, *et al.* Treatment of no-reflow and impaired flow with the nitric oxide donor nitroprusside following percutaneous coronary interventions: initial human clinical experience. J Am Coll Cardiol 2001; **37**(5): 1335–1343.

31. Myers PR, Banitt PF, Guerra R, Jr., Harrison DG. Characteristics of canine coronary resistance arteries: importance of endothelium. Am J Physiol 1989; **257**(2, Pt 2): H603–H610.

32. Kuo L, Chilian WM, Davis MJ. Interaction of pressure- and flow-induced responses in porcine coronary resistance vessels. Am J Physiol 1991; **261**(6, Pt 2): H1706–H1715.

33. Villari B, Ambrosio G, Golino P, *et al.* The effects of calcium channel antagonist treatment and oxygen radical scavenging on infarct size and the no-reflow phenomenon in reperfused hearts. Am Heart J 1993; **125**(1): 11–23.

34. Brogden RN, Benfield P. Verapamil: A review of its pharmacological properties and therapeutic use in coronary artery disease. Drugs 1996; **51**(5): 792–819.

35. Campbell CA, Kloner RA, Alker KJ, Braunwald E. Effect of verapamil on infarct size in dogs subjected to coronary artery occlusion with transient reperfusion. J Am Coll Cardiol 1986; **8**(5): 1169–1174.

36. Werner GS, Lang K, Kuehnert H, *et al.* Intracoronary verapamil for reversal of no-reflow during coronary angioplasty for acute myocardial infarction. Catheter Cardiovasc Interv 2002; **57**(4): 444–451.

37. Pomerantz RM, Kuntz RE, Diver DJ, *et al.* Intracoronary verapamil for the treatment of distal microvascular coronary artery spasm following ptca. Cathet Cardiovasc Diagn. 1991; **24**(4): 283–285.

38. Michaels AD, Appleby M, Otten MH, *et al.* Pretreatment with intragraft verapamil prior to percutaneous coronary intervention of saphenous vein graft lesions: results of the randomized, controlled vasodilator prevention on no-reflow (VAPOR) trial. J Invasive Cardiol 2002; **14**(6): 299–302.

39. Barcin C, Denktas AE, Lennon RJ, *et al.* Comparison of combination therapy of adenosine and nitroprusside with adenosine alone in the treatment of angiographic no-reflow phenomenon. Catheter Cardiovasc Interv 2004; **61**(4): 484–491.

40. Hein TW, Kuo L. cAMP-independent dilation of coronary arterioles to adenosine : role of nitric oxide, G proteins, and K(ATP) channels. Circ Res 1999; **85**(7): 634–642.

41. Sdringola S, Assali A, Ghani M, *et al.* Adenosine use during aortocoronary vein graft interventions reverses but does not prevent the slow-no reflow phenomenon. Catheter Cardiovasc Interv 2000; **51**(4): 394–399.

42. Fischell TA, Carter AJ, Foster MT, *et al.* Reversal of "No reflow" during vein graft stenting using high velocity boluses of intracoronary adenosine. Cathet Cardiovasc Diagn 1998; **45**(4): 360–365.

43. Parikh KH, Chag MC, Shah KJ, *et al.* Intracoronary boluses of adenosine and sodium nitroprusside in combination reverses slow/no-reflow during angioplasty: a clinical scenario of ischemic preconditioning. Can J Physiol Pharmacol 2007; **85**(3–4): 476–482.

44. Ishihara M, Sato H, Tateishi H, *et al.* Attenuation of the no-reflow phenomenon after coronary angioplasty for acute myocardial infarction with intracoronary papaverine. Am Heart J 1996; **132**(5): 959–963.

45. Rawitscher D, Levin TN, Cohen I, *et al.* Rapid reversal of no-reflow using Abciximab after coronary device intervention. Cathet Cardiovasc Diagn 1997; **42**(2): 187–190.

46. Huang RI, Patel P, Walinsky P, *et al.* Efficacy of intracoronary nicardipine in the treatment of no-reflow during percutaneous coronary intervention. Catheter Cardiovasc Interv 2006; **68**(5): 671–676.

47. Fugit MD, Rubal BJ, Donovan DJ. Effects of intracoronary nicardipine, diltiazem and verapamil on coronary blood flow. J Invasive Cardiol 2000; **12**(2): 80–85.

48. Heitzer T, Ollmann I, Koke K, et al. Platelet glycoprotein IIb/IIIa receptor blockade improves vascular nitric oxide bioavailability in patients with coronary artery disease. Circulation 2003; **108**(5): 536–541.

49. Lim SY, Bae EH, Jeong MH, et al. Effect of combined intracoronary adenosine and nicorandil on no-reflow phenomenon during percutaneous coronary intervention. Circ J 2004; **68**(10): 928–932.

50. Skelding KA, Goldstein JA, Mehta L, et al. Resolution of refractory no-reflow with intracoronary epinephrine. Catheter Cardiovasc Interv 2002; **57**(3): 305–309.

51. Carrozza JP, Mumma M, Breall JA, et al. Randomized Evaluation of the TriActiv Balloon-Protection Flush and Extraction System for the Treatment of Saphenous Vein Graft Disease, J Am Coll Cardiol 2005; **46**(9): 1677–1683.

52. Stone GW, Rogers C, Hermiller J, et al. Randomized companison of distal protection with a filter-based catheter and a balloon occlusion and aspiration system during percutaneous intervention of diseased saphenous vein aorto-coronary bypass grafts. Circulation 2003; **108**(5): 548–553.

53. Holmes DR, Coolong A, O'Shaughnessy C, et al. Comparison of the CardioShield filter with the guardwire balloon in the prevention of embolisation during vein graft intervention: results from the CAPTIVE randomised trial. EuroIntervention 2006; **2**(2): 161–168.

54. Dixon SR, O'Neill WW, on behalf of the SPIDER Investigators. Saphenous Vein Graft Protection In a Distal Embolic Protection Randomized Trial (SPIDER). Presented at Transcatheter Cardiovascular Therapeutics (TCT) 2005 in Washington D.C. Available at: http://www.tctmd.com/Show.aspx?id=57712. Accessed April 4 2008.

55. Mauri L, Cox D, Hermiller J, Massaro J, Wahr J, Tay SW, Jonas M, Popma JJ, Pavliska J, Wahr D, Rogers C. The PROXIMAL trial: proximal protection during saphenous vein graft intervention using the Proxis Embolic Protection System: a randomized, prospective, multicenter clinical trial. J Am Coll Cardiol 2007; **50**(15): 1442–1449.

56. Dudek D, Mielecki W, Legutko J, Chyrchel M, Sorysz D, Bartus S, Rzeszutko L, Dubiel JS. Percutaneous thrombectomy with the RESCUE system in acute myocardial infarction. Kardiol Pol 2004; **61**(12): 523–533.

57. Antoniucci D, Valenti R, Migliorini A, Parodi G, Memisha G, Santoro GM, Sciagra R. Comparison of rheolytic thrombectomy before direct infarct artery stenting versus direct stenting alone in patients undergoing percutaneous coronary intervention for acute myocardial infarction. The American Journal of Cardiology 2004; **93**(8): 1033–1035.

58. Napodano M, Pasquetto G, Saccà S, Cernetti C, Scarabeo V, Pascotto P, Reimers B. Intracoronary thrombectomy improves myocardial reperfusion in patients undergoing direct angioplasty for acute myocardial infarction. J Am Coll Cardiol. 2003; **42**(8): 1395–1402.

59. Lefevre T, Garcia E, Reimers B, Lang I, di Mario C, Colombo A, Neumann F-J, Chavarri MV, Brunel P, Grube E, Thomas M, Glatt B, Ludwig J. X-Sizer for Thrombectomy in Acute Myocardial Infarction Improves ST-Segment Resolution: Results of the X-Sizer in AMI for Negligible Embolization and Optimal ST Resolution (X AMINE ST) Trial. J Am Coll Cardiol 2005; **46**(2): 246–252.

60. Burzotta F, Trani C, Romagnoli E, Mazzari MA, Rebuzzi AG, De Vita M, Garramone B, Giannico F, Niccoli G, Biondi-Zoccai GGL, Schiavoni G, Mongiardo R, Crea F. Manual Thrombus-Aspiration Improves Myocardial Reperfusion: The Randomized Evaluation of the Effect of Mechanical Reduction of Distal Embolization by Thrombus-Aspiration in Primary and Rescue Angioplasty (REMEDIA) Trial. J Am Coll Cardiol 2005; **46**(2): 371–376.

61. De Luca L, Sardella G, Davidson CJ, De Persio G, Beraldi M, Tommasone T, Mancone M, Nguyen BL, Agati L, Gheorghiade M, Fedele F. Impact of intracoronary aspiration thrombectomy during primary angioplasty on left ventricular remodelling in patients with anterior ST elevation myocardial infarction. Heart 2006; **92**(7): 951–957.

62. Silva-Orrego P, Colombo P, Bigi R, Gregori D, Delgado A, Salvade P, Oreglia J, Orrico P, de Biase A, Piccalo G, Bossi I, Klugmann S. Thrombus Aspiration Before Primary Angioplasty Improves Myocardial Reperfusion in Acute Myocardial Infarction: The DEAR-MI (Dethrombosis to Enhance Acute Reperfusion in Myocardial Infarction) Study. J Am Coll Cardiol 2006; **48**(8): 1552–1559.

63. Ali A, Cox D, Dib N, Brodie B, Berman D, Gupta N, Browne K, Iwaoka R, Azrin M, Stapleton D, Setum C, Popma J. Rheolytic Thrombectomy With Percutaneous Coronary Intervention for Infarct Size Reduction in Acute Myocardial Infarction: 30-Day Results From a Multicenter Randomized Study. J Am Coll Cardiol 2006; **48**(2): 244–252.

64. Kaltoft A, Bottcher M, Nielsen SS, Hansen HH, Terkelsen C, Maeng M, Kristensen J, Thuesen L, Krusell LR, Kristensen SD, Andersen HR, Lassen JF, Rasmussen K, Rehling M, Nielsen TT, Botker HE. Routine

thrombectomy in percutaneous coronary intervention for acute ST-segment-elevation myocardial infarction: a randomized, controlled trial. Circulation 2006; **114**(1): 40–47.

65. Svilaas T, Vlaar PJ, van der Horst IC, Diercks GFH, de Smet BJGL, van den Heuvel AFM, Anthonio RL, Jessurun GA, Tan E-S, Suurmeijer AJH, Zijlstra F. Thrombus Aspiration during Primary Percutaneous Coronary Intervention. N Engl J Med 2008; **358**(6): 557–567.

66. Cura FA, Escudero AG, Berrocal D, Mendiz O, Trivi MS, Fernandez J, Palacios A, Albertal M, Piraino R, Riccitelli MA, Gruber L, Ballarino M, Milei J, Baeza R, Thierer J, Grinfeld L, Krucoff M, O'Neill W, Belardi J. Protection of Distal Embolization in High-Risk Patients with Acute ST-Segment Elevation Myocardial Infarction (PREMIAR). Am J Cardiol 2007; **99**(3): 357–363.

67. Gick M, Jander N, Bestehorn HP, Kienzle RP, Ferenc M, Werner K, Comberg T, Peitz K, Zohlnhöfer D, Bassignana V, Buettner HJ, Neumann FJ. Randomized evaluation of the effects of filter-based distal protection on myocardial perfusion and infarct size after primary percutaneous catheter intervention in myocardial infarction with and without ST-segment elevation. Circulation. 2005; **112**(10): 1462–1469.

68. Wang HJ, Lo PH, Lin JJ, Lee H, Hung JS. Treatment of slow/no-reflow phenomenon with intracoronary nitroprusside injection in primary coronary intervention for acute myocardial infarction. Catheter Cardiovasc Interv 2004; **63**(2): 171–176.

69. Pasceri V, Pristipino C, Pelliccia F, Granatelli A, Speciale G, Roncella A, Pironi B, Capasso M, Richichi G. Effects of the nitric oxide donor nitroprusside on no-reflow phenomenon during coronary interventions for acute myocardial infarction. Am J Cardiol 2005; **95**(11): 1358–1361.

CHAPTER 29

The Management of Cardiogenic Shock

John Edmond, & Andreas Baumbach

Bristol Heart Institute, University Hospitals Bristol, Bristol, UK

Introduction

Cardiogenic shock is an acute interventional emergency, and can be precipitated by any acute coronary event. Shock is more common in patients with acute ST elevation myocardial infarction, with an incidence in patients with non-ST elevation myocardial infarction of 2.1%, in unstable angina of 2.9% and in acute ST elevation myocardial infarction of around 4.2–7.2% [1–3]. Over the last two decades there have been considerable advances in the treatment of patients with acute coronary syndromes, with associated improved outcomes. However, despite these advances, there has been no significant decrease in the incidence of cardiogenic shock secondary to acute ischemic insults, with one study of patients in a single community in the United States demonstrating that the frequency of cardiogenic shock complicating acute myocardial infarction remained constant over a 23 year period (1975–1997), occurring in 7.1% of presentations [4]. The mortality from cardiogenic shock in this study also remained stable over the majority of the study, with a mortality of 71.7% for patients with cardiogenic shock, compared to 12.0% for those

Interventional Cardiology, First Edition. Edited by Carlo Di Mario, George D. Dangas, Peter Barlis. © 2010 Blackwell Publishing Ltd. Published 2010 by Blackwell Publishing Ltd.

without shock (p < 0.001). An improvement in mortality was noted in this cohort in the mid- to late-1990s, which was mirrored in the 775 hospital National Registry of Myocardial Infarction study which reported that the in-hospital mortality associated with cardiogenic shock decreased from 60.3% in 1995 to 47.9% in 2004 [5].

In patients with ST elevation, shock normally presents early in the course of the admission, with the median time to a diagnosis of shock being made of around 10 hours, and with the vast majority of patients developing shock within 48 hours of their index event [6,7].

The early development of shock following an acute ST elevation infarct is associated with a higher mortality [7]. However, in patients without ST elevation, shock tends to occur later with a median time from admission to the diagnosis of shock of 76.2 hours in Global Use of Strategies to Open Occluded Coronary Arteries (GUSTO) IIb and 94.0 hours in the Platelet Glycoprotein IIb/IIIa in Unstable Angina: Receptor Suppression Using Integrilin (Eptifibatide) Therapy (PURSUIT) trial [1,6]. Patients who present with cardiogenic shock tend to be older, to have a prior history of myocardial infarction, to have a prior history of congestive cardiac failure and to have suffered an anterior infarct at the presentation [2].

Cardiogenic shock is the most extreme presentation of left ventricular dysfunction, and is usually

Table 29.1 Inclusion criteria for randomized trials of revascularization in cardiogenic shock.

	SHOCK[22]	SMASH [19]
Clinical criteria	Cardiogenic shock within 36 hours of index myocardial infarction. Evidence of decreased organ perfusion (urine output <30 mls/hr, or cool and diaphoretic extremities)	Acute myocardial infarction <48 hours prior to randomization
Hemodynamic criteria	Systolic blood pressure of 90 mmHg or less for 30 minutes before inotrope/vasopressor administration, or vasopressors/IABP required to maintain SBP > 90 mmHg Heart rate >60 beats/min Pulmonary capillary wedge >15 mmHg Cardiac index <2.2 l/min/m²	Systolic blood pressure of 90 mmHg or less for 30 minutes despite inotropic support and intravenous volume administration as needed Pulmonary capillary wedge >15 mmHg and cardiac index <2.2 l/min/m² (if measured)

associated with extensive and severe left ventricular dysfunction, involving the loss of 40% or more of the contractile myocardium of the left ventricle in most cases [8]. At autopsy, two thirds of patients who have died of cardiogenic shock have significant disease in all three major coronary vessels.

Definition and Diagnosis

Cardiogenic shock is a clinical syndrome characterized by marked and persistent hypotension, leading to tissue hypoperfusion despite the correction of preload. Although there is no clear definition of the hemodynamic requirements for a diagnosis of cardiogenic shock to be made, cardiogenic shock is usually characterized by systolic arterial pressure <90 mmHg; the diagnosis can also be made in those patients where inotropes or mechanical support are required to maintain a systolic pressure above 90 mmHg (Table 29.1). These depressed hemodynamics lead to the clinical characteristics of cold and clammy skin, mental obtundation or confusion, and oliguria or anuria.

Cardiogenic shock can be the presenting condition in patients with mechanical complications of their infarct, and therefore conditions such as papillary muscle rupture, ventricular septal defect or ventricular rupture must be excluded prior to a diagnosis of cardiogenic shock secondary to left ventricular dysfunction being made.

Echocardiography should be undertaken urgently in patients with cardiogenic shock, especially in cases where a new systolic murmur is noted [9]. Additionally, systemic causes of hypotension such as electrolyte imbalance, hypovolemia, pharmacological side effects and arrhythmias must also be excluded, and non-cardiac causes of collapse such as aortic dissection and massive pulmonary embolus should be considered.

Management of Cardiogenic Shock

Cardiogenic shock caused by ischemia requires urgent revascularization (Table 29.2). Reperfusion therapies, including fibrinolysis and percutaneous intervention (PCI), have been shown to reduce infarct size and alleviate ischemia, but it often takes time for functional recovery to occur following restoration of adequate blood flow to the ischemic myocardium. Accordingly, despite revascularization, patients may develop cardiogenic shock and require hemodynamic support with medical therapy and/or mechanical support until the reperfused myocardium has regained some or all of its function. Additionally, as one third of the patients in the "SHould we emergently revascularize Occluded Coronaries for cardiogenic shocK" trial (SHOCK) had cardiopulmonary resuscitation, sustained ventricular tachycardia or ventricular fibrillation prior to randomization, full

Table 29.2 International guidelines on the management of cardiogenic shock: Class I indications.

European Society of Cardiology [9]	American College of Cardiology/American Heart Association[23]
In cardiogenic shock caused by acute coronary syndromes, coronary angiography and revascularization should be performed as soon as possible. (LoE: A)	Intra-aortic balloon counterpulsation is recommended for STEMI patients when cardiogenic shock is not quickly reversed with pharmacological therapy. The IABP is a stabilizing measure for angiography and prompt revascularization. (LoE: B)
Echocardiography is an essential tool for the evaluation of the functional and structural changes underlying or associated with acute heart failure, as well as in the assessment of acute coronary syndromes. (LoE: C)	Early revascularization, either PCI or CABG, is recommended for patients less than 75 years old with ST elevation or LBBB who develop shock within 36 hours of MI and who are suitable for revascularization that can be performed within 18 hours of shock unless further support is futile because of the patient's wishes or contra-indications/unsuitability for further invasive care. (LoE: A)
Intra-aortic balloon counterpulsation has become a standard component of treatment in patients with cardiogenic shock or severe acute left heart failure that (i) do not respond rapidly to fluid administration, vasodilatation and inotropic support; (ii) is complicated by significant MR or rupture of the intraventricular septum, to obtain hemodynamic stabalization for definitive diagnostic studies or treatment; or (iii) is accompanied by severe myocardial ischemia, in preparation for coronary angiography and revascularization. (LoE: B)	Intra-arterial monitoring is recommended for the management of STEMI patients with cardiogenic shock. (LoE: C) Fibrinolytic therapy should be administered to STEMI patients with cardiogenic shock who are unsuitable for further invasive care and do not have contraindications to fibrinolysis. (LoE: B) Echocardiography should be used to evaluate mechanical complications unless these are assessed by invasive measures. (LoE: C)

resuscitation equipment must be available at all times [10].

Medical therapies are often employed in the initial management of cardiogenic shock, and are tailored to the hemodynamics of the individual. Dopamine or dobutamine in many cases do improve the hemodynamic parameters, but despite extensive study and widespread use neither appears to improve survival to hospital discharge. In most patients with cardiogenic shock there is raised systemic vascular resistance, but in the small number of cases where it is normal or even reduced, norephinepharine, which has both alpha and beta adrenergic agonist properties, may be used to increase diastolic arterial pressure and maintain coronary perfusion.

Intra-aortic Balloon Counterpulsation

The intra-aortic balloon pump (IABP) device comprises of two pieces of equipment; the balloon catheter and the console. Although during its early development the insertion of the balloon catheter required a surgical cut down, the recent IABP catheters can be delivered percutaneously via a Seldinger technique into the femoral artery. The balloon, which has an inflated volume of 30–50 mls, is placed in the descending aorta, with its proximal tip at the distal aortic arch, below the level of the left subclavian artery (Figure 29.1). The console then drives gas, usually helium, into and out of the balloon, triggered by either pressure or ECG traces.

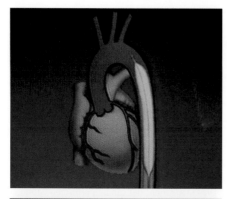

Diastolic IABP inflation

- **Increased coronary perfusion**
- **Increased renal perfusion**
- **Increased carotid blood flow**

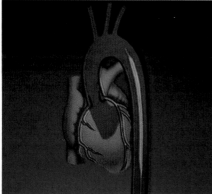

Systolic IABP deflation

- **Decreased afterload**
- **Decreased myocardial oxygen consumption**
- **Increased cardiac output**
- **Decreased cardiac work**

Figure 29.1. Correct placement of an aortic balloon catheter. The tip of the balloon catheter should be 1–2 cm distal to the subclavian artery, and the size of the balloon should be chosen according to the height of the patient, to ensure that renal flow is not compromised by the distal end of the balloon. Image courtesy of Datascope.

The major advantage of helium is its low density and hence rapid diffusion coefficient, which allows for rapid expansion and contraction of the balloon. Inflation and deflation are synchronized to the patient's cardiac cycle; inflation should occur at the onset of diastole, and deflation should occur just prior to the onset of systole (Figure 29.2). This has multiple hemodynamic effects, the most important of which are the decrease in afterload and reduction in myocardial oxygen demand, along with an increase in diastolic aortic pressure and increased coronary flow velocity (Figure 29.1).

Insertion of an IABP device is relatively contraindicated in patients with severe aortic valve insufficiency, known abdominal or aortic aneurysm, or severe aorto-iliac disease. The complications of the

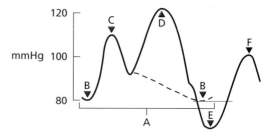

Figure 29.2. Changes in the arterial waveform produced by intra-aortic balloon counterpulsation. The dotted line represents the unassisted arterial waveform. A properly timed balloon will inflate at the dicrotic notch, which will appear as a sharp "V" configuration between the systolic pressure and the diastolic augmentation. A = One complete cardiac cycle; B = Unassisted aortic end diastolic pressure; C = Unassisted systolic pressure; D = Diastolic Augmentation; E = Reduced aortic end diastolic pressure; F = Reduced systolic pressure.

IABP device usually relate to the vascular access, with often prolonged instrumentation of the vessels, with limb ischemia, vascular dissection and thrombus or embolization seen [11]; a higher incidence of major complications is seen in female patients, older patients and those with peripheral vascular disease [12]. Patients with balloon pumps in-situ should be systemically anti-coagulated, although this can be stopped prior to the removal of the balloon. Prolonged IABP use also puts the patient at risk of infection, both local to the site of the insertion of the balloon catheter and respiratory due to immobility.

The main role of IABP therapy in the catheter laboratory in the context of cardiogenic shock is to stabilize patients to allow time for functional recovery. Although there have been clearcut benefits on hemodynamic status and coronary blood flow demonstrated, the best improvements in clinical outcomes with IABP have been seen in conjunction with reperfusion [13].

IABP Assisted Reperfusion

The outcome of patients in cardiogenic shock has been shown to be dependent on the patency of the infarct related artery [14,15]. The success of fibrinolysis depends on the drug delivery to the thrombus, and as blood pressure decreases successful fibrinolysis becomes less likely. The augmentation of diastolic blood pressure by IABP has been demonstrated in experimental studies to increase both the rate and extent of coronary fibrinolysis [16]. Moreover, in patients with acute myocardial infarction complicated by cardiogenic shock, several clinical studies have suggested an improved outcome in those patients treated with the combination of fibrinolysis and IABP; data from the SHOCK registry suggested an improvement in outcomes with a combination of fibrinolytic therapy and IABP, especially with later revascularization [13,17]. There are no data from randomized trials that can accurately answer the question of the role of balloon-assisted thrombolysis in the management of patients with cardiogenic shock. However, it has been suggested that in patients with cardiogenic shock with ST elevation, a fibrinolytic agent should be initiated if the anticipated delay to angiography is more than two hours [10].

Revascularization

Observational studies and clinical trials suggest that an aggressive interventional approach with early revascularization reduces the mortality of patients with cardiogenic shock. In the GUSTO-1 trial, a 30-day mortality of 38% was reported for the 406 patients who underwent early angiography with a view to revascularization, compared to 62% mortality in the 1794 patients with shock who did not undergo early angiography [18]. However, these data were not randomized and it is likely that selection bias would favor those patients taken forward for an interventional approach.

There have been two randomized trials addressing the question of revascularization in cardiogenic shock. Both have been slow to recruit and were underpowered. The first trial, the Swiss Multicenter Trial of Angioplasty in Shock (SMASH), was terminated prematurely as only 55 patients were randomized from nine centers over the course of four years [19]. The second trial, SHOCK, was also underpowered and enrolled 302 patients over a five year period. The SHOCK trial compared immediate revascularization to initial medical stabilization (with revascularization only permitted after 54 hours); 21% of patients in the medical stabilization group were eventually revascularized. Although there was a trend to lower 30-day mortality with revascularization (46.7% vs. 56.0%, p = 0.11), this difference in the primary endpoint did not reach statistical significance. There was, however, a statistically significant improvement in six month and one year mortality, with a one year mortality of 55% in those randomized to revascularization compared to 70% mortality for medical stabilization. It should be noted, however, that almost all the benefit in the SHOCK trial was seen in patients under 75 years of age and those treated within the first six hours of enrolment, although only 56 patients >75 years of age were enrolled.

As patients in cardiogenic shock often have three-vessel coronary artery disease, at the time of intervention the operator is often faced with a decision about treating non-infarct-related arteries. There is no randomized data to help in this decision making, and therefore multivessel intervention needs to be undertaken on a case-by-case basis. Ideally, complete revascularization should be performed but the alternative strategies of mechanical support with urgent surgical revascularization or culprit vessel intervention with later surgery should be considered. The SHOCK trial protocol recommended emergency coronary artery bypass grafting for patients with left main stem or three vessel disease, and these patients had similar outcomes to those patients undergoing PCI despite more severe disease and twice the incidence of diabetes [10].

Left Ventricular Assist Devices

In patients with cardiogenic shock, various mechanical circulatory assist devices including extracorporeal membrane oxygenation, ventricular assist devices and the CardioWest totally artificial heart have been used with variable success. They have predominantly been used in patients in whom the IABP is hemodynamically inadequate to support the failing circulation. These devices are limited by their cost and by the availability of the technical expertise and specialized training required to successfully implant the device and to manage the patient post implantation.

Recent advances have been made with devices designed to support the failing circulation that can be placed percutaneously. Devices such as the Impella percutaneous pump and the TandemHeart percutaneous ventricular assist device have been used in the setting of high risk angioplasty and cardiogenic shock, and appear promising although several technical problems persist [20,21].

Conclusion

In the setting of acute ischemia, the onset of cardiogenic shock heralds a poor prognosis. The primary goal should be to prevent the occurrence of cardiogenic shock with timely reperfusion, ideally with primary PCI. However, if cardiogenic shock does occur the patient should be treated aggressively with pharmacological support, mechanical support and revascularization.

Questions

1. **The most common pathogenic factor for the development of cardiogenic shock is:**

   A Ventricular septal defect

   B Left ventricular failure

   C Myocardial rupture

   D Mitral regurgitation resulting from LV dilation

   E Right ventricular infarction

2. **The Frequency of Cardiogenic Shock**

   A Occurs with a frequency of 3–7% and has been steadily decreasing over time

   B Occurs with a frequency of 7–10% and has been constant over time

   C Occurs with a frequency of 3–7% and has been constant over time

   D Occurs with a frequency of 7–10% and has been decreasing over time

3. **You are at a remote community hospital without a cardiac catheterization laboratory and a 56-year-old patient without a contraindication to thrombolytic therapy presents in cardiogenic shock. The ideal therapy should include the following:**

   A IABP

   B Thrombolytics

   C Transfer for emergency angiography and early revascularization (angioplasty/stent or CABG)

   D All of the above

References

1. Hasdai D, Harrington RA, Hochman JS, et al. Platelet glycoprotein IIb/IIIa blockade and outcome of cardiogenic shock complicating acute coronary syndromes without persistent ST-segment elevation. J Am Coll Cardiol 2000; **36**: 685–692.

2. Hasdai D, Califf RM, Thompson TD, et al. Predictors of cardiogenic shock after thrombolytic therapy for acute myocardial infarction. J Am Coll Cardiol 2000; **35**: 136–143.

3. Hasdai D, Holmes DR, Jr., Topol EJ, et al. Frequency and clinical outcome of cardiogenic shock during acute myocardial infarction among patients receiving reteplase or alteplase. Results from GUSTO-III. Global Use of Strategies to Open Occluded Coronary Arteries. Eur Heart J 1999; **20**: 128–135.

4. Goldberg R, Samad N, Yarzebski J, et al. Temporal trends in cardiogenic shock complicating acute myocardial infarction. N Engl J Med 1999; **340**: 1162–1168.

5. Babaev A, Frederick PD, Pasta DJ, et al. Trends in management and outcomes of patients with acute myocardial infarction complicated by cardiogenic shock. JAMA 2005; **294**: 448–554.

6. Holmes DR, Jr., Berger PB, Hochman JS, et al. Cardiogenic shock in patients with acute ischemic syndromes with and without ST-segment elevation. Circulation 1999; **100**: 2067–2073.

7. Webb JG, Sleeper LA, Buller CE, et al. Implications of the timing of onset of cardiogenic shock after acute myocardial infarction: A report from the SHOCK Trial Registry. SHould we emergently revascularize Occluded Coronaries for cardiogenic shocK? J Am Coll Cardiol 2000; **36**: 1084–1090.

8. Hochman JS, Buller CE, Sleeper LA, et al. Cardiogenic shock complicating acute myocardial infarction—etiologies, management and outcome: A report from the SHOCK Trial Registry. SHould we emergently revascularize Occluded Coronaries for cardiogenic shocK? J Am Coll Cardiol 2000; **36**: 1063–1070.

9. Nieminen MS, Bohm M, Cowie MR, et al. Executive summary of the guidelines on the diagnosis and treatment of acute heart failure: the Task Force on Acute Heart Failure of the European Society of Cardiology. Eur Heart J 2005; **26**: 384–416.

10. Menon V, Hochman J. Management of cardiogenic shock complicating acute myocardial infarction. Heart 2002; **88**: 531–537.

11. Kumbasar SD, Semiz E, Sancaktar O, et al. Mechanical complications of intra-aortic balloon counterpulsation. Int J Cardiol 1999; **70**: 69–73.

12. Ferguson JJ, III, Cohen M, Freedman RJ, Jr., et al. The current practice of intra-aortic balloon counterpulsation: results from the Benchmark Registry. J Am Coll Cardiol 2001; **38**: 1456–1462.

13. Sanborn TA, Sleeper LA, Bates ER, et al. Impact of thrombolysis, intra-aortic balloon pump counterpulsation, and their combination in cardiogenic shock complicating acute myocardial infarction: a report from the SHOCK Trial Registry. SHould we emergently revascularize Occluded Coronaries for cardiogenic shocK? J Am Coll Cardiol 2000; **36**: 1123–1129.

14. Bengtson JR, Kaplan AJ, Pieper KS, et al. Prognosis in cardiogenic shock after acute myocardial infarction in the interventional era. J Am Coll Cardiol 1992; **20**: 1482–1489.

15. Webb JG, Sanborn TA, Sleeper LA, et al. Percutaneous coronary intervention for cardiogenic shock in the

SHOCK Trial Registry. Am Heart J 2001; **141:** 964–970.

16. Nanas JN, Nanas SN, Kontoyannis DA, *et al.* Myocardial salvage by the use of reperfusion and intraaortic balloon pump: experimental study. Ann Thorac Surg 1996; **61:** 629–634.

17. French J, Feldman H, Assmann S, *et al.* Influence of thrombolytic therapy, with or without intra-aortic balloon counterpulsation, on 12-month survival in the SHOCK trial. Am Heart J 2003; **146:** 804–810.

18. Holmes DR, Jr., Bates ER, Kleiman NS, *et al.* Contemporary reperfusion therapy for cardiogenic shock: The GUSTO-I trial experience. The GUSTO-I Investigators. Global Utilization of Streptokinase and Tissue Plasminogen Activator for Occluded Coronary Arteries. J Am Coll Cardiol 1995; **26**(3): 668–674.

19. Urban P, Stauffer JC, Bleed D, *et al.* A randomized evaluation of early revascularization to treat shock complicating acute myocardial infarction. The (Swiss) Multicenter Trial of Angioplasty for Shock-(S)MASH. Eur Heart J 1999; **20:** 1030–1038.

20. Valgimigli M, Steendijk P, Sianos G, *et al.* Left ventricular unloading and concomitant total cardiac output increase by the use of percutaneous Impella Recover LP 2.5 assist device during high-risk coronary intervention. Catheter Cardiovasc Interv 2005; **65:** 263–267.

21. Burkhoff D, Cohen H, Brunckhorst C, *et al.* A randomized multicenter clinical study to evaluate the safety and efficacy of the TandemHeart percutaneous ventricular assist device versus conventional therapy with intraaortic balloon pumping for treatment of cardiogenic shock. Am Heart J 2006; **152:** 469, e1–8.

22. Hochman, Seeper, Godfrey, *et al.* Should we emergently revascularize occluded coronaries for cardiogenic shock: An internatonal randomized trial of emergency PTCA/CABG-trial design. The SHOCK Trial Study Group. Am Heart J 1999; **137:** 313–321.

23. Antman, Anbe, Armstrong, *et al.* ACC/AHA guidelines for the management of patients with ST-elevation myocardial infarcton: A report of the American College of Cardiology/American Heart Association Task Force on Practice Guidelines. Available at www.acc.org/clinical/guidelines/stemi/index.pdf.

Answers

1. B
2. B
3. D

CHAPTER 30

In-stent Restenosis in the DES Era

*Jiro Aoki[1], Adriano Caixeta[2], George D. Dangas[2], &
Roxana Mehran[2]*

[1] Mitsol Memorial Hospital, Tokyo, Japan
[2] Columbia University Medical Center, New York, NY, USA

Introduction

Drug eluting stents (DES) were developed to overcome in-stent restenosis (ISR), which has long been considered the main complication limiting the long-term efficacy of coronary stenting. When the initial clinical trials of the first DES reported the zero-level rates of restenosis [1,2], we expected that we would overcome this powerful enemy and open the doors to a world without ISR. After that, DES vs. bare-metal stents (BMS) randomized pivotal trials showed that DES significantly reduced the ISR rate compared to BMS [3,4]. Nevertheless, a small number of patients with ISR after DES treatment still exists. DES cannot completely unravel the Gordian knot of ISR. The first 2 DES (sirolimus- [SES] and paclitaxel-eluting stents [PES]) have the longest clinical follow-up, and the zotarolimus- (ZES) and everolimus-eluting (EES) stents have been introduced recently into daily practice. Although the low frequency of DES ISR events makes it difficult to fully investigate this syndrome, many studies have been conducted or are ongoing to find the mechanism, incidence, predictors and optimal treatment of DES restenosis. Therefore, in this chapter, we summarize the data

Interventional Cardiology, First Edition. Edited by
Carlo Di Mario, George D. Dangas, Peter Barlis.
© 2010 Blackwell Publishing Ltd. Published 2010 by
Blackwell Publishing Ltd.

relevant to DES restenosis and the perspective on the current treatment of this condition.

Incidence of DES Restenosis

As shown in the pivotal randomized trials comparing DES and BMS, ISR is still observed in a small number of patients (Table 30.1). However, randomized head-to-head DES comparisons have shown higher restenosis rates when compared to the pivotal randomized trials on restenosis in complex lesions [5–10]. It is well known that complex lesions have a higher risk of restenosis even with DES [11], and it should be realized that the real-world performance of DES is not quite the same as that seen in randomized trials, which were largely restricted to *de novo* coronary lesions with visually moderate lesion length and moderate reference vessel diameter. Clinical registries or observational studies have also been conducted by single or multiple centers to ascertain the efficacy of DES in routine clinical settings [12–17]. The potential for under-reporting of clinical events and the low rate of follow-up angiography is the main limitation in using these studies to determine the frequency of restenosis occurring after DES implantation. One study, the *Rapamycin-Eluting Stent Evaluated At Rotterdam Cardiology Hospital* (RESEARCH) registry, included a subgroup with mandatory follow-up angiography in a real world (unselected) setting [18]. In this registry, the rates

Table 30.1. Incidence of restenosis after DES implantation in the randomized trials.

		Number of DES treated patients	Follow-up angiography rate	Follow-up period	In-stent restenosis	In-segment restenosis
SES						
RAVEL [2]		120	89%	6 months	0%	0%
SIRIUS [3]		533	66%	8 months	3.2%	8.9%
E-SIRIUS [49]		175	92%	8 months	3.9%	5.9%
C-SIRIUS [48]		50	88%	8 months	0%	2.3%
SES SMART[a]		129	95%	8 months	4.9%	9.8%
DIABETES[b]		80	93%	9 months	3.9%	7.8%
PES						
TAXUS II SR[c]		131	98%	6 months	2.3%	5.5%
TAXUS II MR[c]		135	96%	6 months	4.7%	8.6%
TAXUS IV [4]		662	44%	6 months	5.5%	7.9%
TAXUS V [11]		577	86%	9 months	13.7%	18.9%
TAXUS V ISR [90]		195	88%	9 months	7.0%	14.5%
TAXUS VI[d]		219	96%	9 months	9.1%	12.4%
SES vs. PES						
REALITY [6]	SES	648	93%	8 months	7.0%	9.6%
	PES	669	91%	8 months	8.3%	11.1%
SIRTAX [7]	SES	503	53%	8 months	3.2%	6.6%
	PES	569	54%	8 months	7.5%	11.7%
ISAR-DIABETIC [8]	SES	180	86%	6–8 months	8.0%	11.4%
	PES	180	88%	6–8 months	14.9%	19.0%
ISAR-SMART 3 [9]	SES	100	91%	6–8 months	11.0%	14.3%
	PES	100	92%	6–8 months	18.5%	21.7%
ISAR-DESIRE [10]	SES	125	82%	6–8 months	4.9%	6.9%
	PES	125	82%	6–8 months	13.6%	16.5%
ZES						
ENDEAVOR II[e]		598	88.5%	8 months	9.4%	13.2%
ZES vs. SES						
ENDEAVOR III	ZES	323	87.3%	8 months	9.2%	11.7%
	SES	113	83.2%	8 months	2.1	4.3%
ZES vs. PES						
ENDEAVOR IV[f]	ZES	770	18.7%	8 months	13.3%	15.3%
	PES	772	17.5%	8 months	6.7%	10.4%
EES vs. PES						
SPIRIT II[g]	EES	223	92%	6 months	1.3%	3.4%
	PES	77	92%	6 months	3.5%	5.8%
EES vs. PES						
SPIRIT III[h]	EES	669	51%	8 months	2.3%	4.7%
	PES	332	50%	8 months	5.7%	8.9%

SES = sirolimus eluting stents, PES = paclitaxel eluting stents, ZES = zotarolimus eluting stents, EES = everolimus eluting stents.

[a] Ardissino D, Cavallini C, Bramucci E, *et al.* Sirolimus-eluting vs uncoated stents for prevention of restenosis in small coronary arteries: A randomized trial. JAMA 2004; **292**(2):2727–2734.

[b] Sabaté M, Jiménez-Quevedo P, Angiolillo DJ, *et al.* Randomized comparison of sirolimus-eluting stent versus standard stent for percutaneous coronary revascularization in diabetic patients: The diabetes and sirolimus-eluting stent (DIABETES) trial. Circulation 2005; **112**(14): 2175–2183.

[c] Colombo A, Drzewiecki J, Banning A, *et al.* Randomized study to assess the effectiveness of slow- and moderate-release polymer-based paclitaxel-eluting stents for coronary artery lesions. Circulation 2003: **108**(7): 788–794.

of ISR and clinically driven target lesion revascularization (TLR) following SES implantation were reported. Patients with acute myocardial infarction, ISR, 2.25 mm diameter SES, left main coronary stenting, chronic total occlusion, stented segment > 36 mm, or bifurcation stenting were selected to comprise the mandatory follow-up angiographic group. The in-segment restenosis rate at 6 months (238 patients, 441 lesions) was 7.9%. Currently, follow-up angiography after DES implantation is usually recommended at 8–9 months. Therefore, the true ISR rate may be underestimated. Furthermore, the TLR rate was 9.5% at 6 months (486 patients, 1,027 lesions) in a large, single-center experience with SES from Milan [13], and the target vessel revascularization (TVR) rate was 8.7% at an average of 6.6 months in the multicenter prospective German Cypher stent registry in which 7,445 patients were enrolled at 122 hospitals [19], and 6.0% at 1 year in the DEScover registry, which collected data on 6,509 patients who underwent DES implantation at 140 medical centers [20]. Considering that there was no mandatory follow-up coronary angiography in these registries, the true angiographic restenosis rates would be even higher than the above figures. In clinical practice, restenosis rates have been higher after implantation of DES in more complex lesions that were excluded from the pivotal randomized trials, probably exceeding 10%.

The Mechanisms of Restenosis After DES Implantation

DES technology enables anti-inflammatory, immuno-modulatory, and/or anti-proliferative agents to be released in appropriate amounts and distributed at the site of arterial injury during the initial 30-day healing period [21]. Unless an appropriate dose of the drug is eluted to the apposite location at the proper times, DES will lose their potential for reducing neointimal growth. Initial reports suggested that SES restenosis was associated with a discontinuity in stent coverage and local barotrauma outside the stent, instead of intrinsic drug-resistance [22]. However, the precise reasons why DES fail in some patients and in some lesions are still controversial. Multiple factors, biological, mechanical, and technical, may all contribute to restenosis after DES implantation (Table 30.2).

Biological Factors
Drug Resistance
Sirolimus (rapamycin) inhibits the function of the mammalian target of rapamycin (mTOR), and potentially suppresses smooth muscle cell migration and proliferation by arresting cells in G1 phase or potentially inducing apoptosis of cells [23]. However, recent data indicate that genetic mutations or compensatory changes influence the sensitivity of rapamycin, conferring rapamycin resistance [24]. Mutations of mTOR or FKBP12 prevent rapamycin from binding to mTOR. Mutations or defects of mTOR-regulated proteins, including S6K1, 4E-BP1, PP2A-related phosphatases, and p27 (Kip1) also contribute to rapamycin insensitivity. In addition, the status of ATM, p53, PTEN/Akt and 14-3-3 are also associated with rapamycin sensitivity.

Laboratory investigations have revealed a wide variety of resistance to the mechanisms of paclit-

---

Table 30.1. *footnote continued*

[d] Dawkins KD, Grube E, Guagliumi G, *et al.* Clinical efficacy of polymer-based paclitaxel-eluting stents in the treatment of complex, long coronary artery lesions from a multicenter, randomized trial: Support for the use of drug-eluting stents in contemporary clinical practice. Circulation 2005; **112**(21): 3306–3313.

[e] Fajadet J, Wijns W, Laarman GJ, *et al.* Randomized, double-blind, multicenter study of the Endeavor zotarolimus-eluting phosphorylcholine-encapsulated stent for treatment of native coronary artery lesions: Clinical and angiographic results of the ENDEAVOR II trial. Circulation 2006; **114**(8): 798–806.

[f] Leon M. The Endeavor DES System: Technical Review and Clinical Trial Updates (ENDEAVOR 1–5 and PROTECT). Paper presented at Transcatheter Cardiovascular Therapeutics conference, Washington, DC, October 2007.

[g] Serruys PW, Ruygrok P, Neuzner J, *et al.* A randomised comparison of an everolimus-eluting coronary stent with a paclitaxel-eluting coronary stent: The SPIRIT II trial. EuroIntervention 2006; **2**: 286–294.

[h] Stone GW, Midei M, Newman W, *et al.* Comparison of an everolimus-eluting stent and a paclitaxel-eluting stent in patients with coronary artery disease: A randomized trial. JAMA 2008; **299**(16): 1903–1913.

Table 30.2. Possible mechanisms of restenosis after DES.

Biological related factors
Drug resistance
Hypersensitivity

Mechanical related factors
Stent underexpansion
Nonuniform stent strut distribution
Stent fracture
Overdilatation of undersized stent
Nonuniform drug deposition
Polymer peeling

Technical related factors
Barotrauma outside the stented segment
Stent gap
Residual uncovered atherosclerotic plaques

axel [25]. Paclitaxel binds specifically to the β-tubulin subunit of microtubules and its principle action is to interfere with microtubule dynamics, preventing their depolymerization [23]. Resistance to paclitaxel is associated with increased expression of the mdr-1 gene and its product P-glyxoprotein, β-tubulin mutation, changes in apoptotic regulatory and mitosis checkpoint proteins, and potentially the over expression of interleukin 6 (IL-6) [26,27]. Currently, however, the relevance of how these drug resistance issues affect restenosis after DES implantation remains unknown.

Hypersensitivity

In the era of bare-metal stents, allergic reactions to nickel and molybdenum released from stents was one of the triggering mechanisms for ISR [28]. In DES the triggers for restenosis are more complex. DES consist of 3 components: the anti-restenotic drug, drug carrier vehicle (polymer), and the stent platform. A hypersensitivity reaction to any one of these components may lead to restenosis after implantation. In the Research on Adverse Drug/Device events And Reports (RADAR) project, 262 patients suffered from hypersensitivity symptoms out of a total of 5,783 reports from the FDA DES database [29]. In those 262 patients, the authors identified 17 cases in which the DES themselves appeared to be a prob-

able cause of hypersensitivity findings. In other studies, pathology findings from 4 autopsies presented the strongest evidence that DES can cause a hypersensitivity reaction. Because the exact incidence is unclear, any patient suspected of having a hypersensitivity reaction after DES implantation should be carefully monitored [30,31].

Mechanical Factors

Stent Under-expansion and Non-uniform Stent Strut Distribution

Intravascular ultrasound (IVUS) permits detailed cross-sectional imaging of the deployed stents, and several factors associated with DES restenosis can be detected through IVUS information. The lack of full stent expansion, IVUS measured stent length (> 40 mm), and non-uniform strut distribution (e.g. non-uniform/circular lumen expansion) contribute to increased risk for ISR after DES implantation [32–36]. The IVUS substudy of the SIRIUS trial showed that a post-procedure minimum stent area (MSA) < 5.0 mm^2 was responsible for the majority of cases of restenosis [34].

Stent Fracture

A stent fracture can be associated with restenosis, due to a decrease in local drug delivery at the fracture point; it may also be a marker of severe non-uniform stent expansion (see above). Initial case reports and small registries detailing SES fractures suggested that implantation of long stents concomitantly with postdilatation using larger balloons at higher pressures was related to coronary stent fractures, and the location of fractured stents was more common in the right coronary artery [37,38,39]. One observational study reported that the incidence of SES fracture was 2.6% [40]. Significant predictors of stent fracture were saphenous vein graft location, length of implanted stent and right coronary artery location. ISR was observed in 37.5% of stent fracture lesions. Stent fracture itself was likely to be induced by mechanical stress provoked by rigid structures and by locations that served as hinges during vessel movement in the cardiac contraction cycle (Figure 30.1); both SES and PES fractures have been reported [41]. In another observational study, Shaikh F *et al.* [42], stent fracture was identified by angiography in

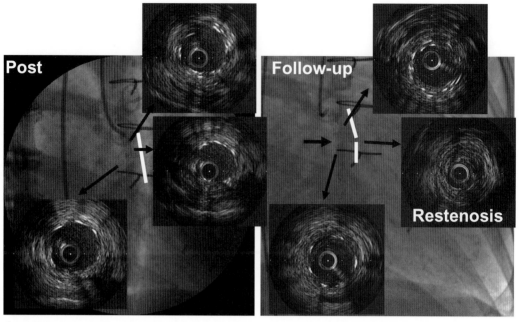

Figure 30.1. Angiographic and IVUS images on fracture stent. Adapted from Aoki *et al.* [98].

19% of all cases of ISR. In this study, stenting on a bend > 75 degrees, SES implantation and overlapping stented segments were independent predictors of stent fracture while larger stent diameter was protective. However, compared to angiography, IVUS can more reliably detect stent fracture during follow-up evaluation [43].

Overdilatation of an Undersized Stent

Stent underexpansion is related to DES restenosis. Paradoxically, overdilatation has also been related to the possibility of increasing the restenosis rate. The supposition is that extreme postdilatation of the stent can impair the effectiveness of DES in different ways: by enhancing tissue proliferation in response to greater vessel injury, by altering the mechanical properties of the stent, by disrupting the polymer coating, and by increasing the distance between the stent struts. However, 2 observational prospective studies concluded that overdilatation of undersized SES with a largely oversized balloon was both safe and effective [44,45]. As it stands despite the rationale of this supposition, to date it remains unsupported by current data.

Non-uniform Drug Deposition

Drug penetration into the tissue is a necessary and sufficient condition for drug efficacy. After a DES is implanted, drug deposition appears not only beneath the regions of arterial contact with the stent strut but also beneath the standing pools of drug created by the strut's disruption of blood flow. Physiological and computational models have shown that local blood flow alternations and the location of drug elution from the strut are more important in determining arterial wall drug deposition and distribution than drug load or arterial wall contact with the drug-coated strut surface [46]. It appears that alterations in the pattern of the blood flow caused by stent strut conditions such as strut thickness, the depth of strut penetration into the arterial wall, and strut overlap may play an important role in the efficacy of DES. In addition, even small amounts of local mural thrombus attached to the stent strut, can affect arterial wall drug uptake and retention (Figure 30.2) [47]. Micro thrombus attachments on DES and stent placement in a clot-laden arterial wall may have an effect on drug distribution in the arterial wall, as well as potential for

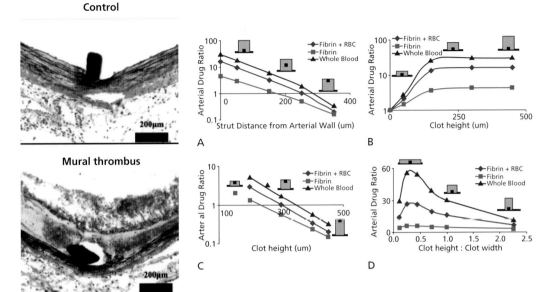

Figure 30.2. Thrombosis Modulates Arterial Drug Distribution for Drug eluting Stents. Adapted from Hwang *et al.* [47].

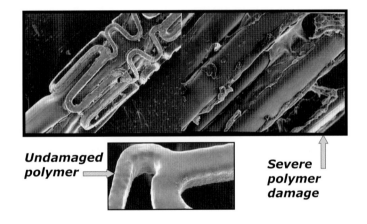

Figure 30.3. DES failed to cross a heavily calcified lesion.

affecting clinical outcome. Furthermore, polymer damage may hamper the uniform drug elution when DES cross a severe calcified lesion (Figure 30.3).

Technical Factors
Barotrauma Outside the Stented Segment
Subgroup analyses in the SIRIUS trial first indicated that the exposed margins of the stents that did not cover the entire region of the balloon injury were the primary sites of restenosis.

Restenosis occurred predominantly at the proximal stent margin after the placement of SES [3]. Today, the recommended technique includes predilatation with shorter balloons, using a longer single stent in order to cover the entire area of balloon injury, and dilatating within the stented regions using short, high-pressure balloons. Following these recommendations, the incidence of proximal margin restenosis rates decreased in subsequent studies that followed a revised implantation protocol: the decreased incidence was 5.9% in E-SIRIUS and 2.3% in C-SERIUS, compared to 5.8% in SIRIUS [48,49]. The use of direct stenting in E-SIRIUS and C-SIRIUS may have also limited proximal edge trauma and subsequent restenosis in some patients.

Stent Gap

Similar to stent fracture, stent gap can cause discontinuity of coverage by drug eluting stents. Theoretically, the amount of local drug deposition to the vessel wall decreases at the gap site. Considering that the safety and efficacy of overlapping drug eluting stents have been reported, stent gap should be avoided in general [22,50].

Residual Uncovered Atherosclerotic Plaques

When treating ostial and bifurcation lesions, it is sometimes difficult to avoid incomplete lesion coverage. In bifurcation lesions, the recent introduction of DES has resulted in a lower incidence of main branch restenosis compared to the historical controls with BMS. However, sidebranch ostial restenosis remains a problem due to the difficulty of full lesion coverage [51,52]. Various techniques using 1 or 2 stents have been developed to optimize the treatment of bifurcation lesions, such as T-stenting, Y-stenting, V-stenting, Crush-stenting, Skirt-stenting, etc. [53]. Kissing balloon post-dilatation after crush-stenting improves stent strut apposition in the carina as much as possible and reduces side branch restenosis, but the best treatment technique to use when treating bifurcation lesions with DES remains controversial [40,54].

The STLLR trial [55] evaluated the frequency and impact of suboptimal percutaneous coronary intervention on long-term outcomes of 1,557 patients treated with SES. The presence of geographic miss during the procedure (injured or diseased segment not covered by SES or balloon-artery size ratio < 0.9 or > 1.3) was associated with increased risk of TVR and myocardial infarction at 1 year.

Predictors of DES Restenosis

In the era of DES, specific characteristics still confer an increased risk for ISR (Table 30.3). The

TAXUS V trial has shown that small-diameter stents (small vessel) and multiple stents are associated with a higher ISR rate [11]. Several studies in daily clinical practice have also investigated predictors of restenosis after DES implantation [18,56–60]. Initial reports from a multivariate logistic regression analysis of 441 lesions indicate that ISR lesions, ostial lesions, diabetes mellitus, total stent length, vessel size and left anterior descending coronary artery are significant predictors of in-segment restenosis after SES implantation [18]. Berenguer *et al* showed that multivariate independent predictors of restenosis after SES implantation in 263 lesions include female patients and lesion length >30 mm [56]. Another study evaluated the significant predictors of SES ISR, including clinical, angiographic, procedural and IVUS predictors [32]. Notably, the independent predictors of restenosis included only IVUS parameters (postprocedural final minimum stent area by IVUS and IVUS-measured stent length).

Recent studies on the predictors of restenosis after coronary implantation of SES and PES have been published by 2 independent centers. Multivariate logistic regression analysis from one, based on angiographic follow-up of 1,703 available lesions, revealed that vessel size, type of DES, and final diameter stenosis were significant predictors of binary angiographic restenosis [57]. The other team indicated that the type of DES used, post-minimal lesion diameter, and lesion length were significant predictors of angiographic restenosis in 2,405 lesions [58]. The predictive factors for DES restenosis identified from the real-world data seem to be similar to those for BMS, such as small vessels, longer stents and stent underexpansion [61–63]. Considering that postminimal lumen diameter is a major factor in restenosis, optimal acute angiographic results are still important after DES implantation.

Morphological Pattern of DES Restenosis

Both the incidence and pattern of restenosis were different between DES and BMS. The most common angiographic restenosis pattern after SES implantation is focal. In the SIRIUS trial, 26 of the 31 (83.9%) restenotic lesions were

Table 30.3. Independent predictors of TLR or ISR after DES implantation.

Randomized trials	Independent predictors of TLR	Observational studies	Independent predictors of restenosis
SES arm in the SIRIUS trial[a]	Post procedure in-stent MLD Total implanted stent length	Lemos et al. [18]	In-stent restenosis lesion Ostial lesion Diabetes Mellitus Vessel size LAD
PES arm in the TAXUS IV trial[b]	No study stents implanted No prior MI Female gender Lesion length	Kastrati et al. [57]	Vessel size Final diameter stenosis DES type
		Lee et al. [58]	DES type Post intervention MLD Lesion length
		Roy et al. [59]	Age Hypertension Procedural length Lack of IVUS guidance Total stented length
		Corbett et al. [60]	Diabetes mellitus Unstable angina Reference vessel diameter Number of stents per lesion

TLR = target lesion revascularization, SES = sirolimus eluting stents, PES = paclitaxel eluting stents, DSE = drug eluting stents, MLD = minimal lumen diameter, MI = myocardial infarction, LAD = left anterior descending coronary artery, IVUS = intravascular ultrasound system.

[a] Holmes DR Jr, Leon MB, Moses JW, et al. Analysis of 1-year clinical outcomes in the SIRIUS trial: A randomized trial of a sirolimus-eluting stent versus a standard stent in patients at high risk for coronary restenosis. Circulation 2004; **109**(5): 634–640.

[b] Stone et al., Circulation 2004; **109**(16); 1942–1947.

focal [64], and this tendency persisted in 2 series from Rotterdam and Milan showing that in "real-world" practice settings, 15 of 20 (75%) and 14 of 14 (100%) restenotic lesions were focal [22,65]. In the TAXUS IV study, the pattern of restenosis after PES implantation was predominantly focal (62.5%), but still a considerable percentage (37.5%) of ISR lesions were non-focal (Table 30.4) [4]. In a series of 977 consecutive patients after PES implantation, 98 lesions were identified as ISR, and half of these were focal [66]. In data from 2 independent centers that reported restenosis patterns after SES and PES implantation in an unselected real-world population, there was a significantly higher incidence of diffuse and occlusive restenosis in the PES cohort when compared

to the SES cohort (Figure 30.4) [67,68]. Therefore, angiographic restenosis patterns following SES and PES implantation may not be identical, and further investigation in large, head-to-head randomized studies is required before we can definitively judge the differences in patterns of restenosis after SES and PES implantation.

Prognostic Implications for Morphologic Patterns of ISR

After BMS implantation, the classification of angiographic patterns of ISR has been shown to be of important prognostic significance. Mehran et al reported that TLR at 1 year after repeat intervention for ISR increased progressively with ISR classification (focal 19%, intra-stent 35%, proliferative

Table 30.4. Morphological pattern of DES vs. BMS restenosis.

	SES (n = 31)	Control (n = 128)	P-value
SIRIUS [64]			
I—focal	83.9%	43.0%	<0.001
II/III—diffuse or proliferative	9.7%	49.2%	<0.001
IV—total occlusion	6.5%	7.8%	0.90
TAXUS IV [4]	PES (n = 16)	Control (n = 65)	P-value
I—focal	62.5%	30.8%	<0.001
II/III—diffuse or proliferative	25.0%	66.2%	<0.001
IV—total occlusion	12.5%	3.1%	0.25

The pattern of restenosis was defined according to the classification of Mehran *et al.* [69].

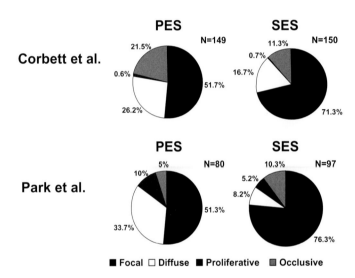

Figure 30.4. Morphological pattern of DES restenosis (SES vs. PES). Adapted from Corbett *et al.* [67] and Park *et al.* [68].

50%, total occlusion 83%, $P < 0.001$) [69]. After DES implantation, it is unknown whether the morphologic pattern of DES ISR has any impact on the outcome of percutaneous re-treatment. Currently, only 1 study in 250 consecutive restenotic lesions in 203 patients showed that the morphologic pattern of DES ISR was predictive [70]. In this study, the rate of re-restenosis was 17.8% in the focal group and 51.1% in the non-focal group ($P = 0.001$); the incidence of TLR at a median of 13.7 months was 9.8% and 23.0%, respectively ($P = 0.007$). Similar to BMS, the morphologic pattern of DES restenosis may have an impact on clinical outcomes (Figure 30.5).

The Issue of Delayed Restenosis

DES dramatically reduce neointimal growth at 6 or 9 months compared to BMS. Although long term follow-up after DES implantation shows a sustained clinical benefit in several trials, little is known about neointimal growth beyond the first 6 to 9 months [71–73]. The issue of a "late catch-up phenomenon" has not been fully investigated with DES. Preclinical porcine studies have consistently demonstrated that the inhibition of neointimal growth after DES implantation does not persist beyond 90 days [74,75]. Previous serial angiographic analysis

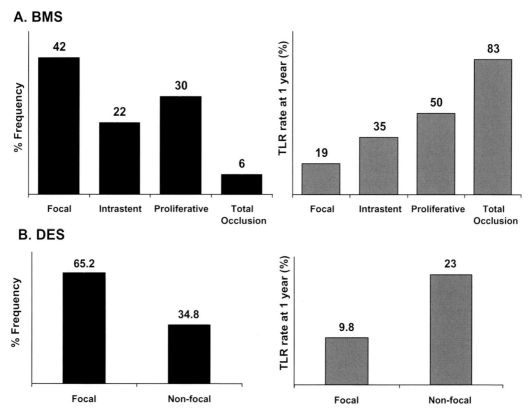

Figure 30.5. Morphological pattern of ISR predicts clinical outcomes after BMS (A) and DES (B) implantation. Adapted from Cosgrave *et al.* [70] and Mehran *et al.* [69].

showed that intimal hyperplasia peaks 12 to 16 weeks after intervention and that restenosis rarely occurs beyond 6 months after BMS implantation in humans [76]. Furthermore, compaction of neointima beyond 6 months after BMS implantation has been described in several reports [77–79]. Histological analyses of post-mortem coronary arteries demonstrate that compaction of neointima occurs due to the replacement of water-trapping proteoglycans by decorin and type I collagen [80,81]. After DES implantation, however, late restenosis and persistent neointimal growth have been reported. Wessely *et al* reported 2 cases of delayed restenosis. Two patients with recurrent angina symptoms were treated with SES at 13 and 19 months [82]. Of note, both patients had undergone follow-up angiography at 7 months, which revealed excellent angiographic results. From Rotterdam, persistence of neointimal growth

was noted 12 months after intervention and occurrences of delayed restenosis were also reported [83]. Fifteen patients with left main coronary artery disease were treated with DES. Average late loss increased from 0.29 mm at 6 months to 0.63 mm after 12 months ($P < 0.001$). One patient with mild hyperplasia at 6 months received a TLR at 12 months due to severe focal restenosis. The finding that neointima may persistently grow beyond 6 months after the index procedure may cast a shadow of doubt on current judgment favoring the efficacy of DES using late loss at 6 to 9 months as an indicator mark. Both serial angiographic analyses and serial IVUS analyses can depict persistent neointimal growth after several kinds of DES implantations [84]. Serial IVUS analyses (up to 2 years) after deployment of BMS and PES were performed in a series of 161 patients in the Taxus II study [85]. Whereas the BMS group showed the compaction of neointima over time, there were only modest increases in neointima in the PES group between 6 months and 2 years. The precise reason for this observation is still unclear, but it may be related to a delayed healing response, a persistent biological reaction caused by the drug soon after implantation, and/ or a hypersensitivity reaction to the polymer carried on the stent. One study showed a 4-year coronary artery response after SES implantation using serial IVUS and computer-assisted grayscale value analysis. Neointima kept growing over 4 years, but no further statistically significant changes occurred between 2 and 4 years. In addition, peri-stent tissue began to shrink with a concomitant increase in echogenicity between 2 and 4 years. These observations may suggest that the biological phenomenon of delayed healing response is beginning to subside [86]. Further study is warranted to investigate the clinical relevance of this persistent neointimal growth and establish the appropriate length of follow-up after DES implantation.

Approaches to DES Restenosis

The optimal treatment for DES restenosis is largely unknown. Although many observational studies have evaluated the clinical and angiographic outcomes after percutaneous treatment for DES restenosis, the numbers of enrolled patients in these studies were too small and the results were not consistent enough to draw any conclusions (Table 30.5). A first report from the team at Rotterdam showed that percutaneous treatment for DES restenosis has a high recurrence rate (42%) [87]. In the randomized SIRIUS trial and the meta-analysis of the TAXUS trials, the TLR rate after percutaneous re-treatment was 22.7% at 1 year and 11.5% at 2 years, respectively. The various treatment options (balloon, cutting balloon, BMS, same DES, different DES, vascular brachytherapy [VBT], or bypass surgery) and various etiologies of DES restenosis (as mentioned previously) make it difficult for interventional cardiologists to find the optimal therapy for DES restenosis.

DES for DES Restenosis

Since the clinical and angiographic results of DES for BMS restenosis were superior to those with conventional therapy (balloon or VBT) in several randomized trials [88–90], DES are used as a re-treatment modality for DES restenosis. Several studies compared the clinical or angiographic effect of re-DES placement with conventional therapies for DES restenosis [91–93]. In the Radiation for Eluting Stents in Coronary FailUrE (RESCUE) trial, TLR rates at 8 months in 112 DES restenotic lesions were not significantly different between repeat-DES and VBT groups (8% vs. 10%, $P = 1.00$) [92]. On the other hand, Kim et al reported that restenosis rates at 6 months in 58 consecutive lesions were 4% with SES treatment and 35% with conventional treatment (cutting balloon angioplasty [CBA] and/or VBT) ($P = 0.006$) [91]. Researchers from Illinois reported similar results in 108 DES failure lesions [93]. The 1 year TLR rate was 28.5% in patients given the same DES, 19.0% with a different DES, and 36.5% with conventional (CBA, BMS, or VBT) treatments. The efficacy of DES re-treatment seems to be feasible compared to conventional percutaneous treatments. However, there has been no study comparing DES re-treatment and bypass surgery for DES restenosis.

Same DES or Different DES

One of the etiologies of DES restenosis is drug resistance. Therefore, the placement of a different DES might be more effective in treating DES restenosis compared with the same DES. There have been few studies to investigate the comparison between same or different DES implantation for DES restenosis; in general, these studies have compared SES vs. PES. There are no data reporting the use of ZES and EES for DES-ISR. Previously mentioned data from Illinois showed that treatment with a different DES tended to result in more favorable outcomes at 12 months than treatment with the same DES [93]. A group from New York also presented data showing that implantation of a different DES resulted in more favorable outcomes compared to using the same DES as the one which failed originally [94]. However, data from Milan [95] and Washington [96] showed no dif-

Table 30.5. Clinical and angiographic outcomes after percutaneous treatment of DES failure.

Author	Restenosis	Treatment	Number of patients (lesions)	Follow-up period	TLR	Angiographic follow-up rate	ISR
Lemos et al. [87]	SES	DES	— (23)	490 days	20.8%*	78% (281 days)	42.0%*
		POBA	— (3)				
		BMS	— (1)				
Moussa et al.[a]	SES	BMS	18 (18)	12 months	16.7%	—	—
		CBA	2 (2)		0%	—	—
		VBT	1 (1)		100%	—	—
		POBA	1 (1)		100%	—	—
Lee et al.[b]	SES	PES	125 (140)	7.2 months	14%	—	—
Nakamura et al.[c]	SES	SES	156 (198)	12 months	6.4%	— (12 months)	7.7%
		PES	152 (161)		15.7%		15.7%
Stone et al.[d]	PES	DES	7 (7)	2 years	0%	—	—
		BMS	12 (12)		17%	—	—
		POBA	13 (13)		23%	—	—
		VBT	9 (9)		11%	—	—
Kim et al. [91]	DES	SES	31 (33)	21.4 months	3.2%	82.8% (6 months)	4%
		CB or VBT	24 (25)		8.3%		35%
Torguson et al. [92]	DES	DES	50 (50)	8 months	8%	—	—
		VBT	61 (62)		10%	—	—
Kwak et al.[e]	DES	DES	—(31)	—	—	67% (6 months)	10.5%
		CBA	— (21)	—	—		53.8%
Mishkel et al. [93]	DES	DES (same)	59 (64)	12 months	28.5%	—	—
		DES (different)	18 (22)		19.0%	—	—
		POBA, BMS, or VBT	15 (22)		36.5%	—	—
Cosgrave et al. [95]	DES	DES (same)	96 (107)	25.7 months	16.7%	69.7% (9 months)	26.4%
		DES (different)	78 (94)		16.7%		25.8%
Solinas et al. [94]	DES	DES (same)	— (61)	13 months	0%	—	—
		DES (different)	— (36)		8.3%	—	—
de Lezo et al.[f]	DES	DES (same)	— (32)	15 months	5.6%*	—	—
		DES (different)	— (47)			—	—
		POBA	— (32)			—	—
Garg et al. [96]	DES	DES (same)	62 (—)	12 months	22.5%	—	—
		DES (different)	54 (—)		21.4%	—	—
Solinas E et al.[g]	DES	DES (same)	37 (—)	12 months	6.7%	—	—
		DES (different)	62 (—)		3.9%	—	—
		POBA	19 (—)		25%		

*Overall incidence.
SES = sirolimus eluting stents, PES = paclitaxel eluting stents, DES = drug eluting stents, BMS = bare-metal stents, POBA = plain old balloon angioplasty, VBT = vascular brachytherapy, CBA = cutting balloon angioplasty, TLR = target lesion revascularization, ISR = in-stent restenosis.

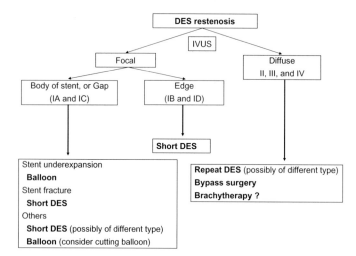

Figure 30.6. Algorithm for the treatment of DES restenosis.

ference between implantation of the same DES vs. a different DES in 201 DES restenotic lesions. The GISE-CROSS trial, which is a randomized study comparing treatment with the same vs. a different DES for DES restenosis, is currently ongoing to further evaluate the strategy of alternate DES therapy [97].

Proposed Treatments of DES Restenosis

It is important to consider that therapy options for DES restenosis are somewhat controversial, as there are few data with interventional modalities (balloon, cutting balloon, BMS, same DES, different DES or VBT) and surgery. The etiologies of DES restenosis are diverse. Therefore, we recommend that treatment of DES restenosis be "indi-

vidualized" using IVUS analysis. Figure 30.6 depicts a proposed algorithm for the current approach to DES restenosis. There are several known etiologies of focal DES restenosis. Percutaneous treatments for focal ISR caused by stent underexpansion or fracture, and focal edge restenosis, have gained general consensus. However, treatments for focal ISR caused by unclear etiology and diffuse DES ISR have not met with widespread agreement.

Summary

Angiographic coronary restenosis rates after DES implantation have fallen below 10% in several randomized trials. However, this rate increases when

Table 30.5. *footnote continued*

[a]Moussa ID, Moses JW, Kuntz RE, *et al.* The fate of patients with clinical recurrence after sirolimus-eluting stent implantation (a two-year follow-up analysis from the SIRIUS trial). Am J Cardiol 2006; **97**(11): 1582–1584.

[b]Lee SS, Price MJ, Wong GB, *et al.* Early- and medium-term outcomes after paclitaxel-eluting stent implantation for sirolimus-eluting stent failure. Am J Cardiol 2006; **98**(10): 1345–1348.

[c]Nakamura S, Bae J-H, Cahyadi YH, *et al.* Impact of sirolimus-eluting stent and paclitaxel-eluting stent on the outcome of patients with sirolimus-eluting stent failure: Multicenter registry in Asia. J Am Coll Cardiol 2007; **49**(9, Suppl. B): 39B.

[d]Stone GW, Colombo A, Grube E, *et al.* Abstract 3251: Long-term outcomes following treatment of in-stent restenosis with drug-eluting stents: Insights from the TAXUS meta-analysis. Circulation 2006; **114**(18, Suppl.): II-689.

[e]Kwak J-J, Kim Y-S, Suh J-W, *et al.* Drug-eluting stent implantation versus cutting balloon angioplasty for in-stent restenosis of drug eluting stent. Am J Cardiol 2006; **98**(Suppl. 8A): 177M.

[f]de Lezo JS, Segura J, Pan M, *et al.* Abstract 3249: Clinical outcome of patients with coronary restenosis after drug eluting stents. Circulation 2006; **114**(18, Suppl): II-689.

[g]Solinas E, Dangas G, Kirtane AJ, *et al.* Angiographic patterns of drug-eluting stent restenosis and one-year outcomes after treatment with repeated percutaneous coronary intervention. Am J Cardiol 2008; **102**(3) 311–315.

treating complex lesions. Whereas predictors of restenosis after BMS deployment such as diabetes mellitus, small vessels, and stenting long lesions are still significant in the era of DES, the morphologic pattern of restenosis is different following BMS vs. DES implantation. The predominant pattern of angiographic restenosis is focal and this pattern is related to better prognosis. However, a diffuse pattern type still exists and is associated with a high incidence of re-restenosis. In addition, the issue of delayed restenosis has not been fully investigated with DES. DES are not a magical cure for resolving restenosis; thus it is important to understand DES restenosis mechanisms and related factors (biological, mechanical, and technical). Further detailed studies are warranted to understand the development of restenosis in DES and the precise treatment for the syndrome. We anticipate that these studies will become more complex with the emergence of new types of DES.

Questions

1. **Which of the following are possible causes to DES restenosis?**

   A Drug resistance

   B Polymer hypersensitivity responses

   C Strut fractures

   D Under expanded stents

   E All of the above

   F None of the above

2. **Which of the following are correct statements concerning the morphologic patterns of DES restenosis?**

   A Compared with BMS, more focal ISR lesions

   B Compared to Cypher, more diffuse patterns with Taxus

   C Diffuse ISR lesions after DES more often recur and recurrence ISR morphology usually remains diffuse

   D All of the above

3. **What is the percentage of total-occlusive PES-ISR in TAXUS-IV trial?**

   A 5%

   B 20%

   C 13%

   D 2%

   E 30%

4. **Which of the following are possible contributing or causative mechanisms of late/very late DES thrombosis?**

   A delayed healing

   B late acquired incomplete stent apposition

   C resistance to anti-platelet agents

   D Pro-inflammatory action of the polymer

   E All of the above

   F None of the above

References

1. Sousa JE, Costa MA, Abizaid AC, et al. Sustained suppression of neointimal proliferation by sirolimus-eluting stents: one-year angiographic and intravascular ultrasound follow-up. Circulation 2001; **104**(17): 2007–2011.

2. Morice MC, Serruys PW, Sousa JE, et al. A randomized comparison of a sirolimus-eluting stent with a standard stent for coronary revascularization. N Engl J Med 2002; **346**(23): 1773–1780.

3. Moses JW, Leon MB, Popma JJ, et al. Sirolimus-eluting stents versus standard stents in patients with stenosis in a native coronary artery. N Engl J Med 2003; **349**(14): 1315–1323.

4. Stone GW, Ellis SG, Cox DA, et al. A polymer-based, paclitaxel-eluting stent in patients with coronary artery disease. N Engl J Med 2004; **350**(3): 221–231.

5. Rogers C, Edelman ER. Pushing drug-eluting stents into uncharted territory: simpler than you think—more complex than you imagine. Circulation 2006; **113**(19): 2262–2265.

6. Morice MC, Colombo A, Meier B, et al. Sirolimus- vs paclitaxel-eluting stents in de novo coronary artery lesions: the REALITY trial: A randomized controlled trial. JAMA 2006; **295**(8): 895–904.

7. Windecker S, Remondino A, Eberli FR, et al. Sirolimus-eluting and paclitaxel-eluting stents for coronary revascularization. N Engl J Med 2005; **353**(7): 653–662.

8. Dibra A, Kastrati A, Mehilli J, et al. Paclitaxel-eluting or sirolimus-eluting stents to prevent restenosis in diabetic patients. N Engl J Med 2005; **353**(7): 663–670.

9. Mehilli J, Dibra A, Kastrati A, et al. Randomized trial of paclitaxel- and sirolimus-eluting stents in small coronary vessels. Eur Heart J 2006; **27**(3): 260–266.

10. Kastrati A, Mehilli J, von Beckerath N, et al. Sirolimus-eluting stent or paclitaxel-eluting stent vs balloon angioplasty for prevention of recurrences in patients with coronary in-stent restenosis: A randomized controlled trial. JAMA 2005; **293**(2): 165–171.

11. Stone GW, Ellis SG, Cannon L, et al. Comparison of a polymer-based paclitaxel-eluting stent with a bare metal stent in patients with complex coronary artery disease: a randomized controlled trial. JAMA 2005; **294**(10): 1215–1223.

12. Lemos PA, Serruys PW, van Domburg RT, et al. Unrestricted utilization of sirolimus-eluting stents compared with conventional bare stent implantation in the "real world": the Rapamycin-Eluting Stent Evaluated At Rotterdam Cardiology Hospital (RESEARCH) registry. Circulation 2004; **109**(2): 190–195.

13. Mikhail GW, Airoldi F, Tavano D, et al. The use of drug eluting stents in single and multivessel disease: results from a single centre experience. Heart 2004; **90**(9): 990–994.

14. Zahn R, Hamm CW, Schneider S, et al. Incidence and predictors of target vessel revascularization and clinical event rates of the sirolimus-eluting coronary stent (results from the prospective multicenter German Cypher Stent Registry). Am J Cardiol 2005; **95**(11): 1302–1308.

15. Urban P, Gershlick AH, Guagliumi G, et al. Safety of coronary sirolimus-eluting stents in daily clinical practice: one-year follow-up of the e-Cypher registry. Circulation 2006; **113**(11): 1434–1441.

16. Abizaid A, Chan C, Lim YT, *et al.* Twelve-month outcomes with a paclitaxel-eluting stent transitioning from controlled trials to clinical practice (the WISDOM Registry). Am J Cardiol 2006; **98**(8): 1028–1032.

17. Russell ME, Friedman MI, Mascioli SR, Stolz LE. Off-label use: An industry perspective on expanding use beyond approved indications. J Interv Cardiol 2006; **19**(5): 432–438.

18. Lemos PA, Hoye A, Goedhart D, *et al.* Clinical, angiographic, and procedural predictors of angiographic restenosis after sirolimus-eluting stent implantation in complex patients: an evaluation from the Rapamycin-Eluting Stent Evaluated At Rotterdam Cardiology Hospital (RESEARCH) study. Circulation 2004; **109**(11): 1366–1370.

19. Zahn R, Hamm CW, Schneider S, *et al.* Predictors of death or myocardial infarction during follow-up after coronary stenting with the sirolimus-eluting stent. Results from the prospective multicenter German Cypher Stent Registry. Am Heart J 2006; **152**(6): 1146–1152.

20. Williams DO, Abbott JD, Kip KE. Outcomes of 6906 patients undergoing percutaneous coronary intervention in the era of drug-eluting stents: report of the DEScover Registry. Circulation 2006; **114**(20): 2154–2162.

21. Kamath KR, Barry JJ, Miller KM. The Taxus drug-eluting stent: a new paradigm in controlled drug delivery. Adv Drug Deliv Rev 2006; **58**(3): 412–436.

22. Lemos PA, Saia F, Ligthart JM, *et al.* Coronary restenosis after sirolimus-eluting stent implantation: morphological description and mechanistic analysis from a consecutive series of cases. Circulation 2003; **108**(3): 257–260.

23. Costa MA, Simon DI. Molecular basis of restenosis and drug-eluting stents. Circulation 2005; **111**(17): 2257–2273.

24. Huang S, Houghton PJ. Mechanisms of resistance to rapamycins. Drug Resist Updat 2001; **4**(6):378–391.

25. Yusuf RZ, Duan Z, Lamendola DE, Penson RT, Seiden MV. Paclitaxel resistance: molecular mechanisms and pharmacologic manipulation. Curr Cancer Drug Targets 2003; **3**(1): 1–19.

26. Orr GA, Verdier-Pinard P, McDaid H, *et al.* Mechanisms of Taxol resistance related to microtubules. Oncogene 2003; **22**(47): 7280–7295.

27. Cabral FR. Isolation of Chinese hamster ovary cell mutants requiring the continuous presence of taxol for cell division. J Cell Biol 1983; **97**(1): 22–29.

28. Koster R, Vieluf D, Kiehn M, *et al.* Nickel and molybdenum contact allergies in patients with coronary in-stent restenosis. Lancet 2000; **356**(9245): 1895–1897.

29. Nebeker JR, Virmani R, Bennett CL, *et al.* Hypersensitivity cases associated with drug-eluting coronary stents: a review of available cases from the Research on Adverse Drug Events and Reports (RADAR) project. J Am Coll Cardiol 2006; **47**(1): 175–181.

30. Virmani R, Guagliumi G, Farb A, *et al.* Localized hypersensitivity and late coronary thrombosis secondary to a sirolimus-eluting stent: should we be cautious? Circulation 2004; **109**(6):701–705.

31. Azarbal B, Currier JW. Allergic reactions after the implantation of drug-eluting stents: is it the pill or the polymer? J Am Coll Cardiol 2006; **47**(1):182–183.

32. Hong MK, Mintz GS, Lee CW, *et al.* Intravascular ultrasound predictors of angiographic restenosis after sirolimus-eluting stent implantation. Eur Heart J 2006; **27**(11): 1305–1310.

33. Mintz GS, Weissman NJ. Intravascular ultrasound in the drug-eluting stent era. J Am Coll Cardiol 2006; **48**(3): 421–429.

34. Sonoda S, Morino Y, Ako J, *et al.* Impact of final stent dimensions on long-term results following sirolimus-eluting stent implantation: serial intravascular ultrasound analysis from the sirius trial. J Am Coll Cardiol 2004; **43**(11): 1959–1963.

35. Fujii K, Mintz GS, Kobayashi Y, *et al.* Contribution of stent underexpansion to recurrence after sirolimus-eluting stent implantation for in-stent restenosis. Circulation 2004; **109**(9): 1085–1088.

36. Takebayashi H, Mintz GS, Carlier, SG, *et al.* Nonuniform strut distribution correlates with more neointimal hyperplasia after sirolimus-eluting stent implantation. Circulation 2004; **110**(22): 3430–3434.

37. Umeda H, Gochi T, Iwase M, *et al.* Frequency, predictors and outcome of stent fracture after sirolimus-eluting stent implantation. Int J Cardiol 2009; **133**(3): 321–326.

38. Sianos G, Hofma S, Ligthart JM, *et al.* Stent fracture and restenosis in the drug-eluting stent era. Catheter Cardiovasc Interv. 2004; **61**(1): 111–116.

39. Halkin A, Carlier S, Leon MB. Late incomplete lesion coverage following Cypher stent deployment for diffuse right coronary artery stenosis. Heart. 2004; **90**(8): e45.

40. Hoye A, Iakovou I, Ge L, *et al.* Long-term outcomes after stenting of bifurcation lesions with the "crush" technique: predictors of an adverse outcome. J Am Coll Cardiol 2006; **47**(10): 1949–1958.

41. Hamilos MI, Papafaklis MI, Ligthart JM, *et al.* Stent fracture and restenosis of a paclitaxel-eluting stent. Hellenic J Cardiol 2005; **46**(6): 439–442.

42. Shaikh F, Maddikunta R, Djelmami-Hani M, *et al.* Stent fracture, an incidental finding or a significant marker of clinical in-stent restenosis? Catheter Cardiovasc Interv. 2008; **71**(5): 614–618.

43. Yamada KP, Koizumi T, Yamaguchi H, *et al.* Serial angiographic and intravascular ultrasound analysis of late stent strut fracture of sirolimus-eluting stents in native coronary arteries. Int J Cardiol 2008; **130**(2): 255–259.

44. Saia F, Lemos PA, Arampatzis CA, *et al.* Clinical and angiographic outcomes after overdilatation of under-sized sirolimus-eluting stents with largely oversized balloons: an observational study. Catheter Cardiovasc Interv. 2004; **61**(4): 455–460.

45. Iakovou I, Stankovic G, Montorfano M, *et al.* Is over-dilatation of 3.0 mm sirolimus-eluting stent associated with a higher restenosis rate? Catheter Cardiovasc Interv. 2005; **64**(2): 129–133.

46. Balakrishnan B, Tzafriri AR, Seifert P, *et al.* Strut position, blood flow, and drug deposition: implications for single and overlapping drug-eluting stents. Circulation 2005; **111**(22): 2958–2965.

47. Hwang CW, Levin AD, Jonas M, *et al.* Thrombosis modulates arterial drug distribution for drug-eluting stents. Circulation 2005; **111**(13): 1619–1626.

48. Schampaert E, Cohen EA, Schluter M, *et al.* The Canadian study of the sirolimus-eluting stent in the treatment of patients with long de novo lesions in small native coronary arteries (C-SIRIUS). J Am Coll Cardiol 2004; **43**(6): 1110–1115.

49. Schofer J, Schluter M, Gershlick AH, *et al.* Sirolimus-eluting stents for treatment of patients with long athero-sclerotic lesions in small coronary arteries: double-blind, randomised controlled trial (E-SIRIUS). Lancet. 2003; **362**(9390): 1093–1099.

50. Kereiakes DJ, Wang H, Popma JJ, *et al.* Periprocedural and late consequences of overlapping Cypher sirolimus-eluting stents: pooled analysis of five clinical trials. J Am Coll Cardiol 2006; **48**(1): 21–31.

51. Tanabe K, Hoye A, Lemos PA, *et al.* Restenosis rates following bifurcation stenting with sirolimus-eluting stents for de novo narrowings. Am J Cardiol 2004; **94**(1): 115–118.

52. Colombo A, Moses JW, Morice MC, *et al.* Randomized study to evaluate sirolimus-eluting stents implanted at coronary bifurcation lesions. Circulation 2004; **109**(10): 1244–1249.

53. Iakovou I, Ge L, Colombo A. Contemporary stent treatment of coronary bifurcations. J Am Coll Cardiol 2005; **46**(8): 1446–1455.

54. Ge L, Airoldi F, Iakovou I, Cosgrave J, Michev I, Sangiorgi GM, Montorfano M, Chieffo A, Carlino M, Corvaja N, *et al.* Clinical and angiographic outcome after implantation of drug-eluting stents in bifurcation lesions with the crush stent technique: importance of final kissing balloon post-dilation. J Am Coll Cardiol 2005; **46**(4): 613–620.

55. Costa MA, Angiolillo DJ, Tannenbaum M, *et al.* Impact of stent deployment procedural factors on long-term effectiveness and safety of sirolimus-eluting stents (final results of the multicenter prospective STLLR trial). Am J Cardiol 2008; **101**(12): 1704–1711.

56. Berenguer A, Mainar V, Bordes P, *et al.* Incidence and predictors of restenosis after sirolimus-eluting stent implantation in high-risk patients. Am Heart J 2005; **150**(3): 536–542.

57. Kastrati A, Dibra A, Mehilli J, *et al.* Predictive factors of restenosis after coronary implantation of sirolimus- or paclitaxel-eluting stents. Circulation 2006; **113**(19): 2293–2300.

58. Lee CW, Park DW, Lee BK, *et al.* Predictors of restenosis after placement of drug-eluting stents in one or more coronary arteries. Am J Cardiol 2006; **97**(4): 506–511.

59. Roy P, Raya V, Okabe T, *et al.* Clinical correlates of restenosis following coronary implantation of drug-eluting stents. J Am Coll Cardiol 2007; **49**(Issue 9 Suppl B): 4B.

60. Corbett SJ, Cosgrave J, Melzi G, *et al.* Clinical, angiographic and procedural predictors of angiographic restenosis after drug-eluting stent implantation. Circulation 2006; **114**(18. Supplement): II-688.

61. Kastrati A, Schomig A, Elezi S, *et al.* Predictive factors of restenosis after coronary stent placement. J Am Coll Cardiol 1997; **30**(6): 1428–1436.

62. Cutlip DE, Chauhan MS, Baim DS, *et al.* Clinical restenosis after coronary stenting: perspectives from multicenter clinical trials. J Am Coll Cardiol 2002; **40**(12): 2082–2089.

63. Cutlip DE, Chhabra AG, Baim DS, *et al.* Beyond restenosis: five-year clinical outcomes from second-generation coronary stent trials. Circulation 2004; **110**(10): 1226–1230.

64. Popma JJ, Leon MB, Moses JW, *et al.* Quantitative assessment of angiographic restenosis after sirolimus-eluting stent implantation in native coronary arteries. Circulation 2004; **110**(25): 3773–3780.

65. Colombo A, Orlic D, Stankovic G, *et al.* Preliminary observations regarding angiographic pattern of restenosis after rapamycin-eluting stent implantation. Circulation 2003; **107**(17): 2178–2180.

66. Iakovou I, Schmidt T, Ge L, *et al.* Angiographic patterns of restenosis after paclitaxel-eluting stent implantation. J Am Coll Cardiol 2005; **45**(5): 805–806.

67. Corbett SJ, Cosgrave J, Melzi G, *et al.* Patterns of restenosis after drug-eluting stent implantation: Insights from a contemporary and comparative analysis of sirolimus- and paclitaxel-eluting stents. Eur Heart J 2006; **27**(19): 2330–2337.

68. Park CB, Hong MK, Kim YH, *et al.* Comparison of angiographic patterns of in-stent restenosis between

sirolimus- and paclitaxel-eluting stent. Circulation 2006; **114**(18, Supplement): II-642.

69. Mehran R, Dangas G, Abizaid AS, et al. Angiographic patterns of in-stent restenosis: classification and implications for long-term outcome. Circulation 1999; **100**(18): 1872–1878.

70. Cosgrave J, Melzi G, Biondi-Zoccai GG, et al. Drug-eluting stent restenosis the pattern predicts the outcome. J Am Coll Cardiol 2006; **47**(12): 2399–2404.

71. Sousa JE, Costa MA, Abizaid A, et al. Four-year angiographic and intravascular ultrasound follow-up of patients treated with sirolimus-eluting stents. Circulation 2005; **111**(18): 2326–2329.

72. Fajadet J, Morice MC, Bode C, et al. Maintenance of long-term clinical benefit with sirolimus-eluting coronary stents: three-year results of the RAVEL trial. Circulation 2005; **111**(8): 1040–1044.

73. Weisz G, Leon MB, Holmes DR, et al. Two-year outcomes after sirolimus-eluting stent implantation: results from the Sirolimus-Eluting Stent in de Novo Native Coronary Lesions (SIRIUS) trial. J Am Coll Cardiol 2006; **47**(7): 1350–1355.

74. Carter AJ, Aggarwal M, Kopia GA, et al. Long-term effects of polymer-based, slow-release, sirolimus-eluting stents in a porcine coronary model. Cardiovasc Res 2004; **63**(4): 617–624.

75. Farb A, Heller PF, Shroff S, Cheng L, Kolodgie FD, Carter AJ, Scott DS, Froehlich J, Virmani R. Pathological analysis of local delivery of paclitaxel via a polymer-coated stent. Circulation 2001; **104**(4): 473–479.

76. Kimura T, Yokoi H, Nakagawa Y, et al. Three-year follow-up after implantation of metallic coronary-artery stents. N Engl J Med 1996; **334**(9): 561–566.

77. Kimura T, Abe K, Shizuta S, Odashiro K, et al. Long-term clinical and angiographic follow-up after coronary stent placement in native coronary arteries. Circulation 2002; **105**(25): 2986–2991.

78. Asakura M, Ueda Y, Nanto S, et al. Remodeling of in-stent neointima, which became thinner and transparent over 3 years: serial angiographic and angioscopic follow-up. Circulation 1998; **97**(20): 2003–2006.

79. Kuroda N, Kobayashi Y, Nameki M, et al. Intimal hyperplasia regression from 6 to 12 months after stenting. Am J Cardiol 2002; **89**(7): 869–872.

80. Farb A, Sangiorgi G, Carter AJ, et al. Pathology of acute and chronic coronary stenting in humans. Circulation 1999; **99**(1): 44–52.

81. Farb A, Kolodgie FD, Hwang JY, et al. Extracellular matrix changes in stented human coronary arteries. Circulation 2004; **110**(8): 940–947.

82. Wessely R, Kastrati A, Schomig A. Late restenosis in patients receiving a polymer-coated sirolimus-eluting stent. Ann Intern Med 2005; **143**(5): 392–394.

83. Valgimigli M, Malagutti P, van Mieghem CA, et al. Persistence of neointimal growth 12 months after intervention and occurrence of delayed restenosis in patients with left main coronary artery disease treated with drug-eluting stents. J Am Coll Cardiol 2006; **47**(7): 1491–1494.

84. Aoki J, Abizaid A, Ong AT, et al. Serial assessment of tissue growth inside and outside the stent after implantation of drug-eluting stent in clinical trials. Does delayed neointimal growth exist? Eurointervention 2005; **1**(3): 253–255.

85. Aoki J, Colombo A, Dudek D, et al. Peristent remodeling and neointimal suppression 2 years after polymer-based, paclitaxel-eluting stent implantation: insights from serial intravascular ultrasound analysis in the TAXUS II study. Circulation 2005; **112**(25): 3876–3883.

86. Aoki J, Abizaid AC, Serruys PW, et al. Evaluation of four-year coronary artery response after sirolimus-eluting stent implantation using serial quantitative intravascular ultrasound and computer-assisted grayscale value analysis for plaque composition in event-free patients. J Am Coll Cardiol 2005; **46**(9): 1670–1676.

87. Lemos PA, van Mieghem CA, Arampatzis CA, et al. Post-sirolimus-eluting stent restenosis treated with repeat percutaneous intervention: late angiographic and clinical outcomes. Circulation 2004; **109**(21): 2500–2502.

88. Alfonso F, Perez-Vizcayno MJ, Hernandez R, et al. A randomized comparison of sirolimus-eluting stent with balloon angioplasty in patients with in-stent restenosis: results of the Restenosis Intrastent: Balloon Angioplasty Versus Elective Sirolimus-Eluting Stenting (RIBS-II) trial. J Am Coll Cardiol 2006; **47**(11): 2152–2160.

89. Holmes DR, Jr., Teirstein P, Satler L, et al. Sirolimus-eluting stents vs vascular brachytherapy for in-stent restenosis within bare-metal stents: the SISR randomized trial. Jama. 2006; **295**(11): 1264–1273.

90. Stone GW, Ellis SG, O'Shaughnessy CD, et al. Paclitaxel-eluting stents vs vascular brachytherapy for in-stent restenosis within bare-metal stents: the TAXUS V ISR randomized trial. JAMA 2006; **295**(11): 1253–1263.

91. Kim YH, Lee BK, Park DW, et al. Comparison with conventional therapies of repeated sirolimus-eluting stent implantation for the treatment of drug-eluting coronary stent restenosis. Am J Cardiol 2006; **98**(11): 1451–1454.

92. Torguson R, Sabate M, Deible R, et al. Intravascular brachytherapy versus drug-eluting stents for the treatment of patients with drug-eluting stent restenosis. Am J Cardiol 2006; **98**(10): 1340–1344.

93. Mishkel GJ, Moore AL, Markwell S, et al. Long-term outcomes after management of restenosis or thrombosis

of drug-eluting stents. J Am Coll Cardiol 2007; **49**(2): 181–184.

94. Solinas E, Kirtane A, Dangas G, *et al.* Long term (one year) follow-up after treatment of drug-eluting stent restenosis (DES-ISR) with repeat DES: to switch or not to switch? *J* Am Coll Cardiol 2007; **49**(Issue 9, Suppl B): 26B.

95. Cosgrave J, Melzi G, Corbett S, *et al.* Repeated drug-eluting stent implantation for drug-eluting stent restenosis: the same or a different stent. Am Heart J 2007; **153**(3): 354–359.

96. Garg S, Smith K, Torguson R, *et al.* Treatment of drug-eluting stent restenosis with the same versus different drug-eluting stent. Catheter Cardiovasc Interv 2007; **70**(1):9–14.

97. Costa MA. Treatment of drug-eluting stent restenosis. Am Heart J 2007; **153**(4): 447–449.

98. Aoki J, Nakazawa G, Tanabe K, *et al.* Incidence and clinical impact of coronary stent fracture after sirolimus-eluting stent implantation. Catheter Cardiovasc Interv 2007, **69**(3): 380–386.

Answers

1. E
2. D
3. C
4. E

CHAPTER 31

Renal Insufficiency and the Impact of Contrast Agents

Carlo Briguori

Clinica Mediterranea, Naples, and "Vita e Salute" University School of Medicine, Milan, Italy

The National Kidney Foundation defines chronic kidney disease (CKD) as either (1) kidney damage for ≥3 months (confirmed by kidney biopsy or markers of kidney damage, with or without a decrease in glomerular filtration rate (GFR), or (2) GFR < 60 mL/min/1.73 m^2 for ≥3 months, with or without kidney damage [1]. The four-variable Modification of Diet in Renal Disease equations (MDRD) equation is the preferred method for estimating GFR, because it does not rely on body weight [2]. This equation is:

$$eGFR = 186.3 \left(\text{serum creatinine}^{-1.154} \right) \times \left(\text{age}^{-0.203} \right)$$

and calculated values are multiplied by 0.742 for women and by 1.21 for black patients.

Other serum markers, such as cystatine C, may be helpful to assess renal function [3] but are not yet used in routine practice.

The prevalence of coronary artery disease (CAD) in CKD patients is high and is a major cause of morbidity and mortality [4]. Revascularization in patients with CKD by either percutaneous and surgical approaches is gravated by an higher rate of complications than in patients without CKD [4–13]. Contrast nephropathy represents one of the most common complications in this subset of patients.

Interventional Cardiology, First Edition. Edited by Carlo Di Mario, George D. Dangas, Peter Barlis.
© 2010 Blackwell Publishing Ltd. Published 2010 by Blackwell Publishing Ltd.

Contrast-induced Nephropathy (CIN)

CIN accounts for 10% of all causes of hospital-acquired renal failure [14–16]. CIN causes a prolongation of hospital stay and represents a powerful predictor of poor early and late outcome. Various cut-off criteria have been proposed to identify a clinically relevant renal function deterioration following contrast agent exposure, ranging from an increase in the serum creatinine concentration at 48 hours ≥25%, ≥50%, ≥0.3 mg/dl or ≥0.5 mg/dl of the baseline value. An increase ≥25% and/or ≥0.3 mg/dl are generally accepted as the recommended threshold [17]. Risk factors for CIN are: pre-existing chronic kidney disease, diabetes mellitus, high volume of contrast media, multiple myeloma, heart failure or other cause of reduced renal perfusion. The risk score proposed by Mehran *et al.* [18] is simple to calculate and very useful for individual patient risk assessment (Figure 31.1). The mechanisms by which CIN occurs are complex and not well understood. It is, however, widely held that a combination of various mechanisms (namely hemodynamic ,toxic, and osmotic) need to act in concert to cause CIN (Figure 31.2) [19]. The deeper portion of the outer medulla, which is particularly exposed to hypoxic damage, is the kidney region where contrast nephrotoxicity take place. Hypoxia derives mainly from decrease in renal medullary flow. Furthermore, contrast media promote reactive oxygen species generation.

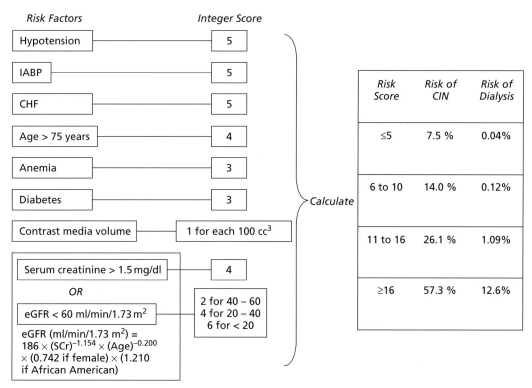

Figure 31.1. Scheme to define CIN risk score. CHF = congestive heart failure classes III–IV by the New York Heart Association classification and/or history of pulmonary edema. eGFR = estimated glomerular filtration rate by Modification of Diet in Renal Disease formula. Anemia: baseline hematocrit value <39% for men and <36% for women. Hypotension: systolic blood pressure <80 mm Hg for at least 1 h requiring inotropic support with medications or intraaortic balloon pump (IABP) within 24 h periprocedurally. Adapted with permission from J Am Coll Cardiol 2004; **44**: 1393–9.

Oxygen radicals are highly reactive and may directly damage renal endothelial-epithelial cells or may induce renal microvessel constriction (e.g. via endothelin-A receptor activation). Contrast media augments fluid viscosity and the resistance to flow in renal tubules; the increase of renal interstitial pressure reduces both renal medullary flow and glomerular filtration rate and may lead to diminished renal perfusion (tubulo-glomerular feedback). Contrast osmolarity seems to have a role, but only if it is high (that is >1000 mOsm/kg of H_2O). In addition to the ischemic changes to the renal tubules, contrast media have a cytotoxic effect on renal tubular cells. Indeed, contrast media induce apoptosis of the tubular epithelial cells by the activation of the intrisinc or "mitochondrial" pathway. This effect seems to be time- and dose-dependent.

The optimal strategy to prevent CIN remains uncertain. At present, recommendations are periprocedural hydration, use of a low- or iso-osmolality contrast, and reduction of the contrast volume used. The use of N-acelytcysteine (NAC), although it is not part of the official recommendations, is also widely used [17]. The role of prophylactic renal replacement therapies (RRT), such as hemofiltration, is still on debate and anyway limited to patients at very high risk.

Volume Supplementation

Volume supplementation prevents CIN mostly via two different mechanisms: (1) the inhibition of arginine-vasopressine (via vagal inputs from the mechanoreceptors located at the atrial-venous junctions and by a direct effect of osmolality on the supra-aortic nuclei), and (2) the increase in

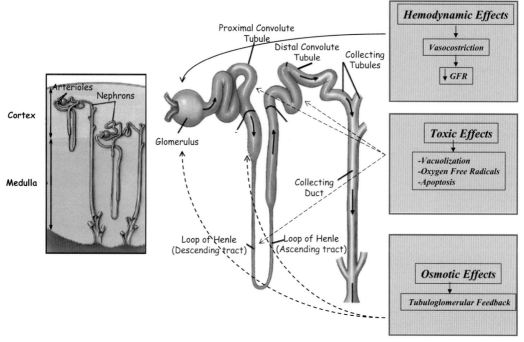

Figure 31.2. Scheme to nephron, the functional unit of the kidney. In the red box on the right are summarized the main pathophysiological mechanisms of CIN.

medullary perfusion and regional pO_2 [19]. The best modalities of hydration to prevent contrast nephropathy (type of solution, total volume, treatment onset before the procedure and duration after) are still unclear. Hydration with isotonic saline is beneficial and strongly recommended [17]. This should be started 12 hours prior to the procedure at a rate of 1 ml/kg/h and should be continued for 12 hours following the procedure. In patients with unstable hemodynamic conditions, where there is a particular concern regarding volume overload, at least 0.5 ml/kg/h of intravenous saline infusion should be received before contrast exposure. The postprocedure hydration target can be adjusted on the urine output which should remain above 150 ml/h. Some evidence, however, suggests that hydration with isotonic saline may be superior to one-half normal saline [20] and hydration with sodium bicarbonate has recently emerged as an effective strategy to prevent CIN [21]. The total volume of intravenous infusion is lower for sodium bicarbonate than for

normal saline. This supports the hypothesis that the mechanism of the effectiveness of sodium bicarbonate in preventing CIN is different from purevolume expansion. The higher amount of bicarbonate (HCO_3^-) in the proximal convoluted tubule may a) buffer the higher amount of H^+ due to cellular hypoxia and b) facilitate Na^+ reabsorption through the electrogenic Na^+/HCO_3^- co-trasposter [22]. Free-radical formation is promoted by an acidic environment typical of tubular urine but is inhibited by the higher pH of normal extracellular fluid [23]. It has been hypothesized that alkalinizing renal tubular fluid with bicarbonate [21] may reduce injury.

Type of Contrast Agents

Osmolality plays an important role in the pathophysiology of CIN [19]. It has been reported that low-osmolality (LOCM) and iso-osmolality (IOCM) contrast agent are less nephrotoxic than high osmolar contrast agents (HOCM). HOCM are highly charged and highly osmolar (approximately 1500 mOsm/kg of H_2O). Osmolality of LOCM is approximately 700–800 mOsm/kg of H_2O. Controversies exist on the lower nephrotoxicity of iso-osmolar contrast agents (that is, osmolality approximately 290 mOsm/kg of H_2O). In the NEPHRIC trial [24], enrolling 126 patients with diabetes mellitus and CKD, CIN occurred in 3% of patients in the IOCM group and 25% in the LOCM group (p = 0.003). This result however has not been confirmed in other observational [25] and randomized trials [26]. In the CARE trial 414 patients with an eGFR between 20 and 59 mL/min and scheduled for a percutaneous coronary procedure have been randomized to the LOCM iopamidol (796 mOsm/kg of H_2O) vs. the IOCM iodixanol (290 mOsm/kg of H_2O). No significant differences overall and in the subgroup of diabetic patients existed in the primary CIN end point (a postprocedural serum creatinine increase ≥0.5 mg/dL) or in the secondary CIN end points (a postprocedural serum creatinine increase ≥25% over baseline, a postdose eGFR decrease ≥25% and the mean peak change in serum creatinine >0.50 mg/dL). While early studies suggested a role for osmolality in the pathogenesis of CIN at high osmolalities (>1000 mOsm/kg of H_2O), it may be that either osmolality in the range of 290 to approximately 800 is not toxic to the kidney, or that for CM within this range of osmolality other characteristics of contrast media, such as viscosity, play a greater role in the development of CIN [27].

Volume of Contrast Agent

The use of a small volume of contrast dye and the avoidance of closely spaced repetitive studies is probably the single most important recommendation to prevent CIN [17]. Low volume has been variably defined as a total absolute volume <70 ml, <125 ml, <140 ml, or a volume adjusted for body weight of <5 ml/Kg (to a maximum of 300 ml) divided by the plasma creatinine concentration [28]. It has been suggested that using the iodine dose/glomerular filtration rate (I/GFR) ratio may be a more expedient way of improving risk assessment of CIN than the most common practice of estimating CM dose from body weight alone [29]. Other

chapters (Angiography, Multivessel, CTO, IVUS) illustrate some of the principles used to minimize contrast use. General recommendations include limitations of the diagnostic angiogram pre-PCI to few essential views, liberal use of staged procedures for complex multivessel disease, especially for urgent unstable patients for whom treatment should be limited to the culprit artery, injections limited to the minimum required to assess proper positioning and final result, filming the balloon during expansion or using fluoroscopic optimization of the stent visualization (stent "boost" modality) or using intravascular ultrasound in the intermediate phases to optimize stent expansion.

Pharmacological Therapy

The generation of reactive oxygen species has been considered an important pathophysiological cause of CIN [19]. In the last years many clinical studies have been conducted with the use of antioxidant compounds in an attempt to prevent CIN. The two most investigated drugs are (a) N-acetylcysteine (NAC) and (b) ascorbic acid.

NAC may prevent CIN by stopping direct oxidative tissue damage and also by improving renal hemodynamics [30–32]. The antioxidant effect of NAC seems to be dose-dependent [33,34]. Although not firmly recommended, NAC administration is suggested especially in high-risk patients [17]. Therefore, high dose of NAC seems to be necessary to prevent CIN expecially in case of high volume of contrast media [33]. Additional evidence of the effectiveness of an antioxidant strategy comes from the observation by Spargias *et al.* [35], who investigated the impact of ascorbic acid in preventing CIN. A combination of different antioxidant compounds was recently tested by Briguori *et al.* [36]. Consecutive patients with chronic kidney disease (eGFR < 40 ml/min/1.73 m²) were randomly assigned to prophylactic administration of (1) 0.9% saline infusion plus N-acetylcysteine (Saline plus NAC group; n = 111), (2) sodium bicarbonate infusion plus NAC (Bicarbonate plus NAC group; n = 108) and (3) 0.9% saline plus ascorbic acid plus NAC (Saline plus Ascorbic Acid plus NAC group; n = 107).

CIN occurred in 11/111 patients (9.9%) in the Saline plus NAC group, in 2/108 (1.9%) in the Bicarbonate plus NAC group (p = 0.019 vs. Saline plus NAC group) and in 11/107 patients (10.3%) in the Saline plus Ascorbic Acid plus NAC group (p = 1.00 vs. Saline plus NAC group). Therefore the combined prophylactic strategy of sodium bicarbonate plus NAC should be utilized to prevent CIN in patients at medium-to-high risk undergoing contrast exposure. The lack of favorable protective effect of the combination of ascorbic acid plus NAC as compared to NAC alone suggests additional and/or alternative mechanism(s) (other than antioxidant effect) which require further investigation. We may hypothesize that NAC and ascorbic acid work through similar pathways while the protective action of bicarbonate may be different in comparison to NAC and therefore additive.

Due to the potential role of focal renal vasoconstriction induced by contrast agents, numerous vasodilators drugs have been tested for prevention of CIN. Theophylline [37], nifedipine [38], adenosine [39], endothelin receptor antagonists [40], atrial natriuretic peptide [41], dopamine and fenoldopam [42–44] do not seem to be effective. Compelling data support that neither mannitol nor furosemide offer additional protection against radiocontrast-induced nephrotoxicity as compared with saline hydration alone in either diabetic or non-diabetic patients [45]. In the study by Solomon et al. [45] there were no beneficial effects of the osmotic diuretic mannitol when added to saline hydration in either diabetic and nondiabetic patients, and there was an actual exacerbation of contrast-induced renal dysfunction with the use of the loop diuretic furosemide with saline hydration [17].

Renal Replacement Therapy

Marenzi et al. [46] compared the effectiveness of hemofiltration, administered as prophylactic therapy in high-risk patients, against volume expansion with intravenous saline in 114 consecutive patients with CKD who required a coronary intervention. Hemofiltration (1000 mL/hour fluid replacement rate) began four to eight hours prior to the procedure, was interrupted during the procedure and resumed and continued for 18

to 24 hours after the procedure. Compared with intravenous saline, hemofiltration was associated with: (a) a lesser likelihood of the serum creatinine rising >25% (5% vs. 50%); (b) a lesser likelihood of requiring dialysis (3% vs. 25%), and (c) a lower in-house (2% vs. 14%) and one-year mortality (10% vs. 30%). It has been pointed out that, however, creatinine removal by the hemofiltration procedure can be sufficient to explain the decreased frequency of elevation in the serum creatinine. The control group had an unusually high incidence of acute renal failure, attributable to the excessive volume of contrast media used and, possibly, to the absence of optimal pharmacological prophylaxis. Patients in the hemofiltration group were cared for in an intensive care unit; their greater intensity of care relative to the control group may explain why hemofiltration was associated with improved short- and long-term survival (with the greatest benefit among patients with higher baseline plasma creatinine ($\geq$4 mg/dL [354 micromol/L]). Similar concerns have been rasied by another study suggesting that the advantage of hemofitration is observed only when it is perfomed pre and post contrast exposure. In contrast, hemofiltration performed only post-contrast exposure is not effective [47]. The applicability of these findings to current clinical practice is unclear. Hemofiltration is expensive, logistically cumbersome and associated with significant risks, its effectivess compared to other less expensive strategies is not well established so that this treatment modality should be reserved for patients who already have fairly advanced renal insufficiency [48]. Figure 31.3 depicts the approach proposed to prevent CIN based on current evidence.

Conclusions

The optimal strategy to prevent CIN remains uncertain. The guidelines [17] recommend (1) intravenous volume expansion with saline solution, (2) use of a low- or iso-osmolality contrast agents, and (3) limiting the volume of contrast agent. Although not firmly recommended, NAC administration is suggested especially in high-risk patients [17]. The combined prophylactic strategy

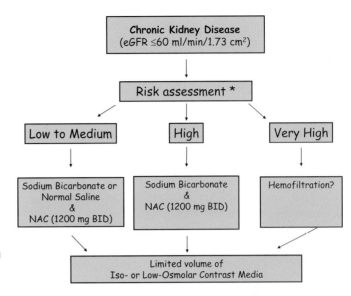

Figure 31.3. Flow chart of suggested preventive measures for CIN* according to the score proposed by Mehran *et al.* [18].

of volume supplementation by sodium bicarbonate plus NAC at high dose (1200 mg BID the day before and the day of the procedure) should be utilized to prevent CIN in patients at medium-to-high risk undergoing coronary or peripheral procedures [36]. Addional data are necessary to clarify the role of hemofiltration in the routine clinical practice.

Questions

1. **The following statements are true regarding contrast induced nephropathy?**
   A The incidence of CIN in the general population receiving contrast is less than 2%
   B In patients considered high risk (e.g., chronic renal failure, diabetes mellitus, chronic heart failure, elderly) the incidence can be as high as 20–30%
   C The total contrast volume used is a major modifiable risk factor for development of CIN.
   D All of the above

2. **Once dye-induced renal dysfunction develops, creatinine levels generally peak at ___ days and remain elevated for ___ days.**
   A 1 and 7–14
   B 2–3 and 7–14
   C 7 and 14–21
   D 4–5 and 7–14

3. **Which of the following statements regarding contrast agents is true?**
   A Low-osmolar agents result in less patient discomfort during internal mammary artery and peripheral angiography
   B Low-osmolar agents have lower iodine content
   C Nonionic agents have greater anticoagulant and antiplatelet activities in vitro
   D High-osmolar agents cause less acute renal failure among patients with baseline renal insufficiency

4. **Which of the following statements about adverse dye reactions is true?**
   A Patients with a previous history of an adverse dye reaction are at highest risk for a subsequent severe reaction
   B Previous anaphylaxis carries a recurrence rate of 40% without premedication.
   C Asthmatics, especially those with nasal polyps, are a high-risk group (6–9 fold risk compared to non-asthmatics)
   D Other predisposing conditions include dehydration, systemic illness, and preexisting heart failure
   E All of the above

5. **A 68-year-old diabetic male develops bronchospasm, laryngeal edema, and profound hypotension immediately after a single contrast injection. The most appropriate initial management of this patient is:**
   A Observation and cool compresses; oral benadryl and atropine (0.5–1.0 mg IV) as needed
   B IV fluids, Benadryl (50 mg IV), steroids (e.g. hydrocortisone 100 mg IV), centrally-acting antiemetics (e.g., Compazine 2 mg IV followed by a 25 mg rectal suppository), and atropine (0.5–2.0 mg for bradycardia or vasovagal reactions).
   C 0.1–0.5 cc of a 1 : 10,000 dilution subcutaneously every 5 minutes
   D 1–5 cc of a 1 : 10,000 dilution intravenously every 5 minutes
   E None of the above

References

1. K/DOQI clinical practice guidelines for chronic kidney disease: Evaluation, classification, and stratification. Am J Kidney Dis 2002; **39**: S1–266.
2. Levey AS, Bosch JP, Lewis JB, *et al.* A more accurate method to estimate glomerular filtration rate from serum creatinine: A new prediction equation. Modification of Diet in Renal Disease Study Group. Ann Intern Med 1999; **130**: 461–70.
3. Shlipak MG, Praught ML, Sarnak MJ. Update on cystatin C: New insights into the importance of mild kidney dysfunction. Curr Opin Nephrol Hypertens 2006; **15**: 270–275.
4. Levey AS, Beto JA, Coronado BE, *et al.* Controlling the epidemic of cardiovascular disease in chronic renal disease: What do we know? What do we need to learn? Where do we go from here? National Kidney Foundation Task Force on Cardiovascular Disease. Am J Kidney Dis 1998; **32**: 853–906.
5. Hillis GS, Croal BL, Buchan KG, *et al.* Renal function and outcome from coronary artery bypass grafting: impact on mortality after a 2.3-year follow-up. Circulation 2006; **113**: 1056–1062.
6. Rubenstein MH, Harrell LC, Sheynberg BV, *et al.* Are patients with renal failure good candidates for percutaneous coronary revascularization in the new device era? Circulation 2000; **102**: 2966–2972.
7. Cooper WA, O'Brien SM, Thourani VH, *et al.* Impact of renal dysfunction on outcomes of coronary artery bypass surgery: Results from the Society of Thoracic Surgeons National Adult Cardiac Database. Circulation 2006; **113**: 1063–1070.

8. Gruberg L, Weissman NJ, Waksman R, *et al.* Comparison of outcomes after percutaneous coronary revascularization with stents in patients with and without mild chronic renal insufficiency. Am J Cardiol 2002; **89**: 54–57.

9. Szczech LA, Reddan DN, Owen WF, *et al.* Differential survival after coronary revascularization procedures among patients with renal insufficiency. Kidney Int 2001; **60**: 292–299.

10. Herzog CA, Ma JZ, Collins AJ. Long-term outcome of dialysis patients in the United States with coronary revascularization procedures. Kidney Int 1999; **56**: 324–332.

11. Hemmelgarn BR, Southern D, Culleton BF, *et al.* Survival after coronary revascularization among patients with kidney disease. Circulation 2004; **110**: 1890–1895.

12. Aoki J, Ong AT, Hoye A, *et al.* Five year clinical effect of coronary stenting and coronary artery bypass grafting in renal insufficient patients with multivessel coronary artery disease: Insights from ARTS trial. Eur Heart J 2005; **26**: 1488–1493.

13. Lemos PA, Arampatzis CA, Hoye A, *et al.* Impact of baseline renal function on mortality after percutaneous coronary intervention with sirolimus-eluting stents or bare metal stents. Am J Cardiol 2005; **95**: 167–172.

14. Tepel M, Aspelin P, Lameire N. Contrast-induced nephropathy: a clinical and evidence-based approach. Circulation 2006; **113**: 1799–1806.

15. Gruberg L, Mehran R, Dangas G, *et al.* Acute renal failure requiring dialysis after percutaneous coronary interventions. Catheter Cardiovasc Interv 2001; **52**: 409–416.

16. McCullough PA, Wolyn R, Rocher LL, *et al.* Acute renal failure after coronary intervention: incidence, risk factors, and relationship to mortality. Am J Med 1997; **103**: 368–375.

17. Solomon R, Deray G. How to prevent contrast-induced nephropathy and manage risk patients: practical recommendations. Kidney Int Suppl 2006: S51–53.

18. Mehran R, Aymong ED, Nikolsky E, *et al.* A simple risk score for prediction of contrast-induced nephropathy after percutaneous coronary intervention: Development and initial validation. J Am Coll Cardiol 2004; **44**: 1393–1399.

19. Persson PB, Hansell P, Liss P. Pathophysiology of contrast medium-induced nephropathy. Kidney Int 2005; **68**: 14–22.

20. Mueller C, Buerkle G, Buettner HJ, *et al.* Prevention of contrast media-associated nephropathy: randomized comparison of 2 hydration regimens in 1620 patients undergoing coronary angioplasty. Arch Intern Med 2002; **162**: 329–336.

21. Merten GJ, Burgess WP, Gray LV, *et al.* Prevention of contrast-induced nephropathy with sodium bicarbonate: a randomized controlled trial. JAMA 2004; **291**: 2328–2334.

22. Boron WF. Acid-base transport by the renal proximal tubule. J Am Soc Nephrol 2006; **17**: 2368–2382.

23. Alpem R. Renal acidification mechanisms. In: Barry M. Brenner, ed. *Kidney*, WB Saunders, Philadelphia, PA, 2000: 455–519.

24. Aspelin P, Aubry P, Fransson SG, *et al.* Nephrotoxic effects in high-risk patients undergoing angiography. N Engl J Med 2003; **348**: 491–499.

25. Briguori C, Colombo A, Airoldi F, *et al.* Nephrotoxicity of low-osmolality versus iso-osmolality contrast agents: impact of N-acetylcysteine. Kidney Int 2005; **68**: 2250–2255.

26. Solomon RJ, Natarajan MK, Doucet S, *et al.* Cardiac Angiography in Renally Impaired Patients (CARE) study: a randomized double-blind trial of contrast-induced nephropathy in patients with chronic kidney disease. Circulation 2007; **115**: 3189–3196.

27. Solomon R. The role of osmolality in the incidence of contrast-induced nephropathy: A systematic review of angiographic contrast media in high risk patients. Kidney Int 2005; **68**: 2256–2263.

28. Cigarroa RG, Lange RA, Williams RH, *et al.* Dosing of contrast material to prevent contrast nephropathy in patients with renal disease. Am J Med 1989; **86**: 649–652.

29. Nyman U, Almen T, Aspelin P, *et al.* Contrast-medium-induced nephropathy correlated to the ratio between dose in gram iodine and estimated GFR in ml/min. Acta Radiol 2005; **46**: 830–842.

30. Tepel M, van der Giet M, Schwarzfeld C, *et al.* Prevention of radiographic-contrast-agent-induced reductions in renal function by acetylcysteine. N Engl J Med 2000; **343**: 180–184.

31. DiMari J, Megyesi J, Udvarhelyi N, *et al.* N-acetyl cysteine ameliorates ischemic renal failure. Am J Physiol 1997; **272**: F292–298.

32. Heyman SN, Goldfarb M, Shina A, *et al.* N-acetylcysteine ameliorates renal microcirculation: studies in rats. Kidney Int 2003; **63**: 634–641.

33. Briguori C, Colombo A, Violante A, *et al.* Standard vs. double dose of N-acetylcysteine to prevent contrast agent associated nephrotoxicity. Eur Heart J 2004; **25**: 206–211.

34. Marenzi G, Assanelli E, Marana I, *et al.* N-acetylcysteine and contrast-induced nephropathy in primary angioplasty. N Engl J Med 2006; **354**: 2773–2782.

35. Spargias K, Alexopoulos E, Kyrzopoulos S, *et al.* Ascorbic acid prevents contrast-mediated nephropathy

in patients with renal dysfunction undergoing coronary angiography or intervention. Circulation 2004; **110**: 2837–2842.

36. Briguori C, Airoldi F, D'Andrea D, *et al.* Renal Insufficiency Following Contrast Media Administration Trial (REMEDIAL): A randomized comparison of 3 preventive strategies. Circulation 2007; **115**: 1211–1217.

37. Katholi RE, Taylor GJ, McCann WP, *et al.* Nephrotoxicity from contrast media: attenuation with theophylline. Radiology 1995; **195**: 17–22.

38. Bakris GL, Burnett JC, Jr. A role for calcium in radio-contrast-induced reductions in renal hemodynamics. Kidney Int 1985; **27**: 465–468.

39. Pflueger A, Larson TS, Nath KA, *et al.* Role of adenosine in contrast media-induced acute renal failure in diabetes mellitus. Mayo Clin Proc 2000; **75**: 1275–1283.

40. Wang A, Holcslaw T, Bashore TM, *et al.* Exacerbation of radiocontrast nephrotoxicity by endothelin receptor antagonism. Kidney Int 2000; **57**: 1675–1680.

41. Kurnik BR, Allgren RL, Genter FC, *et al.* Prospective study of atrial natriuretic peptide for the prevention of radiocontrast-induced nephropathy. Am J Kidney Dis 1998; **31**: 674–680.

42. Stone GW, McCullough PA, Tumlin JA, *et al.* Fenoldopam mesylate for the prevention of contrast-induced nephropathy: A randomized controlled trial. JAMA 2003; **290**: 2284–2291.

43. Briguori C, Colombo A, Airoldi F, *et al.* N-Acetylcysteine versus fenoldopam mesylate to prevent contrast agent–associated nephrotoxicity. J Am Coll Cardiol 2004; **44**: 762–765.

44. Bakris GL, Lass NA, Glock D. Renal hemodynamics in radiocontrast medium-induced renal dysfunction: A role for dopamine-1 receptors. Kidney Int 1999; **56**: 206–210.

45. Solomon R, Werner C, Mann D, *et al.* Effects of saline, mannitol, and furosemide to prevent acute decreases in renal function induced by radiocontrast agents. N Engl J Med 1994; **331**: 1416–1420.

46. Marenzi G, Marana I, Lauri G, *et al.* The prevention of radiocontrast-agent-induced nephropathy by hemofil-tration. N Engl J Med 2003; **349**: 1333–1340.

47. Marenzi G, Lauri G, Campodonico J, *et al.* Comparison of two hemofiltration protocols for prevention of contrast-induced nephropathy in high-risk patients. Am J Med 2006; **119**: 155–162.

48. Klarenbach SW, Pannu N, Tonelli MA, *et al.* Cost-effectiveness of hemofiltration to prevent contrast nephropathy in patients with chronic kidney disease. Crit Care Med 2006; **34**: 1044–1051.

Answers

1. D

2. D—The time course of contrast nephropathy may vary significantly. Porter GA. Am J Cardiol 1989; **64**: 22E–26E.

3. A—In a large study of 337,647 patients, the five most frequent symptoms following intravenous contrast administration (nausea, urticaria, itching, heat sensation, vomiting) were reduced by low osmolar contrast agents. Low osmolar contrast media also result in less patient discomfort during internal mammary artery and peripheral angiography, and have similar iodine contents to high osmolar agents. In-vivo and in-vitro studies have demonstrated greater anticoagulant and antiplatelet activities (prolongation of PTT and clotting time; inhibition of platelet aggregation and degranulation; reduced time to thrombolysis) for ionic compared to nonionic contrast. In earlier prospective trials, ionic contrast was associated with fewer complications than nonionic contrast after PTCA. In one trial, ionic contrast reduced the risk of in-lab abrupt closure, and in others, ionic contrast was associated with a decreased incidence of no-reflow and recurrent ischemia. The EPIC trial demonstrated a decreased incidence of abrupt closure, Q-wave MI and death with ionic contrast compared to nonionic contrast in patients with recent MI, unstable angina, or high-risk lesion morphology suggesting that the presence of preexisting thrombus or hypercoagulable state contributes to the deleterious effects of nonionic agents. In contrast, two recent prospective randomized trials in patients with stable and unable angina showed no difference between ionic and nonionic contrast.

4. E—Despite excellent overall tolerance, contrast media can result in undesirable reactions, ranging from mild nausea to life-threatening anaphylaxis; overall mortality attributable to contrast agents in coronary angiography is 4–23 deaths per million patients. Patients with a previous history of an adverse dye reaction are at highest risk for a subsequent severe reaction; previous anaphylaxis carries a recurrence rate of 40% without premedication. Asthmatics, especially those with nasal polyps, represent another high-risk group (6–9 fold risk compared to non-asthmatics). Other predisposing conditions include dehydration, systemic illness, preexisting cardiac disease, and certain ethnic groups. Grossman W and Baim DS. *Cardiac Catheterization, Angiography and Intervention.* Fourth Edition.

5. D—Symptoms of severe contrast reactions include anaphylaxis (bronchospasm, laryngeal edema, and/or profound hypotension), which may occur immediately with a single contrast injection. Treatment consists of epinephrine (1–5 cc of 1 : 10,000 dilution IV repeated every 2–5 minutes) steroids (e.g. hydrocortisone 100 mg IV or solumedrol 125 mg IV), diphenhydramine (50 mg IV) and possible intubation. Bronchodilators (e.g. Albuterol aerosol 2.5 mg nebulized mist treatments every 1–2 hrs) might be of additional benefit. Prolonged (2–10 hours) infusions of epinephrine or neosynephrine may be necessary for intermittent hypotension.

32 CHAPTER 32

Coronary Artery Dissection and Perforation

Adriano Caixeta[1], Eugenia Nikolsky[1,2], Alexandra J. Lansky[1], Roxana Mehran[1], & George D. Dangas[1]

[1]Columbia University Medical Center, New York, NY, USA
[2]Rambam Health Care Campus, Heart Institute, Haifa, Israel

Coronary dissection and perforation are two of the most dreaded complications occurring in the catheterization laboratory and have been associated with a high rate of major adverse outcomes [1–5]. Although operator experience, equipment and device technology continually improve, major dissection, abrupt closure and arterial perforation remain the primary reasons for failure of percutaneous coronary intervention (PCI). These complications can result in abrupt vessel closure, myocardial infarction, need for urgent coronary artery bypass surgery, pericardial tamponade, and even death. As a result of improvements in PCI technique and equipment, primarily with the widespread use of coronary stents, the incidence of acute closure and the need for emergency revascularization have decreased significantly. Innovative percutaneous approaches to the management of coronary perforation have included microcoil vessel occlusion and the use of covered stents. The current review discusses the risk factors, recognition and contemporary approach of managing dissections and perforation in patients undergoing PCI.

Coronary Artery Dissection

Dissection Following PCI

Separation of the media by hemorrhage with or without an associated intimal tear is termed coronary artery dissection. During the pre-stent era, the incidence of abrupt closure traditionally ranged between 2% and 14%. For a series of patients between 1985 and 1993, the closure rate averaged 8.6% [6–10]. Because of improvements in PCI technique and equipment, primarily the widespread use of coronary stents, acute closure and the need for emergency coronary artery bypass surgery (CABG) have decreased significantly. In contemporary interventional practice, including the use of stents in patients with moderate to high risk acute coronary syndromes the incidence of abrupt vessel closure was only 0.2% [11].

Dissections have been classified by the National Heart, Lung, and Blood Institute (NHLBI) according to their angiographic appearance [12,13]. The modified NHLBI criteria defined dissection as angiographically detectable intimal or medial damage manifesting as a radiolucent area within the vessel or as an extravasation of contrast medium after an interventional procedure. These criteria were refined into a more detailed classification system (Table 32.1). During the angioplasty era, some studies have attempted to distinguish minor dissections from detrimental major ones. Major dissections are characterized by numerous

Interventional Cardiology, First Edition. Edited by Carlo Di Mario, George D. Dangas, Peter Barlis.
© 2010 Blackwell Publishing Ltd. Published 2010 by Blackwell Publishing Ltd.

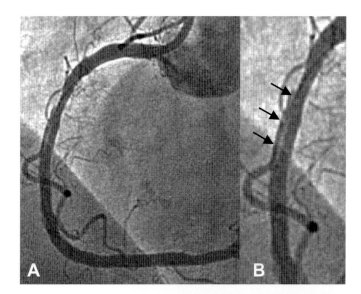

Figure 32.1. An example of type B dissection after balloon dilatation at right coronary artery (A). Notice the radiolucent parallel track at proximal and mid segments of the vessel (arrows) (B).

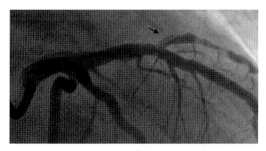

Figure 32.2. Type C dissection at diagonal branch after balloon dilatation. The arrow shows a focal and persistent extraluminal dye contrast.

Table 32.1. Morphologic classification of coronary artery dissection. Classified by the National Heart, Lung and Blood Institute (NHLBI) according to their angiographic appearance.

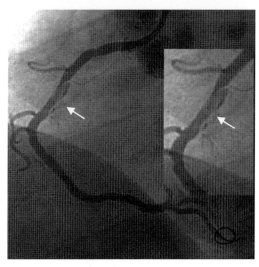

Figure 32.3. This illustration shows a type D dissection at right coronary artery after balloon dilatation for planned stent implantation. Despite the spiral dissection, there is no flow impairment.

Type A	Coronary dissection with only minor radiolucent areas within the coronary lumen without a reduction in coronary flow
Type B	Minimal or no dye persistence in the presence of parallel track or a double lumen separated by a radiolucent area during contrast injection
Type C	Dissection with persistent extraluminal dye after contrast injection
Type D	Spiral dissection
Type E	Dissection with new and filling defects
Type F	This dissection does not fit any of the above types A–E and is associated with impaired flow or total occlusion of the vessel

morphologic features, including (1) a linear intraluminal filling defect or luminal staining evident in 2 projections, (2) a linear filling defect extending greater than 20 mm, and (3) dissection types C to F according to NHLBI criteria [14] (Figures 32.1, 32.2, 32.3, 32.4, and 32.5). Major dissections create intraluminal filling defects of sufficient size to produce a reduction in luminal diameter of at least

50% and/or a reduction in distal coronary flow. Huber *et al.* demonstrated that abrupt closure, myocardial infarction, and bypass grafting occurred in fewer than 3% of patients with NHLBI type B dissections. In contrast, dissection types C to F were associated with complication rates between 12% and 37%. Persistent, extraluminal contrast, new persistent filling defects and spiral dissections portend adverse clinical outcomes.

The dissection can occur following balloon predilatation before the planned stent implantation, or even after stenting. The handling of

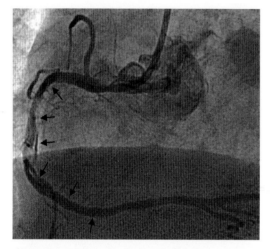

Figure 32.4. An example of a type E dissection. A spiral dissection at the right coronary artery after balloon angioplasty dilatation for stenting. Notice the extensive filling defects (arrows) with lumen narrowing at the mid portion of the artery.

such a complication depends on the severity of the dissection with potential strategies including, (1) stent implantation, (2) bypass surgery, or (3) medical treatment alone. The choice of stenting vs. conservative management or surgery is therefore made on a case-by-case basis. In general, in the vast majority of dissections necessitating treatment, stent implantation is the first choice.

Stent edge dissections are common since the junction between stent metal and reference segment tissue is a site of compliance mismatch. The treatment of coronary edge dissection with stent implantation depends on the combination of angiographic assessment, flow assessment, and signs or symptoms of ischemia. Minor dissections should not be treated unless they result in lumen compromise; the vast majority have sealed when imaged at follow-up. Intramural hematoma is a variant of dissection. By IVUS, intramural hematomas are typically hyperechoic and crescent shaped, with straightening of the internal elastic membrane (Figure 32.6). In general, an intramural hematoma should be treated because of the propensity for propagation and lumen compromise.

Guide Catheter-induced Dissection

The incidence of iatrogenic coronary artery dissection at the time of cardiac catheterization or PCI is not known. Catheter-induced dissection with retrograde extension to the aortic root is rare and has been estimated to occur in approximately 0.008% to 0.02% of diagnostic catheterizations and 0.06% to 0.07% of PCIs [15,16] (Figure 32.7). The natural

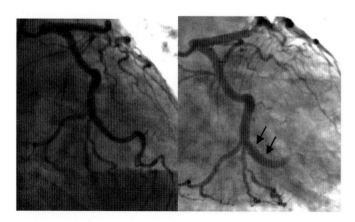

Figure 32.5. This figure illustrates mild disease at circumflex artery by angiogram. Diagnostic IVUS was performed to interrogate the plaque stenosis. During the procedure a type F dissection has been observed; notice the spiral dissection (arrow) associated with total occlusion of the vessel.

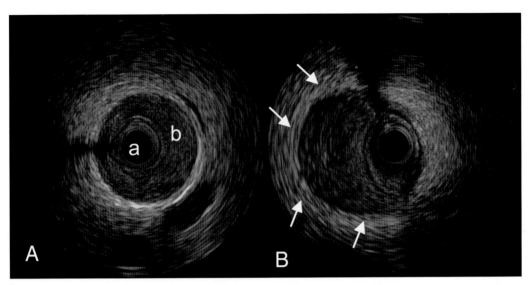

Figure 32.6. This is an example of intramural hematoma with true (a) and false (b) lumen by IVUS (Panel A). Panel B depicts how the false lumen with blood accumulation (arrows) caused true lumen compromise.

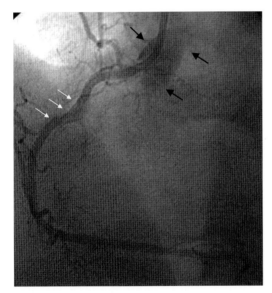

Figure 32.7. Catheter-induced dissection with retrograde extension of the dissection back to involve the aorta root (black arrows). Notice the spiral dissection with narrowing at the right coronary artery (white arrows).

history of catheter-induced coronary artery dissections is varied. In some cases, dissections lead to acute closure of the vessel with myocardial infarction [17]. In other circumstances, retrograde extension of the dissection back to involve the

aorta can occur [18,19], and in other cases, dissections of the coronary artery have been associated with persistently normal (TIMI-3) flow without ischemia, and have healed without any intervention [20]. Several factors are associated with increased risk for catheter-induced artery dissection: (1) left main disease, (2) the use of Amplatz-shaped catheters, (3) catheterization for acute myocardial infarction, (4) catheter manipulations, (5) vigorous contrast media injection, (6) deep intubations of the catheter within the coronary artery, (7) variant anatomy of the coronary ostia, and (8) vigorous, deep inspiration [21]. The management of catheter-induced coronary dissection depends on the patency of the distal vessel and the extent of propagation of the dissection. In general, in the presence of myocardial ischemia or acute closure, PCI or CABG is mandated to prevent AMI. There have been reports of successful outcomes with coronary artery stenting [22] and CABG [17,23]. Nevertheless, in the absence of ischemia the therapeutic options are less clear. Conservative management of guide catheter-induced coronary artery dissection has met with successful outcomes in selected patients [17,20]. The choice of stenting vs. conservative management is therefore made on a case-by-case basis.

Perforation and Rupture

Risk Factors for Coronary Perforation

Coronary artery perforation represents a disruption of the vessel wall through the intima, media, and adventitia. Coronary perforation may engender localized pseudoaneurysm, perivascular hematoma, arterioventricular fistula, or hemopericardium. Risk factors for coronary perforation during standard PCI can be classified as (1) *patient-related*, (2) *procedure-related*, and (3) *device- related* risk factors (Table 32.2).

Patient-related

Patient characteristics that have been associated with a risk of perforation include age [1], female gender [1,24], and history of prior CABG [24]. Several studies have shown this [1,25]. In a multicenter study by Ellis *et al.* [1], patients who developed perforation were almost 10 years older than those who had no perforation. In addition, women represented 46% of the patients with perforation compared with 16% of women among patients without this complication.

Procedure-related

The use of oversized compliant balloons coupled with relatively high inflation pressure to achieve full stent expansion and minimize residual stenosis after stent implantation may cause vessel wall perforation [1,26,27]. Several mechanisms may be involved, including overstretching of the most compliant coronary artery segment, a high-pressure jet due to balloon rupture, and outward pushing of a stent strut through the vessel wall. Procedural success and complication rates as a function of balloon-to-vessel ratio and high inflation pressure have been reported in numerous studies. In a study by Tobis *et al.* [27], the use of a high balloon-to-vessel ratio (1.2:1) with a mean pressure of 12 atm for the treatment of coronary stenosis in 60 patients was associated with a mean final percent stenosis of −8% with 1 case of a coronary rupture. Conversely, usage of a similar balloon-to-vessel ratio with a higher inflation pressure (a mean of 15 atm), applied in the next 300 patients yielded a slight improvement in the final percent stenosis (mean −10%), but at the expense of an increase in the incidence of vessel rupture and major dissection (3.4%). Finally, in a different subgroup, usage of a smaller balloon-to-vessel ratio of only 1.0 but with a higher mean pressure (16 atm), applied in 162 patients, yielded a percent residual stenosis of 1% with a rate of coronary rupture reduced to 0.7%. Similarly, in a series by Ellis *et al.* [1] the mean balloon-to-artery ratio in patients treated with plain balloon angioplasty was significantly higher in those who developed coronary perforation compared with those who did not (1.19 ± 0.17 vs. 0.92 ± 0.16, $p = 0.03$). The same findings were reported by Stankovic *et al.* [28], where a high balloon-to-artery ratio was associated with a 7.6-fold increase in the odds of coronary perforation.

Vessel determinants associated with coronary rupture include lesion severity with American College of Cardiology/American Heart Association (ACC/AHA) type B or C lesions, and the presence of a more highly calcified lesion has also been associated with coronary rupture [24,29,30] (Figure 32.8). Of note, PCI for chronic total occlusions is associated with an increased risk as well [26] (Figures 32.9, 32.10).

Device-related

Coronary perforation may be caused by the guiding catheter, balloon rupture, guidewire, IVUS catheter, embolic protection device, and atheroablative devices [28,31,32]. Dippel *et al.* [33] reported that, of more than 6,000 interventions, ablative procedures were accorded a 6.8-fold risk of perforation. In addition, the perforations with

Table 32.2. Risk factors for coronary perforation.

Patient-related	Procedure-related	Device-related
Female gender	High balloon/ stent-to-artery ratio	Stiff wire
Older age	High inflation pressure	Hydrophilic-coated wire
	Extremely distal location of the guidewire	Cutting balloon
		Atheroablative devices
		IVUS in the false lumen

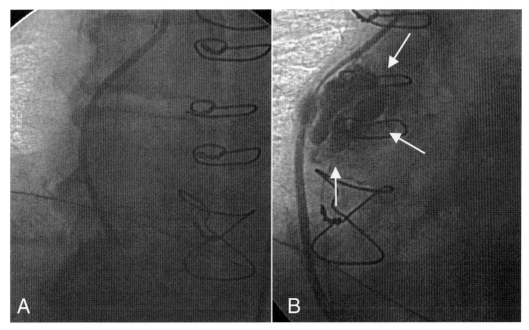

Figure 32.8. (Panel A) An example of type III perforation arrows (Panel B) post-balloon dilatation of a small saphenous vein graft to right coronary artery.

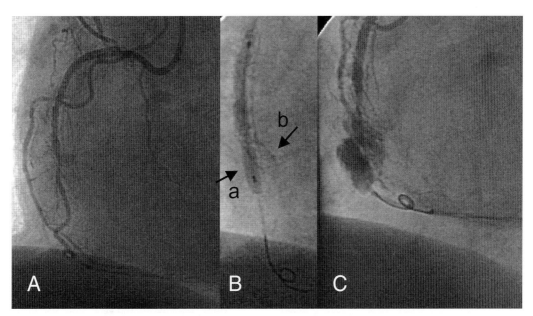

Figure 32.9. An example of type III perforation. This patient underwent a previous stent implantation in the mid right coronary artery. Follow-up catheterization showed restenosis with chronic total occlusion (Panel A). Panel B shows that the guidewire has been crossed and the balloon has been inflated at the origin of the acute marginal branch (a); the distal portion of the stent is shown in Panel B and arrow b. Notice the perforation with contrast extravasation in Panel C.

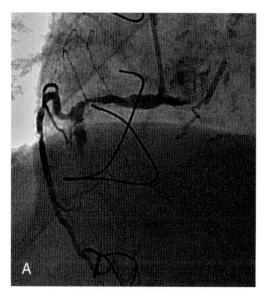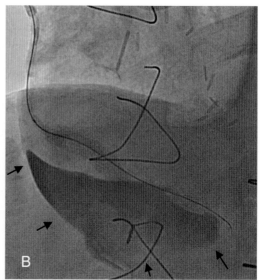

Figure 32.10. This illustration shows a chronic total occlusion at mid right coronary artery (Panel A). Failed attempts leads to vessel dissection and perforation type III with pericardial effusion (Panel B).

these technologies were often Ellis type III. Recently, stiffer wires for chronic total occlusion procedures have been developed to dramatically enhance the ability to cross the lesions. Vessel perforation has become particularly important with the introduction of stiff wires for penetrating the proximal and distal caps of total occlusions. However, dilating a subintimal channel may not only result in vessel occlusion or perforation but also may prohibit future surgical grafting of the coronary artery. Special attention must also be taken when hydrophilic wires are used due to their propensity for subintimal passage and perforation of end capillaries. These wires may easily enter thin-walled vasa vasorum, which are prone to perforation either directly from the wire or from the subsequent dilatations.

Incidence

Limited data are available on the true incidence of coronary perforation with balloon angioplasty alone. Various case series, many of which include the use of atherectomy devices, report an incidence ranging from 0.1% to 0.9% [33,2,14,26,34,35]. Some studies have described the incidence of coronary perforation to be 2–10 times higher in all published series using atheroablative techniques (directional atherectomy, excimer laser, rotablator,

and transluminal extraction catheter) than with balloon angioplasty with or without stenting [36,37]. In 1 study, Ellis *et al.* have reported the incidence of perforations with balloon angioplasty alone to be 0.1%, while that associated with rotablation was 1.3% and with excimer laser was 1.9% [1]. The excimer laser probably carries the highest risk of coronary perforation (up to 3%) [1,38]. However, the device-related learning curve may also explain the higher rates of complications. For example, in 1 series, coronary perforation in conjunction with excimer laser use occurred in 1.2% of 3,000 consecutive patients, but decreased to 0.3% in the last 1,000 patients [38].

The actual incidence of guidewire-related coronary perforation is most likely higher than reported because they remain unrecognized and self-limited in several cases. The incidence of coronary perforation due to guidewire was 0.21% in the series by Dippel *et al.* [33] and 0.36% in the series by Fukutomi *et al.* [34]. In the later series, perforation occurred at the treatment site in 12 cases, in a distal vessel in 10 cases, and could not be localized in 5 cases [34]. In the series by Witzke *et al.* [39], coronary perforation due to guidewire use was observed in 20/39 (51%) cases. Of these cases, perforations occurred while trying to cross the lesion with a guidewire in 11 patients

(55%). Based on these data, the authors emphasized that the distal migration of the guidewire is an important factor contributing to coronary perforation, and that meticulous care of the guidewire should be taken, especially in patients treated with glycoprotein platelet (GP) IIb/IIIa receptor inhibitors.

In cases involving CTOs, perforations due to use of stiff guidewires are the most commonly observed type, mainly divided into (1) perforation of the false lumen while advancing a stiff wire into the false lumen, and (2) distal small branch perforation after crossing a CTO lesion. In general, special treatment is not required for false lumen perforation because they usually disappear after dilatation of another false lumen. In distal small branch perforations, the most important consideration is performing careful observation via angiography. These perforations may cause late tamponade because the operators are often not able to detect them. At the end of the procedure, even in successful cases, final angiography should be carefully performed.

In the past few years, some newer devices (e.g. Tornus, and Frontrunners) have been approved, and rotational atherectomy and excimer laser therapy have been used for PCI of CTO lesions. Although all interventions share some general management principles, newer devices and techniques involve new complications.

Classification

A classification system for coronary perforations related to the angiographic appearance of blood extravasation (Table 32.3) was created based on the analysis of prospectively recorded data from a total of 12,900 PCI procedures from 11 US sites during

Table 32.3. Classification of coronary perforations.

Type I	Extraluminal crater without extravasation
Type II	Pericardial or myocardial blush without contrast jet extravasation
Type III	Extravasation through frank (≥1 mm) perforation
Cavity spilling	Perforation into anatomic cavity chamber, coronary sinus, etc.

a 2-year period [1]. Coronary perforation occurred in 62 patients (0.5%). Type II perforation was the most frequent perforation type in this series (50%), followed by type III (25.8%) and type I (21%); the minority of cases were characterized by cavity spilling (3.2%) [1]. Of note, the NHLBI classification system for coronary dissections overlaps with the Ellis classification model, with NHLBI type C coronary dissections corresponding angiographically with Ellis type I perforations [14].

In addition, other studies have evaluated the proposed classification system as a tool to predict outcome and to serve as the basis of management [1,40–42]. Analysis showed that:

type I perforations rarely result in tamponade or in myocardial ischemia.

type II perforations have high treatment success rates when managed with prolonged balloon inflation, and commonly have low occurrence of persistent contrast extravasation, consequently resulting in a low incidence of adverse sequelae [40].

Type III perforations are associated with the rapid development of hemodynamic compromise and life-threatening complications, including abrupt tamponade, need for emergent bypass surgery, and very high mortality. Notably, type III perforations with contrast spilling into either the left or right coronary ventricle or coronary sinus does not have catastrophic consequences and is commonly benign [41,42].

Management and Treatment of Perforation

Coronary perforation carries a significant mortality risk. Therefore, management and treatment are quite important and should be initiated very rapidly. The strategy for treating coronary perforation is best determined by specific angiographic type and clinical circumstances. Based on angiographic classification, a treatment algorithm for coronary perforations was proposed by Dippel *et al.* [33]. In general, if extravasation is limited (type I) and due to guidewire perforation, the guidewire should be retrieved to a more proximal location in the vessel. In many of these conditions, prolonged proximal balloon inflations may help solve the problem. When limited pericardial effusion occurs, as in type I or II perforations, serial echocardiography may suggest clues to ongoing leakage, as evidenced by changes in the effusion size. Early diastolic right ventricular collapse and late diastolic right atrial collapse are early signs of cardiac tamponade and precede the onset of hypotension.

In type I perforations, management is commonly limited to careful observation for 15 to 30 minutes with repeated injections of contrast media. If the degree of extravasation does not enlarge, intravenous (IV) heparin-neutralizing protamine sulfate should be given (in patients not receiving insulin). In addition, GP IIb/IIIa inhibitors should be discontinued once perforation occurs. The effects of abciximab can be reversed by platelet transfusion; eptifibatide and tirofiban have no antidote but have a relatively short half-life lasting several hours. Direct antithrombin agents (e.g. bivalirudin) may be more problematic, as there is no antidote for this class of agents. Regarding protamine usage, while its effectiveness and safety have been demonstrated following bare-metal stenting, little is known about the risk of protamine administration following drug-eluting stent (DES) implantation.

In type II, the first step in management is placement of a perfusion balloon catheter (or standard balloon) to seal the perforation [33,43]. Echocardiographic assessment should be performed without delay. Reversal of anticoagulation with IV protamine sulfate and platelet transfusion in patients who have received abciximab along with urgent pericardiocentesis should be performed in patients with signs of tamponade [33,34]. Emergent cardiac surgery is reserved for those patients who do not achieve hemostasis with these conservative measures.

In type III, an immediate aggressive treatment strategy is required, including adequate volume resuscitation, administration of catecholamines, and, frequently, urgent pericardiocentesis. Immediate reversal of anticoagulation with IV protamine sulfate and platelet transfusion in abciximab-treated patients is critical. According to the algorithm proposed by Dippel *et al.* [33], treatment of type III perforation should start with standard balloon catheter inflation at the site of perforation for at least 5 to 10 minutes to provide time for preparation of a perfusion balloon catheter and to perform pericardiocentesis. Currently, the strategy for perfusion balloon should be replaced by a standard balloon catheter as the former is no longer commercially available. Subsequent prolonged balloon inflation may successfully seal a type III perforation or can provide time to place a polytetrafluoroethylene (PTFE)-covered stent. The site of coronary perforation must be completely sealed by the covered stent and confirmed by an angiogram performed at least 10 minutes following treatment. Intermittent or continuous pericardial catheter aspiration should be employed overnight. Furthermore, the authors recommend in-hospital observation for an additional 24 hours with repeat echocardiography prior to discharge or on the day following pericardial catheter removal [33].

In limited perforations (types I and II) not caused by guidewire use, maintaining guidewire position across the perforation site is crucial, and careful balloon compression of the perforation site is usually recommended to limit further extravasation. In patients receiving heparin, reversal of the anticoagulant effects should be considered. GP IIb/IIIa inhibitor infusions should be stopped whenever perforation occurs, regardless of the severity. In an analysis of the Mayo Clinic PCI database, administration of protamine sulfate and prolonged balloon inflation were the most common treatments performed after identification of a coronary perforation [24]. In those patients receiving unfractionated heparin, IV protamine sulfate should be given, with subsequent dose titration guided by anticoagulation status to reverse the anticoagulation effects [34]. Reversal of heparin anticoagulation should target an activated clotting time (ACT) of 150 seconds. Protamine may partially neutralize the anti-IIa activity, but not the anti-Xa activity of low-molecular-weight heparin [44,45]. Reversal of heparin anticoagulation is most easily and rapidly achieved through the administration of IV protamine sulfate [46]. Importantly, protamine has been safely administered to facilitate hemostasis following coronary stent deployment without adverse ischemic sequelae [47]. Administration of protamine and/or platelet transfusion may be reserved for patients who have evidence of pericardial effusion, and pericardiocentesis should be performed only in the presence of hemodynamic or echocardiographic cardiac compromise [33].

Devices and Materials for Coronary Perforation

Several devices and materials for sealing the perforation site, such as plugs, coils, glues, beads, and covered-stents have been used. Plugs, coils, glues, and beads are usually used for small (types I or II) or distal perforations caused by the guidewire. These perforations cannot be sealed with covered stents, which are more useful for pinhole perforations. Coil embolization of coronary perforations, especially of the distal vessel, has also been used as a percutaneous bailout treatment [48,49]. In general, most studies report microcolis embolization with platinum or stainless steel coils ranging from 0.014 inches to 0.025 inches in diameter [50,51]. However, larger coils have been used in coronary artery ruptures or in large segment perforations [52,53]. Recently, Japanese operators have used injections of small fragments of adipose tissue via a microcatheter rather than alien substances such as plugs, coils, glues, and beads. Adipose tissue could be absorbed after plugging the small perforation completely. Autologous vein-covered stents have also been described as an effective treatment option for successful percutaneous sealing of perforations [54,55]. However, isolating the graft (typically a cephalic vein) by cutdown and mounting and suturing it onto a metallic stent is time-consuming and an improbable emergency treatment for free-flowing perforation and pericardial tamponade [56]. Successful treatment of 2 cases or perforation with intracoronary injection of thrombin has been described by Fischell *et al.* [50].

After defining the perforation on an angiogram, we recommend reinflating the balloon used in the procedure with low pressure at the perforation site. In general, long balloon inflation ($\geq$ 10 minutes) with 2–3 atm pressure is required to plug the extravasation flow. When the perforation persists, coli embolization is one of the options for treatment. For the distal perforation caused by the guidewire, injection of gel foam strips through an infusion catheter is another option. If cardiac tamponade develops and low blood pressure ensues, pericardiocentesis and drainage with a pigtail catheter are required. One important point to consider is the need to use 2 guiding catheters in order to be able to control the perforation with the inflated balloon while being ready to advance a covered stent if needed. When extravascular flow is observed on angiography despite prolonged balloon inflation, a covered stent should be used to stop the leakage. If a life-threatening perforation occurs while working with a smaller guide requiring the covered stent for sealing, a balloon angioplasty catheter (or stent delivery balloon) should immediately be inflated across the tear in the coronary vessel to provide temporary hemostasis. Another guide catheter should then be introduced via contralateral femoral artery access and used to cannulate the coronary ostium after gently disengaging the other guide. The covered stent should be introduced into the new guide over a second guidewire and passed just proximal to the occluding balloon, which is then deflated and retracted, allowing passage of the new guidewire and the covered stent for definite closure of the perforation [57].

Covered Stent Device Description

The covered stent device was first approved by the US Food and Drug Administation (FDA) in 2001. According to recent reports, the use of the PTFE covered stent can reduce the mortality related to coronary perforation to 10% [28]. The currently available coronary stent graft is a balloon expandable, slotted-tube stent. The Jostent® coronary stent graft device (AbbottVascular Devices, Abbott Park, Illinois) consists of an ultrathin (75 μm), biocompatible, and expandable polytetrafluoroethylene (PTFE) layer sandwiched in between 2 coaxial 316 L stainless steel, slotted-tube, balloon-expandable stents. Available lengths of the stent are 9 mm, 12 mm, and 26 mm, with diameters of 3.0 mm to 5.0 mm. The main limitations of the stent are an enhanced propensity for stent thrombosis, which may be diminished by high-pressure prolonged balloon inflation (for optimal expansion, the recommended inflation pressure is 14–16 atm for at least 30 seconds to allow for complete stent expansion), IVUS evaluation for proper implantation, and prolonged (6-month) antiplatelet therapy that includes aspirin and thienopyridines. Several reports have described the use of the PTFE-covered stent in treating coronary perforations, with favorable results [1,54,57–60].

In a multicenter, retrospective, international registry, Lansky *et al.* [57] reported the use of

Jostent® coronary stent grafts in 41 cases of coronary perforations. Perforations were relatively severe: 16.7% Ellis type I, 54.2% type II, and 29.1% type III. Of the 41 patients, >1/3 (n = 14) experienced life-threatening complications before stent graft implantation, including pericardial tamponade (12.2%), cardiogenic shock (9.8%), and cardiac arrest (2.4%). A total of 52 coronary stent grafts were used to treat the 41 perforations (mean 1.3 per lesion). All coronary stent grafts were placed successfully, with 92.9% of the perforations sealed completely and 7.1% partially. The lesions were predominantly noncomplex (62.9% type A/B1 according to the ACC/AHA classification), with a mean length of 11.97 mm. One patient developed abrupt vessel closure after coronary stent grafts deployment, resulting in an overall procedure success rate of 96.4%. No in-hospital Q-wave myocardial infarctions, emergency coronary bypass surgeries, or deaths resulted. The authors concluded that the coronary stent graft might be a reliable and highly effective treatment option for sealing coronary perforations complicating PCI.

Based on a comparison of outcomes of coronary perforations in 2 Milan centers before and after 1998, Stankovic et al. [28] showed that the use of the covered stent was associated with a significant reduction of in-hospital MACE (death, any myocardial infarction, and target vessel revascularization) in type III perforations (from 91% to 33%), but had no impact on the clinical course of type II perforations. A 2-center study in Europe reported 49 cases of coronary perforation complicating a total of 10,945 PCI procedures (0.45%) [58]. Adequate sealing of the perforation was not achieved by conventional methods (perfusion balloon, reversal of anticoagulation, platelet transfusion with/without pericardiocentesis) in 29 of 49 patients (59%). The first 17 cases of 29 patients in this series were treated with Palmaz-Schatz™ stents (attempted in 5 but successful in only 2 patients) and/or with emergent cardiac surgery (15 patients). In the subsequent 12/29 patients, perforation were treated with PTFE-covered stent: in 11 patients, the stent was uneventfully deployed, and ruptures were successfully sealed. Thrombosis in Myocardial Infarction (TIMI)-3 flow was achieved in all but 1 case; in 1 patient the use of the stent was not feasible following distal location of the ruptured site. Thus, in this series, PTFE-covered stents successfully sealed 91% of coronary perforations after other conservative approaches failed. In the same series, pericardial effusion without hemodynamic impairment was identified less frequently in patients receiving another stent and/or undergoing urgent cardiac surgery. At a mean follow-up of 14 months, 10 of 12 patients treated with PTFE-covered stents were MACE-free. Angiographic restenosis was found in 2 of 7 patients (29%). Although PTFE-covered stents are considered to be the device of choice in the treatment of coronary perforations, in some situations the use of this stent is technically difficult or even impossible due to its limitations, including limited flexibility and tractability, especially in diffusely diseased vessels. Furthermore, the use of covered stents in native coronary arteries must be undertaken with caution, given the potential for sidebranch coverage with subsequent myonecrosis.

Early and Late Clinical Outcome

For the patient with major perforation in hospital, careful observation with frequent hemodynamic monitoring is required after the procedure, and follow-up angiographic examination should be performed the next day. After making sure of no adverse findings, the patient can be discharged.

Sequelae of coronary perforations range in severity from none to devastating, and are fraught with early (often instant) and/or late complications. Based on the series by Ellis et al. [1] a clear correlation exists between the angiographic type of coronary perforation and early complications (Figure 32.11). In this series, mortality and Q-wave myocardial infarction were entirely limited to type III perforations. The majority of cases of emergent CABG and tamponade were also associated with type III perforations (63% for both complications), while emergent CABG and tamponade were remarkably lower in type I and type II coronary perforations.

Other series confirmed the validity of Ellis' classification in relation to early sequelae and treatment modality. In the series described by Dippel et al. [33], clinical outcomes were quite favorable in patients with type II perforations: there were no cases of death or emergency CABG, with only 1 patient (5.3%) requiring pericardiocentesis. Importantly, these outcomes were achieved despite fairly infrequent reversals of procedural

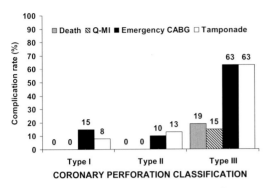

Figure 32.11. Correlation between the angiographic type of coronary perforation and early complications. Adapted from Ellis, Ajluni, Arnold et al. [1].

anticoagulation (21.1%), platelet transfusion (15.8%), or the use of prolonged perfusion balloon catheter inflation (26.3%), although the majority of patients (73.7%) received abciximab during PCI. In contrast, patients with type III perforations had a higher rate of mortality (21.4%), pericardial tamponade (42.9%), and emergent CABG (50.0%), despite more aggressive therapies including the use of protamine (64.3%), platelet transfusions (50.0%), and prolonged perfusion balloon catheter inflations (87.7%). Similarly, in a series by Stankovic et al. [28], all cases of in-hospital death and/or emergency CABG were associated exclusively with type III coronary perforations.

A number of reports have emphasized that pericardial tamponade may develop several hours after coronary perforation. In a series by Ellis et al. [1], there was a 5% to 10% incidence of delayed (24 hours or more post-PCI) tamponade, arguing for careful patient monitoring, especially during that time period. Delayed pericardial tamponade typically results from a guidewire-related perforation and occurs not infrequently in patients undergoing recanalization of a CTO. Fukutomi et al. [34] reported 5 cardiac tamponades occurring in a total of 25 patients; in 12 patients, signs of tamponade emerged immediately after coronary perforation, while a delayed presentation (after a mean time of 4.9 ± 3.4 hours) occurred in 13 patients who were all treated for CTO lesions. In

the same series, a guidewire caused coronary perforations in 8 of 13 patients (61.5%), with a delayed development of pericardial tamponade. Finally, in a series by Fejka et al. [36] analyzing 31 cases of cardiac tamponade occurring in a total of 25,697 procedures (0.12%) during a 7 year period, tamponade was diagnosed during the procedure in 17 patients (55%) at a mean time of 18 minutes from the start of PCI; in 14 patients (45%), tamponade presented later (mean time = 4.4 hours post-PCI, range = 2 to 15 hours). The same study clearly demonstrated that cardiac tamponade related to coronary perforation was associated with high rates of mortality; 13 of 31 patients (42%) in this series died. Mortality was especially high for those patients who developed cardiac tamponade during PCI compared with those who developed delayed tamponade (59% vs. 21% of patients).

Conclusions

Coronary dissection with vessel occlusion and perforation following coronary angiography or PCI are dreaded complications occurring in the catheterization laboratory. These complications can result in acute myocardial infarction, need for urgent coronary artery bypass surgery, pericardial tamponade, and death. The incidence of acute closure following coronary dissection has decreased significantly primarily because of the widespread use of coronary stents. The management of coronary dissection depends on the patency of the distal vessel and the extent of propagation of the dissection. In general, in the presence of myocardial ischemia or acute closure, coronary stenting is mandated. For coronary perforation, the treatment strategy depends on the type of vessel and the location of the injury. Principles include prompt recognition of perforation, immediate balloon tamponade of the injured vessel, rapid reversal of anticoagulation or antiplatelet therapy, addressing hemodynamic instability, involvement of surgeons if appropriate, and specific treatment of the vessel perforation or rupture with a bailout device such as embolization coils or covered stents.

References

1. Ellis SG, Ajluni S, Arnold AZ, *et al.* Increased coronary perforation in the new device era. Incidence, classification, management, and outcome. Circulation 1994; **90**(6): 2725–2730.

2. Ajluni SC, Glazier S, Blankenship L, O'Neill WW, *et al.* Perforations after percutaneous coronary interventions: clinical, angiographic, and therapeutic observations. Cathet Cardiovasc Diagn 1994; **32**(3): 206–212.

3. Elsner M, Zeiher AM. Perforation and rupture of coronary arteries. Herz 1998; **23**(5): 311–318.

4. Holmes DR, Jr., Reeder GS, Ghazzal ZM, *et al.* Coronary perforation after excimer laser coronary angioplasty: the Excimer Laser Coronary Angioplasty Registry experience. J Am Coll Cardiol 1994; **23**(2): 330–335.

5. Kini A, Marmur JD, Duvvuri S, Dangas G, *et al.* Rotational atherectomy: improved procedural outcome with evolution of technique and equipment. Single-center results of first 1,000 patients. Catheter Cardiovasc Interv 1999; **46**(3): 305–311.

6. Detre K, Holubkov R, Kelsey S, *et al.* Percutaneous transluminal coronary angioplasty in 1985–1986 and 1977–1981. The National Heart, Lung, and Blood Institute Registry. N Engl J Med 1988; **318**(5): 265–270.

7. Ellis SG, Roubin GS, King SB, III, *et al.* Angiographic and clinical predictors of acute closure after native vessel coronary angioplasty. Circulation 1988; **77**(2): 372–379.

8. Detre KM, Holmes DR, Jr., Holubkov R, *et al.* Incidence and consequences of periprocedural occlusion. The 1985–1986 National Heart, Lung, and Blood Institute Percutaneous Transluminal Coronary Angioplasty Registry. Circulation 1990; **82**(3): 739–750.

9. de Feyter PJ, van den Brand M, Laarman GJ, *et al.* Acute coronary artery occlusion during and after percutaneous transluminal coronary angioplasty. Frequency, prediction, clinical course, management, and follow-up. Circulation 1991; **83**(3): 927–936.

10. de Feyter PJ, de Jaegere PP, Serruys PW. Incidence, predictors, and management of acute coronary occlusion after coronary angioplasty. Am Heart J 1994; **127**(3): 643–651.

11. Stone GW, Ware JH, Bertrand ME, *et al.* Antithrombotic strategies in patients with acute coronary syndromes undergoing early invasive management: one-year results from the ACUITY trial. JAMA 2007; **298**(21): 2497–2506.

12. Dorros G, Cowley MJ, Simpson J, *et al.* Percutaneous transluminal coronary angioplasty: report of complications from the National Heart, Lung, and Blood Institute PTCA Registry. Circulation 1983; **67**(4): 723–730.

13. Holmes DR, Jr., Holubkov R, Vlietstra RE, *et al.* Comparison of complications during percutaneous transluminal coronary angioplasty from 1977 to 1981 and from 1985 to 1986: the National Heart, Lung, and Blood Institute Percutaneous Transluminal Coronary Angioplasty Registry. J Am Coll Cardiol 1988; **12**(5): 1149–1155.

14. Huber MS, Mooney JF, Madison J, *et al.* Use of a morphologic classification to predict clinical outcome after dissection from coronary angioplasty. Am J Cardiol 1991; **68**(5):467–471.

15. Perez-Castellano N, Garcia-Fernandez MA, *et al.* Dissection of the aortic sinus of Valsalva complicating coronary catheterization: cause, mechanism, evolution, and management. Cathet Cardiovasc Diagn 1998; **43**(3): 273–279.

16. Carter AJ, Brinker JA. Dissection of the ascending aorta associated with coronary angiography. Am J Cardiol 1994; **73**(12): 922–923.

17. Awadalla H, Sabet S, El Sebaie A, *et al.* Catheter-induced left main dissection incidence, predisposition and therapeutic strategies experience from two sides of the hemisphere. J Invasive Cardiol 2005; **17**(4): 233–236.

18. Goldstein JA, Casserly IP, Katsiyiannis WT, *et al.* Aortocoronary dissection complicating a percutaneous coronary intervention. J Invasive Cardiol 2003; **15**(2): 89–92.

19. Dunning DW, Kahn JK, Hawkins ET, *et al.* Iatrogenic coronary artery dissections extending into and involving the aortic root. Catheter Cardiovasc Interv 2000; **51**(4): 387–393.

20. Nikolsky E, Boulos M, Amikam S. Spontaneous healing of long, catheter-induced right coronary artery dissection. Int J Cardiovasc Interv 2003; **5**(4): 211.

21. Boyle AJ, Chan M, Dib J, *et al.* Catheter-induced coronary artery dissection: risk factors, prevention and management. J Invasive Cardiol 2006; **18**(10): 500–503.

22. Kim JY, Yoon J, Jung HS, *et al.* Percutaneous coronary stenting in guide-induced aortocoronary dissection: angiographic and CT findings. Int J Cardiovasc Imaging 2005; **21**(4): 375–378.

23. Gur M, Yilmaz R, Demirbag R, *et al.* Large atherosclerotic plaque related severe right coronary artery dissection during coronary angiography. Int J Cardiovasc Imaging 2006; **22**(3–4): 321–325.

24. Fasseas P, Orford JL, Panetta CJ, *et al.* Incidence, correlates, management, and clinical outcome of coronary perforation: analysis of 16,298 procedures. Am Heart J 2004; **147**(1):140–145.

25. Colombo A, Mikhail GW, Michev I, *et al.* Treating chronic total occlusions using subintimal tracking and reentry: the STAR technique. Catheter Cardiovasc Interv 2005; **64**(4): 407–411; discussion 412.

26. Javaid A, Buch AN, Satler LF, *et al.* Management and outcomes of coronary artery perforation during percutaneous coronary intervention. Am J Cardiol 2006; **98**(7): 911–914.

27. Tobis J, ed. Techiniques in Coronary Artery Stenting. Martin Dunitz, London, 2000.

28. Stankovic G, Orlic D, Corvaja N, *et al.* Incidence, predictors, in-hospital, and late outcomes of coronary artery perforations. Am J Cardiol 2004; **93**(2): 213–216.

29. Gruberg L, Pinnow E, Flood R, *et al.* Incidence, management, and outcome of coronary artery perforation during percutaneous coronary intervention. Am J Cardiol 2000; **86**(6): 680–682, A688.

30. Reimers B, von Birgelen C, van der Giessen WJ, *et al.* A word of caution on optimizing stent deployment in calcified lesions: acute coronary rupture with cardiac tamponade. Am Heart J 1996; **131**(1): 192–194.

31. Pasquetto G, Reimers B, Favero L, *et al.* Distal filter protection during percutaneous coronary intervention in native coronary arteries and saphenous vein grafts in patients with acute coronary syndromes. Ital Heart J 2003; **4**(9): 614–619.

32. Mauser M, Ennker J, Fleischmann D. Dissection of the sinus valsalvae aortae as a complication of coronary angioplasty. Z Kardiol 1999; **88**(12): 1023–1027.

33. Dippel EJ, Kereiakes DJ, Tramuta DA, *et al.* Coronary perforation during percutaneous coronary intervention in the era of abciximab platelet glycoprotein IIb/IIIa blockade: an algorithm for percutaneous management. Catheter Cardiovasc Interv 2001; **52**(3): 279–286.

34. Fukutomi T, Suzuki T, Popma JJ, *et al.* Early and late clinical outcomes following coronary perforation in patients undergoing percutaneous coronary intervention. Circ J 2002; **66**(4): 349–356.

35. Gunning MG, Williams IL, Jewitt DE, *et al.* Coronary artery perforation during percutaneous intervention: incidence and outcome. Heart 2002; **88**(5): 495–498.

36. Fejka M, Dixon SR, Safian RD, *et al.* Diagnosis, management, and clinical outcome of cardiac tamponade complicating percutaneous coronary intervention. Am J Cardiol 2002; **90**(11):1183–1186.

37. Cohen BM, Weber VJ, Relsman M, *et al.* Coronary perforation complicating rotational ablation: the US multicenter experience. Cathet Cardiovasc Diagn 1996; Suppl 3: 55–59.

38. Litvack F, Eigler N, Margolis J, *et al.* Percutaneous excimer laser coronary angioplasty: results in the first consecutive 3,000 patients. The ELCA Investigators. J Am Coll Cardiol 1994; **23**(2): 323–329.

39. Witzke CF, Martin-Herrero F, Clarke SC, *et al.* The changing pattern of coronary perforation during percutaneous coronary intervention in the new device era. J Invasive Cardiol 2004; **16**(6): 257–301.

40. Del Campo C, Zelman R. Successful non-operative management of right coronary artery perforation during percutaneous coronary intervention in a patient receiving abciximab and aspirin. J Invasive Cardiol 2000; **12**(1): 41–43.

41. Korpas D, Acevedo C, Lindsey RL, *et al.* Left anterior descending coronary artery to right ventricular fistula complicating coronary stenting. J Invasive Cardiol 2002; **14**(1): 41–43.

42. Hering D, Horstkotte D, Schwimmbeck P, *et al.* Acute myocardial infarct caused by a muscle bridge of the anterior interventricular ramus: Complicated course with vascular perforation after stent implantation. Z Kardiol 1997; **86**(8): 630–638.

43. Maruo T, Yasuda S, Miyazaki S. Delayed appearance of coronary artery perforation following cutting balloon angioplasty. Catheter Cardiovasc Interv 2002; **57**(4): 529–531.

44. Van Ryn-McKenna J, Cai L, *et al.* Neutralization of enoxaparine-induced bleeding by protamine sulfate. Thromb Haemost 1990; **63**(2): 271–274.

45. Massonnet-Castel S, Pelissier E, Bara L, *et al.* Partial reversal of low molecular weight heparin (PK 10169) anti-Xa activity by protamine sulfate: in vitro and in vivo study during cardiac surgery with extracorporeal circulation. Haemostasis 1986; **16**(2): 139–146.

46. Stoelting RK. Allergic reactions during anesthesia. Anesth Analg 1983; **62**(3): 341–356.

47. Briguori C, Di Mario C, De Gregorio J, *et al.* Administration of protamine after coronary stent deployment. Am Heart J 1999; **138**(1 Pt 1): 64–68.

48. Assali AR, Moustapha A, Sdringola S, *et al.* Successful treatment of coronary artery perforation in an abciximab-treated patient by microcoil embolization. Catheter Cardiovasc Interv 2000; **51**(4): 487–489.

49. Gaxiola E, Browne KF. Coronary artery perforation repair using microcoil embolization. Cathet Cardiovasc Diagn 1998; **43**(4): 474–476.

50. Fischell TA, Korban EH, Lauer MA. Successful treatment of distal coronary guidewire-induced perforation with balloon catheter delivery of intracoronary thrombin. Catheter Cardiovasc Interv 2003; **58**(3): 370–374.

51. Aslam MS, Messersmith RN, Gilbert J, *et al.* Successful management of coronary artery perforation with helical platinum microcoil embolization. Catheter Cardiovasc Interv 2000; **51**(3): 320–322.

52. Dorros G, Jain A, Kumar K. Management of coronary artery rupture: covered stent or microcoil embolization. Cathet Cardiovasc Diagn 1995; **36**(2): 148–154; discussion 155.

53. Mahmud E, Douglas JS, Jr. Coil embolization for successful treatment of perforation of chronically occluded proximal coronary artery. Catheter Cardiovasc Interv 2001; **53**(4): 549–552.

54. Colombo A, Itoh A, Di Mario C, *et al.* Successful closure of a coronary vessel rupture with a vein graft stent: case report. Cathet Cardiovasc Diagn 1996; **38**(2): 172–174.

55. Colon PJ, III, Ramee SR, Mulingtapang R, *et al.* Percutaneous bailout therapy of a perforated vein graft using a stent-autologous vein patch. Cathet Cardiovasc Diagn 1996; **38**(2): 175–178.

56. Satler LF. A revised algorithm for coronary perforation. Catheter Cardiovasc Interv 2002; **57**(2): 215–216.

57. Lansky AJ, Yang YM, Khan Y, *et al.* Treatment of coronary artery perforations complicating percutaneous coronary intervention with a polytetrafluoroethylene-covered stent graft. Am J Cardiol 2006; **98**(3): 370–374.

58. Briguori C, Nishida T, Anzuini A, *et al.* Emergency polytetrafluoroethylene-covered stent implantation to treat coronary ruptures. Circulation 2000; **102**(25): 3028–3031.

59. Ramsdale DR, Mushahwar SS, Morris JL. Repair of coronary artery perforation after rotastenting by implantation of the JoStent covered stent. Cathet Cardiovasc Diagn 1998; **45**(3): 310–313.

60. von Birgelen C, Haude M, Herrmann J, *et al.* Early clinical experience with the implantation of a novel synthetic coronary stent graft. Catheter Cardiovasc Interv 1999; **47**(4): 496–503.

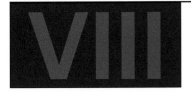

PART VIII
Clinical Trials

CHAPTER 33

Statistical Essentials in the Design and Analysis of Clinical Trials

Stuart J. Pocock
London School of Hygiene and Tropical Medicine, London, UK

Interventional Cardiology is an ever-expanding discipline with continual advances in both drug and device therapies. Such advances require the clinician to keep abreast of the latest developments and to appropriately implement evidence based medicine when making informed clinical decisions. This chapter will address the pertinent role of biostatistics within the discipline of clinical trials and provide the reader with an overview of the fundamentals of statistical analysis while focussing on:
1. Key issues in the design of clinical trials.
2. Additional topics in trial design and analysis.

Coverage is necessarily brief, so that statistical formulae and complex refinements are not included. Examples from real studies are presented to illustrate each issue.

Statistical Analysis: The Fundamentals

Significance Tests and P-values
If a clinical trial is done well, e.g. randomized, etc., there is no bias, so the observed outcome difference between treatment groups is either a genuine effect or due to chance variation. Significance tests enable one to assess the strength of evidence that a real effect is present.

Interventional Cardiology, First Edition. Edited by Carlo Di Mario, George D. Dangas, Peter Barlis.
© 2010 Blackwell Publishing Ltd. Published 2010 by Blackwell Publishing Ltd.

There are three main types of outcome data:
1. *binary* e.g. target lesion revascularization (yes or no)—chi-squared test.
2. *time to event* e.g. time to death—log rank test.
3. *quantitative* e.g. late loss (mm)—t test.
Whilst the calculations differ, the underlying principle is the same for all significance tests. For instance,

TYPHOON trial   (NEJM September 14, 2006)
Drug eluting stents (DES) vs. Uncoated Stents in Primary Percutaneous coronary intervention (PCI)
Primary Endpoint: TV related Death, MI or TVR by 1 year

	Sirolimus	Control
No. of patients	355	357
No. with primary endpoint	26	51
Percentages	7.3%	14.3%

Every test requires *a null hypothesis*, i.e. suppose both sirolimus and control were equally effective.

Then if the null hypothesis is true, what is the *probability P* of getting a difference of 7.3% vs. 14.3% or bigger? The answer from a chi-square test is $P = 0.004$.

The smaller the probability P, the more convincing the evidence to contradict the null hypothesis. Here we have strong evidence that the sirolimus stent reduces the risk of the primary endpoint.

Estimating the Magnitude of Effect

The risk ratio (or relative risk) divides one percentage by other e.g. risk ratio $= \dfrac{7.3\%}{14.3\%} = 0.51$

Risk ratio above or below 1 means the new treatment looks better or worse respectively.

The relative risk reduction = 100 (1 − risk ratio) = 49%

Sometimes people use the odds ratio instead, which here is $\dfrac{7.3}{100-7.3} \div \dfrac{14.3}{100-14.3} = 0.47$

The odds ratio is always further from 1, but if the percentages are small the odds ratio and risk ratio are similar.

It is also important to present the *absolute risk reduction*, i.e. the difference is 14.3 − 7.3 = 7.0%.

The *number needed to treat* is

$$\dfrac{100}{absolute\%difference} = 14 \text{ in this case}$$

Ninety-five Percent Confidence Interval to Express Uncertainty

Any estimate of treatment effect in a clinical trial contains some random error, and calculating a confidence interval enables one to see within what range it is plausible that the true effect lies. For instance, the observed relative risk in TYPHOON is 0.51 whilst the *95% confidence interval* is from 0.33 to 0.80. This means that one is 95% sure that the true relative risk is in this interval. To be precise, whenever one calculates a 95% confidence interval there is a 2½% chance that the truth is below and a 2½% chance that the truth is above the interval.

Now the larger the trial, the tighter the confidence interval (CI) becomes. Specifically, to halve the CI width one needs a trial four times the size.

Interpreting P-values

PASSION trial   (NEJM September 14, 2006)
DES vs. Uncoated Stent in Primary PCI
primary endpoint: cardiac death, MI or TLR by
1 year

	Taxus	Control
N	302	303
primary endpoint	27	39
	(8.8%)	(12.8%)
	P = 0.12	

not significant at 5% level
insufficient evidence of a treatment difference

The PASSION trial also had fewer primary events in the DES group, but with P = 0.12 this is insufficient evidence of a treatment difference.

Use of significance tests is often misleadingly oversimplified by putting too much emphasis on whether P is above or below 0.05. P < 0.05 means the result is statistically significant at the 5% level, but is an arbitrary guideline. It does not mean one has firm proof of an effect. By definition, even if two treatments are truly identical there is a 1 in 20 chance of reaching P < 0.05. Also, P > 0.05, not statistically significant (or n.s.), does not necessarily mean no true difference exists. It could be that the trial was too small. For instance, HORIZONS is a much larger trial (N = 3000) being done to clarify the issues first studied in PASSION.

Link Between P-values and Confidence Intervals

If we have P < 0.05 then the 95% confidence intervals for the risk ratio (or odds ratio) will exclude 1, while if P > .05 is observed then the 95% CI will include 1. Thus, by looking at the confidence interval alone one can infer whether the treatment difference is significant at the 5% level.

Time to Event Data

Many major trials study time to a primary event outcome. For instance, the ACUITY trial studied composite ischaemia: death myocardial infarction or unplanned revascularization over one year's follow-up.

A *Kaplan Meier life table plot* is the main method of displaying such data by treatment group. It displays the cumulative percentage of patients experiencing the event over time for each group. This method takes account of patients having different lengths of follow-up, e.g. any lost to follow-up before the intended one year.

Such a plot is a useful descriptive tool, but one needs to use a logrank test to see if there is evidence of a treatment difference in the incidence of events. For instance, the heparin + IIb/IIIa (N = 4603) and bivalirudin alone (N = 4612) groups had composite ischemia in 15.4% and 16.0% of patients respectively. The logrank test uses the total data by group

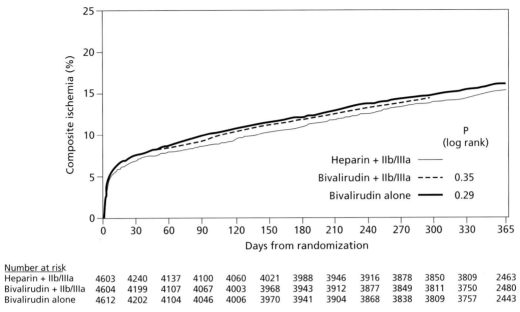

Figure 33.1. Kaplan Meier life-table plot. Shows pattern of treatment difference over time, e.g. ACUITY one year follow-up.

displayed in the Figure 33.1 to obtain P = 0.29, i.e. the data are consistent with the null hypothesis of no treatment difference. The logrank test can be thought of an extension, indeed improvement, to the simpler chi-squared test comparing two percentages since it takes into account the fact that patients have been followed for, and deaths occur at, differing times from randomization.

With time to event data, the *hazard ratio* is used to estimate any relative treatment differences in risk. It is similar to, but more complicated to calculate, than the simple relative risk mentioned above. It effectively averages the instantaneous relative risk occurring at different follow-up times, using what is commonly called a Cox proportional hazards model. In this case the hazard ratio comparing bivalirudin with heparin +IIa/IIIa is 1.06 with 95% CI 0.95 to 1.17. Thus, there is an observed 6% increase in hazard but the 95% CI includes 1 reflecting the lack of statistical significance.

Quantitative Data

For a quantitative measure of patient outcome it is common to compare the mean outcomes in each treatment group.

Quantitative Data   (NEJM January 15, 2004)
TAXUS IV trial: late loss in analysis segment (mm)

	drug eluting stent	bare-metal stent
N	292	267
mean late loss	0.23 mm	0.61 mm
standard deviation (SD)	0.44 mm	0.57 mm
standard error of the mean (SEM)	0.026 mm	0.035 mm

The standard deviation (SD) summarizes the extent of individual patient variation around each mean. If the data are normally distributed then appropriately 95% of individuals will have a value within two standard deviations either side of the mean. This is sometimes called the *reference range*.

However, for a clinical trial outcome measure it is more useful to calculate the *standard error of the mean* (SEM) which is $SD/\sqrt{N}$. That is, precision in the estimated mean increases proportionately with the square root of the number of patients. The 95% confidence for the mean is mean $\pm 1.96 \times SEM$.

However, one is really interested in the difference in means. For TAXUS IV trial, the difference in mean late loss between drug eluting and bare-metal stent groups is $0.23 - 0.61 = 0.38 \, \text{mm}$.

The standard error of this difference in means is:

$$\left(\text{SEM}_1^2 + \text{SEM}_2^2\right)^{1/2} = \left(0.026^2 = 0.035^2\right)^{1/2} = 0.044 \text{ mm}$$

The *two-sample t test* calculates t = difference in means ÷ its standard error = 0.038/0.044 = 8.72 in this case. The P-value for this test can be obtained from statistical tables. Specifically t > 1.96 gives P < .05 and t > 2.58 gives P < 0.01. Here t is so large that P < 0.0000000001. This is remarkably convincing evidence that the drug eluting stent does reduce late loss compared to the bare-metal stent.

The *95% confidence for the difference in means* extends 1.96 standard errors either side of mean difference. That is, 95% CI = 0.38 ± 1.96 × 0.044 = 0.29 to 0.47 mm. In this case, the extreme statistical significance is reflected in the narrowly precise 95% CI for the mean treatment effect.

This is a simple insight into the essentials on quantitative data analysis in clinical trials. If the trial is small further correction for small numbers is needed. There is a variation on the above simplified t test which some people call the real t test. If one has the same quantitative measure also available at baseline for each patient, then one needs to include this information using a method called analysis of covariance. Lastly, if the measure has a very skew distribution, especially in a small trial, it may be better to analyse using medians and distribution-free methods.

Trial Design: The Fundamentals

When planning a clinical trail much energy is devoted to defining exactly what is the *new treatment*, who are the eligible *patients*, and what are the primary and secondary *outcomes*. Then the following statistical design issues need to be considered.

Control Group

One essential is that the trial is *comparative*, i.e. one needs a *control group* of patient receiving a standard treatment who will be compared with patients receiving the new treatment. Such standard treatment may either be an established active treatment or no treatment (possibly a placebo). Of course, all patients in both groups get good medical care in all other respects.

Randomization

One needs a fair (unbiased) comparison between new treatment and control, and *randomization* is the key requirement in this regard. That is each patient has an equal chance of being randomly assigned to new or standard treatment. Furthermore, the method of handling random assignments is such that no-one can predict in advance what each next patient will be assigned to. Thus, randomization ensures there is no selection bias in deciding which patients get new or standard treatment. Such selection bias is a serious problem in any observational (non-randomized) studies comparing treatments, making them notoriously unreliable in their conclusions.

As a consequence randomization ensures that patients in the treatment groups have similar baseline characteristics. This can be guaranteed further if one stratifies the randomization for certain key patients' features, but such stratification is not particularly important if the trial is large.

In addition randomization helps to ensure that all other aspects of patient care, and also the evaluation of patient outcome, is identical in both treatment groups. In this respect it is often also important to make the trial *double blind* whereby neither patients nor those treating them and evaluating their response know which randomized treatment each individual patient is receiving.

If a trial cannot be made double blind one may nevertheless require *blinded evaluation* of outcome by people not aware of which treatment each patient is on.

Trial Size and Power Calculations

For a trial to give a reliably precise answer as to the relative merits of the randomized treatments one needs a sufficiently large number of patients. *Power calculations* are the most commonly used statistical method for determining the required trial size.

Each power calculation entails the following five steps:

1. Choose a *primary outcome* for the trial.

2. Decide on a *level of statistical significance* required for declaring a "positive" trial. Five percent significance is usual chosen.

3. Declare what you expect the *control groups results* to be.

4. Declare the *smallest true treatment difference* that is important to detect. Large treatment effects, if present, can be detected in relatively small trials so it is relevant to focus on what reasonably modest effect one would not wish to miss.

5. Declare with what *degree of certainty* (statistical power) one wishes to detect such a difference as statistically significant. From such information there are statistical formulae that provide the required number of patients.

Let us illustrate the method with the design of the PASSION trial in primary PCI patients mentioned earlier. The primary outcome was a composite of cardiac death, myocardial infarction or target lesion revascularization within one year. The bare-metal stent control group outcome rate was expected to be 21.7% and they wanted to detect a halving of this, down to 10.9%, with the drug eluting stent using a 5% significance level and 90% power. The consequent statistical formula determined that the trial needed around 500 patients.

It is useful to explain some terminology here. The significance level used (5%) is called the risk of a type 1 error (a false positive result). The 90% power refers to the specific alternative hypothesis (21.7% vs. 10.95). The risk of a type 2 error (false negative result) is $1 - \text{power}/100 = 0.1$ in this case. Thus, with around 500 patients there is a 10% risk of failing to reach 5% significance even if in truth the drug eluting stent halves the outcome rate.

This example from the PASSION trial is interesting given the trial's result was not statistically significant (see earlier). This is a common problem reflecting the fact that *most clinical trials are too small*. In this instance the expected control group rate (20.9%) was too high and might more realistically be set at 15%. Also, the hypothesized effect of drug eluting stent (a halving) was too optimistic and to re-set at a 30% reduction, i.e. 15% versus 10.5% would have been more realistic. With the same type 1 and type 2 errors the required number of patients then becomes around 2400.

Often a single clinical trial is neither large nor representative enough to evaluate a particular therapeutic issue. Then, *meta-analyses* can be of value combining evidence from several related trial to reach an overall conclusion.

Additional Topics in Clinical Design and Analysis

This chapter so far has discussed the fundamentals of trial design and statistical analysis. Clearly there are many other important issues that need to be tackled in the design, conduct, analysis and interpretation of clinical trials. All we can do here is briefly alert the reader to these topics and encourage them to pursue further from other courses, textbooks, publications, etc.

In *trial design* we have concentrated on parallel group trial with just two treatments aimed at discovering whether one treatment is superiority to the other. Alternative designs to be aware of include: trials with multiple treatment arms, factorial designs, non-inferiority (equivalence) trials, crossover trials, cluster-randomized trials and adaptive designs.

In the *conduct of trials* of particular concern is patient non-compliance with their randomized treatment, loss to follow-up and other protocol violations. A key ethical, statistical and organizational issue concerns *data monitoring* of interim results with the purpose of stopping a trial early if there is convincing evidence of the new treatments superiority, inferiority (safety concerns) or futility. There exist appropriate statistical guidelines (rules) for assisting Data Monitoring Committees as to when and why they should (or should not) recommend early stopping.

The *analysis of clinical trials* can involve a *multiplicity of data* with multiple outcomes, repeated measures over time, subgroup analyses and alternative methods of data analysis. Accordingly, any trial requires a detailed *Statistical Analysis Plan* that documents all the proposed analyses and any priorities in their interpretation. A particular problem concerns *subgroup analyses* where treatment differences are studies for (often many) different subgroups of patients. Such subgroup analyses require cautious interpretation and should use interaction (heterogeneity) tests rather than subgroup P-values.

Most major trials use *analysis by intention to treat* whereby all patients are included in their randomized groups even though they did not all fully comply with the intended treatments. Such an analysis gives an unbiased comparison of the treatment policies as they were delivered in practice, a so-called *pragmatic trial*. *Per protocol analyses* which exclude any patient follow-up when not on randomized treatment are potentially biased since it may be the sicker patients who opt out.

Reporting of trial findings in medical journals, at conference presentations and to regulatory authorities need to be of the highest standards whereby an unbiased and detailed report of all relevant findings is presented.

The objectives, methods, discussion and conclusions all need to be clearly presented in a balanced report. In particular, results and interpretations should include any safety issues (adverse events) as well as efficacy findings. For publications in medical journal, the CONSORT guidelines are helpful to authors, editors, referees and readers in enhancing the quality-assessment of any trial report.

Questions

1. A randomized study indicated a 4.5% event rate with treatment A vs. a 5.1% event rate with treatment B; p = 0.09. Which of the following is true?

   A There is a >95% likelihood that the result is due to a real difference between A and B.

   B There is a >95% power to support a significant difference between A and B.

   C An increase in the number of study subjects would have definitely shown a statistically significant difference.

   D An increase in the number of study subjects would have definitely shown a statistically significant difference, even with a smaller between-group difference.

   E An increase in the number of study subjects could have shown a statistically significant difference if the between-group difference remained the same.

2. A randomized study of 1000 patients indicated a 13.5% event rate with treatment A versus a 16.0% event rate with placebo; p = 0.08. Another study in a similar patient population with 9000 patients indicated a 14.5% event rate with treatment B compared with 16.0% with placebo; p = 0.02. Which of the following is true?

   A The absolute risk reduction is 2.5% with A and 1.5% with B compared with placebo; this means that A is superior to B.

   B Treatment B is superior to placebo, while A is not; this means that B is superior to A.

   C The number of patients needed to treat with B in order to prevent 1 event that would have occurred with placebo is 67.

   D The number of patients needed to treat with B in order to prevent 1 event that would have occurred with placebo is 11.

   E The number of patients needed to treat with A in order to prevent 1 event that would have occurred with placebo is 6.

3. Which of the following statements is false regarding the results of this trial (image 1105)?

   A The absolute risk reduction with stent is 18%.

   B The relative risk reduction with stent is 42%.

   C There is a <5% likelihood that this result is due to chance.

   D This study had an 80% power; this means that we are 80% certain that the result is accurate.

   E The number of patients that we need to treat with stents in order to prevent 1 event that would have occurred with PTCA is 6.

Answers

1. E—By increasing the number of patients in the study group, we are reducing the possibility that observed difference between the two groups could be due to chance. An increase in the number of study subjects could have shown a statistically significant difference if the between-group difference remains the same—A larger study could have altered the statistically border-line result is if the n was sufficiently high and the difference remained. Mendenhall, Scheaffer and Wackerly, *Mathematical Statistics with Applications.* Second Edition, 1981.

2. C—AAR = 16% − 14.5% = 1.5%, then NNT = 1/ (Absolute Risk Reduction) = 1/1.5% = 66.7.

3. D—ARR = 42 − 24% = 18%, RRR = 18/42 = 42, NNT = 1/ARR = 6, the fact that p value is less than 5%, makes option 3 correct. Thus, option 4 is false. From the data presented we can not determine the power. Type II error is the inability to reject the null hypothesis when the latter is not correct; Study Power = (1-type II error). An 80% study power for a given sample size, indicates an 80% certainty that the absence of a statistical result is not due to chance. Study power does *not* have an important message when a study achieves a statistically significant result; however, it must always be taken under account when the primary objective of a study is negative (i.e. the null hypothesis is not rejected). Mendenhall, Scheaffer and Wackerly, *Mathematical Statistics with Applications.* Second Edition, 1981.

CHAPTER 34

Sirolimus and Paclitaxel Eluting Stent Clinical Studies

Ajay J. Kirtane, Adriano Caixeta, Philippe Généreux,
Rikesh Patel, & Jeffrey W. Moses
Columbia University Medical Center, New York, NY, USA

Over the past three decades, the field of percutaneous coronary intervention (PCI) has been rapidly evolving since the first balloon angioplasty in 1977. Bare-metal stents (BMS) were developed and significantly improved the acute success and reproducibility of PCI results compared to balloon angioplasty [1,2]. As several trials demonstrated the acute and long-term superiority of BMS to balloon angioplasty in the 1990s, the number of procedures incorporating stent placement grew exponentially, accounting for more than 80% of PCI procedures overall [3]. However, the field of PCI remained faced with another challenge: the use of stents resulted in larger final lumen cross-sectional area and abolished arterial remodelling was offset partially by a stent-related increase in neointimal tissue accumulation and in-stent restenosis (ISR). This phenomenon of ISR was observed to occur in roughly 20–40% of lesions, with variation based upon patient, lesion, and technique-specific factors. Whilst some restenosis events were clinically silent, in the majority of cases restenosis was observed to lead to a recurrence of symptoms (including unstable symptoms in up to 35% of cases) necessitating repeat revascularization procedures, increased costs, and substantial patient morbidity [4–6].

Interventional Cardiology, First Edition. Edited by
Carlo Di Mario, George D. Dangas, Peter Barlis.
© 2010 Blackwell Publishing Ltd. Published 2010 by
Blackwell Publishing Ltd.

In order to address the problem of ISR, the field of vascular brachytherapy was developed to treat ISR, but this proved to be time-consuming and was also associated with late stent thrombosis occurring even years after the procedure. Thus, drug eluting stents (DES) with antiproliferative drugs attached via polymer on the stent surface were developed as a logical next step in the evolution of PCI. These devices were designed to maintain the mechanical advantages of BMS over stand-alone balloon angioplasty, while delivering anti-restenotic pharmacologic therapies directly to the arterial wall to combat the neointimal hyperplasia occurring after conventional bare BMS placement.

The development of DES to control in-stent restenosis has been pioneered through a combination of understanding the biology of restenosis, the selection of drugs that would target the pathways in the restenosis process, controlled release drug delivery strategies and the use of the stent as a delivery platform. Of the currently available DES (including both first-generation and second-generation devices), all DES clinical effect is highly dependent on each of the three major components: the stent platform (and delivery system) which are akin to BMS, combined with a drug carrier, usually a polymer, that facilitates intravascular elution and the antiproliferative drug. A plethora of pharmacological approaches have been investigated for the management of clinical restenosis via drug eluting stents. Sirolimus and paclitaxel have shown clear evidence of clinical success with the application of the right dose and release kinetics. This chapter discusses the clinical data on the sirolimus and paclitaxel eluting stents that are currently available.

Initial Studies of First-generation DES

In 2003, the Food and Drug Administration (FDA) approved the use of the two first-generation DES, the CYPHER sirolimus eluting stent (SES, Cordis Corporation, Johnson & Johnson, Miami Lakes, FL), and the TAXUS paclitaxel eluting stent (PES, Boston Scientific Corporation, Maple Grove, MN). The FDA decision was based on the results of pivotal randomized clinical trials comparing a given DES with a comparator BMS in relatively non-complex lesions that constitute the "on-label" indications for DES use. In these early trials, the use of DES was demonstrated to reduce restenosis and repeat revascularization rates by 50–90% compared to BMS across all lesion and patients subsets [7]. These initial trials demonstrating the efficacy of DES were critical to the approval of these devices and the rapid growth of DES utilization.

In addition, DES has shown benefits with respect to reduced repeat revascularization and other restenosis-related endpoints in more complex lesions, including acute myocardial infarction, chronic total occlusions, in-stent restenosis, diffuse disease, saphenous vein grafts, and bifurcation lesions [8–13]. In fact, given the observed relative reductions in restenosis-related endpoints with DES, it follows that as the overall (absolute) risk of restenosis rises—as is observed with more complex lesion subsets—the absolute benefit of DES over BMS should increase. Thus, confidence in DES subsequently swelled, and as positive results from subsequent trials for a variety of expanded indications surfaced, physicians rapidly expanded the patient populations treated with DES to include other "off-label" indications. In the years immediately after DES approval, "off-label" use of these devices was estimated to occur in up to 65% of cases [14,15].

Paclitaxel Eluting Stent

Paclitaxel was approved by the FDA in 1992 as an antineoplastic agent to treat metastatic ovarian malignancies. Paclitaxel is a natural diterpenoid extracted from the bark, roots, and leaves of several Taxus species, including Taxus brevifolia and Taxus media. Its effect has been mainly explained by its ability to stabilize microtubules and thereby inhibit cell division in the G0/G1 and G2/M phases [16]. Several studies have shown that paclitaxel inhibits the development of neointimal hyperplasia in different in vitro and animal models of restenosis [17–20].

Overview of the TAXUS Clinical Trials

The safety and efficacy of the polymer-based paclitaxel eluting TAXUS stent system have been investigated in six studies: TAXUS I [21], TAXUS II [22], TAXUS III [23], TAXUS IV [24,25], TAXUS V de novo [8] and TAXUS VI [26]. All the studies, with the exception of TAXUS III, were randomized, double-blind, multicenter investigations that compared the paclitaxel eluting Taxus™ stent with BMS. TAXUS III was an open-label investigation. Primary endpoints varied by study and included one or more of the following: 30-day major adverse cardiac events (MACE) (TAXUS I and TAXUS III), six-month in-stent volume obstruction caused by neointimal proliferation (TAXUS II), and nine-month ischemia driven target vessel revascularization (TVR) (TAXUS IV, TAXUS V de novo, and TAXUS VI).

TAXUS I enrolled 61 patients and was a feasibility study designed to assess the safety of Taxus™ slow-release vs. BMS. At 12 months, the MACE rates were 10% and three percent in the control and Taxus™, respectively, demonstrating excellent long-term safety. These results were maintained through the four-year follow-up with no new MACE in any TAXUS patient between one and four years.

TAXUS II was a 536-patient, 38-site, randomized, double-blind, controlled study of the safety and efficacy of the Taxus stent system on the NIRx stent platform. In this study, two sequential cohorts (testing the slow- and moderate-release TAXUS formulations) enrolled patients with standard risk, de novo coronary artery lesions. The six-month results showed strong clinical performance as demonstrated by lower MACE and TLR rates in TAXUS patients compared with patients who received a BMS. The six-month MACE rates were reduced from 19.8% in control to 8.5% for the slow-release formulation cohort (p = 0.0035) and 7.8% for the moderate-release formulation cohort (p = 0.0019). At 12 months, the MACE rate in the slow-release cohort remained low at 10.9% compared with the control rate of 21.7% (p = 0.0082) and the TLR rate was 4.7% compared with 14.4% for the control (p = 0.0035). At 12 months, the moderate-release formulation cohort reported a 9.9% MACE rate (p = 0.0048 vs. control) with a 3.8% TLR rate (p = 0.0010 vs. control). The three-year follow-up for TAXUS II results were maintained through the three-year clinical follow-up with no new TLR or stent thromboses occurring in the TAXUS groups.

TAXUS III was a single-arm registry examining the feasibility of implanting Taxus stent for the treatment of in-stent restenosis. The trial enrolled 29 patients, and 28 were treated with the Taxus NIRx stent platform. The trial confirmed safety and reported no stent thromboses, no deaths, and a binary restenosis rate of 16% at six months. From six months to three years, there was only one cardiac death and no stent thromboses.

Similarly, in the large randomized TAXUS-IV trial, randomizing 1314 patients with single, de novo, non-complex coronary lesions, the nine month rate of ischemia-driven target-vessel revascularization was 4.7% with PES vs. 12.0% with BMS, again, a highly significant difference with similar relative effects observed across all subgroups [24].

TAXUS V was a randomized, double-blind trial studying 1156 patients at 66 sites in the United States using the slow-release formulation (Express^2 stent platform). TAXUS V expanded on the TAXUS IV pivotal trial by studying a higher-risk patient population, including patients with small vessels, and long lesions requiring multiple overlapping stents—the most challenging lesions and highest-risk patients ever studied in a randomized, controlled drug eluting stent trial in the United States. The primary endpoint of the trial was nine-month TVR, which was significantly lower in the TAXUS group (12.1%) than in the control group (17.3%) (p = 0.0184). At nine months, the overall MACE rate in the TAXUS group was 15.0%, compared with 21.2% in the control (p = 0.0084). The study also reported a TLR rate of 8.6% in the Taxus™ compared with 15.7% in the control group (p = 0.0003). In addition, stent thrombosis rates were identical between Taxus™ and control stents (0.7% each for the Taxus and the control group). These clinical benefits were maintained at one year with an overall MACE rate of 18.9% in the TAXUS group compared to 25.9% in the control group (p = 0.0052) and a TLR rate of 11.2% in the TAXUS group vs. 19.0% in the control group (p = 0.0003).

TAXUS VI, an international trial studying 446 patients with complex coronary artery disease at 44 sites, was designed to establish the safety and efficacy of the moderate-release formulation (on the Express stent platform) in the treatment of longer lesions. The trial had a primary endpoint of nine-month TVR. The study's TVR rate was 9.1% in the TAXUS group vs. the control rate of 19.4% at nine months (p = 0.0027). Additionally, the Taxus™ group had a TLR rate of 6.8% (compared with 18.9% in the control group, p = 0.0001) and an in-segment binary restenosis rate of 12.4% (compared with 35.7% in the control group, p < 0.0001). The results supported safety as demonstrated by low MACE rates (16.4% MACE rate at nine months in the TAXUS group compared with 22.5% in the control group, p = 0.1208). The two-year follow-up data for TAXUS VI demonstrated that the safety and efficacy benefits associated with a moderate-release formulation of the Taxus™ were maintained at two years; a continued significant reduction in TLR rate (9.7% for the TAXUS group, as compared with 21.0% for the control group, p = 0.0013). Stent thromboses remained low and comparable to control rates (0.9% for both the Taxus™ group and the control group). The two-year results for TAXUS VI support long-term safety with increased local exposure of the vessel to paclitaxel released from the moderate-release formulation compared to the levels released from the slow-release formulation. Even with an in-vitro dosing rate 8–10 times greater than the commercialized slow-release formulation, no compromise in safety was observed.

Recently, longer-term data from the five pivotal PES trials, including 3513 patients, has been

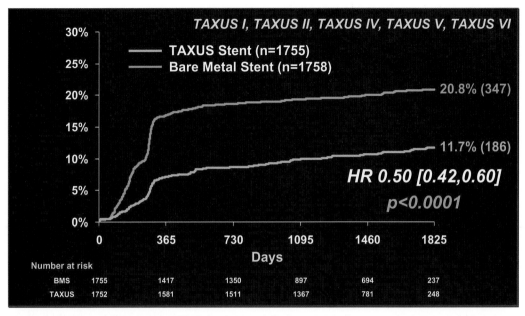

Figure 34.1. Pooled analysis from five TAXUS randomized clinical trials. Kaplan-Meier curves of cumulative rates of target vessel revascularization comparing Taxus™ stent with BMS.

reported; these data demonstrate durable reductions in clinical restenosis endpoints with similar overall safety for Taxus™ vs. BMS [27,28] (Figure 34.1). The cumulative incidence of stent thrombosis was similar between Taxus™ and BMS (2.1% vs. 1.7%, p = 0.46). Subgroup analyses also demonstrated a similar relative benefit of Taxus™ vs. BMS for diabetics, and all vessel sizes (Figure 34.2). From this independent, patient-level meta-analysis from the five principal TAXUS trials it may be concluded that at three–five year follow-up, polymer-based paclitaxel eluting stents compared to BMS stents result in (1) no significant differences in death or myocardial infarction, (2) no significant increase in stent thrombosis, (3) no significant increase in late stent thrombosis by ARC definitions and (4) sustained reduction in target lesion and TVR.

Sirolimus Eluting Stent

First FDA approved in 1999 as prophylaxis for kidney transplant rejection, Sirolimus is a macrolytic lactone produced by *Streptomyces hygroscopicus*. The primary mechanism of action of sirolimus's inhibition of neointimal hyperplasia is probably related to its ability to bind to FK binding protein-12 (FKBP-12) in cells; this complex binds to and inhibits activation of the mammalian target of rapamycin (mTOR), preventing progression in the cell cycle form the G1 phase to the S phase [29]. Its anti-inflammatory and anti-proliferative properties reduce smooth muscle cell proliferation in the arterial wall following stent induced injury [30,31]. With the low-release formulation of the Cypher™, 50% of the drug is released in the first two weeks and most of the sirolimus is released within four weeks after stent implantation.

Overview of the Cypher® Clinical Trials

Following the success of the first pilot study of the SES in 45 patients for suppressing intimal hyperplasia [32,33], the safety and efficacy of the polymer-based sirolimus eluting Cypher® stent system have been investigated in 4 major Studies: Ravel [34], SIRIUS [35], E-SIRIUS [36], and C-SIRIUS [37].

The RAVEL trial, a 238 patients-randomized trial, compared a sirolimus eluting stent with a standard BMS in patients with angina pectoris. At six-month angiographic follow-up, the in-stent late luminal loss was significantly lower in the

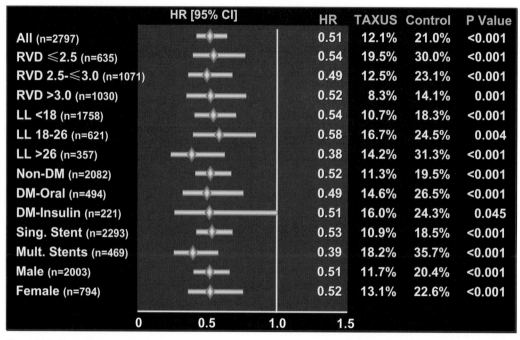

	HR [95% CI]	HR	TAXUS	Control	P Value
All (n=2797)		0.51	12.1%	21.0%	<0.001
RVD ≤2.5 (n=635)		0.54	19.5%	30.0%	<0.001
RVD 2.5-≤3.0 (n=1071)		0.49	12.5%	23.1%	<0.001
RVD >3.0 (n=1030)		0.52	8.3%	14.1%	0.001
LL <18 (n=1758)		0.54	10.7%	18.3%	<0.001
LL 18-26 (n=621)		0.58	16.7%	24.5%	0.004
LL >26 (n=357)		0.38	14.2%	31.3%	<0.001
Non-DM (n=2082)		0.52	11.3%	19.5%	<0.001
DM-Oral (n=494)		0.49	14.6%	26.5%	<0.001
DM-Insulin (n=221)		0.51	16.0%	24.3%	0.045
Sing. Stent (n=2293)		0.53	10.9%	18.5%	<0.001
Mult. Stents (n=469)		0.39	18.2%	35.7%	<0.001
Male (n=2003)		0.51	11.7%	20.4%	<0.001
Female (n=794)		0.52	13.1%	22.6%	<0.001
	0 0.5 1.0 1.5				

Figure 34.2. Target lesion revascularization up to five-year. Subgroup analysis summary from 5 TAXUS pivotal randomized clinical trial. Subgroup analysis shows relative benefit of Taxus™ vs. BMS for diabetics, all vessel sizes and all lesion length.

sirolimus-stent group (−0.01+/−0.33 mm) than in the standard-stent group (0.80+/−0.53 mm, p < 0.001), with a remarkable reduction in the rate of restenosis (0% vs. 26.6%, p < 0.001). The rate of major adverse cardiac events (MACEs), a composite of death, myocardial infarction, coronary artery bypass grafting or target vessel revascularization at one year was 5.8% for SES-treated patients vs. 28.8% for BMS-treated patients (p < 0.001), mostly driven by a higher rate of revascularization of the target vessel in the standard-stent group. At three-year follow-up, these results have been maintained, demonstrating a persistent reduction in MACE with SES compared to BMS (15.5% vs. 33.1%, p = 0.002) [38].

The SIRIUS trial, a 1058-patient randomized trial comparing the Cypher® DES to its uncoated BMS, has led to FDA approval of SES in 2003. More complex than in RAVEL trial, lesions lengths was 15–30 mm with vessel diameters of 2.5–3.5 mm. Both the primary endpoint, the rate of target vessel failure (a composite of cardiac death, myocardial infarction or revascularization of the target vessel)

and the rate of MACE at nine months was markedly lower among SES-treated patients (8.6% vs. 21.0%, p < 0.001 and 7.1% vs. 18.9%, p < 0.001 respectively). The benefit of SES was observed in all tested subgroups in the trial, including diabetic patients, and irrespective of vessel size. Additionally, longer term follow-up from SIRIUS has also demonstrated a persistently maintained benefit of SES over BMS, with 5-year rates of target vessel failure of 22.5% vs. 34.7% (p < 0.0001) and MACE of 20.3% vs. 33.5% (p < 0.0001) respectively [39].

Performed in Canada and Europe, C-SIRIUS and E-SIRIUS have shown similar results than the SIRIUS study. In these trials, the overall rate of angiographic restenosis was markedly lower with SES compared to BMS (in-stent: 3.1% vs. 42.7%, p < 0.001; in-segment: 5.1% vs. 44.2%, p < 0.001). Reductions in MACE with the use of SES compared to BMS were observed as well. A pooled analysis at two-year follow-up of the three SIRIUS studies has shown significant reductions in MACE (10.6% vs. 26.3%, p < 0.001) with SES compared to BMS [40].

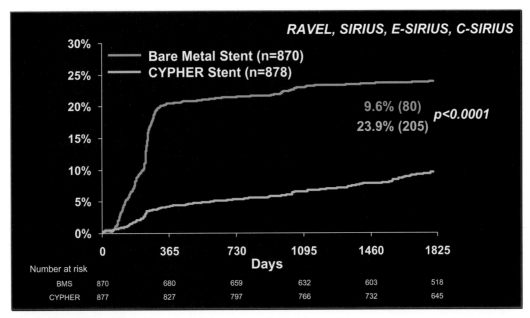

Figure 34.3. Pooled analysis from four Cypher® randomized clinical trials. Kaplan-Meier curves of cumulative rates of target vessel revascularization comparing Cypher® stent with BMS.

Recently, longer-term data from the four pivotal SES trials, including 1748 patients, has been reported; these data demonstrate durable reductions in clinical restenosis endpoints with similar overall safety for Cypher® vs. BMS. (Figure 34.3) [41]. The cumulative incidence of stent thrombosis was similar between Cypher® and BMS (2.1% vs. 2.0%, p = 0.99). Subgroup analyses from the five-year follow-up of the SIRIUS study also demonstrated a similar relative benefit of Cypher® vs. BMS for diabetics and all vessel sizes (Figure 34.4). From this independent, patient-level meta-analysis from the four principal Cypher® trials it may be concluded that at five-year follow-up of patients with single de novo native coronary lesions 2.5–3.5 mm in diameter and ≤30 mm in length, polymer-based sirolimus eluting stents compared to otherwise equivalent bare-metal stents result in: (1) no significant differences in death or myocardial infarction; (2) no significant increase in stent thrombosis; (3) no significant increase in late stent thrombosis by ARC definitions; and (4) sustained reduction in target lesion and target vessel revascularization.

DES in Specific Subgroups: Bifurcations and Acute Myocardial Infarction

Bifurcations

Bifurcations are one of the most challenging subset of lesions in modern interventional cardiology. Currently, there have been no randomized trials comparing the use of DES vs. BMS in patients with bifurcation disease. Previous studies have suggested that stent implantation in the main vessel with stenting of the side branch only when absolutely necessary (provisional approach) is the favoured approach for the treatment of bifurcation disease [42,43–45] (Figure 34.5). These studies have also shown that there is no reduction in the rate of restenosis with the use of two stents. Few studies directly compare the use of SES vs. PES for bifurcation lesions. A recent prospective randomized trial has compared SES to PES in 205 patients where a provisional T-stenting technique has been use [46]. Angiographic follow-up at 24 months shown a lower rate of restenosis in the sirolimus group at the main vessel and the side

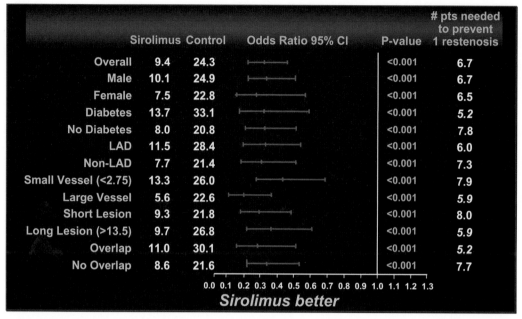

	Sirolimus	Control	Odds Ratio 95% CI	P-value	# pts needed to prevent 1 restenosis
Overall	9.4	24.3		<0.001	6.7
Male	10.1	24.9		<0.001	6.7
Female	7.5	22.8		<0.001	6.5
Diabetes	13.7	33.1		<0.001	5.2
No Diabetes	8.0	20.8		<0.001	7.8
LAD	11.5	28.4		<0.001	6.0
Non-LAD	7.7	21.4		<0.001	7.3
Small Vessel (<2.75)	13.3	26.0		<0.001	7.9
Large Vessel	5.6	22.6		<0.001	5.9
Short Lesion	9.3	21.8		<0.001	8.0
Long Lesion (>13.5)	9.7	26.8		<0.001	5.9
Overlap	11.0	30.1		<0.001	5.2
No Overlap	8.6	21.6		<0.001	7.7

0.0 0.1 0.2 0.3 0.4 0.5 0.6 0.7 0.8 0.9 1.0 1.1 1.2 1.3

Sirolimus better

Figure 34.4. Target lesion revascularization up to five-year. Subgroup analysis from four Cypher® randomized clinical trials. Subgroup analysis shows relative benefit of Cypher® vs. BMS for diabetics and vessel sizes, and all lesion length.

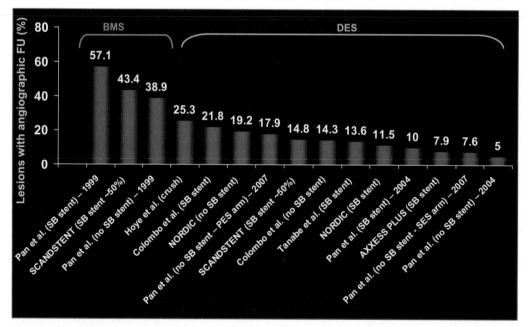

Figure 34.5. Evolution of side branch restenosis in bifurcation series.

branch (9% vs. 29%, p = 0.011), a lower TLR (4% vs. 13%, p = 0.021) and a lower late loss at the main vessel (0.31 mm ± 0.59 mm vs. 0.60 mm ± 0.77 mm, p = 0.027). Another small study comparing SES to PES for bifurcation lesions with the "Crush" technique shown similar results [47]. In this study of 231 patients, angiographic follow-up at 8 months shown lower rate of TVR (7% vs. 16.4%, p = 0.028) and TLR (6.2% vs. 14.5%, p = 0.046) in the SES vs. PES group. According to these data and given the excellent clinical and angiographic results, there appears to be some consensus that strategy of provisional stenting with a DES should be recommended for the initial approach of bifurcation lesions. Current data seem to favour the use of SES over PES in term of restenosis and late loss prevention in this lesion subset.

Acute Myocardial Infarction

The use of DES in acute myocardial infarction has been studied in both observational registries as well as in randomized clinical trials. In a recent meta-analysis of eight randomized trials in 2786 patients with a follow-up up to 24 months, the use of DES compared to BMS was associated with a significantly reduced risk of reintervention, without any difference in the rate of death, recurrent myocardial infarction and stent thrombosis [48]. In recent registry series, DES have shown to decrease significantly the TLR and repeat revascularisation at two years with a significantly decrease of the two-year risk-adjusted mortality rate [49]. These data are quite reassuring regarding the safety of use of DES in acute coronary syndrome.

The TYPHOON trial, a randomized trial of in 712 patients, compared SES vs. BMS in patients undergoing primary PCI. This study has shown a significant reduction in MACE in favor of the SES treatment (5.6% vs. 13.4% with BMS, p < 0.001), largely driven by a lower rate of target vessel revascularization [10]. At eight months, angiographic follow-up demonstrated reductions in late loss and restenosis among patients treated with SES. No differences between the 2 groups were seen in term of rates of death, recurrent myocardial infarction and stent thrombosis. In the SESAMI trial of 320 patients, treatment with a SES was associated with a lower rate of restenosis (9.3% vs. 21.3%, p = 0.032) and with a reductions in target lesion revas-

cularization and MACE [50]. In the MISSION! trial, a randomized trial of SES vs. BMS in 310 patients undergoing primary PCI, treatment with SES was associated with a lower in-segment late luminal loss at 9 months (0.68 ± 0.57 mm vs. 0.12 ± 0.43 mm) and a lower target lesion revascularization rate (3.2% vs. 11.3%; p = 0.006) [51] Rates of death, myocardial infarction, and stent thrombosis were not different. However, IVUS study shown that late stent malapposition at nine months was present in 12.5% BMS patients and in 37.5% SES patients (p < 0.001), raising concern about the long-term safety of SES in STEMI patients. In the other hand, the PASSION trial, a randomized trial of PES vs. BMS in 619 patients undergoing primary PCI, treatment with PES was associated with a nonsignificant trend in the rate of death from cardiac causes or recurrent myocardial infarction (5.5% vs. 7.2%, p = 0.40) and in the rate of target-lesion revascularization (5.3% vs.7.8%, p = 0.23) [9]. There was a trend toward a lower rate of serious adverse events in the PES group than in the uncoated-stent group (8.8% vs. 12.8%, p = 0.09).

Thus, given the design, inclusion criteria, definitions of end points and BMS use in all clinical trials of DES in STEMI were different; it would be hazardous to conclude from these data that one drug eluting stent is better than the other, since no head-to-head comparisons of the two DES in STEMI are available. Data from registry and randomized trials indicate that DES can be used safely in the setting of primary PCI and are likely to reduce the need for repeated revascularization. The HORIZONS AMI (Harmonizing Outcomes with Revascularization and Stents in Acute Myocardial Infarction) [52] randomized 3602 patients from 123 centers in 11 countries. All patients had STEMI with a symptom onset of less than 12 hours. Patients were first randomized in a 1:1 fashion to unfractionated heparin plus a GP IIb/IIIa inhibitor (abciximab or eptifibatide) or to bivalirudin monotherapy plus provisional GP IIb/IIIa inhibitors. The implantation of the paclitaxel eluting Taxus™ stent compared with the BMS Express™ stent resulted in a significant 41% reduction at one year in the primary-efficacy end point of ischemia-driven TLR (4.5% vs. 7.5%, [HR 0.59 (95% CI) 0.43–0.83] and a significant 56% (10.0% vs. 22.9%,

[HR 0.44 (95% CI) 0.33–0.57] reduction in the major secondary efficacy end point of binary restenosis. MACE, a composite of all-cause mortality, reinfarction, stroke, and stent thrombosis, were equivalent with the two stents (8.1% vs. 8.0%, [HR 1.02 (95% CI) 0.76–1.36]. Combining the HORIZONS study with other registries and randomized trials increases the number of MI patients treated with drug eluting stents and provides reassurances about efficacy and safety of DES in this clinical setting.

Randomized trials, Meta-analyses, and Registries

Five-year follow-up data from the pivotal randomized trials has demonstrated durable and sustained reductions in target lesion revascularization and target vessel revascularization with both first-generation DES compared with BMS, with no significant differences in endpoints such as death, MI, or stent thrombosis [53]. These findings have been paralleled in meta-analyses of randomized trials comparing DES with BMS including not only the pivotal trials, but also trials for a variety of other indications, including acute MI [48,54].

One of the most extensive meta-analyses to date comparing BMS and DES included 38 trials, a total of 18,023 patients, at a follow-up of up to four years [55]. There was no significant difference in overall and cardiac mortality in this analysis between BMS, SES, or PES. Moreover, both SES and PES had significantly lower rates of repeat target lesion revascularization compared to BMS. Whilst SES was associated with lower rates of MI when compared to both BMS and PES, the number of patients needed to treat to prevent one MI event was about 100, which as mentioned, did not impact overall or cardiac mortality. With regard to stent thrombosis, there were no differences between BMS, SES, or PES with respect to overall stent thrombosis. Interestingly, there was trend of late temporal separation suggesting that BMS had a lower incidence of definite stent thrombosis at four years. Whilst the reported rate of late stent thrombosis was higher with PES compared to BMS and SES, wide confidence intervals (CI) preclude any definitive conclusions in this regard (Figure 34.6). Although this large collaborative meta-analysis has

clearly demonstrated no worse safety of both first-generation DES (SES and PES) compared to BMS with reductions in revascularization endpoints, head-to-head comparative data of SES with PES have been mixed. In a meta-analysis of 16 randomized trials comparing sirolimus and paclitaxel eluting stents including 8,695 patients, SES reduced the risk of target lesion and stent thrombosis compared to PES, without significant differences in risk of death or MI [56]. However, in the latest randomized trial comparing SES and PES in 2098 patients, there were no differences between SES and PES in the rate of MACE, defined as cardiac death, MI, target lesion revascularization, or target vessel revascularization.

In addition to data from randomized trials and meta-analyses of these trials, there has been a great deal of data presented and published in the last year from "real-world" registries of DES use. Whilst a detailed summary of all these data is beyond the scope of this review, a brief overview of the types of registry data currently available is instructive, and illustrates both the strengths and weaknesses of these types of analyses.

Most of these observational, non-randomized comparisons of BMS and DES fall into two types. The first type consists of a comparison between BMS and DES use occurring during two distinct time periods, a period with predominant use of BMS use (before or in the early stages of DES adoption) and a period with predominant DES use. The second type of analysis consists of a comparison between BMS and DES from a single period of concurrent BMS and DES use. Unlike randomized trials, these types of analyses evaluate both BMS and DES use in "real-world" patients, without restrictions of relatively strict patient and lesion inclusion and exclusion criteria. However, both types of analysis are of course observational, and are limited by differences between patients treated with BMS vs. DES. Whilst the sequential type of comparison attempts to limit selection bias (or decision making swaying the choice of one type of stent over the other), this analysis is subject to bias relating to differences in case selection, adjunctive pharmacology, and procedural factors between two different time periods. Similarly, whilst the concurrent type of registry may be less subject to these latter biases, selection bias can play a major

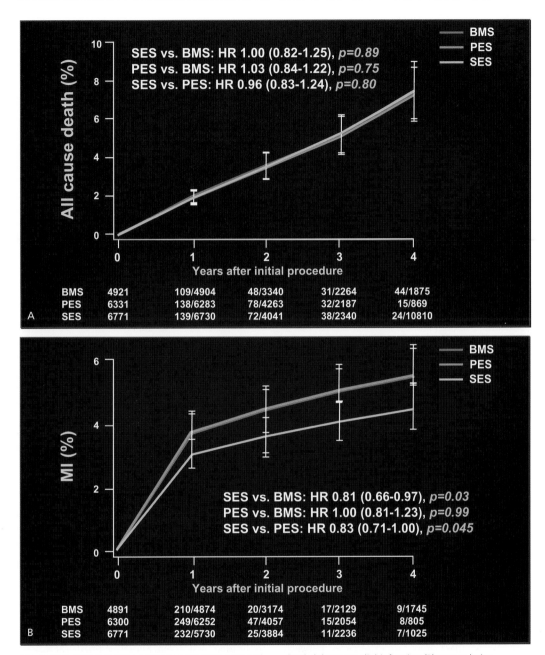

Figure 34.6. Network meta-analyses comparing BMS and DES included 38 trials, a total of 18,023 patients, at a follow-up of up to four years. Kaplan-Meier curve for death (A); myocardial infarction (B); target lesion revascularization (C); and ARC defined stent thrombosis (D).

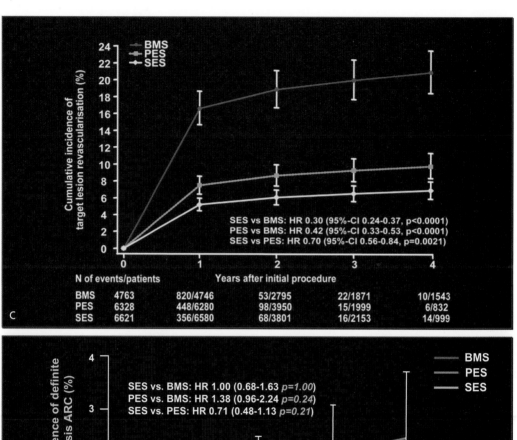

Figure 34.6 *Continued*

role in explaining differences between treatment groups. As a result, observational, non-randomized comparisons between treatment groups are extremely valuable, but must be interpreted with a critical eye despite efforts to statistically adjust for baseline differences between comparator groups.

The majority of registry data presented in the last year has included comparisons of DES vs. BMS with follow-up in some registries of up to four years. Consistent with randomized trial data, these registries all demonstrate significant reductions in target lesion revascularization and other clinical endpoints related to restenosis. In addition, to date, with the exception of the original presentation of the Swedish SCAAR registry that demonstrated increased mortality among DES-treated patients, no other registry (including the re-analysis of SCAAR) has demonstrated a statistically detectable increase in mortality or MI with DES compared to BMS [13,57–61]. In fact, the greater part of these registries have demonstrated up to 20% reductions in all-cause mortality with DES compared to BMS even in adjusted analyses.

Additionally, several registries have assessed the risks and benefits of DES use specifically in "off-label" patients, or patients that would have been excluded from the pivotal DES vs. BMS trials. In a single center registry of 1164 consecutive patients receiving BMS and 1,285 consecutive patients receiving DES, the use of DES was associated with lower all-cause mortality (HR 0.72, 95% CI 0.54–0.94), and non-fatal MI or death (HR 0.78, 95% CI 0.62–0.98) compared to BMS in cases of "off-label" stenting. This study demonstrated an elevated risk associated with "off-label" use independent of stent type, but simultaneously demonstrated a greater relative benefit to DES vs. BMS when "off-label" stenting occurs [13]. Although late stent thrombosis occurred with DES in "off-label" settings, and did not happen with BMS, the relative benefit of reduced target lesion revascularization, non-fatal MI or death, and all-cause mortality would appear to outweigh this risk in "off-label" settings. Similarly, in the NHLBI Dynamic registry, there was no difference in the adjusted risk of death or MI at one year associated with "off-label" DES use compared to BMS use despite a greater prevalence of co-morbid conditions among DES-treated patients. Consistent with other randomized trial and registry data, the risk of repeat revascularization was significantly lower with DES, regardless of the setting (Figure 34.7) [57].

In summary, the preponderance of both randomized and registry data, now including greater than 150,000 patients (including unpublished but presented data) with follow-up in some cases out to five years, supports the use of DES in reducing restenosis-related events with no untoward effects related to death or MI, and in fact a possible reduction in mortality observed in registry series. Despite these reassuring data, newer generation technolo-

gies are needed, as the current generation DES do appear to be associated with a risk of late stent thrombosis, as discussed above. Additionally, issues such as incomplete delayed re-endotelization and neointimal growth, enhanced platelet aggregation and inflammation, late-acquired incomplete stent apposition and localized hypersensitivity reaction have been observed to occur with the current generation DES. Novel DES systems have been introduced with the aim to improve outcomes whilst diminishing adverse events.

Safety Concerns with DES

In late 2006, safety concerns were raised about of these first-generation DES. Two meta-analyses and a large observational registry study that individually suggested increases in adverse clinical endpoints with DES largely emerging following the first year of stent implantation [62–64]. These initial data, combined with additional data that has demonstrated that DES are associated with a small but measurable risk of late stent thrombosis (stent thrombosis occurring beyond 30 days) [65,66], were widely reported in the media and lay press, and generated considerable controversy and concern for patients, physicians, device companies, and regulatory bodies alike.

Data from numerous trials and registries have shown that the overall rate of acute and subacute stent thrombosis (occurring within 24 hours or within 30 days after stent placement, respectively), appears to be no different for DES or BMS [25,35]. However, in analyses incorporating long-term follow-up, there is a small but finite risk of late stent thrombosis (occurring beyond 30 days) associated with DES use [27,65]. In theory, this occurrence of late stent thrombosis would be expected to increase mortality and non-fatal myocardial infarction (MI) rates for DES-treated patients, but most studies, including meta-analyses inclusive of the early cautionary data, found no differences in death and MI at extended follow-up [27,54]. Moreover, subsequent re-analysis of the large Swedish registry study that initially raised concerns over DES safety with additional follow-up to four years and the addition of more patients have demonstrated no differences in hard clinical endpoints between DES and BMS.

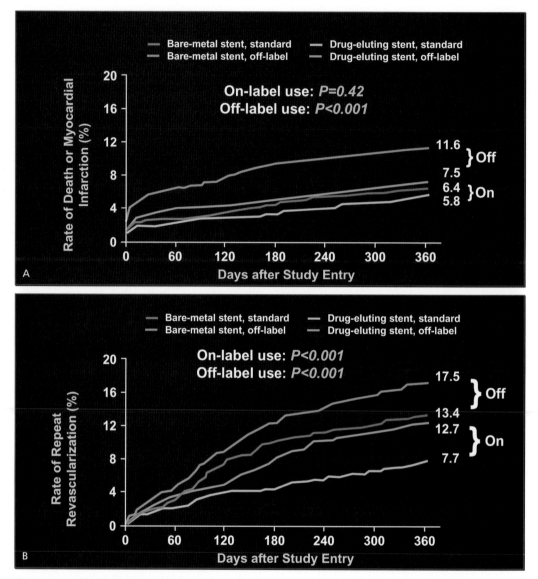

Figure 34.7. NHLBI Registry. Kaplan-Meier curves of death or myocardial infarction (A) and for target vessel revascularization (B) between "on-label" vs. "off-label" use.

A critical issue that has been consistently manifest in analyses of DES safety relates to the danger of examining underpowered endpoints such as death or MI in relatively small DES studies due to statistical variability in low event-rate clinical outcomes. A good example of this is demonstrated by examining the data of SES vs. BMS in diabetic patients. A widely-heralded analysis of the four pivotal SES trials demonstrated improvements in restenosis-related endpoints but greater mortality among diabetic patients treated with SES [10]. However, closer examination of this data demonstrates that in these trials there was far better than expected survival among BMS-treated patients, which may have accounted for the observed differences between DES and BMS. Indeed, a recent and similarly-performed analysis of PES vs. BMS from the five pivotal PES trials has demonstrated similar mortality outcomes with both stents with durable reductions in target vessel and target lesion revascularization [28].

Whilst the lack of an observed difference between hard clinical endpoints among DES and BMS-treated patients in most studies may be due to inadequate statistical power to detect these differences, there may be other explanations for the relative equipoise that currently exists. First, the assessment of stent thrombosis in the major randomized trials of DES vs. BMS censored stent thrombosis events occurring after intervening revascularizations. Because intervening revascularizations occurred far more frequently among BMS-treated patients (largely due to greater restenosis among these patients), this effectively under-counted thromboses occurring in this group [7]. To corroborate this, a subsequent intention-to-treat based analysis using Academic Research Consortium definitions of stent thrombosis without censoring of "secondary" thrombosis events demonstrated that the occurrence of stent thrombosis was similar for both DES and BMS at 4-year follow-up [67]. Second, it appears that at least with the current length of follow-up available, the incremental risk of stent thrombosis may be offset by the other benefits of DES with respect to reductions in restenosis-related endpoints, including repeat revascularization and its subsequent sequelae. For example, a detailed analysis of four pivotal PES trials elegantly demonstrated the offsetting competing risks of restenosis and stent thrombosis with respect to death/MI events in these trials [68].

At present, there appears to be some consensus that whilst DES are likely associated with a slightly increased rate of late stent thrombosis compared to BMS, at least with "on-label" DES use, these risks appeared to be offset by reductions in restenosis-related outcomes, and thus, there are no observed increases in hard safety endpoints such as death or MI with the use of DES compared to BMS. Data from the combined Bern-Rotterdam registries demonstrate a consistent linear risk over follow-up out to four years [65]. However, a recent study from the large Mayo Clinic PCI database demonstrated a measurable risk of late stent thrombosis with *BMS* over a follow-up period of up to 10 years [69]. Finally, whilst it appears that premature discontinuation of dual antiplatelet therapy is a profound risk factor for stent thrombosis [70,71], the optimal duration of dual antiplatelet therapy to prevent thrombosis events remains unclear. Finally, it remains unclear whether modifications of DES design (e.g. changes to the polymer or elimination of the polymer) or newer generation DES will be associated with similar concerns regarding late thrombotic events.

Conclusion

Current approaches to sirolimus- and paclitaxel eluting stent development and clinical data were reviewed in this chapter. The first-generation DES have overcome the obstacle of restenosis and consequent need for repeat revascularization. However, long-term safety issues have arisen. Whilst there is a likely greater risk of late stent thrombosis with DES, the preponderance of current data suggests that current DES are not associated with increases in death, MI, or other "hard clinical endpoints" compared to BMS, and are durably associated with reductions in restenosis-related endpoints, with potentially even greater absolute benefits (and risks) in "off-label" utilization.

As PCI continues to adapt and evolve, new developments in DES technology are clearly on the horizon. The third and the fourth DES available in the United States was recently approved by the FDA. Aside from these second-generation stents, a whole host of new DES technologies are currently under active investigation. Bifurcation DES systems, DES with bioabsorbable polymers, non-polymer DES approach with surface modification to obviate the use of a polymer, and even wholly bioabsorbable DES are all currently in preclinical or clinical trials.

References

1. Leon MB, Baim DS, Popma JJ, *et al*. A clinical trial comparing three antithrombotic-drug regimens after coronary-artery stenting. Stent Anticoagulation Restenosis Study Investigators. N Engl J Med 1998; **339**(23): 1665–1671.

2. Serruys PW, de Jaegere P, Kiemeneij F, *et al*. A comparison of balloon-expandable-stent implantation with balloon angioplasty in patients with coronary artery disease. Benestent Study Group. N Engl J Med 1994; **331**(8): 489–495.

3. Serruys PW, Kutryk MJ, Ong AT. Coronary-artery stents. N Engl J Med 2006; **354**(5): 483–495.

4. Nayak AK, Kawamura A, Nesto RW, *et al*. Myocardial infarction as a presentation of clinical in-stent restenosis. Circ J 2006; **70**(8): 1026–1029.

5. Chen MS, John JM, Chew DP, *et al*. Bare metal stent restenosis is not a benign clinical entity. Am Heart J 2006; **151**(6): 1260–1264.

6. Schuhlen H, Kastrati A, Mehilli J, Hausleiter J, Pache J, Dirschinger J, Schomig A. Restenosis detected by routine angiographic follow-up and late mortality after coronary stent placement. Am Heart J 2004; **147**(2): 317–322.

7. Jeremias A, Kirtane A. Balancing efficacy and safety of drug-eluting stents in patients undergoing percutaneous coronary intervention. Ann Intern Med 2008; **148**(3): 234–238.

8. Stone GW, Ellis SG, Cannon L, *et al*. Comparison of a polymer-based paclitaxel-eluting stent with a bare metal stent in patients with complex coronary artery disease: a randomized controlled trial. JAMA 2005; **294**(10): 1215–1223.

9. Laarman GJ, Suttorp MJ, Dirksen MT, *et al*. Paclitaxel-eluting versus uncoated stents in primary percutaneous coronary intervention. N Engl J Med 2006; **355**(11): 1105–1113.

10. Spaulding C, Henry P, Teiger E, *et al*. Sirolimus-eluting versus uncoated stents in acute myocardial infarction. N Engl J Med 2006; **355**(11): 1093–1104.

11. Lemos PA, Serruys PW, van Domburg RT, Saia F, Arampatzis CA, Hoye A, Degertekin M, Tanabe K, Daemen J, Liu TK, McFadden E, Sianos G, Hofma SH, Smits PC, van der Giessen WJ, de Feyter PJ. Unrestricted utilization of sirolimus-eluting stents compared with conventional bare stent implantation in the "real world": The Rapamycin-Eluting Stent Evaluated At Rotterdam Cardiology Hospital (RESEARCH) registry. Circulation 2004; **109**(2): 190–195.

12. Urban P, Gershlick AH, Guagliumi G, *et al*. Safety of coronary sirolimus-eluting stents in daily clinical practice: one-year follow-up of the e-Cypher registry. Circulation 2006; **113**(11): 1434–1441.

13. Applegate RJ, Sacrinty MT, Kutcher MA, *et al*. "Off-label" stent therapy 2-year comparison of drug-eluting versus bare-metal stents. J Am Coll Cardiol 2008; **51**(6): 607–614.

14. Kip KE, Hollabaugh K, Marroquin OC, *et al*. The problem with composite end points in cardiovascular studies: the story of major adverse cardiac events and percutaneous coronary intervention. J Am Coll Cardiol 2008; **51**(7): 701–707.

15. Win HK, Caldera AE, Maresh K, *et al*. Clinical outcomes and stent thrombosis following off-label use of drug-eluting stents. JAMA 2007; **297**(18): 2001–2009.

16. Rowinsky EK, Donehower RC. Paclitaxel (taxol). N Engl J Med 1995; **332**(15): 1004–1014.

17. Sollott SJ, Cheng L, Pauly RR, *et al*. Taxol inhibits neointimal smooth muscle cell accumulation after angioplasty in the rat. J Clin Invest 1995; **95**(4): 1869–1876.

18. Drachman DE, Edelman ER, Seifert P, *et al*. Neointimal thickening after stent delivery of paclitaxel: change in composition and arrest of growth over six months. J Am Coll Cardiol 2000; **36**(7): 2325–2332.

19. Heldman AW, Cheng L, Jenkins GM, *et al*. Paclitaxel stent coating inhibits neointimal hyperplasia at 4 weeks in a porcine model of coronary restenosis. Circulation 2001; **103**(18): 2289–2295.

20. Axel DI, Kunert W, Goggelmann C, *et al*. Paclitaxel inhibits arterial smooth muscle cell proliferation and migration in vitro and in vivo using local drug delivery. Circulation 1997; **96**(2): 636–645.

21. Grube E, Silber S, Hauptmann KE, *et al*. TAXUS I: six- and twelve-month results from a randomized, double-blind trial on a slow-release paclitaxel-eluting stent for de novo coronary lesions. Circulation 2003; **107**(1): 38–42.

22. Colombo A, Drzewiecki J, Banning A, *et al*. Randomized study to assess the effectiveness of slow- and moderate-release polymer-based paclitaxel-eluting stents for coronary artery lesions. Circulation 2003; **108**(7): 788–794.

23. Tanabe K, Serruys PW, Grube E, *et al*. TAXUS III Trial: in-stent restenosis treated with stent-based delivery of paclitaxel incorporated in a slow-release polymer formulation. Circulation 2003; **107**(4): 559–564.

24. Stone GW, Ellis SG, Cox DA, *et al*. A polymer-based, paclitaxel-eluting stent in patients with coronary artery disease. N Engl J Med 2004; **350**(3): 221–231.

25. Stone GW, Ellis SG, Cox DA, *et al*. One-year clinical results with the slow-release, polymer-based, paclitaxel-eluting TAXUS stent: the TAXUS-IV trial. Circulation 2004; **109**(16): 1942–1947.

26. Dawkins KD, Grube E, Guagliumi G, *et al.* Clinical efficacy of polymer-based paclitaxel-eluting stents in the treatment of complex, long coronary artery lesions from a multicenter, randomized trial: support for the use of drug-eluting stents in contemporary clinical practice. Circulation 2005; **112**(21): 3306–3313.

27. Stone GW, Moses JW, Ellis SG, *et al.* Safety and efficacy of sirolimus- and paclitaxel-eluting coronary stents. N Engl J Med 2007; **356**(10): 998–1008.

28. Kirtane AJ, Ellis SG, Dawkins KD, *et al.* Paclitaxel-eluting coronary stents in patients with diabetes mellitus: pooled analysis from 5 randomized trials. J Am Coll Cardiol 2008; **51**(7): 708–715.

29. Marx SO, Marks AR. Bench to bedside: the development of rapamycin and its application to stent restenosis. Circulation 2001; **104**(8): 852–855.

30. Marx SO, Jayaraman T, Go LO, *et al.* Rapamycin-FKBP inhibits cell cycle regulators of proliferation in vascular smooth muscle cells. Circ Res 1995; **76**(3): 412–417.

31. Poon M, Marx SO, Gallo R, *et al.* Rapamycin inhibits vascular smooth muscle cell migration. J Clin Invest 1996; **98**(10): 2277–2283.

32. Sousa JE, Costa MA, Abizaid A, *et al.* Lack of neointimal proliferation after implantation of sirolimus-coated stents in human coronary arteries: a quantitative coronary angiography and three-dimensional intravascular ultrasound study. Circulation 2001; **103**(2): 192–195.

33. Sousa JE, Costa MA, Abizaid AC, Rensing BJ, *et al.* Sustained suppression of neointimal proliferation by sirolimus-eluting stents: one-year angiographic and intravascular ultrasound follow-up. Circulation 2001; **104**(17): 2007–2011.

34. Morice MC, Serruys PW, Sousa JE, *et al.* A randomized comparison of a sirolimus-eluting stent with a standard stent for coronary revascularization. N Engl J Med 2002; **346**(23): 1773–1780.

35. Moses JW, Leon MB, Popma JJ, *et al.* Sirolimus-eluting stents versus standard stents in patients with stenosis in a native coronary artery. N Engl J Med 2003; **349**(14): 1315–1323.

36. Schofer J, Schluter M, Gershlick AH, *et al.* Sirolimus-eluting stents for treatment of patients with long atherosclerotic lesions in small coronary arteries: double-blind, randomised controlled trial (E-SIRIUS). Lancet 2003; **362**(9390): 1093–1099.

37. Schampaert E, Cohen EA, Schluter M, *et al.* The Canadian study of the sirolimus-eluting stent in the treatment of patients with long de novo lesions in small native coronary arteries (C-SIRIUS). J Am Coll Cardiol 2004; **43**(6): 1110–1115.

38. Fajadet J, Morice MC, Bode C, *et al.* Maintenance of long-term clinical benefit with sirolimus-eluting coronary stents: three-year results of the RAVEL trial. Circulation 2005; **111**(8): 1040–1044.

39. Leon MB. Unpublished data. Paper presented at: American College of Cardiology Scientific Meeting, 2007.

40. Schampaert E, Moses JW, Schofer J, *et al.* Sirolimus-eluting stents at two years: a pooled analysis of SIRIUS, E-SIRIUS, and C-SIRIUS with emphasis on late revascularizations and stent thromboses. Am J Cardiol 2006; **98**(1): 36–41.

41. Kirtane A. Unpublished data. Paper presented at Transcatheter Cardiovascular Therapeutics, 2007; Washington DC.

42. Colombo A, Moses JW, Morice MC, *et al.* Randomized study to evaluate sirolimus-eluting stents implanted at coronary bifurcation lesions. Circulation 2004; **109**(10): 1244–1249.

43. Pan M, de Lezo JS, Medina A, *et al.* Rapamycin-eluting stents for the treatment of bifurcated coronary lesions: a randomized comparison of a simple versus complex strategy. Am Heart J 2004; **148**(5): 857–864.

44. Steigen TK, Maeng M, Wiseth R, *et al.* Randomized study on simple versus complex stenting of coronary artery bifurcation lesions: the Nordic bifurcation study. Circulation 2006; **114**(18): 1955–1961.

45. Kelbaek H, Helqvist S, Thuesen L, *et al.* Sirolimus versus bare metal stent implantation in patients with total coronary occlusions: subgroup analysis of the Stenting Coronary Arteries in Non-Stress/Benestent Disease (SCANDSTENT) trial. Am Heart J 2006; **152**(5): 882–886.

46. Pan M, Suarez de Lezo J, Medina A, *et al.* Drug-eluting stents for the treatment of bifurcation lesions: a randomized comparison between paclitaxel and sirolimus stents. Am Heart J 2007; **153**(1): 15 e11–e17.

47. Hoye A, Iakovou I, Ge L, *et al.* A. Long-term outcomes after stenting of bifurcation lesions with the "crush" technique: Predictors of an adverse outcome. J Am Coll Cardiol 2006; **47**(10): 1949–1958.

48. Kastrati A, Dibra A, Spaulding C, *et al.* Meta-analysis of randomized trials on drug-eluting stents vs. bare-metal stents in patients with acute myocardial infarction. Eur Heart J 2007; **28**(22): 2706–2713.

49. Mauri L, Silbaugh TS, Garg P, *et al.* Drug-eluting or bare-metal stents for acute myocardial infarction. N Engl J Med 2008; **359**(13): 1330–1342.

50. Menichelli M, Parma A, Pucci E, *et al.* Randomized trial of Sirolimus-Eluting Stent Versus Bare-Metal Stent in Acute Myocardial Infarction (SESAMI). J Am Coll Cardiol 2007; **49**(19): 1924–1930.

51. van der Hoeven BL, Liem SS, Jukema JW, *et al.* Sirolimus-eluting stents versus bare-metal stents in

patients with ST-segment elevation myocardial infarction: 9-month angiographic and intravascular ultrasound results and 12-month clinical outcome results from the MISSION! Intervention Study. J Am Coll Cardiol 2008; 51(6): 618–626.

52. Stone GW. Unpublished data. Paper presented at: Transcatheter Cardiovascular Therapeutics, 2008; Washington, DC.

53. Caixeta A, Leon MB, Lansky MDA, et al. Five-year clinical outcomes after sirolimus-eluting stent implantation: Insights from a patient-level pooled analysis of four randomized trials comparing sirolimus-eluting stents with bare-metal stents. J Am Coll Cardiol 2009 (in press).

54. Kastrati A, Mehilli J, Pache J, et al. Analysis of 14 trials comparing sirolimus-eluting stents with bare-metal stents. N Engl J Med 2007; 356(10): 1030–1039.

55. Stettler C, Wandel S, Allemann S, et al. Outcomes associated with drug-eluting and bare-metal stents: a collaborative network meta-analysis. Lancet 2007; 370(9591): 937–948.

56. Schomig A, Dibra A, Windecker S, et al. A meta-analysis of 16 randomized trials of sirolimus-eluting stents versus paclitaxel-eluting stents in patients with coronary artery disease. J Am Coll Cardiol 2007; 50(14): 1373–1380.

57. Marroquin OC, Selzer F, Mulukutla SR, et al. A comparison of bare-metal and drug-eluting stents for off-label indications. N Engl J Med 2008; 358(4): 342–352.

58. Abbott JD, Voss MR, Nakamura M, et al. Unrestricted use of drug-eluting stents compared with bare-metal stents in routine clinical practice: findings from the National Heart, Lung, and Blood Institute Dynamic Registry. J Am Coll Cardiol 2007; 50(21): 2029–2036.

59. Marzocchi A, Saia F, Piovaccari G, et al. Long-term safety and efficacy of drug-eluting stents: two-year results of the REAL (REgistro AngiopLastiche dell'Emilia Romagna) multicenter registry. Circulation 2007; 115(25): 3181–3188.

60. Jensen LO, Maeng M, Kaltoft A, et al. Stent thrombosis, myocardial infarction, and death after drug-eluting and bare-metal stent coronary interventions. J Am Coll Cardiol 2007; 50(5): 463–470.

61. Tu JV, Bowen J, Chiu M, et al. Effectiveness and safety of drug-eluting stents in Ontario. N Engl J Med 2007; 357(14): 1393–1402.

62. Camenzind E, Steg PG, Wijns W. Stent thrombosis late after implantation of first-generation drug-eluting stents: a cause for concern. Circulation 2007; 115(11): 1440–1455; discussion 1455.

63. Nordmann AJ, Briel M, Bucher HC. Mortality in randomized controlled trials comparing drug-eluting vs. bare metal stents in coronary artery disease: a meta-analysis. Eur Heart J 2006; 27(23): 2784–2814.

64. Lagerqvist B, James SK, Stenestrand U, et al. Long-term outcomes with drug-eluting stents versus bare-metal stents in Sweden. N Engl J Med 2007; 356(10): 1009–1019.

65. Daemen J, Wenaweser P, Tsuchida K, et al. Early and late coronary stent thrombosis of sirolimus-eluting and paclitaxel-eluting stents in routine clinical practice: data from a large two-institutional cohort study. Lancet 2007; 369(9562): 667–678.

66. Pfisterer M, Brunner-La Rocca HP, et al. Late clinical events after clopidogrel discontinuation may limit the benefit of drug-eluting stents: an observational study of drug-eluting versus bare-metal stents. J Am Coll Cardiol 2006; 48(12): 2584–2591.

67. Mauri L, Hsieh WH, Massaro JM, et al. Stent thrombosis in randomized clinical trials of drug-eluting stents. N Engl J Med 2007; 356(10): 1020–1029.

68. Stone GW, Ellis SG, Colombo A, et al. Offsetting impact of thrombosis and restenosis on the occurrence of death and myocardial infarction after paclitaxel-eluting and bare metal stent implantation. Circulation 2007; 115(22): 2842–2847.

69. Doyle B, Rihal CS, O'Sullivan CJ, et al. Outcomes of stent thrombosis and restenosis during extended follow-up of patients treated with bare-metal coronary stents. Circulation 2007; 116(21): 2391–2398.

70. Jeremias A, Sylvia B, Bridges J, et al. Stent thrombosis after successful sirolimus-eluting stent implantation. Circulation 2004; 109(16): 1930–1932.

71. Iakovou I, Schmidt T, Bonizzoni E, et al. Incidence, predictors, and outcome of thrombosis after successful implantation of drug-eluting stents. JAMA 2005; 293(17): 2126–2130.

CHAPTER 35

Zotarolimus Eluting Stent Clinical Studies

William Wijns[1], & Marco Valgimigli[2]

[1] Cardiovascular Center Aalst, Moorselbaan, Aalst, Belgium
[2] Cardiovascular Institute, University of Ferrara, Ferrara, Italy

Challenges for New-Generation Drug Eluting Stents

Considerable efforts have gone into the development of new-generation drug eluting stent (DES) that would retain the powerful anti-restenosis properties of sirolimus and paclitaxel eluting stents, yet provide improved deliverability and regain safety profiles comparable or superior to bare-metal stents (BMS). The components of a DES can be divided into a platform (the stent), a carrier (usually a polymer), and an agent (a drug) to prevent restenosis. The choice of a suitable carrier to transport an appropriate agent has been challenging, since it must have mechanical resistance to abrasion during implantation, be suitable for sterilization, allow time- and dose-controlled drug release, be non-thrombogenic and not be the cause of inflammation of the vessel-wall and tissue [1]. Various types of coatings have been developed, including biocompatible non-erodable, biodegradable, or bioabsorbable polymers as well as ceramic layers. A drug that is successfully eluted should inhibit the complex cascade of events that leads to neointimal forma-tion after stent implantation. The inflammatory and proliferative mechanisms of the general tissue-healing response and specific blood and vessel-wall components of the vascular reparative processes are potential targets for therapeutic approaches aimed at reducing neointimal proliferation (Figure 35.1).

The success of eluting devices is highly dependent on each component of the complex, as well as on the interactions among these elements. Therefore different DES brands will not share a class effect, since there is a myriad of possible iterations on each component of the drug-device combinations that may have significant therapeutic implications (Table 35.1). Many proposed devices failed to show efficacy profile over BMS and different DES show different abilities to inhibit neointimal proliferation. Because the results of short term experiments in animal models cannot be directly translated to humans, specific clinical trials are required in order to establish the efficacy and safety for any newer drug-device combination. Numerous drug-device combinations have been tested, of which over 20 have received the CE certificate that is necessary for use in the European Union [2]. So far, however, only two of the newer generation DES have received positive reviews by the Food and Drug Administration, namely the zotarolimus [3–5] and the everolimus eluting stents [6].

Interventional Cardiology, First Edition. Edited by Carlo Di Mario, George D. Dangas, Peter Barlis.
© 2010 Blackwell Publishing Ltd. Published 2010 by Blackwell Publishing Ltd.

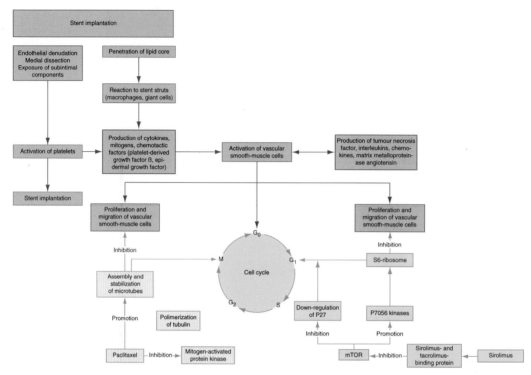

Figure 35.1. Mechanisms of restenosis after stent implantation and targets of therapy with sirolimus including other "limus" agents and paclitaxel. Sirolimus analogues act through the same pathway as sirolimus.

The restenosis casade that is initiated after stent implantation is shown in red. The mechanism of action of sirolimus (and analogues including zotarolimus) is shown in blue. Reproduced from Serruys , Kutryk, Ong [1].

Table 35.1. Features of the "Optimal"DES.

- High deliverability in complex and difficult anatomy.
- Eliminate restenosis at least to the extent first-generation DES did.
- Improve durability of the results of PCI thereby justifying expanding indications.
- Limit the release/presence of cytotoxic drugs and/or poorly biocompatible components to the necessary minimum (in time and dose).
- Allow vessel healing and endothelialization, without interfering with vessel biology.
- Avoid any systemic side effects of the drug-device combination.
- Avoid the need for extended duration of dual antiplatelet therapy.

Technical Characteristics of the Zotarolimus Eluting Stents

Initially two different iterations of the zotarolimus eluting DES have been developed in parallel, i.e. the Endeavor DES by Medtronic and the ZoMaxx DES by Abbott Vascular. Evaluation of the latter device was interrupted because initial studies showed reduced antiproliferative properties compared to existing DES [7]. Components of the Endeavor stent are illustrated on Figure 35.2. Zotarolimus is a novel pharmacologic therapy that shares similar structure and biologic activity with the antirestenotic agent sirolimus, i.e. it blocks the function of mTOR (Figure 35.1). The Endeavor stent is a cobalt-based alloy stent with a phosphorylcholine polymer loaded with zotarolimus at dose concentration of $10\,\mu g/mm$ stent length. It has been shown in preclinical studies that approxi-

Driver Cobalt Alloy Stent

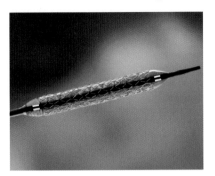

Stent Delivery System

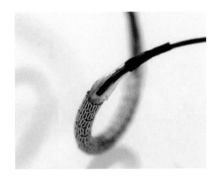

Phosphorylcholine Polymer

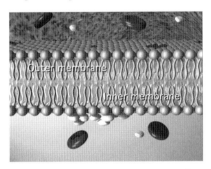

Zotarolimus ABT-578

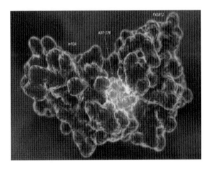

Figure 35.2. Components of the Endeavor zotarolimus eluting stent.

mately 95% of zotarolimus is eluted from the stent within 15 days of implantation, although drug concentrations within surrounding vascular tissue may be detected as late as 30 days after stent deployment [8]. Zotarolimus is equivalent to sirolimus in terms of antiproliferative power (IC50 at 0.3 nM) but is more lipophilic: logD >4.5, as compared to 3.6 for sirolimus. Phosphorylcholine is a durable polymer primarily comprised of hydrophilic monomers that mimic the chemical structure of phospholipid headgroups, similar to the outer membrane of red blood cells (90% of phospholipids in the outer membrane of a red blood cell contain the phosphorylcholine headgroup). This polymer has a broad history of use in medical devices including coronary stents (Figure 35.3). At the time of Endeavor development, >150.000 stent implants had taken place world wide (BiodivYsio PC Coated Stent, approved September 29, 2000). Biocompatibility of phos-

phorylcholine polymer is well studied in preclinical models indicating thrombo-resistance in shunt models and preserved endothelialization of metallic stent struts at 30 days [9].

Anti-restenosis Efficacy of the Endeavor Zotarolimus Eluting Stent

The clinical evaluation program of the Endeavor stent (Table 35.2) is exhaustive as it includes over 22,000 patients so far. This particular drug-device combination has undergone the evaluation pathways of both first- and new-generation DES, being compared to a contemporary BMS as well as to the established Cypher and Taxus stents (Figure 35.4). Following the first-in-man study [3], the pivotal ENDEAVOR II trial has demonstrated sustained and highly significant reduction in all metrics of restenosis, as compared to the Driver BMS [4,5,10].

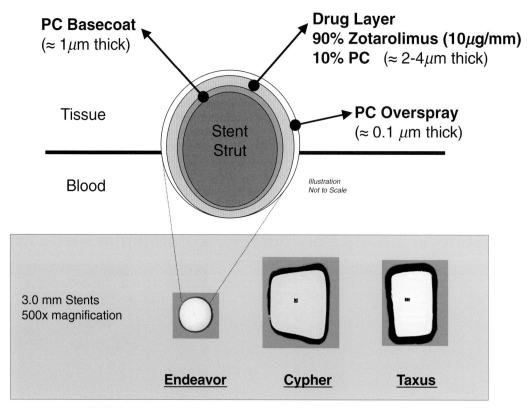

Figure 35.3. Details of stent platform and phosphorylcholine coating. Strut thickness and geometry likely are important factors for re-endothelialization and restenosis propensity.

Table 35.2. Endeavor Clinical Program.

ENDEAVOR I	First In Man study (n = 100)	5 years
ENDEAVOR II	Randomized (1:1) Trial vs Driver BMS (n = 1.197)	4 years
ENDEAVOR II PK	Pharmacokinetics study (106 patients subset of E II)	4 years
ENDEAVOR II CA	Continued access single arm (n = 296)	3 years
ENDEAVOR III	Randomized (3:1) Trial vs Cypher (n = 636)	3 years
ENDEAVOR IV	Randomized (1:1) Trial vs Taxus (n = 1.548)	3 years
ENDEAVOR Japan	Single arm registry (n = 99)	2 years
ENDEAVOR PK	Pharmacokinetics study (n = 43)	1 year
PROTECT	Randomized (1:1) Trial vs Cypher (n = 8.800)	enrolling
e-FIVE	Single arm registry (n = 8.000)	enrolling
US post-approval	Single arm registry (sample to be defined)	proposed

For instance, target vessel revascularization rate at 1440 days was significantly (p < 0.001) reduced from 18.8% with Driver to 9.8% with Endeavor (97.5 and 97.2% completeness of follow-up, respectively). A comparison of the essential characteristics and results of the three main pivotal randomized trials shows a striking difference between Endeavor and the first-generation DES (Table 35.3). Whilst similar reductions in *clinical* restenosis were observed, *angiographic* metrics of

Evaluation Pathways for DES

1st Generation

- Pre-clinical
- First In Man
- (Dose-response & kinetics)
- Pivotal Randomised Trial
- Superiority vs BMS
- Powered for combined clinical / angio endpoints
- Complex Lesion / patient subsets
- Real life registry

2nd Generation

- Pre-clinical
- First In Man
- (Dose-response & kinetics)
- Pivotal Randomised Trial
- Non inferiority vs 1st DES
- Powered for angiographic efficacy endpoints
- Complex Lesion / patient subsets
- Real life registry

Figure 35.4. Design of pre-clinical and clinical evaluation schemes of DES. New drug-devices combinations are tested for non-inferiority against first-generation DES (Cypher or Taxus). The Endeavor stent has been tested for superiority against BMS and non-inferiority against both Cypher and Taxus. None of the published stent trials are powered for clinical outcome (death, non fatal myocardial infarction).

Table 35.3. Comparison of pivotal DES trials.

	ENDEAVOR II	TAXUS IV	SIRIUS
N patients	598	662	533
Vessel diameter (mm)	2.74	2.75	2.78
Lesion length (mm)	14.0	13.4	14.4
B2 / C lesions (%)	78	51	59
Diabetes (%)	18	24	25
Dual antiplatelet (months)	3	6	3
LAD stenosis (%)	43	40	44
Clinical follow-up (%)	99	97	98
Target vessel failure (%)	8.1	7.6	8.6
MACE (%)	7.4	8.5	7.1
In-stent late loss (mm)	0.62	0.39	0.17
In-segment late loss (mm)	0.36	0.23	0.24

LAD = left anterior descending coronary artery; MACE = major adverse cardiac events.
Numbers represent mean values. Duration of dual antiplatelet therapy refers to the prescription.

anti-restenosis efficacy, such as in-stent and in-segment late loss, were superior for Cypher and Taxus. To date, following the pivotal ENDEAVOR II study, four additional clinical trials evaluating the safety and efficacy of Endeavor DES have been completed. The most recent ENDEAVOR IV study compared zotarolimus eluting stent to paclitaxel eluting stent in 1578 patients presenting with single de-novo lesion in 2.5–3.5 diameter vessels with an overall lesion length of less than 28 mm [4,5]. The primary endpoint of the study was target vessel failure at nine months with pre-specified non-inferiority absolute margin of 3.8%. A subset of 328 patients underwent angiographic follow-up at eight months. Whilst in-stent late loss was significantly higher in the Endeavor stent (0.67 ± 0.49 mm vs. 0.42 ± 0.50 mm, $p < 0.001$), this did not translate into a difference in terms of the primary endpoint (6.6% in the Endeavor vs. 7.2% in the Taxus group), which satisfied the non-inferiority endpoint ($p < 0.001$) for non-inferiority of the Endeavor compared to the Taxus stent. Recently, at the 2009 TCT Conference in San Francisco, the 3 year results were presented and demonstrated a statistically significant relative risk reduction in target vessel failure with the Endeavor stent (12.3% versus 15.9% for Taxus, $p = 0.049$).

There is no consensus on the minimal strength of antiproliferative effect that limits neointimal growth to a degree that is sufficient to prevent clinically relevant luminal re-narrowing. Antiproliferative power of stents can be estimated from quantitative metrics derived from angiography (in-stent late loss) or intravascular ultrasound (percentage in-stent neointimal proliferation). The zotarolimus eluting stent is one that has been associated with good clinical outcome, yet anatomic metrics of antiproliferative efficacy are clearly inferior to both the sirolimus and paclitaxel eluting stent. Critics argue that use of this particular DES in lesion/patients subsets at higher risk for restenosis (small vessels, long lesions, diabetes) will not portend efficacy results that are equivalent to those achievable with first-generation DES (Figure 35.5). Post-hoc analysis of pooled data from over 2000 patients included in the Endeavor series of trials shows consistent median in-stent late loss values (ranging between 0.57 mm and 0.67 mm) across high-risk subsets such as vessel diameter smaller than 2.7 mm, lesion length above 13 mm or the presence of diabetes [4,11,12]. Confidence intervals of the corresponding target lesion revascularization

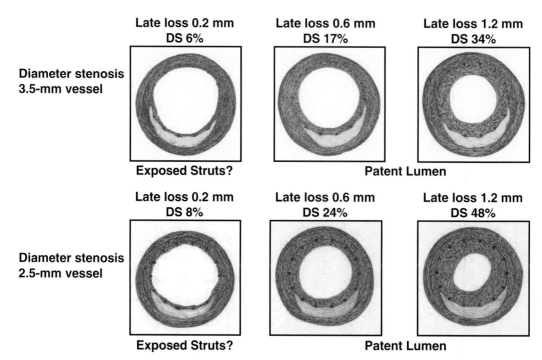

Figure 35.5. This cartoon attempts to illustrate how much late loss is clinically relevant, both from the efficacy and the safety viewpoints. Stent struts are indicated by blue dots. The upper and lower rows pertain to reference vessel diameters of 3.5 mm and 2.5 mm, respectively. From the efficacy viewpoint, it is obvious that higher late loss is more likely to become an issue as vessel size decreases.

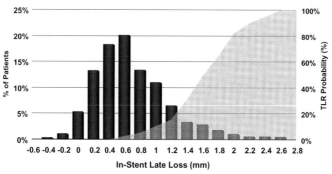

Figure 35.6. Relationship between in-stent late loss and probability of target lesion revascularization. Data represent a post-hoc analysis of the pooled ENDEAVOR I to III trials and are obviously restricted to patients undergoing repeat angiography. The curvilinear relationship shows that the probability of target lesion revascularization increases once the luminal loss reaches 0.8 mm. Lower values of late loss are less likely to narrow the coronary lumen to an extent that is sufficient to cause ischemic symptoms.

rates at 270 days did overlap, consistent with the hypothesis that neointimal proliferation only needs to be constrained below a threshold value of ~0.8 mm in order to prevent clinical restenosis (Figure 35.6). The currently ongoing PROTECT randomized trial (1:1) will test both efficacy and safety of zotarolimus vs. sirolimus eluting stents in a large population of patients drafted from daily practice, therefore enriched with high-risk patient and lesion subsets.

Late Stent Thrombosis and DES Safety

Whilst all four FDA-approved DES have shown superiority in terms of angiographic recurrence and clinical re-intervention rates compared to un-coated stents, there is evidence for both sirolimus and paclitaxel eluting stents that late adverse events related to abrupt stent closure (i.e. late or very late stent thrombosis) are more frequent than with the use of BMS [13]. These thrombosis events are rare but clinically severe, associated with sudden death or myocardial infarction in half of the cases [14]. Absolute rates are difficult to capture because death and myocardial infarction can be the expression of the disease process itself. Definitions and criteria have varied from very specific to more inclusive, resulting in a range of under- to over-estimated figures [15]. The most conservative estimates indicate a 0.6 % yearly incidence up to four years, corresponding to an incidence density of one case/100 patient years [16]. Comparisons between DES and BMS will require the use of standardized definitions, such as provided by the Academic Research Consortium [17]. Data up to four years following implant of the Endeavor stent seem to indicate that no such incremental risk is present with use of this specific drug-device combination [3–5]. Pooled data were presented at ACC 2008 by L. Mauri on a cohort of 2131 patients treated with Endeavor compared to 596 patients randomised to Driver in ENDEAVOR II trial. Cumulative incidence of definitive/probable stent thrombosis at 1.080 days was 0.7% for Endeavor vs. 1.5% for Driver (log rank = 0.059). The incidence of late stent thrombosis (beyond 12 months) was 0.08% with Endeavor. Importantly, dual antiplatelet therapy was continued in 26.3% at one year, 9.9% at two years and 8.3% at three years. Rates of hard events at four years in ENDEAVOR II trial were presented at EuroPCR 2008 by J. Fajadet. All-cause mortality was 5.0 vs. 5.1%, and myocardial infarction rate was 3.3 vs. 4.5%, for Endeavor and Driver respectively (all non significant). In the ENDEAVOR IV 3 year results recently presented at TCT 2009, there was a 93% relative risk reduction in very late stent thrombosis with Endeavor (0.1%) versus Taxus (1.5%), p = 0.004.

Whether this specific safety profile of Endeavor is related to its weaker antiproliferative effect or to the use of a more biocompatible polymer remains speculative. Delayed healing and impaired endothelialization are common features of most cases of late and very late stent thrombosis [18]. Preclinical studies fail to show delayed endothelialization with Endeavor [8] and intravascular imaging in humans typically shows regular strut coverage, without much evidence for late incomplete stent apposition since only two such cases have been identified out of 541 intravascular ultrasound studies analysed in the core-laboratory by Fitzgerald and colleagues [19].

Systemic Dual Antiplatelet Therapy

With the use of first-generation DES, an empirical approach in order to reduce stent thrombosis has been to prolong the duration of dual antiplatelet effect as to match the presumed window of increased risk. A retrospective analysis of the Duke database suggested that there is possibly benefit associated with extension of dual antiplatelet therapy from six months to one year [20]. This practice is now endorsed by international guidelines [21,22]. Available data would suggest that this recommendation is less relevant for Endeavor and instructions for use recommend three months of dual antiplatelet therapy. At the same time, it should be acknowledged that the exact duration of the period "at risk" is not known and likely to differ by patient and lesion subset depending on variable healing properties.

Next Generation Zotarolimus Eluting Stent: The Endeavor Resolute DES

Whilst attempting to design a zotarolimus eluting DES with stronger antiproliferative properties for use in more complex and high-risk patient/lesion subsets, it became apparent that drug release kinetics needed to be modified, i.e. the period of drug elution extended. A new blend of hydrophilic and hydrophobic polymers was designed (BioLynx) and attached to the stent struts via a primer. Preclinical data show that high biocompatibility and complete healing by 28 days seem to be maintained [23]. Drug release kinetics were indeed altered with lower systemic exposure and slower zotarolimus release profiles compared to Endeavor. First-in-man data show reduced late loss values at four and nine months [24] and the large RESOLUTE III trial has started enrolment in May 2008. Trial design encourages inclusion of all-comer cases and will randomize 2300 patients (1:1) to either Endeavor Resolute or Xience-V. The primary hypothesis is non-inferiority between tested DES for a combined target-lesion failure endpoint, including cardiac death, target lesion revascularization and myocardial infarction at 12 months. Subsets will undergo repeat angiography and intracoronary imaging using optical coherence tomography for examination of stent apposition and strut tissue coverage (25).

Conclusion

Until the concerns with late stent thrombosis were recognized, attention was primarily, if not exclusively focused on the anti-restenosis properties of DES. Today, the emphasis is placed on their efficacy-safety ratio which appears to depend on the balance between the early benefit, namely the desired anti-restenosis effect, and the late hazard, driven by the rare but severe complication of stent thrombosis. During early human evaluation, intermediate mechanistic endpoints that might be relevant for safety, such as the degree of endothelial coverage, are being collected using high definition intracoronary imaging of stent struts with optical coherence tomography [25] or angioscopy [26]. In this way, claims regarding increased biocompatibility of new or bioerodable materials can be tested at an early stage of the evaluation plan of these novel devices. The assessment plan that has been applied so far to DES has allowed robust evaluation of efficacy, rapid identification of many inefficacious iterations and relatively rapid patient access, at least in Europe (Figure 35.4). However, this approach has been primarily device-oriented aiming to address the superiority or equivalence of one device vs. the other. Given today's knowledge base, new-generation DES, among which are the zotarolimus eluting stents, are aimed at achieving reconciliation between powerful efficacy and retained safety [27]. Data on follow-up periods extending up to three–five years as well as performance evaluation in all-comer populations will be required to establish to which extent newer generation DES convey the features of the "optimal" DES.

References

1. Serruys PW, Kutryk MJ, Ong AT. Coronary-artery stents. N Engl J Med 2006; **354**: 483–495.
2. Silber S, Borggrefe M, Böhm M, et al. Positionspapier der DGK zur Wirksamkeit und Sicherheit van Medikamente freisentzenden Koronarstents (DES). Der Kardiologe 2007; **1**: 84–111.
3. Meredith IT, Ormiston J, Whitbourn R, et al. ENDEAVOR I Investigators. Four-year clinical follow-up after implantation of the endeavor zotarolimus-eluting stent: ENDEAVOR I, the first-in-human study. Am J Cardiol 2007; **100**: 56M–61M.
4. Pinto Slottow TL, Waksman R. Overview of the 2007 Food and Drug Administration Circulatory System Devices Panel meeting on the endeavor zotarolimus-eluting coronary stent. Circulation 2008; **117**: 1603–1608.
5. US FDA/CDRH: New Device Approval—Endeavor Zotarolimus-Eluting stent. Access at: http://www.fda.gov/cdrh/pdf6/p060033b.pdf-02-12-2008.
6. US FDA/CDRH: New Device Approval- Xience-V Everolimus Eluting Coronary Stent System. Access at: htp//www.fda.gov/ohrms/dockets/ac/07/slides/Presentation.pdf-01-17-2008.
7. Abizaid A, Lansky AJ, Fitzgerald PJ, et al. Percutaneous coronary revascularization using a trilayer metal phosphorylcholine-coated zotarolimus-eluting stent. Am J Cardiol 2007; **99**: 1403–1408.
8. Burke SE, Kuntz RE, Schwartz LB. Zotarolimus (ABT-578) eluting stents. Adv Drug Deliv Rev. 2006; **58**: 437–446.
9. Hayward JA, Chapman D. Biomembrane surfaces as models for polymer design: the potential for haemocompatibility. Biomaterials 1984; **5**: 135–142.
10. Fajadet J, Wijns W, Laarman GJ, et al. Randomized, double-blind, multicenter study of the Endeavor zotarolimus-eluting phosphorylcholine-encapsulated stent for treatment of native coronary artery lesions: clinical and angiographic results of the ENDEAVOR II trial. Circulation 2006; **114**: 798–806.
11. Gershlick A, Kandzari DE, Leon MB, et al. ENDEAVOR Investigators. Zotarolimus-eluting stents in patients with native coronary artery disease: Clinical and angiographic outcomes in 1,317 patients. Am J Cardiol 2007; **100**: 45M–55M.
12. Mehta RH, Leon MB, Sketch MH Jr. ENDEAVOR II Continued Access Registry. The relation between clinical features, angiographic findings, and the target lesion revascularization rate in patients receiving the endeavor zotarolimus-eluting stent for treatment of native coronary artery disease: An analysis of ENDEAVOR I, ENDEAVOR II, ENDEAVOR II Continued Access

Registry, and ENDEAVOR III. Am J Cardiol 2007; **100**: 62M–70M.

13. Camenzind E, Steg PG, Wijns W. Stent thrombosis late after implantation of first-generation drug-eluting stents. A cause for concern. Circulation 2007; **115**: 1440–1455.

14. Kuchulakanti PK, Chu WW, Torguson R, *et al.* Correlates and long-term outcomes of angiographically proven stent thrombosis with sirolimus- and paclitaxel-eluting stents. Circulation 2006; **113**: 1108–1113.

15. Mauri L, Hsieh W, Massaro JM *et al.* Stent thrombosis in randomized trials of drug-eluting stents. N Engl J Med 2007; **356**: 1020–1029.

16. Daemen J, Wenaweser P, Tsuchida K, *et al.* Early and late coronary stent thrombosis of sirolimus-eluting and paclitaxel-eluting stents in routine clinical practice: data from a large two-institutional cohort study. Lancet 2007; **369**: 667–678.

17. Cutlip DE, Windecker S, Mehran R, *et al.* Academic Research Consortium. Clinical endpoins in coronary stent trials: a case for standardized definitions. Circulation 2007; **115**: 2344–2351.

18. Joner M, Finn AV, Farb A, *et al.* Pathology of drug-eluting stents in humans: delayed healing and late thrombotic risk. J Am Coll Cardiol 2006; **48**: 193–202.

19. Sakurai R, Hongo Y, Yamasaki M, et al; ENDEAVOR II Trial Investigators. Detailed intravascular ultrasound analysis of Zotarolimus-eluting phosphorylcholine-coated cobalt-chromium alloy stent in de novo coronary lesions (results from the ENDEAVOR II trial). Am J Cardiol 2007; **100**: 818–823.

20. Eisenstein EL, Anstrom KJ, Kong DF, *et al.* Clopidogrel use and long-term clinical outcomes after drug-eluting stent implantation. JAMA 2007; **297**: 159–68.

21. Spencer B. King, III, Sidney C. Smith, Jr, Hirshfeld John W., Jr, *et al.* 2007 Focused Update of the ACC/AHA/SCAI 2005 Guideline Update for Percutaneous Coronary Intervention. A Report of the American College of Cardiology/American Heart Association Task Force on Practice Guidelines: 2007 Writing Group to Review New Evidence and Update the ACC/AHA/SCAI 2005 Guideline Update for Percutaneous Coronary Intervention, Writing on Behalf of the 2005 Writing Committee. Circulation 2008; **117**: 261–295.

22. Silber S, Albertsson P, Avilés FF, *et al.* Guidelines for percutaneous coronary interventions. The Task Force for Percutaneous Coronary Interventions of the European Society of Cardiology. Eur Heart J 2005; **26**: 804–847.

23. Udipi K, Chen M, Cheng P, *et al.* Development of a novel biocompatible polymer system for extended drug release in a next-generation drug-eluting stent. J Biomed Mater Res A. 2007 October 15. (Epub ahead of print.)

24. Meredith I, Worthley S, Whitbourn R, *et al.* The next-generation Endeavor Resolute stent: 4-month clinical and angiographic results from the Resolute first-in-man trial. EuroIntervention 2007; **3**: 50–53.

25. Takano M, Yamamoto M, Inami S, *et al.* Long-term follow-up evaluation after sirolimus-eluting stent implantation by optical coherence tomography: do uncovered struts persist? J Am Coll Cardiol 2008; **51**: 968–969.

26. Kotani J, Awata M, Nanto S, et al. Incomplete neointimal coverage of sirolimus-eluting stents: angioscopic findings. J Am Coll Cardiol 2006; **47**: 2108–2111.

27. Daemen J, Simoons ML, Wijns W *et al.* ESC Forum on Drug Eluting Stents, Meeting Report at the European Heart House, September 27–28, 2007. Eur Heart J 2009; **30**(2): 152–161.

Everolimus Eluting Coronary Stents: Clinical Trials

Neville Kukreja[1], Yoshinobu Onuma[2], & Patrick W. Serruys[2]

[1] Lister Hospital, Stevenage, UK

[2] Thoraxcenter, Erasmus Medical Center, Rotterdam, The Netherlands

Introduction

Cobalt chromium everolimus eluting stents (EES) are now available for clinical use. After initial studies using a biodegradable polymer, the EES design was changed in favor of a biostable polymer with a long previous history of medical use and large randomized trials have compared the new EES with the paclitaxel eluting TAXUS stent, and found a similar reduction in restenosis and repeat revascularization rates. There were no significant differences in mortality, myocardial infarction or stent thrombosis rates. Several registries of unselected ("real world") patients are currently evaluating the efficacy and safety of everolimus eluting stents in high-risk complex cases.

In 2002–2003, drug eluting stents were approved by regulatory bodies in Europe and the USA after initial studies showed significant reduction of restenosis rates compared with BMS. The Cypher and Taxus stents are stainless steel stents covered by permanent polymer eluting sirolimus, an antiproliferative macrolide used to prevent rejection of renal transplantation, and paclitaxel an antimitotic microtubule inhibitor which suppresses cell division widely used to treat neoplastic diseases [1]. Delayed healing and hypersensitivity reactions

have been described in animals and postmortem examinations for both stents, attributed to the permanent polymer or to the toxic effects of the drug used. Furthermore, both stents were designed in the late 1990s, have strut thickness >150 μm (Cypher, Taxus Express) or >100 μm (Taxus Liberte) when the polymer thickness is added to the metallic strut and lack the flexibility required for the insertion of long stents in distal positions. Despite its excellent results in restenosis prevention, the closed cell design of the Cypher stent limits strut opening in the treatment of bifurcation lesions and confers a small but definite risk of stent fracture when long stents are implanted at flexing points, such as in the right coronary artery or in saphenous vein grafts.

Everolimus Eluting Stents

Everolimus eluting stents are commercialized under different names (XIENCE V, Abbott Vascular, Santa Clara, California and PROMUS, Boston Scientific, Natick, MS) but consists of the same platform. In June 2009, the Xience Prime stent (Abbott Vascular, Santa Clara, CA) received CE mark approval in the European Union. In this iteration of the Xience stent, the design has been modified for greater flexibility and deliverability and is now available in a 38 mm length. The Multi-link Vision Cobalt Chromium (CoCr) balloon-mounted stent is coated with a nonerodable polymer and loaded with 100 μg/cm² everolimus,

Interventional Cardiology, First Edition. Edited by Carlo Di Mario, George D. Dangas, Peter Barlis.
© 2010 Blackwell Publishing Ltd. Published 2010 by Blackwell Publishing Ltd.

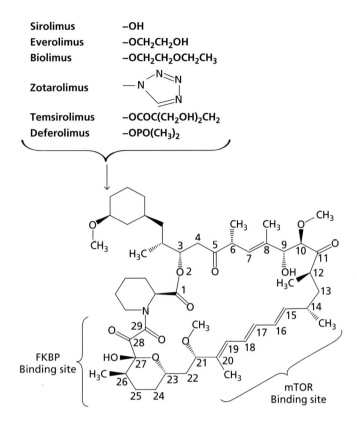

Sirolimus	–OH
Everolimus	–OCH₂CH₂OH
Biolimus	–OCH₂CH₂OCH₂CH₃
Zotarolimus	
Temsirolimus	–OCOC(CH₂OH)₂CH₂
Deferolimus	–OPO(CH₃)₂

Figure 36.1. The chemical structures of sirolimus and its analogues.

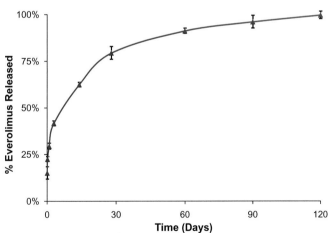

Figure 36.2. Release kinetics of everolimus from the Xience V stent. *In vivo* data in a porcine model.

a synthetic analogue of sirolimus [40-O-(2-hydroxyethyl)-rapamycin] (Figure 36.1). Approximately 75% of the drug is released within 30 days (Figure 36.2).

The indications for use in Europe are for use in *de novo* native coronary artery lesions (length ≤28 mm) with reference vessel diameters of 2.5–4.25 mm. Currently available stent sizes in Europe are 2.25, 2.5, 2.75, 3.0, 3.5 or 4.0 mm diameter and 8, 12, 15, 23 or 28 mm length. The nominal inflation pressure of its compliant balloon is 8 atmospheres with a rated burst pressure of 16 atmospheres. As with other DES, dual antiplatelet therapy with aspirin and clopidogrel is recommended for 12 months after implantation [2].

Stent Platform

The initial DES were composed of 316 L stainless steel since this material is radiopaque with adequate radial strength to maintain adequate arterial scaffolding and low degrees of acute recoil. However, Cobalt Chromium (CoCr) exhibits superior radial strength and improved radiopacity allowing for thinner stent struts which may reduce restenosis and target lesion revascularization (TLR) whilst reducing device profile and hence improving its deliverability to the target lesion [3–5]. The Multi-link Vision L-605 CoCr stent consists of serpentine rings connected by links. The results of a registry of 297 patients treated with the thin strut (0.0032 inches) bare metal Multi-link Vision stent demonstrated a six-month binary angiographic restenosis rate of 15.7% and mean late lumen loss of 0.83 ± 0.56 mm. The six-month rates of mortality, myocardial infarction, target vessel revascularization (TVR) and TLR were 1.2%, 0.4%, 5.1% and 4.3% respectively [4].

Polymer

The $7.8 \mu m$ polymer coating of the Xience V stent is a fluorinated copolymer consisting of vinylidene fluoride and hexafluoropropylene, compounds which have proven biocompatibility, having been used clinically in permanent surgical sutures.

Everolimus

Everolimus is a synthetic analogue of sirolimus (40-O-(2-hydroxyethyl)-rapamycin), which was initially developed for use in transplantation (Figure 36.1). Everolimus has a similar mode of action to sirolimus: it binds to FK506-binding protein 12 (FKBP-12) and subsequently binds to and inhibits the mammalian target of rapamycin (mTOR). The drug acts as a cytostatic inhibitor of cellular proliferation, by arresting cells in the late G1 phase of the cell cycle and preventing them entering the S phase [6]. Everolimus inhibits cytokine-mediated and growth-factor–mediated proliferation of lymphocytes and smooth-muscle cells, thereby acting as an immunosuppressant. It has successfully been used in combination with other drugs to prevent rejection in recipients of heart transplants. Furthermore, as a result of its effects on growth-factor stimulated vascular smooth muscle cell proliferation, everolimus also reduces the severity and incidence of cardiac-allograft vasculopathy [7].

Preclinical Trials

Orally administered everolimus proved to be effective in reducing neointimal hyperplasia in a rabbit iliac artery model. Following balloon injury and implantation of a bare metal Multi-link Vision stent, oral everolimus (1.5 mg/kg the day before the procedure followed by 0.75 mg/kg/day for 28 days) reduced the neointimal thickness from 0.12 ± 0.03 mm to 0.07 ± 0.03 mm (p = 0.005) [8]. After 28 days, $86.7 \pm 6.8\%$ of the stent surface was endothelialised in the everolimus-treated animals (versus $96.8 \pm 5.4\%$ in the control animals, p < 0.006). The results of histological assessment in a porcine model, comparing the EES with the bare Multi-Link Vision and the Cypher SES after 28 days are shown in Table 36.1 [9]. The results were similar for the EES and SES.

The Future 1 and 2 Trials

Everolimus has previously been evaluated in the poly-L-lactic acid-coated stainless steel S stent (Biosensors International, Singapore), which was effective in the first-in-man trial of 42 patients randomized 2:1 to EES (27 patients) vs. BMS (15 patients). The six-month late lumen loss was 0.10 mm vs. 0.85 mm (p < 0.0001) for the bare metal stent, with binary angiographic restenosis of 0% vs. 9.1% (p = ns) [10,11]. This stent releases 70% of the $197 \mu g/cm^2$ everolimus within 30 days and 85% within 90 days. A pooled analysis of 106 randomized patients enrolled in both the Future 1 and Future 2 clinical trials demonstrated the beneficial effect of EES regardless of vessel size [12].

The SPIRIT I First-in-man Trial

In the first-in-man study of the cobalt chromium everolimus eluting stent, 60 patients were randomized at nine medical centers in Europe to either the EES (n = 28) or the bare metal Vision stent (n = 32). The study included patients with stable

Table 36.1. Histological results at 28 days in porcine coronary arteries.

	Everolimus eluting stent	Sirolimus eluting stent	Bare metal stent
Neointimal thickness (mm)	0.13 ± 0.07*	0.13 ± 0.08*	0.20 ± 0.07
Area stenosis (%)	20.8 ± 6.9*	20.8 ± 7.6*	26.9 ± 7.8
Vessel injury score	0.08 ± 0.11	0.15 ± 0.25	0.18 ± 0.25
Struts with fibrin (%)	76.9 ± 31.5**	88.4 ± 7.7**	5.4 ± 5.9
Fibrin score	1.36 ± 0.66**	1.61 ± 0.61**	0.08 ± 0.15
Inflammation score	0.75 ± 0.29	0.75 ± 0.29	0.89 ± 0.57
Struts with ganulomas (%)	0.4 ± 1.3	0	1.9 ± 6.4
Endothelialization (%)	100	99.3	100

* = p < 0.05 vs. BMS.

** = p < 0.001 vs. BMS.

or unstable angina or silent ischemia with a single *de novo* significant coronary lesion (50–99% stenosis) in a 3.0 mm vessel which could be covered with an 18 mm stent. Patients with an evolving myocardial infarction, unprotected left main stem disease, ostial lesion or within 2 mm of a bifurcation, moderate to heavy calcification, visible thrombus, LV ejection fraction <30% or hypersensitivity to aspirin, clopidogrel, heparin, cobalt, chromium, nickel, tungsten, everolimus, polymer coating or contrast were excluded. The angiographic results at 6 months and one year are shown in Table 36.2 with clinical results up to four years shown in Table 36.3 [13–15]. Since this study was powered for angiographic outcomes (primary outcome: instent late lumen loss), any differences in clinical outcomes did not reach statistical significance. There were no cases of stent thrombosis by any of the Academic Research Consortium (ARC) criteria [16].

The SPIRIT II Randomized Trial

This was a multicenter (28 centers in Europe, India and New Zealand) trial of 300 patients randomized 3 : 1 to EES (n = 223) vs. PES (n = 77). The primary endpoint was late lumen loss after six months. The trial was powered to demonstrate non-inferiority of the EES. More complex patients and lesions were permitted compared to SPIRIT 1: the patients could have up to two *de novo* lesions in different arteries, the reference vessel diameter had to be between 2.5 mm and 4.25 mm and lesion length

≤28 mm. Patients with an acute myocardial infarction within three days, left ventricular ejection fraction <30%, aorto-ostial or left main lesion, heavy calcification, visible thrombus or hypersensitivity reaction as defined in SPIRIT 1 were excluded [17]. The angiographic and clinical results of the SPIRIT II trial are shown in Tables 36.4 and 36.5. Detailed analysis of the 6-month angiographic data confirmed the benefit of the EES across all subgroups (Figure 36.3) [18]. After two years, despite an increase in late loss in the EES cohort, clinical events were non-significantly lower than the PES cohort (PW Serruys, American College of Cardiology annual conference, Chicago, March 2008).

The SPIRIT III Randomized US Trial

This US trial recruited 1002 patients who were randomized 2 : 1 to EES (n = 669) vs. PES (n = 333). Patients with up to two *de novo* lesions (maximum in each vessel) were allowed. The lesion criteria for enrolment were diameter between 2.5 mm and 3.75 mm and length ≤28 mm. The primary endpoint was late lumen loss on eight-month follow-up angiography. The angiographic results confirmed the findings in SPIRIT II (Table 36.4). Furthermore, EES resulted in a significant reduction in the secondary endpoint of composite major adverse cardiac events (cardiac death, myocardial infarction or target lesion revascularization) both at nine months (4.6% vs. 8.1%, relative risk = 0.56 [95% CI 0.34–0.94], p = 0.03) and at one year

Table 36.2. Angiographic results of the SPIRIT 1 first-in-man trial.

Time	In-stent						In-segment					
	Late lumen loss (mm)		Diameter Stenosis (%)		Binary angiographic restenosis		Late lumen loss (mm)		Diameter stenosis (%)		Binary angiographic restenosis	
	EES	BMS	EES	BMS	EES	BMS	EES	BMS	EES	BMS	EES	BMS
6 months	0.10 ± 0.21**	0.87 ± 0.37	16 ± 8**	39 ± 14	0.0%*	25.9%	0.07 ± 0.19**	0.61 ± 0.37	22 ± 11**	41 ± 14	4.3%*	33.3%
12 months	0.24 ± 0.27**	0.84 ± 0.45	18 ± 13**	37 ± 17			0.14 ± 0.24**	0.59 ± 0.42	22 ± 15**	40 ± 16		

EES = everolimus eluting stent.
BMS = bare metal stent.
* = p < 0.05 vs. BMS.
** = p < 0.001 vs. BMS.

Table 36.3. Cumulative incidence of adverse clinical events in the SPIRIT 1 trial.

	6 months		12 months		24 months		36 months		48 months	
	EES	BMS	EES	BMS	EES	BMS	EES	BMS	EES	BMS
Death	0%	0%	0%	0%	0%	0%	0%	0%	0%	0%
Myocardial infarction	3.8%	0%	7.6%	0%	7.6%	0%	7.6%	0%	7.6%	0%
Target lesion revascularization	3.8%	17.9%	7.7%	17.9%	7.7%	25.0%	7.7%	25.0%	7.7%	25.0%
Major adverse cardiac events†	7.7%	21.4%	15.4%	21.4%	15.4%	25.0%	15.4%	25.0%	15.4%	25.0%

† = death, myocardial infarction or target lesion revascularization.

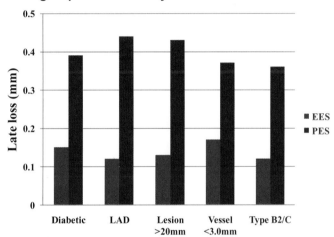

Figure 36.3. Subgroup late lumen loss analysis from the SPIRIT II trial.

(6.0% vs. 10.3%, relative risk = 0.58 [95% CI 0.37–0.90], p = 0.02) (Table 36.5) [19]. A pooled analysis of nine-month clinical events in SPIRIT II and III are shown in Figures 36.4 and 36.5. Overall, the EES was associated with significant reductions in TLR, target vessel revascularization (TVR), MACE (composite major adverse cardiac events: cardiac death, nonfatal myocardial infarction or TLR) with no difference in safety endpoints, including death, myocardial infarction and stent thrombosis.

Ongoing and Future Trials

SPIRIT IV

This US randomized trial commenced enrolment in August 2006. Patients with up to three *de novo* lesions (maximum two per vessel) were included. In total, 3690 patients were randomized 2:1 to EES

(n = 2640) vs. PES (n = 1230). With lesion lengths ≤28 mm and vessel diameter between 2.5 mm and 4.25 mm. At the 2009 TCT, Greg Stone presented the 1 year results. The rate of target lesion failure was 3.9% in the Xience V group versus 6.6% in the Taxus group (p = 0.0008) with a further statistically significant difference in ischemia driven TLR (2.3% for Xience versus 4.5% for Taxus, p = 0.0008). Investigators also found a statistically significant difference in stent thrombosis between the two arms at one year: 1.06% for Taxus vs 0.29% for Xience V (p = 0.003). Interestingly, there was no difference in outcomes for both stents in the sub-group of patients with diabetes mellitus.

SPIRIT V

Starting recruitment in October 2006, this international study consists of two arms. In the diabetic

Table 36.4. Angiographic results from the SPIRIT II and III trials.

Trial	Time	In-stent						In-segment					
		Late lumen loss (mm)		Diameter Stenosis (%)		Binary angiographic restenosis (%)		Late lumen loss (mm)		Diameter Stenosis (%)		Binary angiographic restenosis (%)	
		EES	PES	EES	PES	EES	PES	EES	PES	EES	PES	EES	PES
SPIRIT II	6 months	0.12 ± 0.29**	0.37 ± 0.38	16 ± 10**	21 ± 12	1.3	3.5	0.07 ± 0.33	0.15 ± 0.38	24 ± 12*	27 ± 13	3.4	5.8
	24 months	0.33	0.34	19	19	2.0	2.9	0.20	0.17			5.1	8.6
SPIRIT III	8 months	0.16 ± 0.41*	0.30 ± 0.53	5.9 ± 16.4*	10.3 ± 21.4	2.3*	5.7	0.14 ± 0.39*	0.26 ± 0.46	18.8 ± 14.4*	22.8 ± 16.4	4.7	8.9

EES = everolimus eluting stent.
PES = paclitaxel eluting stent.
* = p < 0.05 vs. PES.
** = p < 0.001 vs. PES.

Table 36.5. Cumulative incidence of adverse clinical events in the SPIRITII and III trials.

	SPIRIT II		SPIRIT III		SPIRIT II	
	6 months		12 months		24 months	
	EES	PES	EES	PES	EES	PES
Cardiac death	0%	1.3%	0.8%	0.9%	0.5%	1.4%
Myocardial infarction	0.9%	2.6%	2.8%	4.1%	2.8%	5.5%
Target lesion revascularization	2.7%	6.5%	3.4%	5.6%	4.6%	9.1%
Major adverse cardiac events†	2.7%	6.5%	6.0%*	10.3%	6.6%	11.0%
Stent thrombosis	0.5%	1.3%	0.8%	0.6%	0.9%	1.4%

† = death, myocardial infarction or target lesion revascularization.
* = p < 0.05 vs. PES.

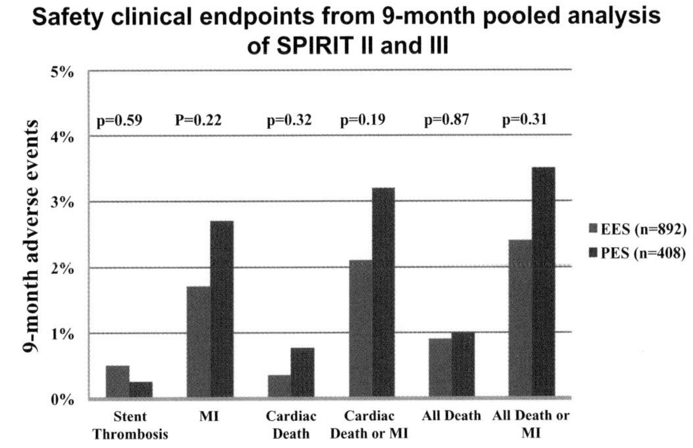

Figure 36.4. Safety clinical endpoints from nine-month pooled analysis of SPIRIT II and III: rates of stent thrombosis, myocardial infarction, cardiac death, cardiac death or myocardial infarction, all-cause death and all-cause death or myocardial infarction.
EES = everolimus eluting stent;
PES = paclitaxel eluting stent;
MI = myocardial infarction.

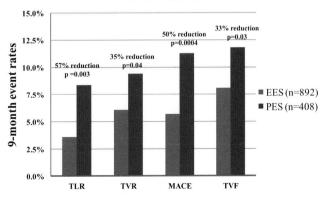

Safety clinical endpoints from 9-month pooled analysis of SPIRIT II and III

Figure 36.5. Revascularization endpoints from the pooled analysis of SPIRIT II and III: rates of target lesion revascularization, target vessel revascularization, major adverse cardiac events and target vessel failure.
EES = everolimus eluting stent;
PES = paclitaxel eluting stent;
TLR = target vessel revascularization;
TVR = target vessel revascularization;
MACE = major adverse cardiac events, defined as cardiac death, myocardial infarction or TLR; TVF = target vessel failure.

Revascularization endpoints from the pooled analysis of SPIRIT II and III.

randomized arm, 300 patients were randomized 2:1 to EES (n = 200) vs. PES (n = 100). A further 2700 patients have been recruited into the non-randomized multinational registry arm, including sites in Europe, Australia, Canada and Asia. The 30-day results were presented (E Grube, European Society of Cardiology Conference, Munich, September 2008). The registry included 30% diabetics, 42% with multivessel disease and 33% with unstable angina. The mean lesion length was 15.6 mm. Device success was 99%, with procedural success of 98%. After 30 days, all-cause mortality was 0.5% with MACE (all-cause death, TVR or MI) of 2.6%. The one year results were presented at the EuroPCR in Barcelona, 2009 demonstrating a TLR rate of 1.8%, a 0.7% rate of stent thrombosis and a 5.1% of MACE.

SPIRIT V Women

This trial also is split into two arms: 450 patients will be randomized 2:1 to EES (n = 300) vs. PES (n = 150). A further 1550 women will be recruited into the non-randomized registry arm.

The Resolute III All-comers Trial

This is a randomized European trial comparing the Medtronic Zotarolimus eluting Endeavor Resolute stent with the Xience V EES. 2300 patients have been randomized 1:1 to the ZES or EES. This "real-world" trial has broad inclusion criteria, including patients with ST-elevation MI and vessel reference diameter 2.25–4.0 mm. The only exclusion criteria are pregnancy, a known intolerance or allergy to any of the stent component materials or radiopaque contrast or planned surgery within six months of enrolment. Twenty percent of patients are scheduled for angiographic follow-up at 13 months (after the 12-month primary clinical end-point) with a further subgroup also undergoing optical coherence tomography (OCT) follow-up to assess stent strut apposition and coverage in addition to standard volumetric measurements (minimum lumen area, lumen area/volume and stent area/volume).

The Xience Stent Evaluated At Rotterdam Cardiology Hospital (X-SEARCH) Registry

Since March 1, 2007, our institution commenced the use of EES (Xience V; Abbott Vascular) as the default strategy for every percutaneous coronary intervention (PW Serruys, American College of Cardiology annual conference, Chicago, March 2008). Between March 1 and October 31, 2007, 649 consecutive patients presenting with *de novo* lesions were treated exclusively with EES. These patients were compared to three historical cohorts of consecutive patients from the RESEARCH and T-SEARCH registries; 450 patients treated with bare metal stents (BMS) between December 2002 and April 2003, 508 with sirolimus eluting stents (SES) treated from April to October 2002 and 576 with paclitaxel eluting stents (PES) treated February to September 2003 [20,21]. Survival data for all patients was obtained at one month from Municipal Civil Registries. All living patients were subsequently contacted by questionnaire or by telephone with specific enquiries on adverse clinical events. As the principal regional cardiac referral center, repeat procedures (percutaneous and surgical) are normally performed at our institution and recorded prospectively in our database. For patients who suffered an adverse event at another center, medical records or discharge summaries from the other institutions were systematically reviewed. General practitioners, referring cardiologists, and patients were contacted as necessary if further information was required.

The patients in the EES cohort were significantly older than the historical controls (64 ± 12 years old for EES patients vs. 61 ± 11 BMS, 61 ± 11 SES and 62 ± 11 PES, $p < 0.05$) and more often presented with ST-elevation Myocardial Infarction (39% EES vs. 18% BMS, 18% SES and 21% PES, $p < 0.001$). The Left main stem was also more frequently treated in the EES group (7.4% EES vs. 1.7% BMS, 2.2% SES and 3.2% PES, $p < 0.05$) and the total stented length was longer (57 ± 26 mm EES vs. 30 ± 20 BMS, 39 ± 28 SES and 43 ± 31 PES, $p < 0.001$). After 1 month, the crude all-cause mortality rate was higher in the EES group (4.2% vs. 2.0% BMS, 1.6% SES and 2.1% PES, $p = 0.02$). Multivariable logistic regression to account for differences in baseline and angiographic variables indicated no difference in adjusted mortality between SES (adjusted HR 1.27, 95% CI 0.34–4.73) and PES (adjusted HR 1.69, 95%CI 0.58–4.97) when compared to EES. The BMS group had a higher adjusted mortality (adjusted HR 4.67, 95%CI 1.45–15.01). The multivariable analysis suggested a higher incidence of adjusted composite major adverse cardiac events (MACE: all-cause death, nonfatal myocardial infarction or target vessel revascularization) rates in the historical cohorts (BMS adjusted HR 2.52, 95%CI 1.24–5.10; SES adjusted HR 1.80, 95%CI 0.89–3.61; PES adjusted HR 1.99, 95%CI 1.07–3.71). Further follow-up is planned at 6 and 12 months, then annually, and will provide essential real-world data on the use of these stents in high-risk complex patients.

Conclusion

The Xience V thin strut cobalt chromium everolimus eluting stent is a second-generation drug eluting stent: all aspects of the stent design are an improvement on the 1st generation DES. The stent platform allows great deliverability to the target lesion, even in tortuous vessels; the polymer is biocompatible with a long history of clinical use in surgical sutures and the drug has proven ability to suppress neointimal formation to an equivalent degree reported with sirolimus and more than paclitaxel. The SPIRIT III and IV trials suggest clinical superiority over first-generation paclitaxel eluting stents. Further developments and the availability of longer stent lengths (up to 38 mm for the Xience Prime) will ensure these "next generation" stents continue to play an integral part in modern interventional cardiology practice.

References

1. Serruys PW, Kutryk MJB, Ong ATL. Coronary-Artery Stents. N Engl J Med 2006; **354**(5): 483–495.
2. King SB, III, Smith SC, Jr., Hirshfeld JW, Jr. et al. 2007 focused update of the ACC/AHA/SCAI 2005 guideline update for percutaneous coronary intervention: a report of the American College of Cardiology/American Heart Association Task Force on Practice guidelines. J Am Coll Cardiol 2008; **51**(2): 172–209.
3. Kastrati A, Mehilli J, Dirschinger J, et al. Intracoronary Stenting and Angiographic Results: Strut Thickness Effect on Restenosis Outcome (ISAR-STEREO) Trial. Circulation 2001; **103**(23): 2816–2821.
4. Kereiakes DJ, Cox DA, Hermiller JB, et al. Usefulness of a cobalt chromium coronary stent alloy. American Journal of Cardiology 2003; **92**(4): 463–466.
5. Pache Ju, Kastrati A, Mehilli J et al. Intracoronary stenting and angiographic results: strut thickness effect on restenosis outcome (ISAR-STEREO-2) trial. Journal of the American College of Cardiology 2003; **41**(8): 1283–1288.
6. Schuler W, Sedrani R, Cottens S, et al. SDZ RAD, a new rapamycin derivative: pharmacological properties in vitro and in vivo. Transplantation 1997; **64**(1): 36–42.
7. Eisen HJ, Tuzcu EM, Dorent R, et al. Everolimus for the Prevention of Allograft Rejection and Vasculopathy in Cardiac-Transplant Recipients. 10.1056/NEJMoa022171. N Engl J Med 2003; **349**(9): 847–858.
8. Farb A, John M, Acampado E, Kolodgie FD, Prescott MF, Virmani R. Oral everolimus inhibits in-stent neointimal growth. Circulation 2002; **106**(18): 2379–2384.
9. Carter AJ, Brodeur A, Collingwood R et al. Experimental efficacy of an everolimus eluting cobalt chromium stent. Catheter Cardiovasc Interv 2006; **68**(1): 97–103.
10. Grube E, Sonoda S, Ikeno F, et al. Six- and Twelve-Month Results From First Human Experience Using Everolimus-Eluting Stents With Bioabsorbable Polymer. Circulation 2004; **109**(18): 2168–2171.
11. Costa RA, Lansky AJ, Mintz GS, et al. Angiographic results of the first human experience with everolimus-eluting stents for the treatment of coronary lesions (the FUTURE I trial). The American Journal of Cardiology 2005; **95**(1): 113–116.
12. Tsuchiya Y, Lansky AJ, Costa RA, et al. Effect of everolimus-eluting stents in different vessel sizes (from the pooled FUTURE I and II trials). Am J Cardiol 2006; **98**(4): 464–469.
13. Serruys PW, Ong ATL, Piek JJ, et al. A randomized comparison of a durable polymer Everolimus-eluting stent with bare metal coronary stent: the SPIRIT first trial. Eurointervention 2005; **1**(1): 58–65.
14. Tsuchida K, Piek JJ, Neumann F, et al. One-year results of a durable polymer everolimus-eluting stent in de novo coronary narrowings (The SPIRIT FIRST Trial). Eurointervention 2005; **1**: 266–272.
15. Beijk MA, Neumann F, Wiemer M, et al. Two-year results of a durable polymer everolimus-eluting stent in de novo coronary artery stenosis (the SPIRIT FIRST Trial). Eurointervention 2007; **3**: 206–212.
16. Cutlip DE, Windecker S, Mehran R, et al. Clinical End Points in Coronary Stent Trials: A Case for Standardized Definitions. Circulation 2007; **115**(17): 2344–2351.
17. Serruys PW, Ruygrok P, Neuzner J, et al. A randomised comparison of an everolimus-eluting coronary stent with a paclitaxel-eluting coronary stent: the SPIRIT II trial. Eurointervention 2006; **2**: 286–294.
18. Khattab A, Richardt G, Verin V, et al. Differentiated analysis of an everolimus-eluting stent and a paclitaxel-eluting stent amonghigher risl subgroups for restenosis: results from the SPIRIT II trial. EuroInterv 2008; **3**: 566–573.

19. Stone GW, Midei M, Newman W, *et al*. Comparison of an everolimus-eluting stent and a paclitaxel-eluting stent in patients with coronary artery disease: a randomized trial. JAMA 2008; **299**(16): 1903–1913.

20. Ong ATL, Serruys PW, Aoki J, *et al*. The unrestricted use of paclitaxel- versus sirolimus-eluting stents for coronary artery disease in an unselected population: One-year results of the Taxus-Stent Evaluated at Rotterdam Cardiology Hospital (T-SEARCH) registry. Journal of the American College of Cardiology 2005; **45**(7): 1135–1141.

21. Lemos PA, Serruys PW, van Domburg RT, *et al*. Unrestricted utilization of sirolimus-eluting stents compared with conventional bare stent implantation in the "real world": the Rapamycin-Eluting Stent Evaluated At Rotterdam Cardiology Hospital (RESEARCH) registry. Circulation 2004; **109**(2): 190–195.

CHAPTER 37

Novel Drug Eluting Stent Systems

Adriano Caixeta[1], Alexandre Abizaid[2],
George D. Dangas[1], & Martin B. Leon[1]

[1] Columbia University Medical Center, New York, NY, USA
[2] Institute Dante Pazzanese of Cardiology, São Paulo, Brazil

Introduction

Since the introduction of percutaneous transluminal coronary angioplasty and stenting, restenosis has been a major factor limiting its long-term success [1–4]. Drug eluting stents (DES) with antiproliferative drugs attached via polymers on the stent surface have reduced restenosis and rates of target lesion revascularization (TLR) by 50% to 90% compared with bare-metal stent (BMS) across nearly all lesion and patient subsets [5–14]. More recently, safety concerns were raised about these first generation DES, particularly regarding late thrombosis [15–22]. Necropsy and clinical studies have clearly demonstrated delayed re-endothelialization and neointimal growth, enhanced platelet aggregation and inflammation, late-acquired incomplete stent apposition and localized hypersensitivity reactions to DES that can be associated with late thrombosis [23–25]. Novel DES systems have been introduced that aim to improve outcomes while diminishing adverse events. This chapter focuses on a novel generation of DES, discussing new programs, including new antiproliferative agents, novel polymeric and non-polymeric stents.

Interventional Cardiology, First Edition. Edited by
Carlo Di Mario, George D. Dangas, Peter Barlis.
© 2010 Blackwell Publishing Ltd. Published 2010 by
Blackwell Publishing Ltd.

Rationale

The clinical effects of DES are highly dependent on each of the components of the complex platform/drug/polymer, as well as the interactions among these elements.

Stent Platform

Metallic alloys available for the stent platform include 316 L stainless steel, cobalt chromium (CoCr), nitinol and tantalum. For BMS and the first-generation of DES struts—including Cypher® (sirolimus eluting stent; Cordis Corporation, Johnson & Johnson, Miami Lakes, FL) and Taxus® (paclitaxel eluting stent; Boston Scientific Corporation, Maple Grove, MN), the predominant material used has been 316 L stainless steel. The platform material used in novel DES designs is CoCr, which can provide superior radial force and better radiopacity, with significantly thinner struts [26,27]. Cobalt chromium appears to lack the adverse proliferative response that accompanies the incorporation of other alloys (e.g., gold, nickel, molybdenum and chromium) [28,29], while enhancing visibility and flexibility. For novel self-expandable DES, nitinol has been used as the predominant material, offering better deliverability by means of a lower crossing profile. There is some evidence that the strut thickness of BMS can influence rates of restenosis and TLR [30–35]. It is unclear, however, whether this association applies in a similar manner to DES. In DES systems, stent thickness may have more of an effect on deliverability than on efficacy. Currently, new stent platform are under investigation in humans. The Conor™ platform (Cordis Corporation, Johnson & Johnson, Miami Lakes, FL), specifically designed for DES, consists of a CoCr laser-cut stent with hundreds of small holes that serve as drug-polymer reservoirs. It is believed that this reservoir design, can greatly enhance control over the rate and direction of drug release and enable a wider range of drug therapies. CardioMind™ is a stent-on-a-wire nitinol self-expanding system designed for tortuous anatomy and small vessels (Figure 37.1) [36]. Several dedicated stents for bifurcation lesions are currently under investigation [37,38].

Drugs

The first-generation DES drugs sirolimus and paclitaxel are both associated with impaired endothelial cell function [25], incomplete neointimal coverage [39,40] and incomplete stent apposition [41,42]. The ideal agent would be one that could suppress excessive neointimal growth while maintaining endothelial cell proliferation and function. Seven Limus related drugs, sirolimus, everolimus, biolimus A9, zotarolimus, tacrolimus, pimecrolimus and novolimus, are currently under investigation. The family of mTOR (mammalian Target Of Rapamycin) inhibitors, sirolimus, everolimus, biolimus A9, zotarolimus, and novolimus, all bind to the FKBP12 binding protein, which subsequently binds to the mTOR and thus blocks the cell cycle of the smooth muscle cell (SMC) from the G1 to S phase [43,44].

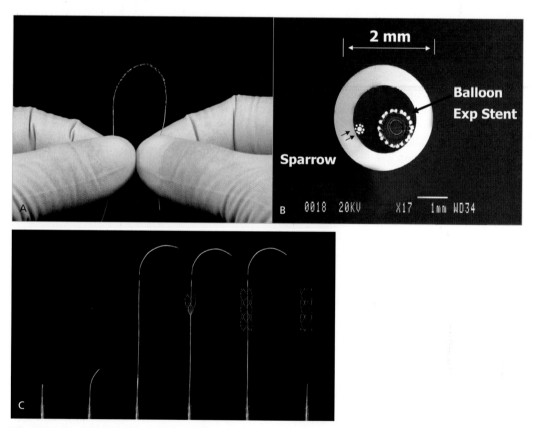

Figure 37.1. CardioMind™ stent-on-a-wire nitinol self-expanding system (Panel A). In Panel B a transversal profile comparison between CardioMind™(small arrows) and another balloon-expandable stent (bigger arrow). The sequence of a self-expandable stent system is shown in Panel C.

The calcineurin inhibitor family, tacrolimus and pimecrolimus, have different mechanisms of action. Both drugs bind to FKBP506. The tacrolimus/pimecrolimus-FKBP506 complex subsequently inhibits the calcineurin receptor, preventing dephosphorylation of NK-AT, which leads to decreased cytokine expression on the cell surface membrane and results in an inhibition of T-cell activation and lower SMC selectivity. A non-Limus related drug widely studied in coronary stents is paclitaxel. Its effect have been mainly explained by its ability to stabilize microtubules, thereby inhibiting cell division in the G0/G1 and G2/M phases [45–47].

The combination of different agents with distinct mechanism of action—one with antiproliferative effects and the other with pro-healing/anti-inflammatory properties—may be an alternative to improve efficacy and safety. Another option, demonstrated by the REDOX study, involves reducing the of sirolimus eluted by the Cypher® stent without affecting efficacy [48].

Polymer/Coatings

The stent coating serves as the interface between the stent and vascular tissue and functions as the drug carrier. Nonbiodegradable polymer coating technology has been used in most clinically available DES and is considered partly responsible for late adverse events and pathologic reactions, including inflammation and hypersensitivity [39,49]. Research is now focusing on polymers that are biomimetic or biodegradable. The goal is to achieve a more controlled release of drug from a stable, less thrombogenic and biocompatible coating with less polymer mass, and preferably bioabsorbable.

In addition, novel non-polymeric DES and the use of an endothelial progenitor cell (EPC)-capture stent are under investigation [50,51].

New DES Programs

Polymeric Approach
Sirolimus
Sirolimus (rapamycin) is a naturally occurring macrolide antibiotic produced by the fungus Streptomyces. Sirolimus was the first mTOR family related drug used on an endovascular prosthesis. The first-generation Cypher® sirolimus eluting

stents (SES) are coated with a thin layer of a poly-*n*-butyl methacrylate and polyethylene-vinyl acetate copolymer containing 140 μg of sirolimus (Wyeth-Ayers). Several successive studies proved the efficacy of this first-generation SES in populations that ranged from highly selected patients with single lesions to unselected all-comers [5,6,52–57].

The Supralimus™ Core (Sahajanand Medical Technologies, India), and Excel™ stents (JW Medical Co. Ltd, China) are composed of CoCr and stainless steel alloys, respectively, with a biodegradable polymer containing sirolimus. Registries have shown efficacy and safety with both systems [58,59]. Multicenter and randomized studies are pending to confirm long-term follow-up results.

A new program from Sahajanand Medical Technologies, a dual sirolimus/genistein eluting stent, is currently under investigation. This dual drug eluting stent is composed of a CoCr/stainless steel alloy and coated with five different layers of biodegradable heparinized polymers containing both sirolimus and genistein. Genistein is a soy-derived isoflavone and phytoestrogen with antioxidant, antiplatelet and antiproliferative activities that inhibits collagen-induced platelet aggregation related to primary thrombosis. Genistein and sirolimus each block the cell cycle between G2/M and G1/S phases. This novel DES allows a combination of two drugs with a lower dose of sirolimus [46].

A new DES with the Conor™ platform that elutes will be tested by Cordis Corporation in a randomized trial sirolimus.

Everolimus
Everolimus is a sirolimus analog with a single minimal alteration in its molecular structure (position 40). In cells, everolimus generates an immunosuppressive complex that binds to and inhibits the activation of the mTOR, resulting in cell arrest in the late G1 stage [60]. Everolimus is used as immunosuppressive therapy following heart and renal transplant, and has been shown to retard cardiac allograft vasculopathy. In an experimental model, a more rapid endothelialization was observed with the everolimus eluting stent as compared with sirolimus, zotarolimus, or paclitaxel eluting stents [61].

The feasibility of using everolimus on a DES was initially demonstrated in the FUTURE-I and FUTURE II studies [62]. More recently, the series of SPIRIT trials were planned to assess the efficacy and safety of the Xience™ Vision everolimus eluting coronary stent (Xience™ V; Abbott Vascular, CA, USA). This new-generation Xience™ V DES is composed of the Multi-Link™ Vision stent (Abbott Vascular, Santa Clara, CA), with CoCr alloy, coated with a durable polymer containing 100 µg of everolimus/cm^2 of stent surface area. Due to its chemical structure, everolimus has a less extensive tissue penetration as compared to sirolimus, which is believed to be desirable in terms of local application of an antiproliferative agent via a DES system. Additionally, the matrix is designed to release more than 75% of the everolimus dose during the first 28 days poststenting, with approximately 25% released during the first 24 hours [63].

The SPIRIT FIRST [64] study randomized 60 patients to receive Xience™ V or BMS. The angiographic in-stent late loss observed with Xience™ V was 0.10 mm at six months and 0.24 mm at 12 months, a reduction of 88% and 71% relative to BMS, respectively.

In the recently randomized SPIRIT II and SPIRIT III trials [65], Xience™ V proved to be superior to Taxus® for reduction of both late loss and binary restenosis. In a pooled meta-analysis of the SPIRIT II (n = 300) and SPIRIT III (n = 1002) trials, which had similar inclusion and exclusion criteria, Xience™ V resulted in significantly less in-stent late loss (0.14 mm vs. 0.33 mm; p < 0.001; a reduction of 58%) and less in-segment late loss (0.11 mm vs. 0.22 mm; p = 0.0004; reduction of 50%). There was also a 57% reduction in total TLR (3.6% vs. 8.4%; p = 0.003) and a 50% reduction in total MACE (5.7% vs. 11.3%; p = 0.0004) at nine months for the group treated with Xience™ V. The rate of stent thrombosis per Academic Research Consortium (ARC) criteria [66] and per protocol were similar between Xience™ V (0.5%) and Taxus® (0.3%).

In the SPIRIT III intravascular ultrasound (IVUS) subanalysis, Xience™ V (107 lesions) was more effective at reducing neointimal hyperplasia than Taxus® (42 lesions). The percentage of neointimal hyperplasia volume obstruction (% NIH) was 6.9% for Xience™ V and 11.2% for Taxus® (p = 0.01) [65].

Additional SPIRIT studies are in progress. In the United States, the SPIRIT IV, a modified extension of SPIRIT III, intends to enroll 3,690 patients to provide additional data on safety and efficacy in patients with up to three *de novo* native coronary artery lesions. Again, patients will be randomized to receive Xience™ V or Taxus® to obtain data in a more complex coronary anatomy, bringing the research population closer to "real-world" situations. The study started in August 2006 and initial results are expected to be shown in 2009.

The SPIRIT V International Evaluation Trial plans to enroll 3,000 patients and consists of both a randomized study of diabetic patients as well as a registry of "real world" patient use of Xience™ V. SPIRIT WOMEN will evaluate patient and disease characteristics specific to women and study clinical outcomes following Xience™ V implantation.

Abbott Vascular has also proposed a 5,000-patient registry study, dubbed Xience™ V USA, which will evaluate stent thrombosis as its primary endpoint.

Xience™ V is commercially available, having been approved by the FDA in 2008. An identical stent, named Promus™, made by Abbott but distributed on a private-label basis by Boston Scientific, is also available.

Zotarolimus

Zotarolimus (Abbott Pharmaceuticals, Abbott Park, Ill) is a newly synthesized rapamycin analogue (change on position 40) developed specifically for elution from intravascular stents, which likewise contains antiproliferative [67] and anti-inflammatory effects. The zotarolimus chemical and molecular structural confers the potential advantage of marked lipophilicity and low aqueous solubility. These properties may be useful for elution from the stent surface, because theoretically it provides both preferential uptake by the vessel wall and minimal loss of drug to the systemic circulation [67,68], leading to a higher tissue retention compared with SES. Importantly, recent data on endothelial function after stent placement in an experimental model demonstrated a normally functioning endothelium 1 and three months after zotarolimus eluting stent implantation [69].

The Endeavor™ stent system that has been used combines the CoCr-alloy Driver™ (Medtronic Vascular, Santa Rosa, CA) stent (strut thickness of

91 µm; 0.0036 in) with a 10 µg zotarolimus/mm stent length and a biocompatible phosphorylcholine polymer coating. The phosphorylcholine coating is a synthetic copy of the predominant phospholipid in the outer membrane of red blood cells and therefore has a high biovascular compatibility. The polymer is very thin—less than 5 µm in total thickness—which means it is almost a quarter of the thickness of the Taxus® polymer and less than half the thickness of the Cypher® polymer.

In ENDEAVOR I, the first in-man (FIM) study of 100 patients, the Endeavor™ stent was associated with a low cumulative incidence of MACE— 2% at four months, 2% at one year, 3% at two years, 6.1% at three years, and 7.2% at four years [70]. In the pivotal ENDEAVOR II [71] study, a prospective, randomized, double-blind, multicenter trial of 1,197 patients, Endeavor™ significantly reduced the rates of clinical and angiographic restenosis at 9 months compared with a BMS. The rate of MACE was reduced from 14.4% with BMS to 7.3% with Endeavor™ (p < 0.001).

ENDEAVOR III [72,73] was a prospective, multicenter, 3:1 randomized trial conducted to evaluate the safety and efficacy of Endeavor™ (n = 323) relative to Cypher® (n = 113). Endeavor™ failed to achieve its primary endpoint of noninferiority for in-segment late lumen loss at eight months when compared with Cypher® (0.34 mm vs. 0.13 mm; p < 0.001). Also in-stent late loss was greater with Endeavor™ compared to Cypher® (0.15 mm vs. 0.62 mm; p < 0.001). In-hospital MACE events were significantly lower among patients treated with Endeavor™ (0.6% vs. 3.5%, p < 0.04). However, neither clinically driven TLR (6.3% vs. 3.5%, p = 0.34) nor target vessel failure (TVF) (12.0% vs. 11.5%, p = 1.0) differed significantly. Importantly, newly observed incomplete late stent apposition with abnormal remodeling and vessel expansion occurred in four patients (5.9%) treated with Cypher® and in only one (0.5%) patient receiving Endeavor™ (p = 0.02). Two-year follow-up from the ENDEAVOR III trial suggests that Endeavor™ may be equivalent to Cypher® for clinical endpoints (MACE of 9.3% vs. 11.6%) [74].

The ENDEAVOR IV trial is a randomized, single-blind trial evaluating the safety and efficacy of Endeavor™ compared to Taxus®. ENDEAVOR IV evaluated 1,548 patients at 80 clinical centers in the United States, with a primary endpoint of TVF (a composite of cardiac death, myocardial infarction and target vessel revascularization) at nine months. In this study, the Endeavor™ stent was noninferior to Taxus® with respect to TVF (6.6% vs. 7.2%, p = NS for noninferiority). In addition, the investigators showed that TVF noninferiority was maintained at 12 months, and for all other clinical endpoints there were no differences between the two stent types. Nonetheless, eight-month angiographic results in a subset of patients (less than 300 of the 1,548 randomized in the trial) showed that there were clear, statistically significant differences between the two stents. In-segment late lumen loss was 0.36 mm for Endeavor™ and 0.23 mm for Taxus® (p = 0.023) (unpublished data from Leon MB, Transcatheter Cardiovascular Therapeutics 2007).

The reasons for higher late lumen loss observed with Endeavor™ compared with Cypher® and Taxus® are incompletely understood. One potential reason is that the more rapid elution kinetics of zotarolimus from the phosphorylcholine polymer compared with the slower release of sirolimus and paclitaxel might significantly influence biological efficacy. After considering ENDEAVOR IV clinical trial data, an FDA panel approved the stent for clinical use in the United States in 2008.

A novel generation—the Endeavor™ Resolute stent received CE (Conformité Européenne) approval in October 2007. Endeavor™ Resolute shares the same CoCr alloy stent platform as Endeavor™, with the same concentration of zotarolimus. Endeavor™ Resolute adds the BioLinx non-inflammatory polymer to improve biocompatibility and extend drug elution. This new polymer is designed to help match the duration of drug delivery with the longer healing duration often experienced by first-generation DES. BioLinx is different from other polymers in that it combines a hydrophilic component that is in direct contact with the vessel wall (outer surface), which leads to high biocompatibility, with a hydrophotic inner surface which helps to precisely control the drug release (Figure 37.2). With Endeavor™ Resolute, the tissue concentration of zotarolimus is more sustained and effective than with the first-generation Endeavor™ [75,76].

The recently published RESOLUTE trial [77] enrolled 130 patients at 12 clinical centers in

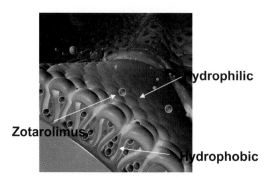

Figure 37.2. Endeavor Resolute Polymer BioLinx. Hydrophilic polymer: Polyvinyl pyrrolidinone (PVP) for initial drug burst and enhanced biocompatibility (outer surface in blue color). Hydrophobic polymer: based upon hydrophobic butyl methacrylate (C10) for combining with zotarolimus and uniform drug dispersion (inner surface in pink color). Combination polymer: hydrophobic hexyl methacrylate, hydrophilic vinyl pyrrolidinone and vinyl acetate (C19) to support delayed drug elution and biocompatibility.

Australia and New Zealand, with a primary endpoint of in-stent late lumen loss at nine months and customary angiographic, IVUS and clinical secondary endpoints. In 30 patients the in-stent late lumen loss was 0.22 mm and the binary restenosis rate was 1%. IVUS results showed % NIH of 2.2% at four months. At 12 months, only one patient required clinically driven TLR or TVR and the incidence of MACE was 8.5%. The Endeavor™ Resolute stent showed better angiographic and intravascular findings compared to those with Endeavor™, probably due to the slower drug release from the new BioLinx polymer.

Biolimus

Biolimus A9™ is a highly lipophilic sirolimus analog that inhibits T cell and SMC proliferation, exhibiting similar immunosuppressive and anti-inflammatory properties. Biolimus A9™ is a new drug designed specifically for DES which shows promise in preventing restenosis due to its expected ability to interrupt cell migration and proliferation by arresting cell cycle in the late G1 phase.

The Stent Eluting A9 Biolimus Trial in Humans (STEALTH) trial was the FIM study to assess the safety and efficacy of the poly-lactic acid (PLA) bioabsorbable-polymer-coated Biolimus A9–eluting BioMatrix™ stent (Biosensors Interna-

tional, Singapore). The polymer degrades into CO_2 and H_2O over a 6–9 month period leaving only a bare stainless steel stent. The STEALTH-I [78] trial randomized 120 (2:1 ratio) patients to receive BioMatrix™ or a control uncoated stent. At six-month follow-up, the primary endpoint of in-stent late lumen loss was significantly decreased with BioMatrix™ (0.26 mm vs. 0.74 mm, p < 0.001); by IVUS, BioMatrix™ was associated with a 100% reduction in %NIH (3.2% vs. 32%, p < 0.0001) (Figure 37.3). The MACE rates at 30 days (3.8% vs. 2.5%) and 720 days (6.55% vs. 8.1%) were similar between BioMatrix™ and BMS groups, respectively (unpublished data from Grube E, Transcatheter Cardiovascular Therapeutics 2007).

Two ongoing trials have compared BioMatrix™ with Cypher® and Taxus®. The STEALTH II Pivotal study was designed to compare BioMatrix™ with Taxus® in 1,340 US patients. The LEADERS Trial was recently published [79], randomizing 1,700 European "all-comer" patients to BioMatrix™ vs. Cypher Select ®. At nine-month follow-up, there were no significant differences in MACE, TLR and stent, thrombosis rates between the two stents, with the trial meeting its non-inferiority objective. Follow-up is continuing out to five years and will provide greater insights into the potential advantages of a biodegradable polymer with respect to late thrombotic events.

The Nobori™ (Terumo Corporation, Tokyo, Japan) coronary stent comprises three components: the stainless steel stent, a bioabsorbable PLA polymer, and Biolimus A9. The Nobori-I trial [80] randomized (2:1) patients to receive the Nobori™ (85 patients) or Taxus® (35 patients) stents. At nine months, the primary endpoint of in-stent late loss was 0.11 mm for Nobori™ and 0.32 mm for Taxus® (p = 0.006 for noninferiority). By IVUS, %NIH was 2.2% and 8.9% for the Nobori™ and Taxus® stents respectively (p = 0.017). The rates of MACE and stent thrombosis at nine months were similar for both groups. In the Nobori Core study, 107 patients were treated with either Nobori™ or Cypher®. The in-stent late loss at nine months was similar between groups (0.10 mm vs. 0.13 mm, p = 0.66) [81].

A novel dedicated Biolimus A9 drug-eluting bifurcation stent, used in conjunction with the self-

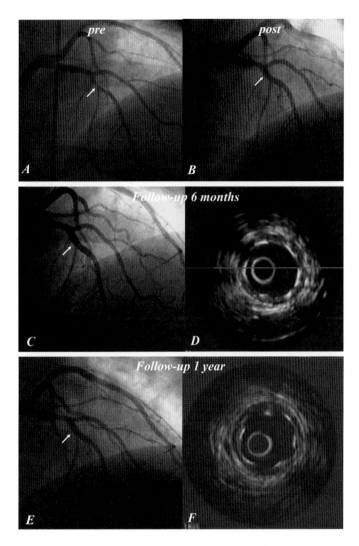

Figure 37.3. This patient presented lesion at mid left anterior descending pre procedure (arrow, Panel A) treated with BioMatrix Biolimus A9 stent with optimal angiographic result (arrow, Panel B). At six-month follow-up, both angiography (Panel C) and IVUS (Panel D) show no intimal hyperplasia, with no changes at 12-month follow-up (Panel E and Panel F).

expanding, nitinol alloy Axxess™ (Devax, Irvine, California) stent was evaluated in a prospective single arm FIM study. The Axxess™ design allows it to expand into the irregular anatomy of a bifurcation lesion at the level of the carina. The drug is loaded in a bioabsorbable PLA polymer. The nominal drug loading is 22 μg/mm of stent length for all sizes. The Axxess Plus trial[38] enrolled 139 patients from 13 sites located in Germany, Belgium, The Netherlands, UK, Brazil, and New Zealand. The primary endpoint, angiographic in-stent late loss with the Axxess stent, was 0.09 mm, which is comparable to the results with sirolimus, or everolimus-eluting stents in nonbifurcated *de novo* lesions. The incidence of angiographic in-stent res-

tenosis was 7.1% with the parent vessel stents and 9.2% in the group receiving stents in the side branch, compared with 25% for balloon angioplasty treatment and 12% for no treatment. Six-month IVUS follow-up [82] analysis was available in 49 cases where %NIH was only 2.3%.

The investigational Xtent® Custom NX™ DES system (XTENT, Inc., Menlo Park, CA) is designed to enable the treatment of long and multiple lesions of varying lengths and diameter in one or more arteries with a single device. The stent is composed of multiple interdigitated CoCr stent modules, each 6mm in length. The number of stent segments can be adjusted *in situ* to deliver up to 36mm or 60mm of stent length. The stents are coated with biodegradable PLA polymer loaded with Biolimus A9 [83]. The CUSTOM I and II trials showed promising early results, and the CUSTOM III trial is ongoing [84].

Pimecrolimus

Pimecrolimus is an ascomycin macrolactam derivative. It has been shown *in vitro* that pimecrolimus binds to macrophilin-12 and inhibits calcineurin. Pimecrolimus does not block mTOR and inhibits endothelial cell proliferation to a much lesser degree [85]. The active pharmaceutical ingredient of pimecrolimus is Elidel, an FDA-approved drug (Novartis Pharmaceuticals Corp, East Hanover, NJ) for the treatment of atopic dermatitis.

A new DES Symbio™ paclitaxel/pimecrolimus eluting stent system, using the Conor™ platform was tested in the recently presented GENESIS trial. The study randomized 230 patients to be treated with Conor™ Symbio with three different drug approaches: (1) paclitaxel alone, (2) paclitaxel/pimecrolimus or (3) pimecrolimus alone. Designed as a noninferiority trial, the study was terminated before reaching its planned enrollment due to the poor angiographic and clinical outcomes in the pimecrolimus group, nearly 40% six-month rate of MACE (unpublished data from Stefan Verheye, American College of Cardiology 2008 Scientific Sessions).

Tacrolimus

Tacrolimus is widely used to prevent allograft rejection after organ transplantation. It binds to the FKBP12 protein, but its mechanism of action differs from sirolimus. In contrast to sirolimus, tacrolimus demonstrates far more potent smooth muscle cell inhibition rather than endothelial cell inhibition. The Jupiter II randomized controlled trial, using a tacrolimus-Janus™ Carbofilm™ coated stent, failed to show angiographic or clinical benefits compared to BMS [86]. A study with a new tacrolimus eluting Nahoroba™ stent, which combines a thin, flexible CoCr metal stent platform (strut thickness of 75 μm) with a PLGA polymer coating, is ongoing in Europe.

Novolimus

Novolimus is a novel mTOR inhibiting macrocyclic lactone with antiproliferative and immunosuppresive properties designed for DES therapy.

The Novolimus™ stent is manufactured from a CoCr alloy and designed with durable polymer coating technology.

The four-month results for EXCELLA, a FIM clinical trial with the Novolimus™ eluting coronary stent (Elixir Medical), validate the safety and effectiveness profile demonstrated in preclinical studies. The trial enrolled 15 patients and showed an in-stent lumen loss of 0.15 mm and a %NIH of only 2.7%. There were no MACE events reported through the four-month follow-up period (Figure 37.4) (unpublished data from Abizaid A, Transcatheter Cardiovascular Therapeutics 2007).

Bioabsorbable Stents

Despite technological progress with metallic stents, safety concerns remain associated with their use as permanent devices. On one hand, metallic stents are extremely effective in preventing acute and chronic recoil and late restenosis, but on the other hand, remaining in the coronary arteries, they have the potential for evoking biologic responses along with the risk of long-term endothelial dysfunction or inflammation [87] and may be associated to thrombosis [88]. The first bioabsorbable stents were made of PLA and recently studied in porcine models [89]. PLA has been used in a variety of medical applications and the final products of its degradation are carbon dioxide and water.

The FIM ABSORB trial using the BVS (Bioabsorbable Vascular Solutions, Abbott Vascular) stent is the first fully absorbable DES, consisting of a bioabsorbable PLA polymer that contains everolimus ($98 g/cm^2$ of surface area). The bioabsorbable BVS, has shown promising results. ABSORB, a prospective open-label trial, was designed to enroll up to 60 patients in Europe. Nine-month results for the first 30 patients are promising, with 100% procedural success, no stent thrombosis, and a 4% rate of MACE. In-stent late loss and restenosis were greater with the BVS stent than with current DES (0.44 mm and 11.5%, respectively). In addition, the 15% elastic recoil was slightly greater than with a metallic platform. Of concern is the higher incidence of late-acquired incomplete stent apposition of 27% [90].

Other BVS stents using an absorbable magnesium alloy stent platform have been tested in humans with potential future applications as a DES [91].

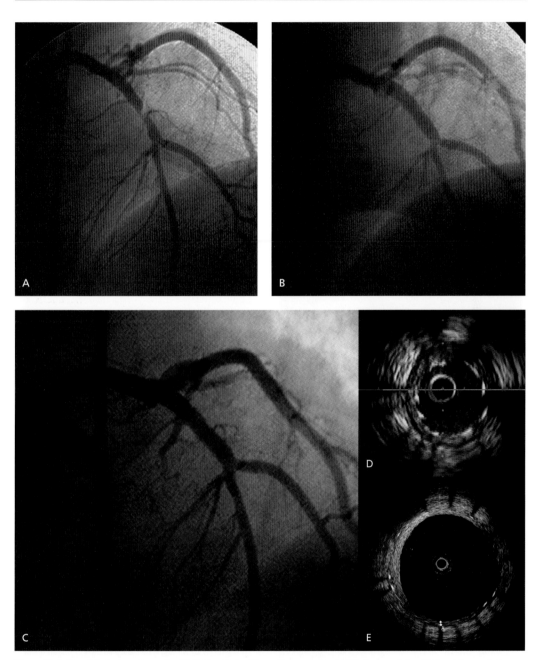

Figure 37.4. Panel A: lesion at proximal LAD treated with Novolimus™ stent (Panel B). At 6-month follow-up angiography (Panel C) and IVUS (Panel D) showed no restenosis with optimal results. Panel E: Optical Coerence Tomography (OCT) shows minimal intimal hyperplasia covering all the stent struts at this site; the minimal thickness is 0.09 mm which is not detectable by IVUS.

Non-polymer Approach

Because of long-term safety concerns with polymeric material, some researchers have developed a theoretically safer non-polymeric approach for drug delivery. A new technology using a porous stent surface was designed to function as reservoirs for a polymer surrogate for continuous drug release. Pore sizes range from 1–100 nm in a nanoporous stent prototype (Setagon™, Medtronic, Inc., Charlottesville, VA) and approximately

$2 \mu m$ in a microporous stent system (Yukon™ stent; Translumina™, Hechingen, Germany) [92].

Initial randomized trials have shown similar angiographic results between the polymer free sirolimus-Translumina™ stent and polymer-based Taxus® stent. However, in the ISAR-TEST-3, the polymer-free sirolimus-Translumina™ stent demonstrated inferior efficacy compared to both a sirolimus-biodegradable stent and the sirolimus-non biodegradable Cypher® stent [93].

New platforms have been developed and tested in clinical studies, including a 3D microporous nanofilm, a drug elution mechanism from biodegradable nanoparticles (Sahajanand Medical, India) and the BioMatrix™ Freedom stent with Biolimus A9 (Figure 37.5). One of the most promising non-polymeric approaches is the MIV system

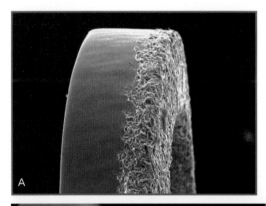

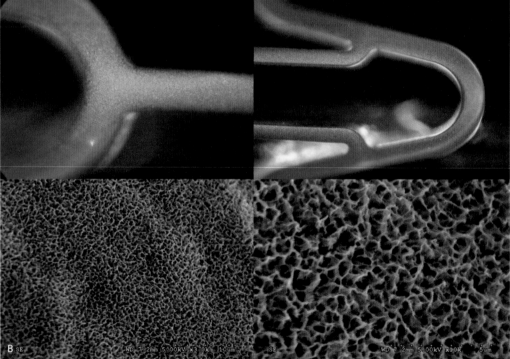

Figure 37.5. Two examples of non-polymeric stents. The Biomatrix Freedom (Panel A) with selectively micro-structured surface holds drug in abluminal surface structures; and (Panel B) the 3D microporous nanofilm with hidroxyhepatite coating (HAp).

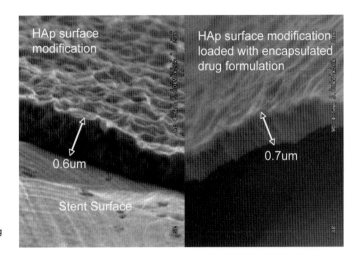

Figure 37.6. Examples of a non-polymeric stent. The MIV system that uses hidroxyhepatite coating (HAp) with a thickness of 0.7 μm after loading with encapsulated drug formulation.

that uses hidroxyhepatite coating. This technology allows the drug to be embedded on the stent surface with a more controlled release (Figure 37.6) (unpublished data from Abizaid A, Transcatheter Cardiovascular Therapeutics 2007).

Conclusion

Current approaches to DES development were reviewed in this report. Although first-generation DES placed great emphasis on efficacy, long-term safety issues have arisen. Nevertheless, there is no doubt that DES will continue to play a pivotal role in the treatment of coronary artery disease, yet future designs need to incorporate features that reduce thrombosis and promote endothelialization. Through the integration of mechanical, pharmacologic, and manufacturing endeavors, the development of an ideal DES is within our reach.

Questions

1. The REALITY trial

    A Included patients with 1 or 2 lesions treated with DES in non-urgent PCI and STEMI.

    B Had greater acute gain and higher delivery success with Taxus stent.

    C Had significantly lower late loss in-stent and in-segment with Cypher stent.

    D Had significantly lower binary restenosis but similar TLR and MACE with Cypher vs Taxus

    E None of the above.

2. The SIRTAX trial

    A Included patients with any type of lesion treated with DES, but excluded STEMI.

    B Had significantly lower late loss in-stent and in-segment binary restenosis, TLR and MACE with Cypher vs Taxus stent.

    C Had greater acute gain and higher delivery success with Taxus stent.

    D Had significantly lower stent thrombosis with Cypher.

    E All of the above.

3. In the SIRIUS trial, which clinical outcomes in the SES group were not significantly reduced at 4 years, when compared with the BMS group?

    A TLR.

    B TVR.

    C Composite of death and MI.

    D TVF.

    E MACE.

References

1. Gruntzig AR, Senning A, Siegenthaler WE. Nonoperative dilatation of coronary-artery stenosis: percutaneous transluminal coronary angioplasty. N Engl J Med 1979; **301**(2): 61–68.

2. Serruys PW, de Jaegere P, Kiemeneij F, et al. A comparison of balloon-expandable-stent implantation with balloon angioplasty in patients with coronary artery disease. Benestent Study Group. N Engl J Med 1994; **331**(8): 489–495.

3. Fischman DL, Leon MB, Baim DS, et al. A randomized comparison of coronary-stent placement and balloon angioplasty in the treatment of coronary artery disease. Stent Restenosis Study Investigators. N Engl J Med 1994; **331**(8): 496–501.

4. Brophy JM, Belisle P, Joseph L. Evidence for use of coronary stents. A hierarchical bayesian meta-analysis. Ann Intern Med 2003; **138**(10): 777–786.

5. Morice MC, Serruys PW, Sousa JE, et al. A randomized comparison of a sirolimus-eluting stent with a standard stent for coronary revascularization. N Engl J Med 2002; **346**(23): 1773–1780.

6. Moses JW, Leon MB, Popma JJ, et al. Sirolimus-eluting stents versus standard stents in patients with stenosis in a native coronary artery. N Engl J Med 2003; **349**(14): 1315–1323.

7. Stone GW, Ellis SG, Cox DA, et al. One-year clinical results with the slow-release, polymer-based, paclitaxel-eluting TAXUS stent: the TAXUS-IV trial. Circulation. 2004; **109**(16): 1942–1947.

8. Stone GW, Ellis SG, Cox DA, et al. A polymer-based, paclitaxel-eluting stent in patients with coronary artery disease. N Engl J Med 2004; **350**(3): 221–231.

9. Grube E, Dawkins KD, Guagliumi G, et al. TAXUS VI 2-year follow-up: randomized comparison of polymer-based paclitaxel-eluting with bare metal stents for treatment of long, complex lesions. Eur Heart J 2007; **28**(21): 2578–2582.

10. Kastrati A, Dibra A, Spaulding C, et al. Meta-analysis of randomized trials on drug-eluting stents vs. bare-metal stents in patients with acute myocardial infarction. Eur Heart J 2007; **28**(22): 2706–2713.

11. Weisz G, Leon MB, Holmes DR, Jr., et al. Two-year outcomes after sirolimus-eluting stent implantation: Results from the Sirolimus-Eluting Stent in de Novo Native Coronary Lesions (SIRIUS) trial. J Am Coll Cardiol. 2006; **47**(7): 1350–1355.

12. Stettler C, Allemann S, Wandel S, et al. Drug eluting and bare metal stents in people with and without diabetes: collaborative network meta-analysis. BMJ. 2008; **337**: a1331.

13. Kirtane AJ, Ellis SG, Dawkins KD, et al. Paclitaxel-eluting coronary stents in patients with diabetes mellitus: pooled analysis from 5 randomized trials. J Am Coll Cardiol 2008; **51**(7): 708–715.

14. Pucelikova T, Mehran R, Kirtane AJ, et al. Short- and long-term outcomes after stent-assisted percutaneous treatment of saphenous vein grafts in the drug-eluting stent era. Am J Cardiol 2008; **101**(1): 63–68.

15. McFadden EP, Stabile E, Regar E, et al. Late thrombosis in drug-eluting coronary stents after discontinuation of antiplatelet therapy. Lancet 2004; **364**(9444): 1519–1521.

16. Stone GW, Moses JW, Ellis SG, et al. Safety and efficacy of sirolimus- and paclitaxel-eluting coronary stents. N Engl J Med 2007; **356**(10): 998–1008.

17. Kastrati A, Mehilli J, Pache J, et al. Analysis of 14 trials comparing sirolimus-eluting stents with bare-

metal stents. N Engl J Med 2007; **356**(10): 1030–1039.

18. Pfisterer M, Brunner-La Rocca HP, Buser PT, *et al.* Late clinical events after clopidogrel discontinuation may limit the benefit of drug-eluting stents: an observational study of drug-eluting versus bare-metal stents. J Am Coll Cardiol. 2006; **48**(12): 2584–2591.

19. Daemen J, Wenaweser P, Tsuchida K, *et al.* Early and late coronary stent thrombosis of sirolimus-eluting and paclitaxel-eluting stents in routine clinical practice: data from a large two-institutional cohort study. Lancet 2007; **369**(9562): 667–678.

20. Spaulding C, Daemen J, Boersma E, *et al.* A pooled analysis of data comparing sirolimus-eluting stents with bare-metal stents. N Engl J Med 2007; **356**(10): 989–997.

21. Lagerqvist B, James SK, Stenestrand U, *et al.* Long-term outcomes with drug-eluting stents versus bare-metal stents in Sweden. N Engl J Med 2007; **356**(10): 1009–1019.

22. Mauri L, Hsieh WH, Massaro JM, *et al.* Stent thrombosis in randomized clinical trials of drug-eluting stents. N Engl J Med 2007; **356**(10):1020–1029.

23. Virmani R, Guagliumi G, Farb A, *et al.* Localized hypersensitivity and late coronary thrombosis secondary to a sirolimus-eluting stent: should we be cautious? Circulation 2004; **109**(6): 701–705.

24. Nebeker JR, Virmani R, Bennett CL, *et al.* Hypersensitivity cases associated with drug-eluting coronary stents: A review of available cases from the Research on Adverse Drug Events and Reports (RADAR) project. J Am Coll Cardiol. 2006; **47**(1): 175–181.

25. Hofma SH, van der Giessen WJ, van Dalen BM, *et al.* Indication of long-term endothelial dysfunction after sirolimus-eluting stent implantation. Eur Heart J. 2006; **27**(2): 166–170.

26. Ako J, Bonneau HN, Honda Y, *et al.* Design criteria for the ideal drug-eluting stent. Am J Cardiol 2007; **100**(8B): 3M–9M.

27. Kereiakes DJ, Cox DA, Hermiller JB, *et al.* Usefulness of a cobalt chromium coronary stent alloy. Am J Cardiol. 2003; **92**(4): 463–466.

28. vom Dahl J, Haager PK, Grube E, *et al.* Effects of gold coating of coronary stents on neointimal proliferation following stent implantation. Am J Cardiol. 2002; **89**(7):801–805.

29. Koster R, Vieluf D, Kiehn M, *et al.* Nickel and molybdenum contact allergies in patients with coronary in-stent restenosis. Lancet 2000; **356**(9245): 1895–1897.

30. Kastrati A, Mehilli J, Dirschinger J, *et al.* Intracoronary stenting and angiographic results: strut thickness effect on restenosis outcome (ISAR-STEREO) trial. Circulation 2001; **103**(23): 2816–2821.

31. Pache J, Kastrati A, Mehilli J, *et al.* Intracoronary stenting and angiographic results: strut thickness effect on restenosis outcome (ISAR-STEREO-2) trial. J Am Coll Cardiol. 2003; **41**(8): 1283–1288.

32. Rittersma SZ, de Winter RJ, Koch KT, *et al.* Impact of strut thickness on late luminal loss after coronary artery stent placement. Am J Cardiol 2004; **93**(4): 477–480.

33. Kastrati A, Mehilli J, Dirschinger J, *et al.* Restenosis after coronary placement of various stent types. Am J Cardiol 2001; **87**(1): 34–39.

34. Briguori C, Sarais C, Pagnotta P, *et al.* In-stent restenosis in small coronary arteries: impact of strut thickness. J Am Coll Cardiol 2002; **40**(3): 403–409.

35. Kereiakes D, Linnemeier TJ, Baim DS, *et al.* Usefulness of stent length in predicting in-stent restenosis (the MULTI-LINK stent trials). Am J Cardiol 2000; **86**(3): 336–341.

36. Yamasaki M, Ako J, Honda Y, *et al.* Novel guidewire-based stent delivery system: Examination by intravascular ultrasound. Catheter Cardiovasc Interv 2008; **72**(1): 47–51.

37. Sukhija R, Mehta JL, Sachdeva R. Present status of coronary bifurcation stenting. Clin Cardiol 2008; **31**(2): 63–66.

38. Grube E, Buellesfeld L, Neumann FJ, *et al.* Six-month clinical and angiographic results of a dedicated drug-eluting stent for the treatment of coronary bifurcation narrowings. Am J Cardiol 2007; **99**(12): 1691–1697.

39. Joner M, Finn AV, Farb A, *et al.* Pathology of drug-eluting stents in humans: delayed healing and late thrombotic risk. J Am Coll Cardiol 2006; **48**(1): 193–202.

40. Kotani J, Awata M, Nanto S, *et al.* Incomplete neointimal coverage of sirolimus-eluting stents: angioscopic findings. J Am Coll Cardiol 2006; **47**(10): 2108–2111.

41. Hoffmann R, Morice MC, Moses JW, *et al.* Impact of late incomplete stent apposition after sirolimus-eluting stent implantation on 4-year clinical events: intravascular ultrasound analysis from the multicentre, randomised, RAVEL, E-SIRIUS and SIRIUS trials. Heart 2008; **94**(3): 322–328.

42. Siqueira DA, Abizaid AA, Costa J de R, *et al.* Late incomplete apposition after drug-eluting stent implantation: Incidence and potential for adverse clinical outcomes. Eur Heart J 2007; **28**(11): 1304–1309.

43. Braun-Dullaeus RC, Mann MJ, *et al.* Cell cycle progression: new therapeutic target for vascular proliferative disease. Circulation 1998; **98**(1): 82–89.

44. Marx SO, Marks AR. Bench to bedside: the development of rapamycin and its application to stent restenosis. Circulation 2001; **104**(8): 852–855.

45. Giannakakou P, Robey R, Fojo T, *et al.* Low concentrations of paclitaxel induce cell type-dependent p53, p21 and G1/G2 arrest instead of mitotic arrest: molecular determinants of paclitaxel-induced cytotoxicity. Oncogene 2001; **20**(29): 3806–3813.

46. Daemen J, Serruys PW. Drug-eluting stent update 2007: Part II: Unsettled issues. Circulation 2007; **116**(8): 961–968.

47. Blagosklonny MV, Darzynkiewicz Z, Halicka, HD, *et al.* Paclitaxel induces primary and postmitotic G1 arrest in human arterial smooth muscle cells. Cell Cycle 2004; **3**(8): 1050–1056.

48. Nakamura M, Abizaid A, Hirohata A, *et al.* Efficacy of reduced-dose sirolimus-eluting stents in the human coronary artery: serial IVUS analysis of neointimal hyperplasia and luminal dimension. Catheter Cardiovasc Interv 2007; **70**(7): 946–951.

49. Luscher TF, Steffel J, Eberli FR, *et al.* Drug-eluting stent and coronary thrombosis: biological mechanisms and clinical implications. Circulation 2007; **115**(8): 1051–1058.

50. Caixeta A, Abizaid A, Aoki J, *et al.* Future stent drug delivery systems. Minerva Cardioangiol 2008; **56**(1): 155–166.

51. Aoki J, Serruys PW, van Beusekom H, *et al.* Endothelial progenitor cell capture by stents coated with antibody against CD34: The HEALING-FIM (Healthy Endothelial Accelerated Lining Inhibits Neointimal Growth-First In Man) Registry. J Am Coll Cardiol 2005; **45**(10): 1574–1579.

52. Schofer J, Schluter M, Gershlick AH, *et al.* Sirolimus-eluting stents for treatment of patients with long atherosclerotic lesions in small coronary arteries: double-blind, randomised controlled trial (E-SIRIUS). Lancet 2003; **362**(9390): 1093–1099.

53. Schampaert E, Cohen EA, Schluter M, *et al.* The Canadian study of the sirolimus-eluting stent in the treatment of patients with long de novo lesions in small native coronary arteries (C-SIRIUS). J Am Coll Cardiol 2004; **43**(6): 1110–1115.

54. Lemos PA, Lee CH, Degertekin M, *et al.* Early outcome after sirolimus-eluting stent implantation in patients with acute coronary syndromes: insights from the Rapamycin-Eluting Stent Evaluated At Rotterdam Cardiology Hospital (RESEARCH) registry. J Am Coll Cardiol 2003; **41**(11): 2093–2099.

55. Kirtane AJ, Chieffo A, Magni V, *et al.* Revascularization of unprotected left main coronary artery disease with percutaneous coronary intervention: the role of drug-eluting stents. Minerva Cardioangiol. 2008; **56**(1): 43–53.

56. Kirtane AJ, Leon MB. Clinical use of sirolimus-eluting stents. Cardiovasc Drug Rev 2007; **25**(4): 316–332.

57. Aoki J, Abizaid AC, Serruys PW, *et al.* Evaluation of four-year coronary artery response after sirolimus-eluting stent implantation using serial quantitative intravascular ultrasound and computer-assisted gray-scale value analysis for plaque composition in event-free patients. J Am Coll Cardiol 2005; **46**(9): 1670–1676.

58. Ramcharitar S, Vaina S, Serruys PW. The next generation of drug-eluting stents: what's on the horizon? Am J Cardiovasc Drugs 2007; **7**(2): 81–93.

59. Han Y, Jing Q, Chen X, *et al.* Long-term clinical, angiographic, and intravascular ultrasound outcomes of biodegradable polymer-coated sirolimus-eluting stents. Catheter Cardiovasc Interv. 2008; **72**(2): 177–183.

60. Grube E, Sonoda S, Ikeno F, Honda Y, *et al.* Six- and twelve-month results from first human experience using everolimus-eluting stents with bioabsorbable polymer. Circulation 2004; **109**(18): 2168–2171.

61. Joner M, Nakazawa G, Finn AV, *et al.* Endothelial cell recovery between comparator polymer-based drug-eluting stents. J Am Coll Cardiol 2008; **52**(5): 333–342.

62. Tsuchiya Y, Lansky AJ, Costa RA, *et al.* Effect of everolimus-eluting stents in different vessel sizes (from the pooled FUTURE I and II trials). Am J Cardiol 2006; **98**(4): 464–469.

63. Kirchner GI, Meier-Wiedenbach I, Manns MP. Clinical pharmacokinetics of everolimus. Clin Pharmacokinet 2004; **43**(2): 83–95.

64. Tsuchida K, Piek JJ, Neumann F, *et al.* One-year results of a durable polymer everolimus-eluting stent in de novo coronary narrowing (The SPIRIT FIRST Trial). EuroInterv 2005; **1**: 266–272.

65. Stone GW, Midei M, Newman W, *et al.* Comparison of an everolimus-eluting stent and a paclitaxel-eluting stent in patients with coronary artery disease: a randomized trial. JAMA. 2008; **299**(16): 1903–1913.

66. Cutlip DE, Windecker S, Mehran R, *et al.* Clinical end points in coronary stent trials: a case for standardized definitions. Circulation. 2007; **115**(17): 2344–2351.

67. Garcia-Touchard A, Burke SE, *et al.* Zotarolimus-eluting stents reduce experimental coronary artery neointimal hyperplasia after 4 weeks. Eur Heart J 2006; **27**(8): 988–993.

68. Burke SE, Kuntz RE, Schwartz LB. Zotarolimus (ABT-578) eluting stents. Adv Drug Deliv Rev 2006; **58**(3): 437–446.

69. Whelan DM, van der Giessen WJ, Krabbendam SC, *et al.* Biocompatibility of phosphorylcholine coated stents in normal porcine coronary arteries. Heart 2000; **83**(3): 338–345.

70. Meredith IT, Ormiston J, Whitbourn R, *et al.* Four-year clinical follow-up after implantation of the endeavor zotarolimus-eluting stent: ENDEAVOR I, the first-in-human study. Am J Cardiol 2007; **100**(8B): 56M–61M.

71. Fajadet J, Wijns W, Laarman GJ, et al. Randomized, double-blind, multicenter study of the Endeavor zotarolimus-eluting phosphorylcholine-encapsulated stent for treatment of native coronary artery lesions: Clinical and angiographic results of the ENDEAVOR II trial. Circulation 2006; **114**(8): 798–806.

72. Kandzari DE, Leon MB, Popma JJ, et al. Comparison of zotarolimus-eluting and sirolimus-eluting stents in patients with native coronary artery disease: a randomized controlled trial. J Am Coll Cardiol 2006; **48**(12): 2440–2447.

73. Mehta RH, Leon MB, Sketch MH, Jr. The relation between clinical features, angiographic findings, and the target lesion revascularization rate in patients receiving the endeavor zotarolimus-eluting stent for treatment of native coronary artery disease: an analysis of ENDEAVOR I, ENDEAVOR II, ENDEAVOR II Continued Access Registry, and ENDEAVOR III. Am J Cardiol 2007; **100**(8B): 62M–70M.

74. Gershlick A, Kandzari DE, Leon MB, et al. Zotarolimus-eluting stents in patients with native coronary artery disease: clinical and angiographic outcomes in 1,317 patients. Am J Cardiol. 2007; **100**(8B):45M–55M.

75. Udipi K, Chen M, Cheng P, et al. Development of a novel biocompatible polymer system for extended drug release in a next-generation drug-eluting stent. J Biomed Mater Res A 2008; **85**(4): 1064–1071.

76. Udipi K, Melder RJ, Chen M, et al. The next generation Endeavor Resolute stent: role of the BioLinx polymer system. EuroIntervention 2007; **3**: 137–139.

77. Meredith IT, Worthley S, Whitbourn R, et al. On behalf of the Endeavor Resolute Investigator. EuroIntervention 2007; **3**: 5053.

78. Costa RA, Lansky AJ, Abizaid A, et al. Angiographic results of the first human experience with the Biolimus A9 drug-eluting stent for de novo coronary lesions. Am J Cardiol 2006; **98**(4): 443–446.

79. Windecker S, Serruys PW, Wandel S, et al. Biolimus-eluting stent with biodegradable polymer versus sirolimus-eluting stent with durable polymer for coronary revascularisation (LEADERS): a randomised non-inferiority trial. Lancet 2008; **372**(9644): 1163–1173.

80. Chevalier B, Serruys PW, Silber S, et al. Randomised comparison of Nobori, biolimus A9-eluting coronary stent with Taxus, paclitaxel-eluting coronary stent in patients with stenosis in native coronary arteries: The Nobori I trial. EuroInterv 2007; **2**: 426–434.

81. Ostojic M, Sagic D, Beleslin B, et al. First clinical comparison of Nobori-Biolimus A9 eluting stent with Cypher sirolimus-eluting stents: NOBORI CORE nine months angiographic and one year clinical outcomes. EuroInterv 2008; **3**: 574–579.

82. Miyazawa A, Ako J, Hassan A, et al. Analysis of bifurcation lesions treated with novel drug-eluting dedicated bifurcation stent system: intravascular ultrasound results of the AXXESS PLUS trial. Catheter Cardiovasc Interv 2007; **70**(7): 952–957.

83. Evans LW, Doran P, Marco P. XSTENT Custom NX drug eluting stent systems. EuroInterv 2007; **3**: 158–161.

84. Stella PR, Mueller R, Pavlakis G, et al. One year results of a new in situ length-adjustable stent platform with a biodagradable Biolimus A9 eluting polymer: results of the CUSTOM -II trial. EuroInterv 2007; **4**: 200–207.

85. Zollinger M, Waldmeier F, Hartmann S, et al. Pimecrolimus: absorption, distribution, metabolism, and excretion in healthy volunteers after a single oral dose and supplementary investigations in vitro. Drug Metab Dispos 2006; **34**(5): 765–774.

86. Morice MC, Bestehorn HP, Carrie D, et al. Direct stenting of de novo coronary stenosis with tacrolimus-eluting versus carbon-coated carbostents. The randomized JUPITER II trial. EuroInterv 2006; **2**: 45–52.

87. Virmani R, Farb A. Pathology of in-stent restenosis. Curr Opin Lipidol. 1999; **10**(6): 499–506.

88. Tepe G, Wendel HP, Khorchidi S, et al. Thrombogenicity of various endovascular stent types: an in vitro evaluation. J Vasc Interv Radiol. 2002; **13**(10): 1029–1035.

89. Vogt F, Stein A, Rettemeier G, Krott N, et al. Long-term assessment of a novel biodegradable paclitaxel-eluting coronary polylactide stent. Eur Heart J 2004; **25**(15): 1330–1340.

90. Ormiston JA, Serruys PW, Regar E, et al. A bioabsorbable everolimus-eluting coronary stent system for patients with single de-novo coronary artery lesions (ABSORB): a prospective open-label trial. Lancet 2008; **371**(9616): 899–907.

91. Erbel R, Di Mario C, Bartunek J, et al. Temporary scaffolding of coronary arteries with bioabsorbable magnesium stents: a prospective, non-randomised multicentre trial. Lancet 2007; **369**(9576): 1869–1875.

92. Tsujino I, Ako J, Honda Y, et al. Drug delivery via nano-, micro and macroporous coronary stent surfaces. Expert Opin Drug Deliv. 2007; **4**(3): 287–295.

93. Mehilli J, Byrne RA, Wieczorek A, et al. Randomized trial of three rapamycin-eluting stents with different coating strategies for the reduction of coronary restenosis. Eur Heart J 2008; **29**(16): 1975–1982.

Answers

1. C—The REALITY trial was the first large multicenter prospective head to head comparison of paclitaxel eluting stents (PES) and sirolimus eluting stents (SES) in *de novo* coronary artery lesions. The primary endpoint of binary stenosis at 8 month angiographic follow-up proved not significantly different between the groups, with SES (n = 684) displaying 9.6% and PES (n = 669) 11.1% binary restenosis, p = 0.31. SES did, however, demonstrate a significantly (1) increased MLD, (2) decreased late lumen loss and (3) decreased diameter stenosis, all with p values <0.001. Although there was also no difference in MACE at 1 year, of concern was the increased stent thrombosis in PES group at one month 1.9% vs. 0.7% in the SES group). JAMA 2006; **295**: 895–904.

2. B—The goal of this trial was to evaluate treatment with sirolimus eluting stents (SES) compared with paclitaxel eluting stents (PES) among patients with coronary artery disease, with no exclusions based on presenting syndrome or lesion site, complexity, or length. The trial enrolled 509 patients, of whom 49% presented in stable angina, and 51% in ACS, with a subset of 22% STEMI. The trial primary endpoint was MACE at 9 months, which was significantly decreased in the SES group, 6.2% vs. 10.8% in the PES arm, p = 0.009. This was driven by difference in TVR, 4.8% vs. 8.3% in SES and PES respectively. No significant difference was noted in MI or death, and notably, no significant difference was observed between stent thrombosis rates [2.0% for SES and 1.6% for PES]. SES had significantly lower in-stent late lumen loss (0.13 mm vs. 0.25 mm for SES and PES, respectively, p = 0.001) and binary restenosis (3.2% vs. 7.6%, p = 0.013). N Engl J Med 2005; **353**: 6530–662.

3. C

Index

Note: page numbers in *italics* indicate figures and those in **bold** indicate tables.

Interventional Cardiology, First Edition. Edited by
Carlo Di Mario, George D. Dangas, Peter Barlis.
© 2010 Blackwell Publishing Ltd. Published 2010 by
Blackwell Publishing Ltd.